Fashions in Hair

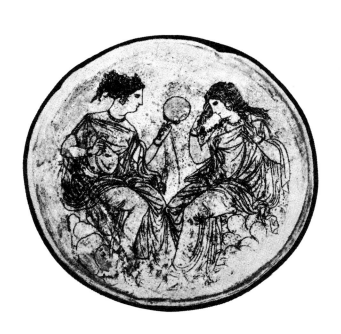

Richard Corson

Fashions in Hair

THE FIRST FIVE THOUSAND YEARS

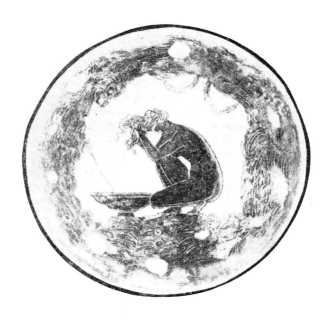

PETER OWEN · LONDON

ISBN 0 7206 3283 8

PETER OWEN LIMITED
73 Kenway Road London SW5 ORE

First published 1965
Second impression 1966
Third impression with supplement 1971
Fourth impression 1977
Fifth impression with revised supplement 1980
Sixth impression 1984
Seventh impression 1991
Eighth impression 1995
© Richard Corson 1965, 1980

Book designed by Beatrice Musgrave
Composition and original printing by
R&R Clark Ltd Edinburgh
Reprinted 1995 by St Edmundsbury Press Limited
Bury St Edmunds Suffolk

To V. L. C.

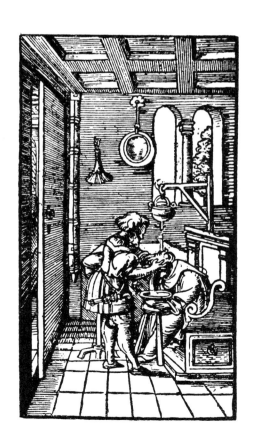

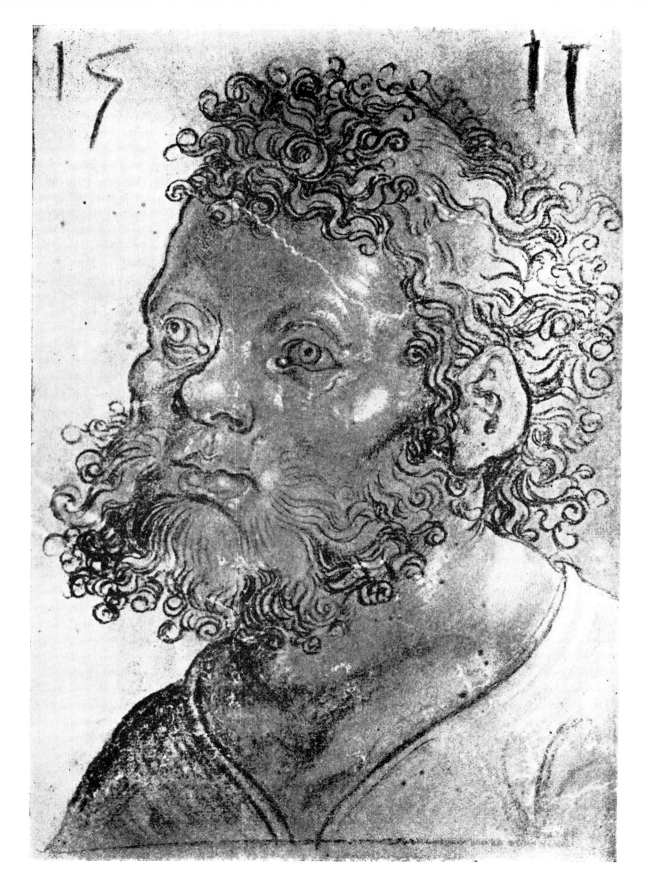

Preface

My original intention was to make this a book of illustrations of hair styles, to be used as a practical guide in producing historical plays, with perhaps a page of explanation for each plate. But the fascinating information that kept turning up during the course of research proved irresistible, and the book has grown. Although it is still designed to serve as a practical handbook, I like to think that it may possibly be of interest—in a more general way, of course—to all people with hair.

There are three main elements in the book: first, and by far the most important, the illustrations; secondly, the page of brief factual data accompanying each plate; and thirdly, the text of each chapter, which includes information on the development of the styles and, as often as possible, pertinent and illuminating comments by contemporary writers.

The book attempts to cover, in as much detail as possible, five thousand years of western civilization. Strictly speaking, these are not the *first* five thousand years, since from the beginning of time men and women, faced with the problem of keeping their hair out of their eyes, have originated or followed a fashion of some sort. And there is evidence that wigs were worn ten thousand years ago. But since even the archaeologists know relatively little about these early people, the ancient Egyptians seem to provide, for all practical purposes, a logical starting-point.

There have been two major problems in selecting material to include. One is the scarcity of information available on certain periods in history; the other is the overwhelming amount of it in more recent times. Both problems make it impossible for such a book ever to be complete; and I regret all of the omissions, voluntary and involuntary. But every attempt has been made to include sufficient material to make the book useful as a practical guide to hair fashions in Western countries for almost any period in history. I am deeply indebted to Mitchell Erickson for reading the manuscript and making numerous invaluable suggestions, and to Miss Elizabeth Roth and Mr Wilson Duprey of the Print Division of the New York Public Library for putting both the collection and their own vast knowledge of prints at my disposal. I also wish to acknowledge my debt to the New York Public Library Picture Collection, which has provided the material for many of the illustrations in this book.

R. C.

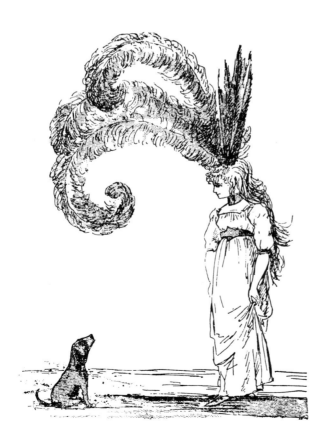

Contents

Illustrations

Plates

Figures

Fig. 48 is reproduced by courtesy of the Spencer Collection, Prints Division, New York Public Library; Fig. 77 by courtesy of the British Museum, London; Figs. 70, 72, 74, 78, 83, 85, 86, 87, 88, 89, 91, 95 by courtesy of the Prints Division, New York Public Library.

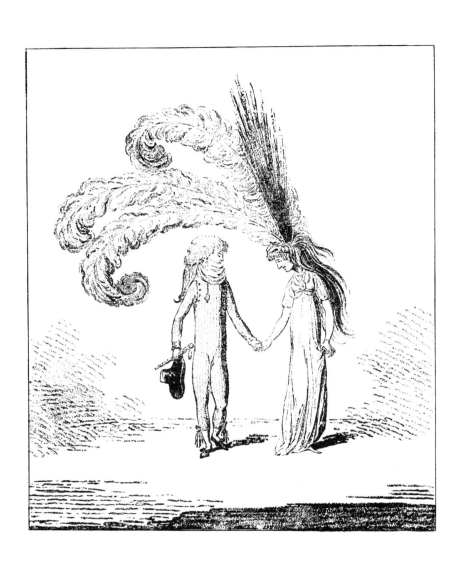

1 · The Wheel of Fashion

The acorns of the forest or the wild bees
of Hybla cannot surpass in number the
infinite variety of women's coiffures.

OVID

The capriciousness of fashion, which, after all, is merely a reflection of the caprice of a relatively small number of influential individuals, is nowhere more evident than in the manner of wearing the hair. As with fashions of any kind, there are the leaders and the followers. The leaders have included the court, the social élite, and, more recently, film stars and famous hairdressers. The Church and the lawmakers have tried desperately in times past to influence styles through threats and pronouncements and legislation, but their meagre success has been hard won.

It is true that the Church arranged to cut a few beards (and at other times to nourish them, according to its whim); and the Law did finally manage to tax hair powdering out of existence. But in the main, fashions flow from year to year and from century to century, reflecting climate (the Egyptians shaved their heads and wore wigs), customs (Romans consecrated their first beards and sometimes their hair to the gods), religious beliefs (the Jews were forbidden to round the corners of their heads or mar the corners of their beards), accidents (Hadrian grew a beard to cover scars on his chin), the personal tastes of the powerful (Henry VIII liked beards but not long hair, so that's the way it was), or the unbridled imagination of enthusiastic —or in some cases desperate—hairdressers.

It was the appearance of the professional hairdresser in eighteenth-century France which speeded up the turnover in hair fashions. A hair arrangement which would be good for centuries in ancient Egypt might easily be out of style in a few months in the twentieth century.

But whatever the century, the so-called leaders of fashion have been those who were first to follow the latest styles, not necessarily those who created them. Whether this is done to curry favour with royalty, to express one's own individuality, or to outdo one's friends, it becomes a sort of status symbol. And then eventually the less privileged classes imitate the style changes, destroying their value to those who promulgated them, and necessitating new styles. This happened very slowly in ancient times; it happens very quickly today.

But we are concerned here not only with the ebb and flow of fashion from year to year and from century to century, but with the specific problem of relating the individual to the fashion of his day. Although the variety of individuals is infinite, the arrangement of their hair seems to fall very roughly into four groups as related to fashion—the *Fashionable*, the *Conservative*, the *Individual*, and the *Eccentric*.

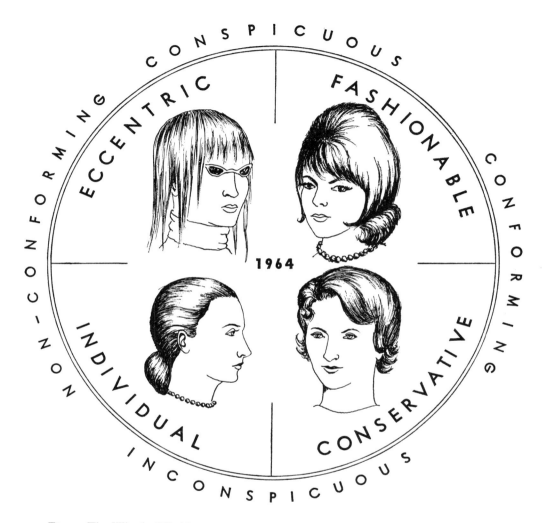

The circular diagram contains the following labels arranged around the wheel:

CONSPICUOUS · ECCENTRIC · FASHIONABLE · NON-CONFORMING · CONFORMING · INDIVIDUAL · CONSERVATIVE · INCONSPICUOUS · 1964

Fig. 1 : The Wheel of Fashion

The categories can be defined or explained as follows:

Fashionable. This is the standard to which all other styles are compared. It is established by a very small minority and followed to a greater or lesser extent by the vast majority. In some periods the variety of styles considered fashionable is fairly wide. In others it may be quite small. This group includes not only high fashion but slight modifications which clearly conform to the pattern set by fashion leaders.

Conservative. This style conforms generally to the fashionable line and form but in a simplified way, or to the simplest of the fashionable styles if there are several. Or it may conform to the fashionable style of a previous period. The latter is usually the result of an increasing conservatism which often comes with age. As people grow older, they tend less and less to imitate slavishly the latest fashions but out of habit maintain a style they have grown accustomed to.

Individual. This is a nonconformist group. Although the hair may be carefully styled, the objective is to suit the hair to the individual, not to copy the fashions. In other words, one wears what is convenient or becoming (or what one believes to be becoming) whether or not it happens to be fashionable.

Eccentric. The style is based solely on individual taste (or lack of it) or on a desire to be different, to show off, and to be noticed. If the individual happens to be royalty or of considerable importance in the social world, then he may establish new fashions. High fashion is quite often eccentric until it has gained some degree of acceptance.

The accompanying diagram (Figure 1) should help to clarify and relate the categories. As we have pointed out, the Conservative is a modification of the Fashionable; the Individual is related to the Conservative; the Eccentric is an exaggeration of the Individual; and the line between the Eccentric and the Fashionable may be very thin.

It is also possible to jump across the wheel. A fashion which has been kept long enough to be considered Conservative may, if clung to for a very long time, become decidedly Eccentric. For example, the women's high powdered coiffures of 1780 would, if worn in 1790, be considered old-fashioned or Conservative. But if worn in 1810, they would be wildly Eccentric. Also, a style which is Individual may, if worn by the right people, become Fashionable. This happened regularly in the days when the slightest royal whim of fashion was slavishly copied by court sycophants. If a queen had her hair cut short because of illness, as did Marie Antoinette, then all the ladies of the court followed suit. If a monarch wore a wig to hide his baldness, as did Louis XIII, wigs became fashionable.

Frequently a style may not quite fit one of the four categories provided. It may be basically Fashionable but also somewhat Conservative, in which case it will fall between the two quadrants and should be considered Fashionable-Conservative. Or, by the same token, it may be Fashionable-Eccentric, Individual-Eccentric, or Individual-Conservative. For that matter, it may be located at any point on the wheel; but so far as terminology is concerned, eight categories are probably sufficient.

The circle can also be divided in half vertically and horizontally. The two sections in the right half are basically conformist, whereas the two in the left half are non-conformist. The division between them is, however, gradual, not abrupt.

The two sections in the upper half are relatively exhibitionistic or, at least, conspicuous. Those in the lower half are not. In other words, the nearer the top of the circle an individual falls, the more he wishes to be noticed. Near the bottom of the circle he either wishes to remain inconspicuous or lacks the courage to make himself noticed.

The classification of a particular style depends largely on the social group in which it is found as well as on the period. An enormous white wig on a kitchen maid would be highly eccentric (if not intolerable) even in 1780. In 1880 it would be eccentric on anyone.

In the diagram are shown four styles worn in 1964. The Fashionable style is fairly extreme and therefore conspicuous. Anyone wearing it would be conforming to the trend of the year, which ran to straight hair, at least partially covering the forehead, and a high crown.

The Conservative style shown is also somewhat fashionable (and therefore conformist), but it is relatively inconspicuous—or was in 1964. In 1864 it would have been considered shockingly eccentric.

The Individual style does not conform to the current fashion and it is not an outmoded style which has been retained through habit. Rather, it is a simple, inconspicuous style which the young woman likes either because it is becoming or because it is practical—or both; and she is not interested in going along with the current fashions unless they happen to suit her.

The Eccentric girl (sketched in Greenwich Village) is also unconcerned with current fashions—aggressively unconcerned, one might say; but she clearly does not wish to remain inconspicuous. It may be argued that in a sense her hair style is really conformist since she is conforming to the practices of a group of people who make a fetish of not conforming to the customs of the majority. However, for our purposes she must be judged on the basis of the generally accepted pattern in 1964; and in that respect she would clearly fall into the category of Eccentric, which is presumably where she would choose to be.

It should be emphasized that the purpose of the wheel is, first, to account for individual differences in hair styles within any given period of history and secondly, to make it possible to select for a specific character a suitable style.

The illustration of hair styles in the plates at the end of each chapter are arranged and dated, in so far as possible, according to the date of the work of art or photograph from which they were taken. Thus, some of the portraits may represent fashionable styles of the period, and some may not. In interpreting the style shown, it is helpful to keep in mind the relationship of the individual to current fashions, as shown graphically on the fashion wheel.

In selecting a style to be used for an individual (such as a character in a play, a film, a story, or an illustration) it is essential to decide to what extent, if any, he would follow the latest fashion of his day. This decision can be simplified by placing the individual at the appropriate spot on the wheel. The decision will, of course, be influenced by various factors—age, temperament, social status, and, in particular, personality. If he is a conformist, he will automatically fall in the right half; if a non-conformist, in the left. If he wishes to be conspicuous, he belongs in the top half; if he does not, he belongs in the bottom. That automatically places him in the correct quadrant. Then adjustments can be made within the quadrant to fit the individual.

Once the character is placed on the wheel, the next step is to determine which styles within the correct period fit the classification. All four groups will not usually be found illustrated for every period. By far the greatest number of styles shown will be Fashionable or Fashionable-Conservative, especially for women. In that case, it will be necessary either to modify the fashionable style as the character might do or, in recent centuries, when style changes have been relatively frequent, to return to a style of the preceding few years.

The ultimate objective in choosing a style to fit a particular character is to select that style which he would be most likely to choose for himself at that particular moment in history in which we are to meet him.

2 · Ancient Civilizations

Ye shall not round the corners of your
heads, neither shalt thou mar the
corners of thy beard.

LEVITICUS 19 : 27

The category includes the Egyptians, Assyrians, Sumerians, Chaldeans, and others from about 3200 B.C. to as late as A.D. 400. The Greeks and the Romans are treated in succeeding chapters. Although written records of these early centuries are relatively scarce, we do have, especially from the Egyptian tombs, a wealth of ornaments, jewellery, wall paintings, and mummies which provide a reasonably accurate picture of the hair styles. In the case of the Hebrews of Biblical times, however, the problem is considerably more difficult. Since it was against their religion to make graven images, we must rely on descriptions.

EGYPTIANS (Plates 1-6)

Although the earliest Egyptians wore their own hair, wigs for both men and women became almost universal and were worn until the Roman influence infiltrated into their culture. All of the drawings, except as otherwise indicated, represent wigs. The precise reason for the adoption of wigs is not known; but it may very well have been a combination of the religious custom of shaving the head and the practical problem of keeping the hair clean and free of vermin in the hot Egyptian climate, especially since they had a taste for elaborate hair styles which could not be combed out frequently.

Ancient shaving sets have been found, dating from 2000 B.C. or earlier, containing bronze razors, bronze tweezers mounted on wooden blocks, bronze hair curlers, grit stone hones, bronze mirrors with ivory handles, tubes for kohl and rods for applying it, shaving mugs of obsidian, combs, and other instruments (see Plate 6).

Priests and certain high officials shaved the entire body, including the head, and did not wear wigs. Labourers also are often seen with shaved heads; and even women (Queen Nefert-iti, for example) are sometimes shown with head-dresses but no wigs on their shaved heads. Although it appears that shaving the head was practically universal among men (except when they were away from their own country), women sometimes wore wigs over their own hair, which was parted in the middle and combed flat, often showing below the wig in front. Herodotus believed that shaving the head from childhood toughened the skull.

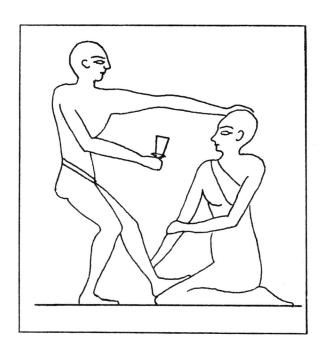

Fig. 2: An Egyptian barber

When making the wigs, which were usually large and well ventilated, there was no attempt to imitate natural hair. They were decorative—often indicative of rank—and they served the same function as any head covering in protecting it from the sun. Members of the upper classes, especially women, often had several wigs in different styles. Some women added braids to their own hair instead of wearing wigs.

At first, wigs were worn only by the upper classes; but as in all civilizations to follow, the fashion eventually spread. The people of rank then adopted longer and more elaborate wigs. There are several periods (see plates) during which high-ranking women wore exceedingly large wigs.

The best wigs were made of human hair; but various substitutes, such as wool and palm-leaf fibres, were also used. Natural dark brown hair was sometimes worn, but the wigs were frequently dyed. Black was the favourite colour, though around the twelfth century B.C., red, blue, green, and other colours apparently were worn. Both henna and indigo were used as hair dyes.

As can be seen from the drawings, braids of assorted sizes were very common and were used in various ways. They were usually set with beeswax or some similar substance and consequently were rather stiff. The wig shown in Figure 3, unearthed during the past century, was reportedly still sticky and quite stiff when found.

Although the wigs were ventilated and did give protection against the burning rays of the sun, they could be uncomfortably warm indoors. At dinner parties cakes of perfumed wax were frequently placed on the wigs of the guests. The melting wax was supposed to provide a pleasantly cooling effect.

Boys' heads were shaved except for a long, braided or twisted lock on one side (usually the right). Although this is less commonly seen on girls, Plate 5-J shows a princess with the 'lock of youth'. The form shown in 2-I for the child god is,

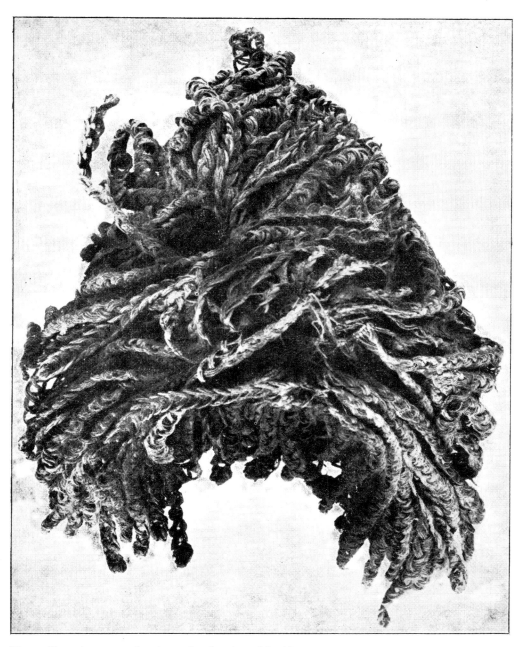

Fig. 3 : Egyptian woman's wig made of curls and braids

however, somewhat more usual. Ordinarily, there would be only the one lock on the side, none at the back. Priests and gods were also represented with the lock of youth. In these cases the lock was attached to a short wig. These locks were also worn by other peoples, as shown in Figure 6.

The wigs for men and women were similar, the women's often being more voluminous and sometimes longer. The very large and elaborate wigs or the ones with very long hair were worn by women of rank, never by the common people, though serving women to ladies of high rank often wore long wigs. During the Roman period the Egyptians let their hair grow and copied the Roman hair styles.

Archaeologists have uncovered a remedy for baldness used by the mother of King Chata in about 4000 B.C. The head was to be rubbed vigorously with a preparation made of dogs' paws, dates, and asses' hooves ground up and cooked in oil. Since there are no records of the results obtained, and since the king's mummy has not been found (or his mother either, for that matter), it is not possible to say how effective the remedy was.

Beards, originally real, later largely false, were worn by men of rank, the rank being signified by the length of the beard. An upward curl at the end was usually reserved for gods. Beards were sometimes braided; later these braided beards were copied in metal, often gold, and worn by kings. To complicate still further the distinction between the sexes, false beards were also sometimes worn by queens. A number of enormous statues of Hat-shepsūt (*c.* 1480 B.C.) show her with a long, turned-up beard. The statues were broken up by her son-in-law, who succeeded her; but some of them were later excavated and pieced together and can now be seen in the Metropolitan Museum of Art (New York).

OTHER ANCIENT PEOPLES (Plates 7-11)

The Assyrian styles were similar to the Egyptian in that wigs and false beards were worn. The wigs, however, were not so voluminous as the larger Egyptian ones; and the shape was quite different, as can be seen on Plate 9. The crimped hair, real or false, was usually parted in the centre, pulled back behind the ears, and allowed to hang down on to the shoulders. The ends were often tightly curled. Women's hair styles were similar. Men of lower status sometimes wore shorter and less elaborate hair styles. Beards, however, were more indicative of rank than wigs; and kings and high officials wore them long and elaborately curled. Slaves, on the other hand, shaved off their beards; and soldiers either shaved or wore short beards. Both hair and beard were given great care—treated with perfumed ointments, curled with tongs, dyed black or henna, and, for special occasions, powdered with gold dust.

Styles of other peoples are closely related (see Plates 7-10). Among the Phoenecians, the hair is usually seen bound up in back, but beards are similar to those of the Assyrians. The Phoenecian ladies who sacrificed their hair to the gods found wigs a great convenience. Among the Sumerians, wigs and false beards were some-times extremely elaborate.

The Persians, though wearing tightly curled hair and beards, can be distinguished by the length and general shape of the coiffure as well as the shorter, pointed beards (Plate 10). The beards were sometimes plaited with golden threads. Unbearded men, according to Reynolds, were considered ridiculous.

Since it was believed among many superstitious peoples that the guardian spirit of the head might be injured or inconvenienced, the hair was not frequently washed; and when it was, the occasion often became a ceremonial one, especially among royalty. According to Herodotus, the head of the king of Persia was washed only on his birthday. The Egyptian custom of letting the hair grow when away from one's own country apparently was grounded not so much in a desire to conform to foreign customs as to avoid possible dangers arising from unfamiliar and presumably evil spirits who might get at one in a foreign land through clippings of the hair.

Speight tells us that 'Mausolus, King of Caria, the same Monarch to whose memory Artenisia erected the celebrated tomb, also ordered a universal shave among his subjects. . . . The King, being badly in want of money, had a large quantity of wigs manufactured, and these he compelled his shorn subjects to buy at his own price to recruit his exhausted treasury.' According to Dr John Doran (*Habits and Men*), the Lycians, having been shorn by the order of the conquering Mausolus, imported wigs from Greece and started a new fashion.

Various tribes followed their own fashions and could frequently be identified from their hair styles. The ancient Moabites of Biblical times shaved the forehead halfway back to the crown, combing the remaining hair back and allowing it to fall to the shoulders. The front hairline was concealed by a fillet or narrow band bound around the head (see Figure 6a).

The Amorites (Figure 6c) wore their hair and beard long, the hair being bound with a fillet tied in a bow in back with two long lappets.

The Tyrians, according to Osburn, usually had flaxen beards, blue eyes, and florid complexions. The hair, worn in much the style of the Amorites, was often heavily dusted with a white powder and covered with a net decorated with blue beads. Sometimes the hair was entirely covered by a cap.

The Hittites at one time, or at least certain groups among them, apparently shaved the beard, moustache, and eyebrows and, most curious of all, they also shaved a spot above the ear, as shown in Figure 6d. But the side-whiskers remained and were braided into an Egyptian-style lock. That this was not universally practised is indicated by the Hittites shown in Plate 8 A-B-C. They also are clean shaven; but the hair styles differ radically from the one in Figure 6 and, in fact, appear to be wigs. No doubt the shaved spot and the side-lock had some special significance. The Philistines also shaved off their beards.

Certain of the Hamathites shaved a spot above the ear and wore the braided side-lock (Figure 6b). The hair was also braided in the Egyptian style. Other Hamathites,

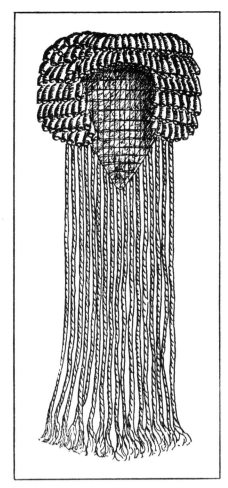

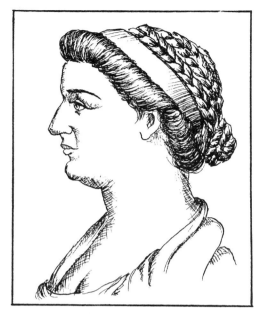

Fig. 5 : Cleopatra (69–30 B.C.). From a portrait by Meunier, based on ancient bronze medals

Fig. 4 : Wig of Entiu-ny, probably the daughter of King Pay-nudjem, buried 1049 B.C.

though they wore long beards, shaved the side-whiskers and the forehead like the Moabites (Figure 6a). But the hair was worn rather bushy behind.

Among the Sidonians, statesmen and merchants wore their hair long and bound it with a fillet, whereas warriors cut the hair and the beard short.

The Etruscan hair and beards (Plate 11) appear to be natural and are much more like some of the late medieval and early Renaissance styles than those of contemporary civilizations. Beards were allowed to grow, but frequently the upper lip was shaved (11-E-L).

Although the Jews were specifically forbidden to shave, there are frequent allusions to razors in the books of the Pentateuch. The Israelites, who preferred black hair, used hair dyes as well as perfumed oils. Hair powder was occasionally used. Solomon's horse guards reportedly powdered their hair with gold dust. Cutting the hair was a form of punishment; and although beards were always worn at home, they were sometimes shaved in other countries to conform to the customs there—

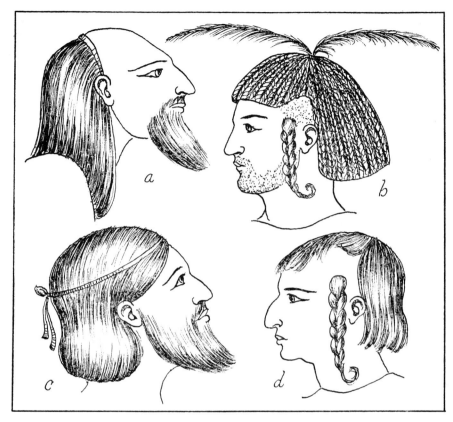

Fig. 6: Ancient Biblical tribes: (a) Moabite; (b) Hamathite; (c) Amorite; (d) Hittite. Based on Osburn

for example, Joseph in Egypt. They might also be shaved at home as a sign of mourning.

'The Jews in Moses's time,' according to James Stewart, writing in the eighteenth century, 'had innumerable rules as to the mode of wearing the hair, though most of them seem to have been devised by their lawgiver to keep them from mingling with the neighbouring nations; even at this day the women do not, or should not, wear their hair in sight after marriage, but this, with many other of their forms, are wearing out.'

According to Speight, the Jewish priests had their hair cut every fortnight while they were waiting at the temples. This was done with scissors, not razors. 'The Jewish women generally wore their hair long, dressed in a variety of ways, and adorned with gold, silver, pearls, and other ornaments. The Jewish men, however, in turn took to wearing their hair cut short, as did the Greeks and Romans.'

Little is known about the barbaric peoples of the times except that, as would be expected, hair styles were relatively simple in conformity with the simpler, more rugged life they led. We do know that among many of them there was a tendency to shave the beard and let the moustache grow, which offended both the bearded and the shaven peoples exceedingly. The early Franks (8-Q) are known to have shaved the chin and the back of the head while letting the moustache and the rest of the hair grow long. Plate 8-L shows the long hair, long moustaches, and shaved chin of the Celtic peoples.

Stewart mentions that 'it was esteemed a peculiar honour among the ancient Gauls to have long hair; for this reason Julius Caesar, upon subduing the Gauls, made them cut off their hair as a token of submission. It was with a view to this that such as afterwards quitted the world to go and live in cloisters, procured their hair to be shaved off, to show that they bid adieu to all earthly ornaments, and made a vow of perpetual subjection to their superiors.'

PLATE 1 : ANCIENT EGYPTIAN MEN 2700 – 1400 B.C.

A *c.* 2700 B.C. The hair is braided and the braids stitched to a woven foundation to keep them firmly in place. The ends of the braid are fringed.

B *c.* 2650 B.C. High official. The wig is constructed of human, animal, or artificial hair tightly curled and stitched in rows on to a woven foundation. The curls were usually smaller than this, as shown in I below. The pencil moustache is found occasionally but is not common.

C *c.* 2650 B.C. Wig of spiral curls.

D *c.* 2600 B.C.

E *c.* 2500 B.C. Re'-Hotpe, Royal Scribe, Keeper of the Documents, and Promulgator of the Edicts of the King. The centre parting is formed simply by stitching down the hair (see also F, H, J, and P below).

F *c.* 2500 B.C.

G *c.* 2500 B.C. Courtier. This tile-like arrangement of the curls in back is quite common.

H *c.* 2500 B.C. The false beard is attached with a band or a ribbon over the ears (see also J below).

I *c.* 2500 B.C. Senodem, a magistrate. This style was very common. Rows of small, tight, spiral curls were stitched on to a well-ventilated cap or woven foundation. Drawing B above shows a similar wig covering the back of the neck.

J *c.* 2400 B.C. The false beard is held on by a gold band over the ears. Usually only gods were depicted with turned-up beards.

K *c.* 1875 B.C. Sehetep-Ib-Rē'-'Ankh, steward and 'true intimate of the king'. The body of the hair is very slightly waved and is curled only at the ends, as shown in the detail. The beard is presumably real (see also Plate 2-J).

L *c.* 1940 B.C. Official. Compare with I above, which is of the same general size and shape. There were many variations in the pattern of the curls.

M *c.* 1450 B.C. Wig of spiral curls. A hole for the ears is left in the wig.

N *c.* 1450 B.C. Priest with forelock of youth (see also Plate 2-O). Usually the lock was real ; here it becomes part of a wig.

O *c.* 1400 B.C. Official. Wig of spiral curls. Drawing Q shows a similar tile-like arrangement of the curls at the side.

P, R *c.* 1400 B.C. Horemheb, general of Akhenaten and Tutankhamen, later last Pharaoh of the eighteenth dynasty.

Q *c.* 1400 B.C. Army officer. The ends of the side curls are very tightly bound and permanently set with beeswax or some other waxy substance. The style is quite common (see Plate 2-A).

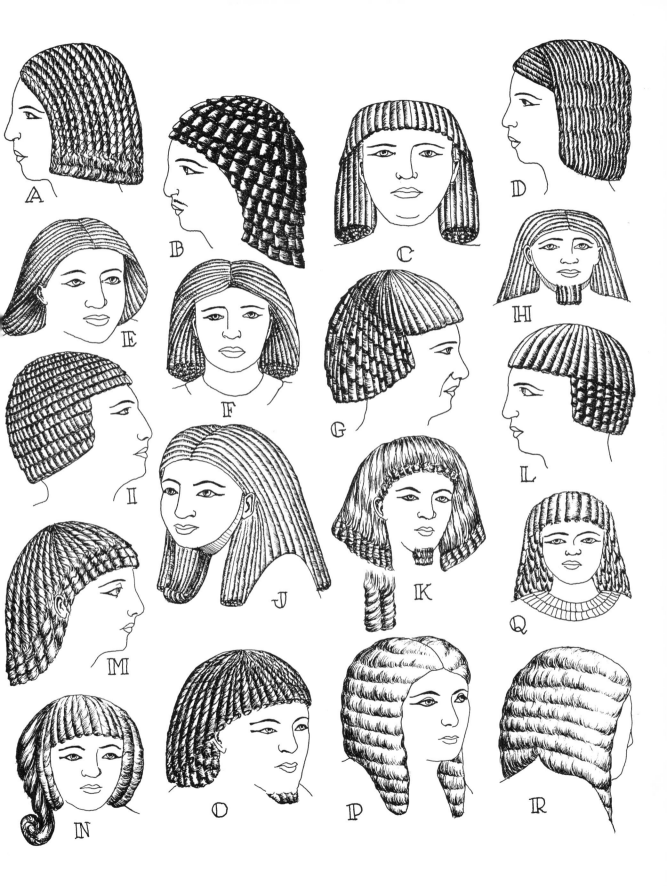

PLATE 2 : ANCIENT EGYPTIAN MEN 1400 B.C.–A.D. 200

A c. 1400 B.C. The body of the hair may have been crimped to give it fullness. The ends were formed into very tight curls and permanently set with bees-wax (see D below and Plate 1-Q).

B c. 1400 B.C. The hair was stitched down from forehead to crown to form a centre parting.

C Ramses II. Notice especially the extravagant and decorative development of the lock of youth.

D c. 1250 B.C. Notice that the hair radiates from a central point. The lower side sections are formed of tile-like layers of tiny curls, as in A above.

E c. 1250 B.C.

F c. 1250 B.C. The hair is crimped and the ends tightly curled. The beard is real. Since the beard is short, the man is not of high rank.

G c. 1250 B.C. (compare with F above).

H Ramses IX, 1137–1113 B.C.

I Child God with locks of youth.

J c. 700 B.C. Official. (Note similarity to much earlier wig shown in 1-K.)

K c. 650 B.C. High official. The construction of the wig is similar to that of B above except that there is no centre stitching to represent a parting (see also Plate 4-F).

L c. 600 B.C. Priest. Priests and labourers did not usually wear wigs.

M Nefertum. The long beard was permitted only to kings and to gods. Often gold threads were woven into the beard.

N c. 450 B.C. A very simple wig with stitching to indicate a centre parting.

O A.D. 60. Priest with forelock of youth attached to his wig (see also Plate 1-N and C above).

P c. A.D. 200. The short natural hair is a result of the Roman influence.

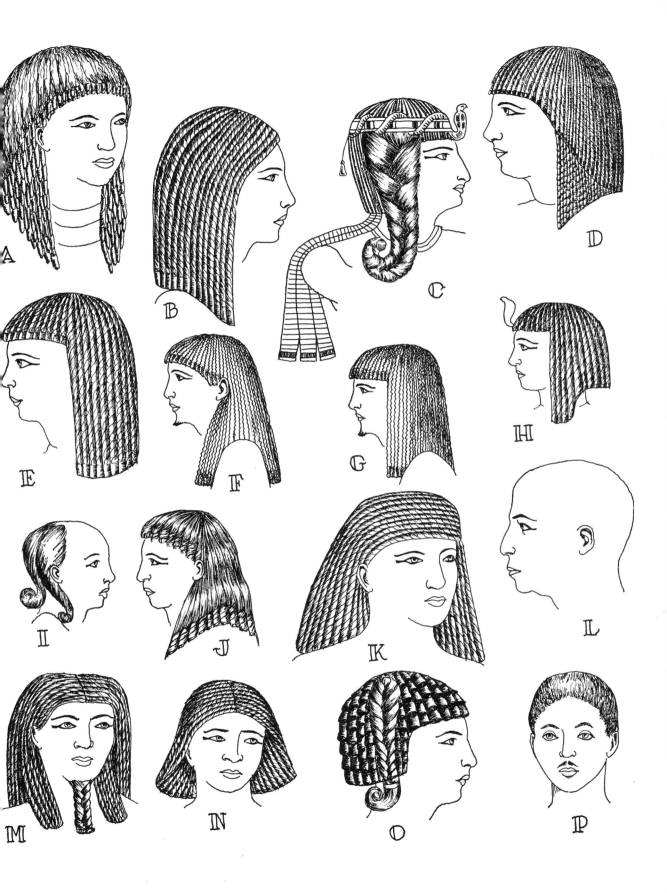

A   B   C   D

E   F   G   H

II   J   K   L

M   N   O   P

PLATE 3 : ANCIENT EGYPTIAN MEN AND WOMEN 3200 B.C.–A.D. 400

MEN

A *c.* 2500 B.C. Mitry, Province Administrator. Natural hair. Another wood carving shows Mitry in a wig like the one in Plate 1-I.

B *c.* 3200 B.C. Warrior from Lower Egypt. This is the earliest style shown on these plates. The beard is probably real.

C Ha'je. Ends of the curls are set with a wax-like substance.

D *c.* 1450 B.C. Kha'-Em-Wēset. Black wig in typical tile-like arrangement of hundreds of tiny curls.

E *c.* 1420 B.C. Roy, Scribe and Steward of the Queen. Notice the size of the wig, resulting from many layers of curls.

F Fourth century A.D. Natural hair and beard.

G Last half, second century A.D. Natural hair and beard.

H Second century A.D. Natural hair, resulting from the Roman influence.

WOMEN

I *c.* 2900 B.C. The braids of hair are stitched firmly on to a foundation. Braids were not always so large.

J *c.* 2500 B.C. Wife of Mitry. Notice the three rows of tiny curls across the forehead.

K *c.* 3000 B.C. The hair was stitched down from forehead to crown to form an artificial centre parting.

L *c.* 1615 B.C. Queen Tetisheri. Ends of the small braids were tightly bound and set with wax.

M Between 2475 and 2000 B.C. Uhk-Mūt, wife of Indy, Bearer of the Seal of Lower Egypt. The elaborateness of the wig is indicative of her status. The hair showing in front of the ear is presumably real.

N Between 2400 and 2280 B.C. Girl with close-cropped, wavy hair.

O Fourth century A.D. Natural hair, showing the Roman influence.

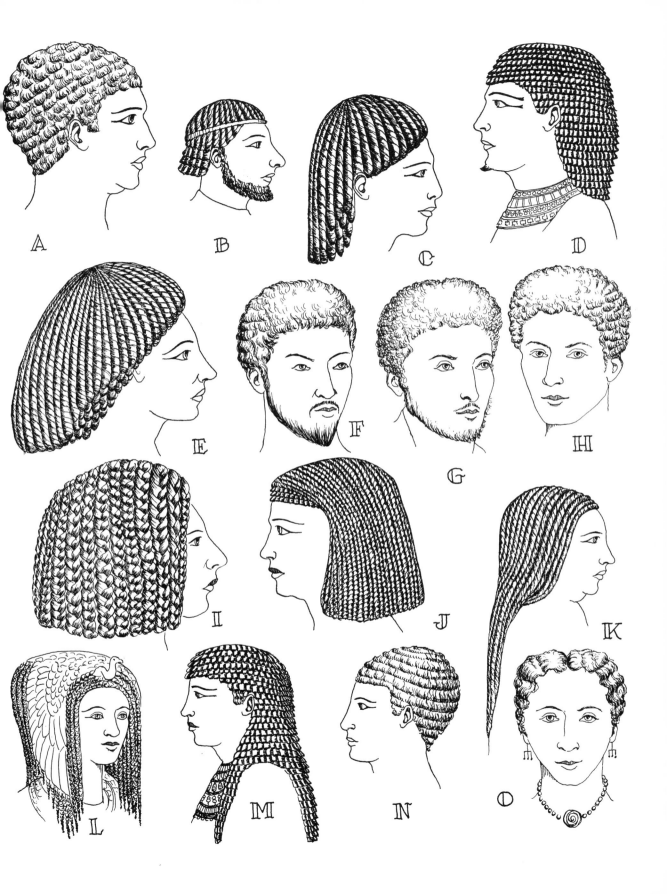

A

B

C

D

E

F

G

H

I

J

K

L

M

N

O

A   *c.* 2700 B.C. Notice the tile-like arrangement of the end curls. Hair is stitched down to form a centre parting.

B   Fourth dynasty. Nofret. When the head was not shaved, the natural hair was often allowed to show on the forehead beneath the fillet or head band, as it does here (see also C and O below).

C   *c.* 2500 B.C. Lady of high rank. Centre parting is formed by stitching down the hair from forehead to crown.

D   *c.* 2350 B.C. Hair emanates from a central point.

E   *c.* 2200 B.C.

F   *c.* 2200 B.C. Servant. Notice the lack of a centre parting, as in Plate 2-K.

G   Hathor. Wig of spiral curls.

H   *c.* 2000 B.C.

I   *c.* 2030 B.C. Hair is stitched down to form a centre parting.

J   *c.* 2000 B.C. Servant. Wig of spiral curls.

K   *c.* 2000 B.C. The hair is decorated with gold ornaments and a woven circlet of gold wire which belonged to the Lady Senebtisi.

L   *c.* 1450 B.C. Metal headband decorated with blossoms and belonging to a lady of the court. The body of the hair is frizzed and puffed out and the curled ends tightly bound and waxed.

M   *c.* 1500 B.C. Compare with the simpler, less decorative braided wig shown in Plate 3-I.

N   *c.* 1450 B.C. Metal headband. Hair is crimped for fullness and the ends tightly curled.

O   Eighteenth dynasty. Centre hair below the headband is real.

P   *c.* 1350 B.C. Queen Mutnezemt.

Q   *c.* 1400 B.C. A lady of rank. Back hair is plaited below crown, whereas the side hair is crimped for fullness and the ends tightly curled.

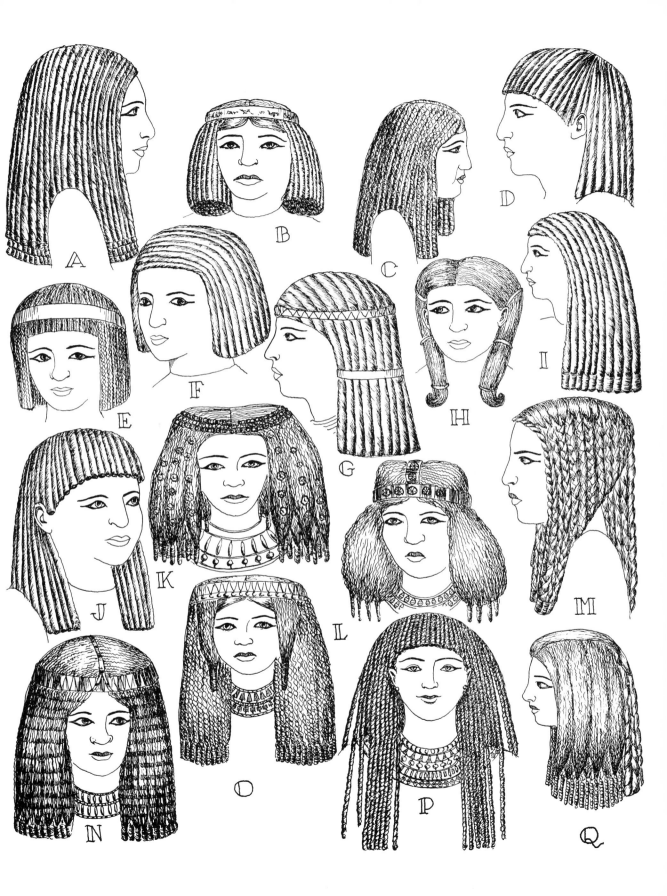

A

B

C

D

E

F

G

H

I

J

K

L

M

N

O

P

Q

PLATE 5 : ANCIENT EGYPTIAN WOMEN 1385 B.C.–A.D. 200

A   *c.* 1385 B.C.

B   *c.* 1300 B.C. The same style of wig can be found composed entirely of braids.

C   *c.* 1320 B.C. Metal headpiece.

D   *c.* 1250 B.C. Queen or princess.

E   *c.* 1250 B.C.

F   *c.* 1250 B.C. Young girl.

G, H   *c.* 1250 B.C. A wig belonging probably to an Egyptian lady of high rank. It is made of human hair, and the small plaits are set with a bituminous substance. The wig is in the British Museum. The top hair is a mass of tiny curls, now light brown, undoubtedly darker originally. The stiff braids, of which there are several hundred, are dark brown, less than ¼ inch in width, and of varying lengths (see also Figure 4).

I   *c.* 1025 B.C. Princess Na-ny, daughter of King Pinedjem. The wig is in the Metropolitan Museum of Art. It consists of a long, narrow braid of human hair over linen thread, from which numerous plaits, set with bees-wax, hang. The braid is sewn together loosely with a faggoting stitch to form a skull cap or caul. The size was adjusted by linen drawstrings fastened at each temple, which also held the plaits at the forehead in place.

J   *c.* 1200 B.C. Young girl, probably a princess. The lock of hair is natural.

K   *c.* 700 B.C.

L   *c.* 350 B.C.

M   Queen Arsinoë, wife of Ptolemy II, 285–247 B.C.

N   *c.* 600 B.C. Queen.

O   *c.* 240 B.C. Natural hair shows below wig.

P   Between 206 and 30 B.C. One of the Cleopatras (see also Figure 5).

Q   Second century A.D. Natural hair, showing Roman influence.

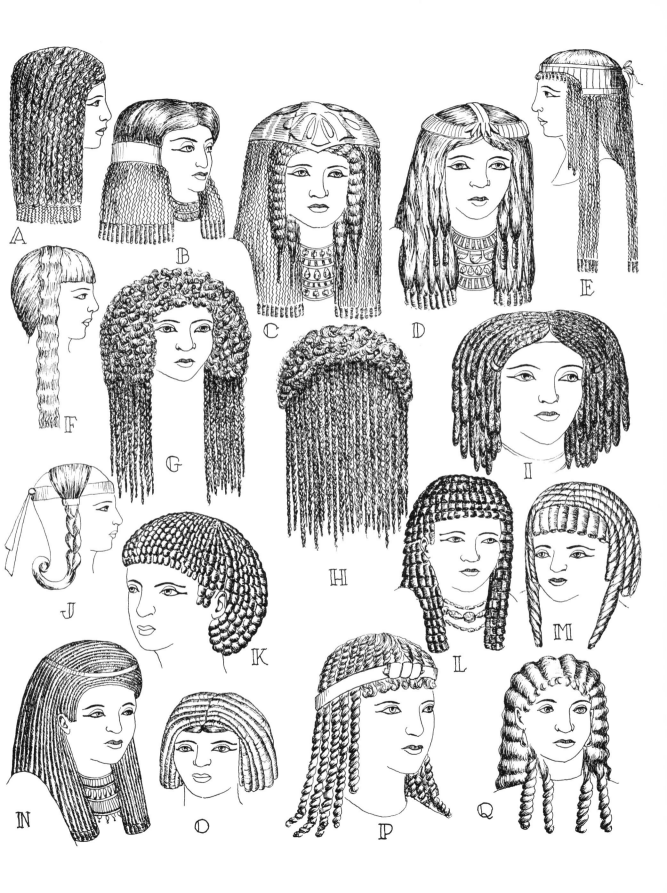

A

B

C

D

E

F

G

H

I

J

K

L

M

N

O

P

Q

PLATE 6 : ANCIENT EGYPTIAN HAIR AND BEARD IMPLEMENTS

A   Braid of hair to add to the natural hair when a wig was not worn. The braids varied in size and length, but the one on which the drawing is based was about $\frac{3}{8}$ inch at the widest point and between $\frac{1}{16}$ and $\frac{1}{8}$ at the narrowest. The length was about 10 inches. The braids were sometimes kept in a basket with sweet-smelling wood.

B   *c.* 1200 B.C. Hairpins of bone. The longest one shown is about 4 inches. Hairpins were also made of wood.

C   *c.* 1450 B.C. Rotating type of bronze razor with wooden handle, about 6 inches long. Arrows indicate the sharp edges.

D, E   *c.* 1450 B.C. Hair curlers. According to the British Museum, they were probably used for setting the small curls on wigs. One end was used as the curling tongs and the other end, flattened into a blade, was used to trim loose ends of hair. Actual size, about 4 inches long. D is inscribed with the name of Tuthmosis III.

F, G   Combs.

H   *c.* 1450 B.C. Bronze razor of the scraping type.

I, J, K, L   Combs, made of wood or bone (see also Figure 2).

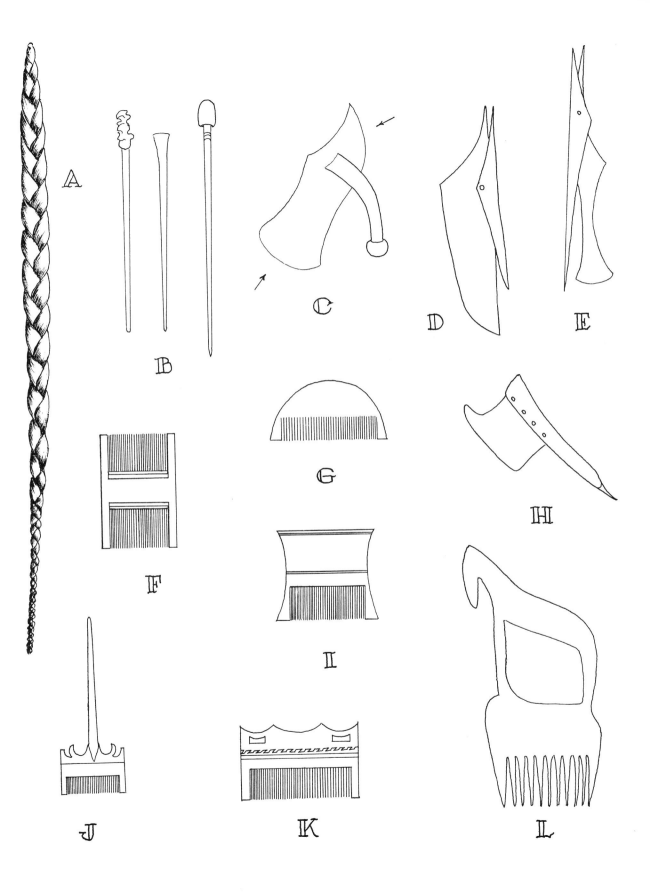

A

B

C

D

E

F

G

H

I

J

K

L

PLATE 7 : ANCIENT CIVILIZATIONS, MEN AND WOMEN 2800–870 B.C.

A, B   *c.* 2800 B.C. Sumerian woman with wig.

C   *c.* 2800 B.C. Sumerian woman.

D   *c.* 2800 B.C. Sumerian man. The bundle of hair at the back is typical of the Sumerian hairdo.

E   *c.* 2500 B.C. Sumerian. Wig and false beard. The beard style strongly resembles both the Assyrian and the Greek, but the hair seems more closely related to the Phoenician and the Semitic Akkadian.

F   Semitic Akkadian. False beard, shaved head.

G   Semitic Akkadian. False beard and wig of spiral curls similar to the Egyptian style.

H, I   *c.* 2500 B.C. Semitic Akkadian woman with wig.

J   Mesopotamian. Both hair and beard appear to be real.

K   Mesopotamian woman.

L, M   Phoenician priests. The false beards are less elaborate than those of kings would be.

N   *c.* 860 B.C. Phoenician. The binding up of the hair in back is typical and distinguishes the hair style from that of the Assyrian, which it otherwise resembles.

O   Ninth century B.C. Assyrian.

P   *c.* Eighth century B.C. Assyrian woman (for an Assyrian queen see Plate 9-D).

Q   *c.* 870 B.C. Assyrian.

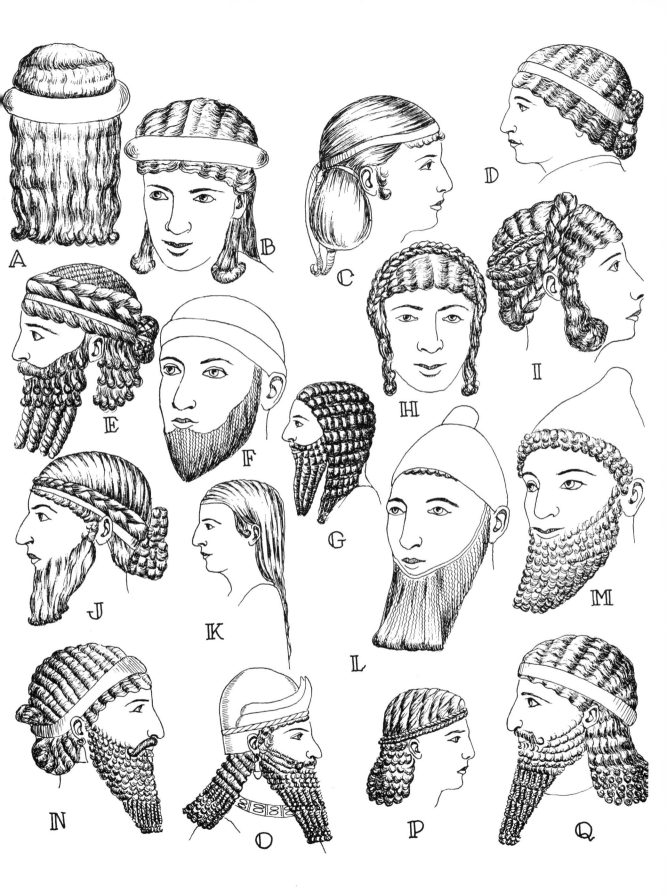

A   B   C   D   E   F   G   H   I   J   K   L   M   N   O   P   Q

PLATE 8 : ANCIENT CIVILIZATIONS, MEN 1500 B.C.–A.D. 400

A   *c.* 1500 B.C. Hittite king (see also Figure 6-d).

B   *c.* 1500 B.C. Hittite prince.

C   *c.* 1500 B.C. Hittite warrior from Carchemish.

D   883–859 B.C., Assyrian.

E   Late eighth century B.C., Phoenician.

F   883–859 B.C., Assyrian (for other Assyrian styles see Plate 9).

G   *c.* Seventh century B.C., Assyrian.

H   Late seventh century B.C., Persian.

I   Etruscan.

J   485–460 B.C., Persian.

K   Late second century A.D., Syrian. Hairan, son of Marion.

L   Celtic. The shaved chin with long moustaches and long hair are typical.

M   Late second century A.D., Syrian (for other Syrians see Plate 10).

N   240–200 B.C. A Gaul captured by the Romans. His long hair has been cut as a symbol of his subjugation. The moustache with no beard was considered by the Romans to be the epitome of barbarism.

O   *c.* A.D. 400., Syrian.

P   Third century A.D., Syrian.

Q   Early Frank. (*Speculative drawing.*) In common with the Gauls, the Franks shaved their chins and let their moustaches and hair grow long. Although the shaving of the back of the head is typical of the early Franks, the style was reportedly followed by other tribes as well (for other barbaric tribes see Plates 24-B-C-D and 25-G).

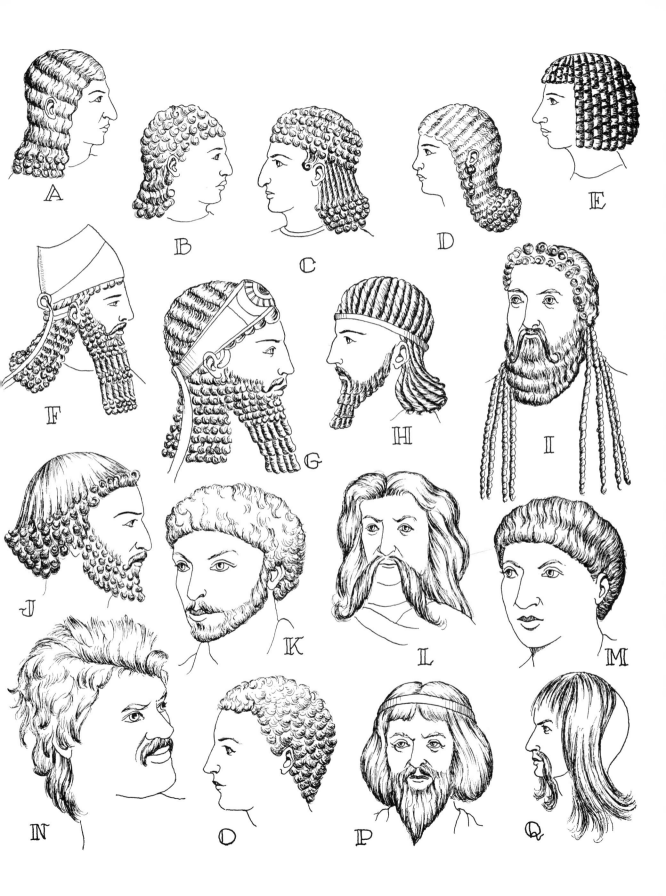

A

B

C

D

E

F

G

H

I

J

K

L

M

N

O

P

Q

PLATE 9 : ASSYRIAN MEN AND WOMEN 800–700 B.C.

A   Royal attendant. The crimped hair, parted in the centre and curled at the ends, was typical of the Assyrian style. The ears were always exposed.

B, C   Assyrian king. The beard is false and shows some similarity to the Egyptian wigs of spiral curls.

D   Assyrian queen (for another Assyrian woman see Plate 7-P).

E   *c.* 740 B.C. Assyrian king. Note the variation in beard styles on this plate.

F   *c.* 740 B.C. Bearer of the king's bow.

G   *c.* 710 B.C. Eunuch of King Sargon.

H   *c.* 700 B.C.

I   *c.* 700 B.C. Servant.

J   *c.* 700 B.C.

K   *c.* 700 B.C. Bearer of the king's bows and arrows.

L   Ruler of Khorsabad.

M   Ruler of Khorsabad. The beard, with its decorative border across the cheek, is obviously false.

N   Assyrian king. The beard is bound with metal bands.

O, P   From Khorsabad. The straight hair and the spiral curls are typical of Khorsabad (see L and M above). Usually spiral curls are found only in the beard.

Q   *c.* 700 B.C. Chaldean.

R   Razor of the type used in Assyria and Persia (for other Assyrian styles see Plate 7-O-P-Q and 8-D-F-G).

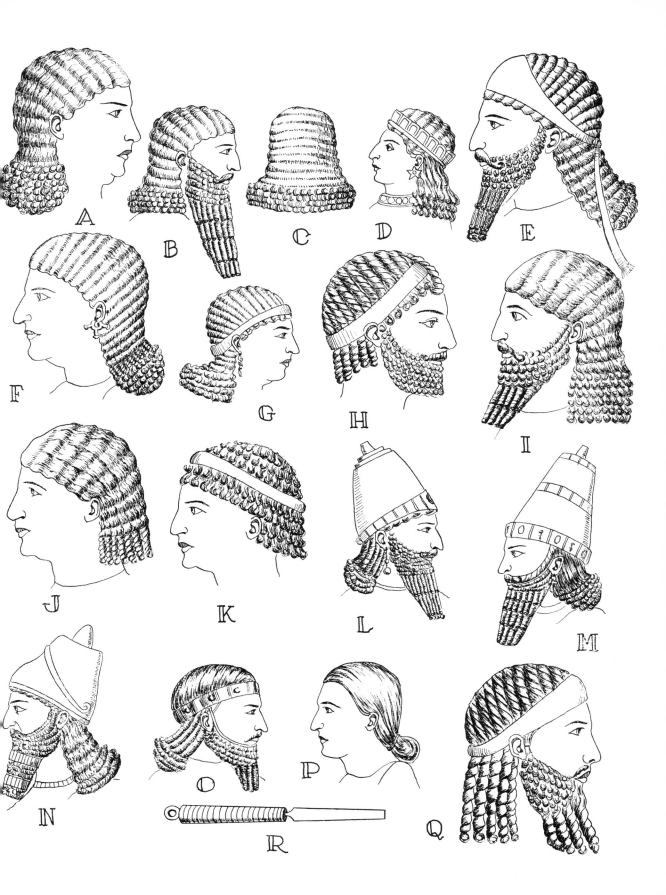

A   B   C   D   E

F   G   H   I

J   K   L   M

N   O   P   Q

R

PLATE 10 : ANCIENT CIVILIZATIONS, MEN AND WOMEN 700 B.C.—A.D. 200

A   Ancient Gaul. The authenticity of the hair style cannot be guaranteed, but the long moustaches, beardless face, and long hair with partially shaved head are typical (see also Plate 8-L-N-Q).

B   Elanite woman.

C   *c.* 500 B.C., Persian. High officer of Darius.

D   *c.* 500 B.C., Persian (see also Plate 8-J).

E   *c.* 500 B.C., Persian.

F   Persian.

G   Median lady.

H   Syrian (Judean) woman (for other Syrians see Plate 8).

I   Syrian (Judean).

J, K, L, M   Syrian (Judean) women.

N   Late second century A.D., Syrian. Young man.

O   Late second century A.D. Syrian woman.

P   Late second century A.D., Syrian.

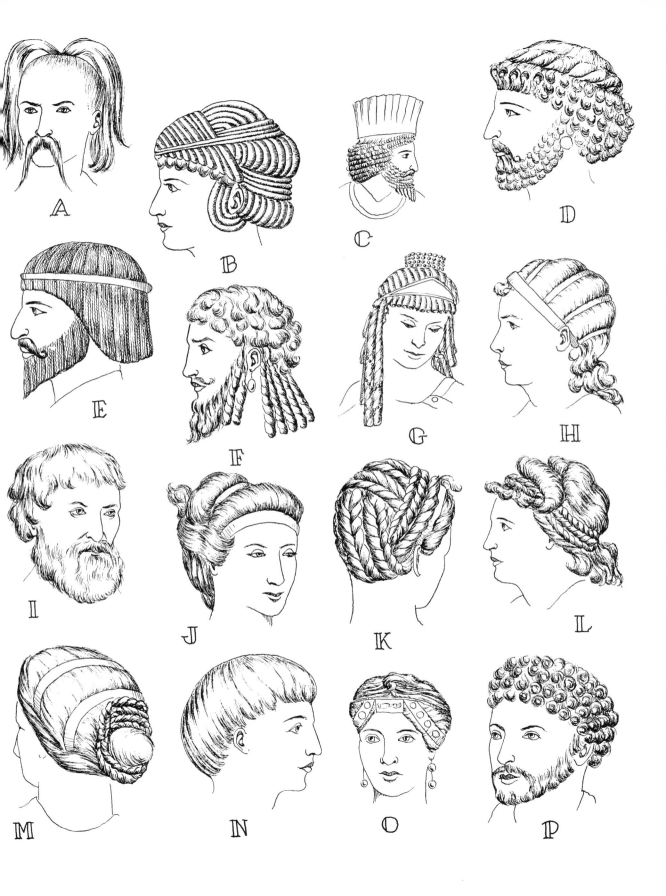

A

B

C

D

E

F

G

H

I

J

K

L

M

N

O

P

Plate 11 : Etruscan Men and Women

A   Late seventh century B.C. Man.

B   *c.* 600 B.C. Man.

C   *c.* 550 B.C. Girl.

D   Late sixth century B.C. Youth.

E   *c.* 525 B.C. The shaved upper lip was not uncommon among bearded men (see also L below).

F   Late sixth century B.C. Youth.

G   *c.* 520 B.C. Young man.

H   Apollo.

I   *c.* 525 B.C. Young man.

J   Late sixth century B.C. Girl.

K   Late sixth century B.C. Young man.

L   *c.* 500 B.C.

M   *c.* 500 B.c. Athlete.

N   *c.* 470 B.C. Young man.

O   *c.* 480 B.C. Young man.

P   Early fifth century B.C.

Q   Fourth century B.C.

R   Early fourth century B.C. Man.

S   Fourth century B.C. Woman.

T   Fourth century B.C. Youth.

U   *c.* 350 B.C. Youth.

V   Late fourth century B.C. Youth.

W   Third century B.C. Youth.

X   Third Century B.C. Youth.

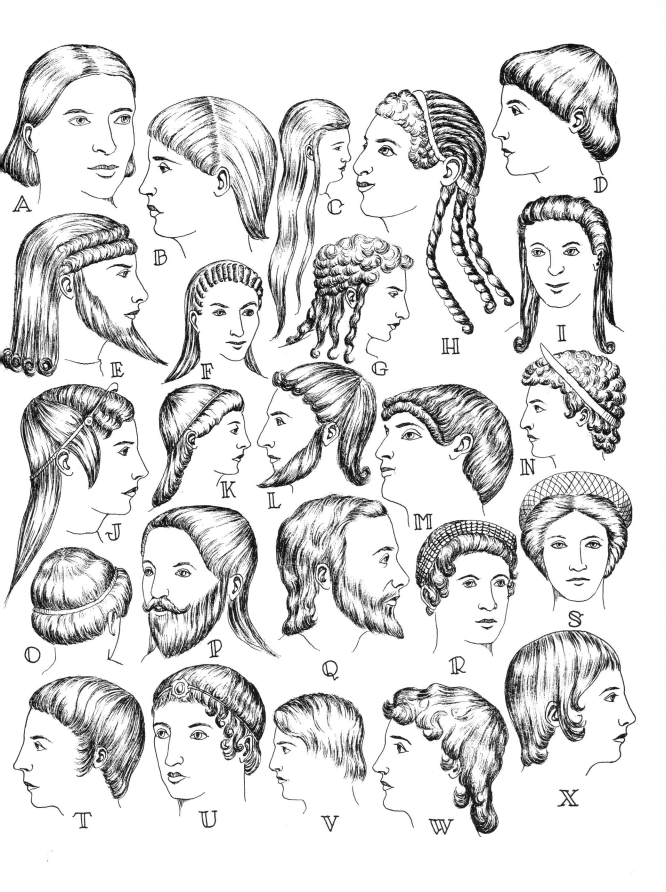

A

B

C

D

E

F

G

H

I

J

K

L

M

N

O

P

Q

R

S

T

U

V

W

X

3 · Ancient Greek Times

What can we women do wise or brilliant, who
sit with hair dyed yellow, outraging the
character of gentlewomen, causing the
overthrow of houses, the ruin of nuptials, and
accusations on the part of children?

MENANDER

Among the early Greeks, hair styles for men and women were remarkably similar.
Later, men wore the hair short, whereas women kept theirs long. The natural hair
was preferred by both sexes, though wigs were not unknown. Hannibal, for example,
had a number of them in various styles and colours. In both sexes the hair differs
notably from that of other ancient civilizations in its naturalness. Although it was
often curled, the curls were usually soft rather than stiff, and there were no great
exaggerations or distortions of the general shape of the head.

The Greeks attached great importance to the hair beyond its decorative value. It
was customary, according to Speight, for them 'to hang the hair of the dead on their
doors previous to interment, and the mourners not infrequently tore, cut off, or
shaved their own hair, which they laid upon the corpse, or threw into the pile to be
consumed along with the body of the relation or friend whose loss they lamented'.

MEN (Plates 12-14)

Although the early styles show some slight similarity to those of the Egyptians,
Assyrians, Sumerians, and other ancient peoples, the stiffness and artificiality eventually disappeared; and by the end of the sixth century B.C., the hair, especially among
young men, was cut shorter or worn up. Once short hair was firmly established, only
some older men and elegant young men wore their hair long. Alcibiades (Figure 7)
perfumed, dyed, and painted his hair, eyebrows, and beard. He is believed to have
been the inspiration for most of the statues of Hermes.

Pythagoras, while travelling in Egypt, is said to have been so plagued by insects
and vermin in his hair that he cut it off and wore an Egyptian wig. It is also said,
though perhaps the story is apocryphal, that Thespis, observing the remarkable
change in his appearance made by the wig, conceived the idea of acting.

Children usually did not cut their hair until their beards began to grow, at which
time they sacrificed their hair to Apollo.

Shaving was not commonly practised in Greece until the fourth century B.C., when
Alexander ordered his armies to shave lest the Persian armies use their beards as

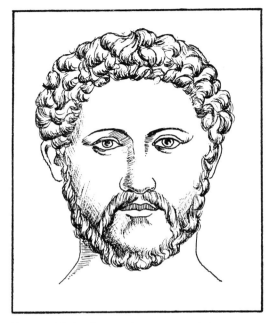

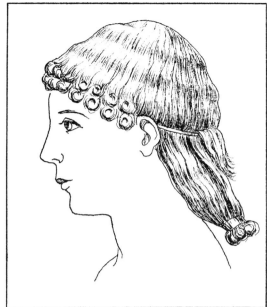

Fig. 7 : Alcibiades (450?–404 B.C.), Athenian politician and general

Fig. 8 : Apollo of Piombino. About 500 B.C.

handles. That, at least, is the reason usually given. They continued to shave until the time of Justinian.

Philosophers and scholars, however, wore beards. Slaves also were bearded, though their heads were shaved. When they were freed, they let their hair grow and shaved their beards. Late in the fifth century there was a fad of letting only the moustache grow. A crescent-shaped razor was used (Plate 13); and the barbers' shops, which were equipped with special chairs, were popular gathering places for the intellectuals as well as those who wished merely to exchange gossip.

WOMEN (Plates 15-17)

The early Greek women usually let the hair fall loosely over the shoulders; and even as late as the seventh and sixth centuries B.C., it was bound only by a band, a ribbon, a diadem, or a string of pearls (see Plate 15). Usually the hair was parted in the centre, waved, and pulled back, exposing the ears. Often three or four locks or spiral curls were separated from the rest of the hair and allowed to hang down the front, while the remainder hung down loosely behind.

Since low foreheads were considered more beautiful than high ones, the front hair was usually dressed forward so as to decrease the height of the forehead. By the

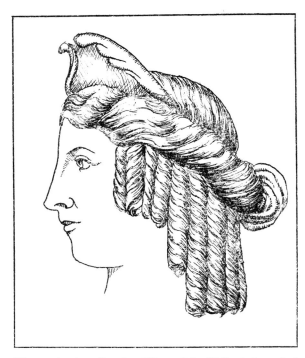

Fig. 9 : Ancient Greek coiffure of the Hellenistic period
(c. first century B.C.)

fifteenth century A.D., tastes had changed so radically that women plucked or shaved the hairline to make the forehead higher.

In the fifth century B.C., women began to pull up the back hair and loop it over the fillet. Sometimes the front hair was also turned up over the fillet, but this style was less popular than with the men. In the second half of the century there appeared a sort of melon-shaped hairdo which was still being worn in the fourth century and was later popular in Rome. At the same time, the older and simpler styles were worn, especially by young girls, who usually let their hair hang more or less free.

Until the time of Alexander, in the fourth century B.C., the hair was often bound with ribbons, triangular fabrics, or folded kerchiefs, waved, pulled back, and tied at the crown or sometimes lower (Plate 16). After Alexander, the hair was usually waved off the temples and knotted behind, the knots or chignons being held in place with ornamental pins. Quite a different style of the Hellenistic period shows ringlets and corkscrew curls, sometimes combined with the chignon.

The hair was oiled and perfumed, and a special mud and various pomades and unguents were used to set curls. Coloured powders (gold, white, and red), dyes, and false hair were used. The earliest evidence we have of the hair being coloured dates from 444 B.C. As in all periods of history, there were those who objected. Clement of Alexandria, who died in A.D. 215, was one of them:

'Additions of other people's hair are entirely to be rejected, and it is a most sacrilegious thing for spurious hair to shade the head, covering the skull with dead locks. For on whom does the Presbyter lay his hand? Whom does he bless? Not the woman decked out, but another's hair, and through them another head. . . . They deceive the men by the excessive quantity of their hair and shame the Lord as far as in them lies, by adorning themselves meretriciously, in order to dissemble the truth. And they defame the head, which is truly beautiful. . . . The woman who dyes her head yellow, Menander, the comic poet, expels from the house: "Now get out of this house, for no chaste woman ought to make her hair yellow", nor, I would add, stain her cheeks nor paint her eyes. Unawares, the poor wretches destroy their own beauty by the introduction of what is spurious. . . . Wherefore they are seen to be yellow from the use of cosmetics and susceptible to disease, their flesh, which has been shaded with poisons, being now in a melting state. So they dishonour the Creator of men, as if the beauty given by Him were nothing worth. As you might expect, they become lazy in housekeeping, sitting like painted things to be looked at, not as if made for domestic economy.' In succeeding centuries the cry of outrage was to be repeated again and again, never with the slightest effect.

PLATE 12 : ANCIENT GREEK MEN 700–400 B.C.

A   Sixth century B.C. Note the similarity to the styles of other ancient peoples.

B   Sixth century B.C. The centre parting later disappeared for men but continued to be worn by women. The fillet continued to be worn in various forms by both sexes throughout their history.

C   *c.* Sixth century B.C.

D, E   *c.* Sixth century B.C. Athlete.

F   *c.* Sixth century B.C. Athlete.

G   Late sixth century B.C. Young men were beginning to wear shorter hair, though older ones often let theirs grow. A braid sometimes replaced the fillet and was arranged in various ways (see K, N, P, and S below). Here the ends of the braid are concealed under the front hair.

H   *c.* 490 B.C. The ends of the hair in front are artificially curled.

I   *c.* 470 B.C.

J   Sixth century B.C.

K   *c.* 475 B.C. The ends of the braid are concealed under the front curls.

L   *c.* Fifth century B.C. The style of turning the hair over the fillet was followed by both men and women. The long, hanging ends come from both the front and the back hair.

M   *c.* Fifth century B.C. Spiral curls of false hair were attached to the fillet. The elaborate hairdress suggests that either Zeus or a king was being represented.

N   Fifth century B.C. The braids, starting on either side, cross in back and are tied in front, as in P below.

O   *c.* Fifth century B.C. Sometimes, instead of being wrapped neatly around the fillet, the back ends of the hair were simply allowed to hang down (see also Figure 8).

P   Fifth century B.C. The front hair is cut short and the long back hair braided (see N above).

Q   *c.* Fifth century B.C.

R   Fifth century B.C. Zeus. Note particularly how the hair falls forward from the crown, then is draped over the fillet.

S   Fifth century B.C. Zeus. The braids are tied in front (see P above).

T   *c.* 450 B.C.

U   Fifth century B.C.

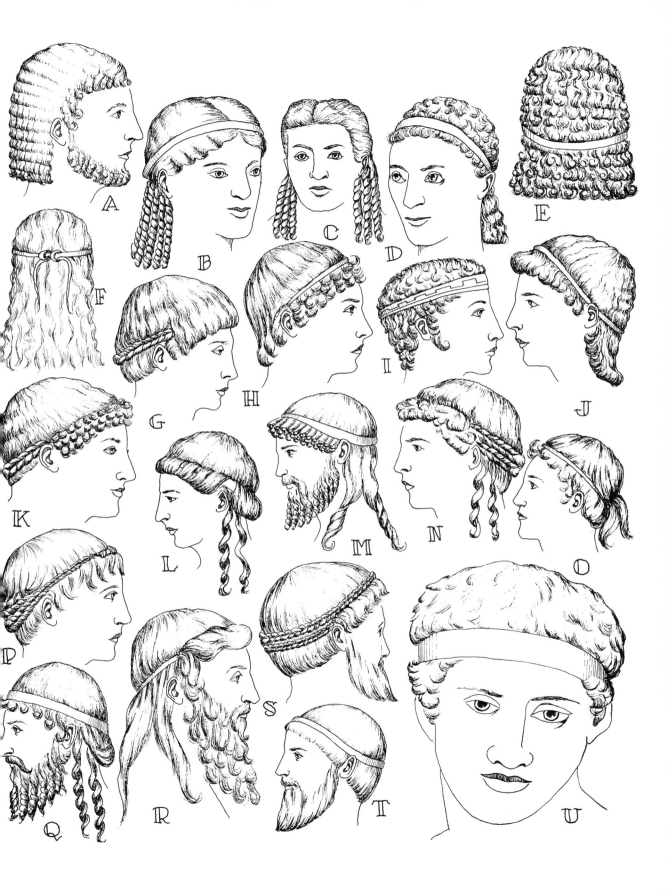

PLATE 13 : ANCIENT GREEK MEN 650 B.C.–A.D. 200

A   *c.* 540–500 B.C. Votary.

B   *c.* 575–550 B.C. Note the similarity to other ancient styles, such as those of the Assyrians and Sumerians.

C   *c.* 500–450 B.C.

D   Late seventh century B.C. Attic. Wig.

E   Plato, 427?–347? B.C. (see J below). The hair is turned over a fillet, which is completely concealed; and the long hanging ends are curled.

F   Dionysius the Elder, 430?–367 B.C. Tyrant of Syracuse. The hair spreads out from the crown in all directions, as in C above, and the ends are curled.

G   470–440 B.C. Votary. Hair and beard are artificially curled.

H   Euripides, 485 or 480–406 B.C. Athenian dramatist.

I   *c.* 325 B.C. Razor.

J   Plato, 427?–347? B.C. (see E above).

K   The god Pan. He is usually depicted with horns.

L   Zeus. The front hair is wrapped around the fillet. Zeus was always depicted with a beard, usually curled.

M   First century A.D. Pedanius Dioscorides. Botanist. Beards were again being generally worn.

N   Early comb.

O   *c.* 300 B.C. Apollo. He was usually depicted with his hair tied in front and falling loose on his neck in back.

P   Galen, *c.* A.D. 130–200. Physician and philosophical writer.

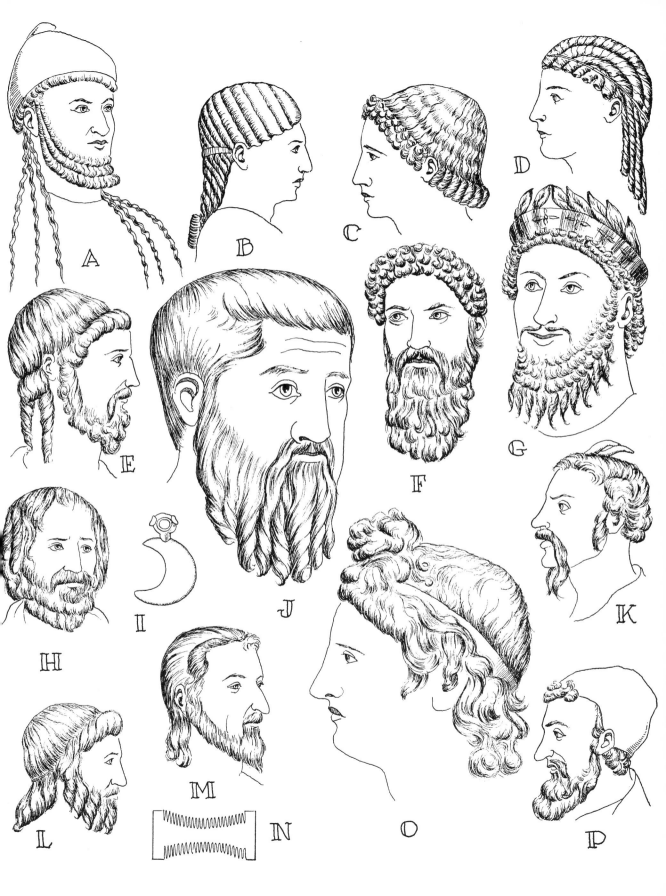

A   B   C   D

E   F   G

H   I   J   K

L   M   N   O   P

PLATE 14 : ANCIENT GREEK MEN 600–90 B.C.

A   Fifth century B.C. Young men were clean shaven, but older ones often wore beards. Fillets were not worn when the hair was as short as this.

B   *c.* 457 B.C. The back hair is pulled up smoothly over the fillet.

C   440–400 B.C.

D   Fifth century B.C. Fillets were worn by both sexes and adults of all ages.

E   470–450 B.C. The fillet here is in the form of a braided cord.

F   *c.* 420 B.C. Euripides.

G   *c.* 400 B.C. Hippocrates.

H   *c.* 400 B.C. Socrates.

I   Fourth century B.C.

J   Fourth century B.C.

K   *c.* 330 B.C. Alexander. Other portraits show the hair shorter.

L   *c.* 300 B.C. Menander.

M   Third century B.C. Young boy.

N   Fourth century B.C.

O   Hellenistic period. Child.

P   *c.* 290 B.C. Epicurus. Philosophers were customarily bearded.

Q   Third century B.C.

R   Second century B.C.

S   *c.* 90 B.C.

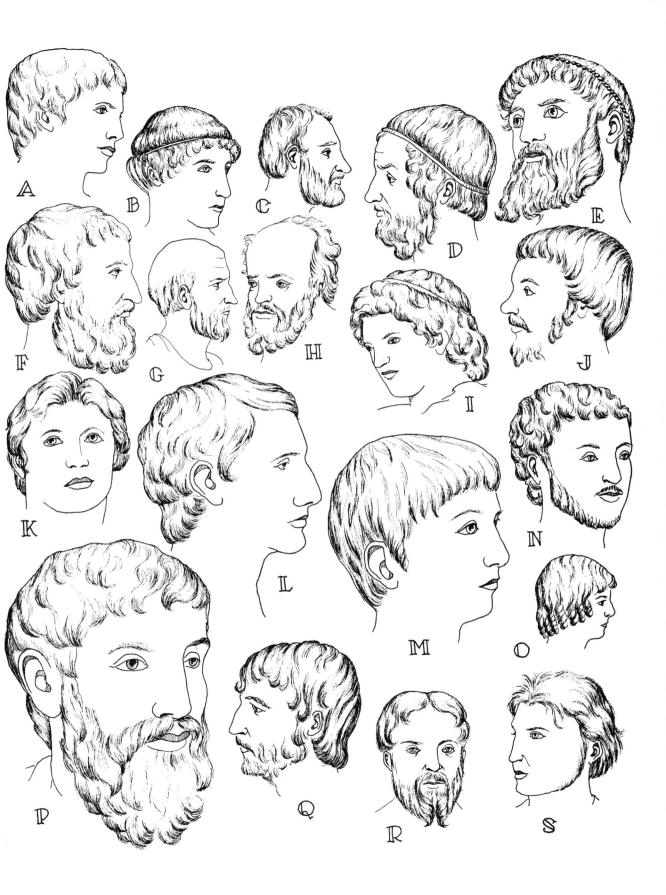

A

B

C

D

E

F

G

H

I

J

K

L

M

N

O

P

Q

R

S

PLATE 15 : ANCIENT GREEK WOMEN 800–450 B.C.

A   Before the seventh century B.C.

B   Sixth century B.C.

C   Fifth century B.C.

D   Sixth century B.C.

E   Sixth century B.C.

F   Late sixth or early fifth century B.C.

G   Fifth century B.C.

H   Amazon of Ephesus.

I   Date uncertain.

J   Persephone.

K   Date uncertain.

L   Fifth century B.C.

M   *c.* 460 B.C.

N   Early fifth century B.C. Old woman.

O   Date uncertain.

P   Date uncertain.

Since the Greeks always considered low foreheads a mark of beauty, the hair was usually arranged to decrease the height in one way or another.

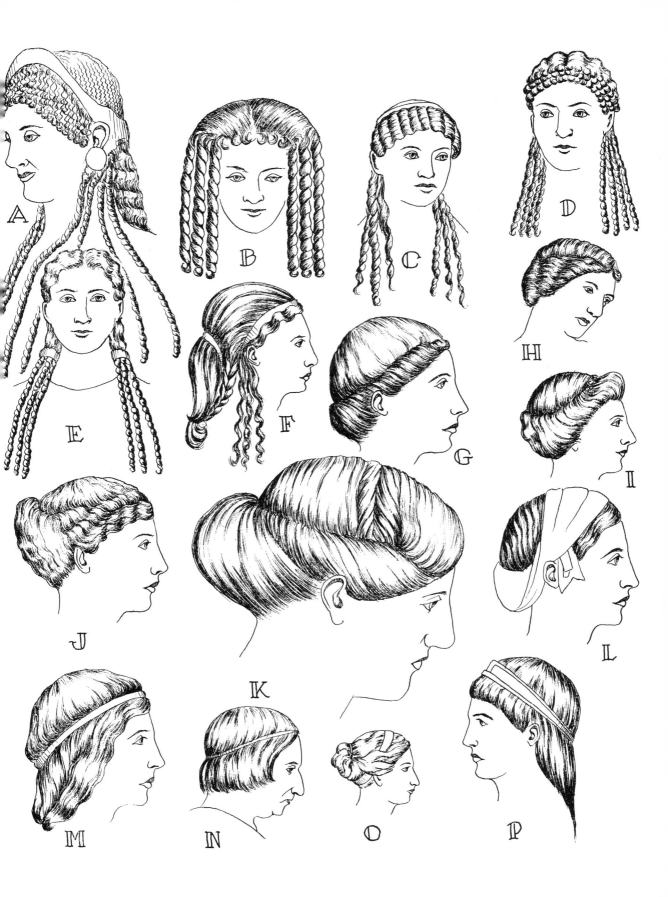

A   B   C   D

E   F   G   H

I

J   K   L

M   N   O   P

PLATE 16 : ANCIENT GREEK WOMEN 450–100 B.C.

A   Mid-fifth century B.C. The ribbons and kerchiefs binding the hair, as shown here and in C, D, and G, below, were popular until the time of Alexander (see also 17-J-K-L).

B   Late fifth or fourth century B.C.

C   Late fifth or fourth century B.C.

D   Late fifth or fourth century B.C.

E   Late fifth or fourth century B.C.

F   Fourth century B.C.

G   Fourth century B.C.

H   Fourth century B.C.

I   Fourth century B.C. A modification of the melon-shaped hairdo shown in Plate 17-E.

J   Second century B.C.

K   Hellenistic period.

L   Hellenistic period.

M   The goddess Artemis.

N   Post-Alexandrian.

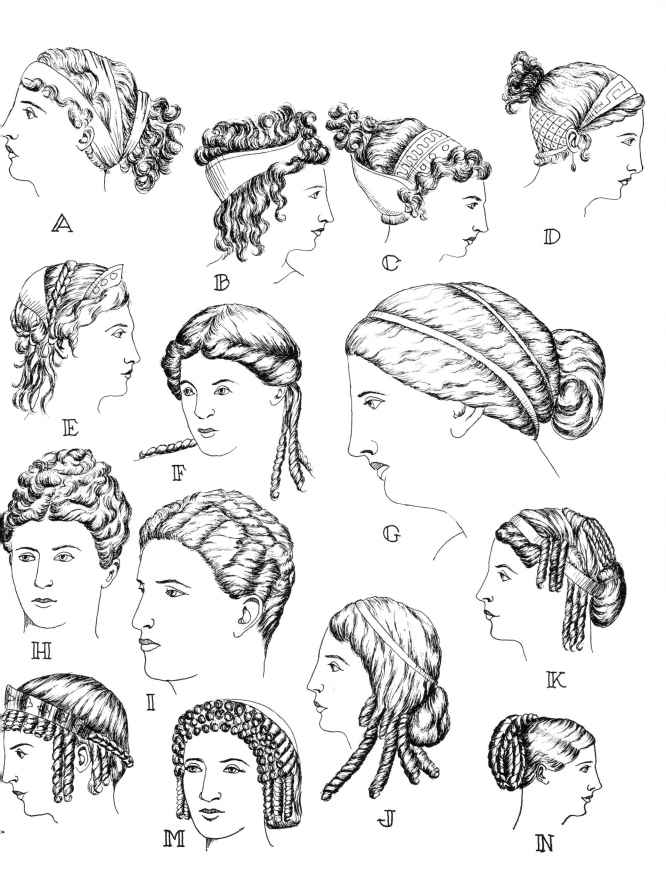

A

B

C

D

E

F

G

H

I

J

K

M

N

Plate 17 : Ancient Greek Women 500 b.c.–a.d. 100

A   Fifth century B.C. The short locks reaching upward toward the crown gradually became longer and longer and eventually developed into the knots and bows shown in F, G, and H below.

B   *c.* 450 B.C.

C   Fifth century B.C. According to Koester, 'The hair is not parted but is combed down from the crown equally on all sides in the manner of the latter end of the sixth century. The mass of hair thus drawn toward the front is then divided above the middle of the forehead, twisted slightly, and then wound round a ribbon laid rather low down across the brow and head in such a manner that it is only visible in the center of the forehead, being concealed as far as the ears by the hair which falls over it in loose waves, and is then drawn through the ribbon behind the ears and allowed to fall in long flowing curls over the shoulders. Another ribbon encircles the head a little higher up than the first, binding the hair combed down from the crown on all sides, which then hangs down from the nape of the neck in twisted locks. We might regard the older front roll of hair as a forerunner of this style, only that the front hair rolled around the head is much firmer and tighter and has consequently a more severe and conventional effect.'

D   Early fifth century B.C.

E   Second half of the fifth century B.C. Sections of the hair running the length of the head are separated and curled, then arranged in parallel rows. The style was still worn in the fourth century and was later popular in Rome (see also Plate 16-I).

F   Fifth century B.C. (see A above).

G   Probably late fifth century B.C. (see A above).

H   Probably late fifth century B.C. (see A above).

I   Probably late fifth century B.C.

J   *c.* Fifth century B.C.

K   *c.* Fifth century B.C.

L   The goddess Hera.

M   Date uncertain.

N   Late period.

O   The goddess Artemis.

P, Q   Between 300 B.C. and A.D. 100. The higher forehead and the knot behind were popular after Alexander.

R   Late period.

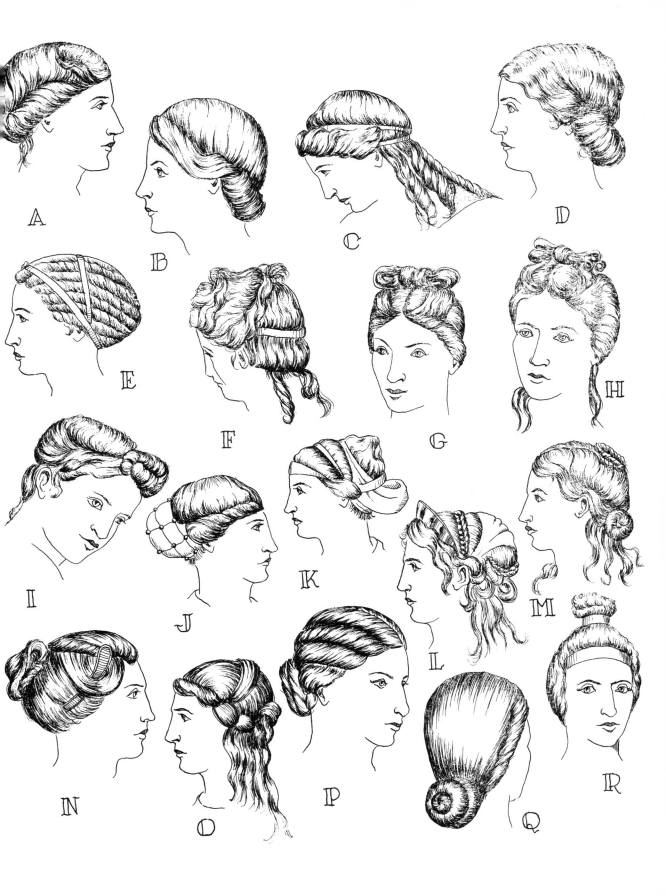

A

B

C

D

E

F

G

H

I

J

K

L

M

N

O

P

Q

R

4 · Ancient Roman Times

Did I not tell you to leave off dyeing
your hair? Now you have no hair left
to dye.

OVID

Styles for both men and women showed marked similarity to those of the Greeks; but whereas the men throughout the period of the empire maintained relatively simple styles, women taxed their ingenuity in thinking up an unending parade of new and increasingly complex arrangements.

MEN (Plates 18, 19)

As can be seen from Plates 18 and 19, the hair was for the most part worn relatively short and combed forward. Fashionable young men often curled or frizzed their hair, and until A.D. 268, sometimes wore gold dust or other coloured powders on it. Nero, of course, followed this fashion.

In the seventeenth century, William Prynne, of whom we shall hear more later, delved into the writings of ancient Romans for material to feed his violent campaign against long and 'unnatural' hair; and he reported with enormous gratification that 'Clemens Romanus enjoynes men to pole their Heads, and not to suffer their Haire to grow long, least the nourishing and perfuming of their Haire should be a meanes to inflame their lusts, and to illaqueate or inamour women with them: yeah, hee saith expressely that it is unlawfull for any Christian, or Man of God, to frizell, or trounce, to powder or coloure his Haire, to suffer it to grow long, or to fold it together, or tye it up with an haire-lace, because it is effeminate and contrary to the Law of God'.

He was apparently equally pleased to report that Clement of Alexandria 'doeth utterly condemne Colouring, Poudring, Frizeling, Curling, and Effeminate and Meretricious dressing, Adorning, and Composing of the Haire, both in the male and female sexe: so he likewise commands men to weare their Haire of a moderate and decent length, and not to suffer it to grow long, nor yet to binde it up in fillets like women, as the Frankes and Scythians doe'.

Since churchmen spoke so feelingly about long hair, clearly there must have been the temptation on the part of some men to wear it so; and we do know that it was allowed to grow long as a sign of mourning and for other special reasons. Martial, in describing the fashionable young man of his day, said that

A beau is one who with the nicest care,
In parted locks divides his curling hair;
One who with balm and cinnamon smells sweet,
Whose humming lips some Spanish air repeat.

Wigs were occasionally worn by men either as a disguise or, as in the case of Hadrian (18-M), to conceal baldness. It is said that bald Romans who preferred not to wear a wig sometimes had hair painted on with special essences and perfumes. There is evidence of this in lines addressed to Phoebus: 'Your counterfeit hair is a falsehood of the perfume which imitates it; and your sense, disgracefully bald, is covered with painted locks; you may shave much better with a sponge.'

James Stewart, writing in the latter part of the eighteenth century, says that 'it is doubted whether or no the use of what we call perukes was known among the ancients, although it is true they used false hair. Martial and Juvenal make merry with the women of their time, for making themselves look young with this borrowed hair; with the men, who changed their colour according to the seasons: and the dotards, who hoped to deceive the destinies by their white hair. But what they describe seems to have had scarce anything in common with our perukes, and were at best composed of hair painted and glued together. Nothing can be more ridiculous than the description Lanprideses gives of the emperor Commodus's peruke; it was powdered with scrapings of gold and oiled, if we may use the expression, with glutinous perfumes for the powder to hang by.'

The early Romans were bearded, but in 297 B.C. a Sicilian arrived in Rome with a troop of barbers, who cropped beards at first and eventually shaved them. The fashion caught on; and from then until the time of Hadrian, most men were beardless. Young men, however, let the beard grow until they reached their majority, at which time it was consecrated to a god. This was an important and festive day for the young man and his family. When Nero dedicated his first beard, he encased it in a golden box encrusted with pearls and consecrated it at the Capitol.

Superstitions regarding the hair, which we have already mentioned in connection with other ancient peoples, had obviously not died out. According to Plutarch, Roman women washed their heads annually on the birthday of Diana, the thirteenth day of August. Too frequent washing was believed to disturb the spirit guarding the head. And if the spirit was disturbed by washing, it can be imagined what dangers lay in cutting the hair. According to Petronius, Romans believed the hair should not be cut on board ship except during a storm, the theory being that when there was a storm, whatever mischief the evil spirits might do had already been done and a little hair cutting couldn't make things any worse.

During shaven periods, beards were allowed to grow as a sign of mourning. And when free men shaved, as they did early in the first century, slaves were required to wear beards as a sign of their subjugation. When free men were bearded, as they were in the second and third centuries, slaves were required to shave off their beards for the same reason.

The upper classes were shaved by their slaves, whereas the rest of the populace went to the public barbers' shops. Some men plucked their beards instead of shaving them. The Romans initiated the practice of using warm water for shaving, and beards were frequently softened with an oily substance before shaving. The razors were flat and straight. Scipio Africanus is believed to have been the first Roman to shave daily.

In the time of Cicero, although the beard was not generally worn, a very small beard was sometimes grown by ultra-fashionable young men. Marcus Livius was not permitted to take his seat in the senate until he had shaved off his beard. Caligula, upon occasion, wore a false gold beard.

Hadrian is generally credited with being the first Roman emperor to resume wearing the beard, which he found convenient for concealing scars. Antoninus Pius and Marcus Aurelius followed his example. But, as an article in Charles Dickens's *All the Year Round* points out, after them came Commodus; and 'as this exemplary monarch found the time hang so heavily upon his hands that he was obliged to kill flies of an afternoon, it was not likely that he would discard the precious means afforded him by shaving or making half-hours go by; barbers had a new time of it, and thenceforth continued to have the Roman emperors for patrons until Edoard overturned Romulus Augustulus, the last imperator, and inaugurated the kingdom of Italy, and with it the reign of moustaches'. It is also said that Commodus, to while away the time, would commandeer a barber's shop and cut off the noses of the customers.

WOMEN (Plates 20-23)

A Roman writer, addressing himself to the women, admonished them for their fickleness: 'You are at a loss what to be at with your hair. Sometimes you put it into a press; at others you tie it negligently together or set it entirely at liberty. You raise or lower it according to your fancy. Some keep it closely twisted up into curls, while others choose to let it float loosely on the wind.'

The Republic. Prior to the Empire, the hair was dressed rather simply at first. Married women often wore a coil on top of the head. Later the hair was parted and combed back with a knot low at the back of the head, and sometimes a slight roll over the ear. In early times elaborate coiffures were looked upon with disfavour and were associated with foreigners and courtesans. One of Plautus's characters says: 'Unless you go away from here at once, by heaven I will tear from your head those curly perfumed false locks you have so carefully arranged!' In the time of Fulvia and Octavia, during the late Republic, it was the fashion to wear the hair in a puff at the

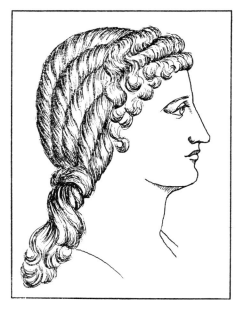

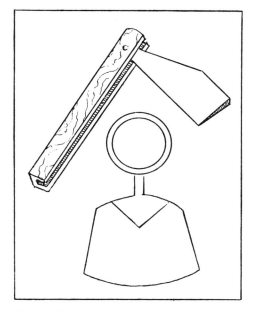

Fig. 10 : Poppaea, wife of Nero (Emperor A.D. 54–68)

Fig. 11 : Roman razors

forehead, both sides being pulled loosely back and coiled low on the head. Braids were frequently incorporated into the hairdo, as shown on Plate 20. The hair was not elaborately waved or curled.

Early Empire (27 B.C.–A.D. 69). In the time of Livia, wife of Augustus, instead of the puff and braid on top, we find the hair parted in the middle and waved, brought together in the back, and allowed to fall in waves or curls or a loose roll quite low on the neck. Sometimes a fringe of curls was worn on the forehead. The simple coiffure worn by Livia, though maintaining its basic form, gradually became more and more complicated; as a result, wigs were frequently worn. Messalina had a variety of them and always wore a blonde one as a disguise in setting off on her nocturnal adventures. But apparently nobody was fooled, especially since she often arrived back at the palace without it. It was usually gallantly returned the following day.

It is interesting to note that at one time prostitutes were required either to dye their hair yellow or to wear yellow wigs. Later—perhaps due at least partially to the influence of Messalina—yellow hair became fashionable. As for Messalina herself, Martial wrote: 'Her toilet table contained a hundred lies; and while she was in Rome, her hair was blushing by the Rhine. A man was in no condition to say he loved her, for what he loved in her was not herself, and that which was herself was impossible to love.'

Pliny handed down a formula for a black hair dye consisting of leeches and vinegar which had fermented for two months in a lead vessel. This was to be applied to the hair in the sunlight, and the lady was instructed to hold oil in her mouth to keep her teeth from turning black.

Women who wanted their hair blonde, like that of the Germans, either wore blonde wigs (made from German hair) or bleached their hair with ashes of plants, elderberries, nutshells, vinegar sediment, etc. The Germans used a mixture of goat's fat and beechwood ashes to redden their hair; and the same formula, called Hessian soap, was used by the Romans to colour their hair or their wigs. Later, Galen tells us that some ladies of his time used saffron to make their hair yellow, whereas others tried to bleach it by sitting in the sun. Martial touched on the matter in verse:

> The golden hair that Galla wears
> Is hers—who would have thought it?
> She swears 'tis hers, and true she swears,
> For I know where she bought it.

At another time he says to a lady no longer young, 'I know very well that the baldness of your head can easily be concealed; but as to your blind eye, the case is not the same. There are wigs in the shops, but there are no eyes.' Wigs continued to be found in the shops until A.D. 672.

The better wigs were usually made on a goatskin foundation. The *galerus* or half-dress wigs were worn at home or as a disguise outside. Messalina would have worn this type on her adventures. The *capillameus* (worn by Caligula, for example) was a fuller wig, more carefully constructed. Sometimes only false curls were added to the natural hair.

It was in this period that Ovid, in his *Art of Love*, advised women to arrange their hair with art. 'All its charm will depend on how much or how little care you bestow on it. There are a thousand styles of hairdressing. Each woman must know how to choose that which suits her best; and as to this matter, her mirror will be her wisest counsellor.'

Flavian Period (A.D. 69–96). Later in the first century the fringe of forehead curls got out of hand. This is the period of the striking arrangement known as an *orbis*, in which the front hair, the ends tightly curled, was arranged on a crescent-shaped wire frame (Plate 22). There were many variations of this; and Plotina, wife of Trajan, later modified the basic style. Juvenal describes a tense session of arranging the *orbis*:

> Another, trembling on the left, prepares
> To open and arrange the straggling hairs
> In ringlets trim; meanwhile the council meet
> And first the nurse, a personage discreet,
> Late from the toilet to the wheel removed
> (The effect of time) yet still of taste approved,

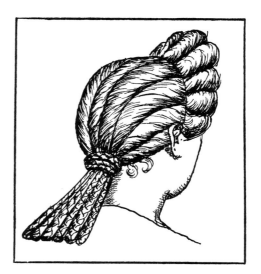

Fig. 12 : Plotina, wife of Trajan
(Emperor A.D. 98–117),
wearing her own version
of the *orbis*

Gives her opinion; then the rest in course
As age or practice lends their judgment force;
So warm they grow and so much pains they take,
You'd think her life, or honour, was at stake.
So high they pile her head, such tiers on tiers
With wary hands they pile, that she appears
Andromache before—and what behind?
A dwarf, a creature of another kind!

The iron for curling the hair was called a *calamistrum*, and the slaves who used it were the *ciniflones*. Women of quality spent great sums on oils and perfumes for the hair. The principal ingredients of most of these were the root of the Indian kostum plant and the leaf of the spikenard.

Second Century. With Matidia, niece of Trajan, the *orbis* was replaced by an equally complex arrangement in the nature of a diadem (Plate 22-K-L), usually composed of several metal bands wound with hair. Behind this, braids were wound about the head several times, leaving the crown uncovered. Later, in Hadrian's reign, the circle of braids developed to such an extent that the diadem was crowded out.

In the time of Faustina the Elder (Plate 23-B), who is said to have worn three hundred wigs in nineteen years, the circle of braids was much smaller and lower. With Lucilla, Faustina the Younger, and Crispina, it disappeared completely, the hair being parted and waved and brought together at the back and arranged with coiled braids or hair loosely coiled without being braided.

Third Century. At the end of the second century and early in the third, in the time of Septimus Severus and his wife, Julia Domna (Plate 23-J-K), the coiffures were padded to make them more massive, with heavy waves around the face and masses of coiled braids on the back of the head. Wigs were frequently worn. In many cases portrait busts of women were made with detachable marble hair so that the coiffure could be kept in style. Christian writers were highly displeased with the wigs and said so regularly. 'Ye annex I know not what enormities of Periwiges and counterfeite Haire', complained Tertullian (in a seventeenth-century translation), 'sometimes upon the crowne of the head like an Hat, sometimes behind in the poll'.

During most of the third century the ears were exposed; and the hair at first was lower in back, falling on to the shoulders. Later it rose again. Intricate braid arrangements were often worn on the back of the head. At the close of the century and into the next the weight of the hair moved upward to the crown of the head. Braids, as usual, were an important part of the coiffure (see Plate 23).

The Vestal Virgins wore a special style, described by Palmerlee:

'We see a cloth in six folds wound around the head and over this a hood-like drapery. Examining the back, we find that the hair was divided into six parts, these being made into six braids, three on each side. These braids were crossed and so wound about the head that there were six braids on top, under the six folds of cloth. This cloth, called the *infula*, was fastened at the back by the narrower *vitta*, the ends of which are seen falling on the shoulders in front. Over all this was placed the hood-like drapery before mentioned. In early times, the hair of the newly married women was parted into six locks with a spear and the style adapted by the Vestals may be a relic of that custom.'

The hairpins used were single-pronged, of gold, silver, jet, bone, and ivory and usually had decorative or jewelled heads, often several inches long (Plate 21 and Figure 13). Nets and ribbons were worn as well as flowers, leaves, pearls, and precious stones.

Wigs continued to be worn into the third century, and the Church railed against them. The wearing of them was even designated by some churchmen a mortal sin. Cyprian is said to have declared that 'adultery is a grievous sin; but she who wears false hair is guilty of a greater'. Dr John Doran suggests that it must have been a comfortable state of society when two angry ladies could exclaim to each other, 'You may say of me what you please; you may charge me with breaking the seventh commandment; but, thank Heaven and Cyprian, you cannot accuse me of wearing a wig!'

Tertullian declared that 'all personal disguise is adultery before God. All perukes, paint, and powder are such disguises and inventions of the devil.' And he pointed out to his listeners that 'the fake hair you wear may have come not only from a criminal but from a very dirty head, perhaps from the head of one already damned'. If this didn't work, he reminded people that they were not born with wigs. 'God did not give them to you', he thundered. 'God not giving them, you must necessarily have received them from the devil.'

Clement of Alexandria went a step further and declared in all seriousness that when wig wearers were blessed, the benediction remained on the wig and did not penetrate to the wearer. The timid may have been frightened into conformity by this; but there were those, as there always are, who preferred to keep their wigs and take their chances.

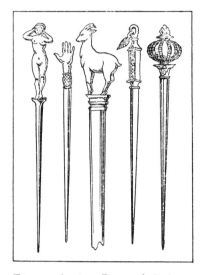

Fig. 13 : Ancient Roman hairpins

PLATE 18 : ANCIENT ROMAN MEN 50 B.C.–A.D. 250

A   Marcus Junius Brutus, 85–42 B.C.

B   Julius Caesar, 102?–44 B.C. (see also Plate 19-D).

C   Pompey, 106–48 B.C.

D   Augustus as a boy, *c.* 50 B.C.

E   Lucius Augustus.

F   *c.* A.D. 10. Boy.

G   Claudius, 10 B.C.–A.D. 54. Emperor, A.D. 41–54.

H   Lucius Annaeus Seneca, 3? B.C.–A.D. 65.

I   A.D. 50.

J   Vespasian, A.D. 9–79. Emperor, A.D. 69–79.

K   Titus, A.D. 40?–81. Son of Vespasian. Emperor, A.D. 79–81.

L   *c.* A.D. 100. Boy.

M   Hadrian, A.D. 87–138. Emperor, A.D. 117–38. He wore a wig to cover his baldness, and he revived the beard to conceal scars.

N, O   *c.* A.D. 130. Antinous, favourite of Hadrian. Noted for his beauty. Drawing O represents his usual hair style. The coiffure in N is indicative of special honours and achievements, as in P below.

P   Second century A.D.

Q   Septimus Severus, 146–211. Emperor, 193–211.

R   Caracalla, 188–217. Emperor, 211–17.

S   Third century A.D.

T   Tweezers.

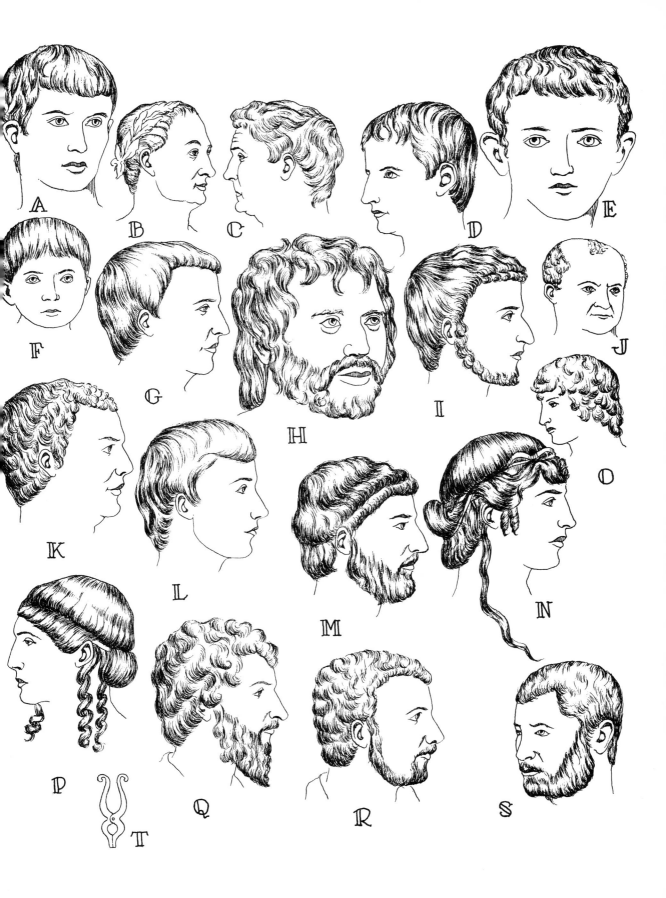

A

B

C

D

E

F

G

H

I

J

K

L

M

N

O

P

Q

R

S

T

PLATE 19 : ANCIENT ROMAN MEN 50 B.C.–A.D. 395

A   Marcus Salvius Otho, A.D. 32–69. Emperor A.D. 69.

B   *c.* 30 B.C. Child.

C   The young Nero, A.D. 37–68. Emperor, A.D. 54–68.

D   Caius Julius Caesar, 102?–44 B.C. (see also Plate 18-B).

E   End of the first century A.D.

F   A.D. 100.

G   Marcus Aurelius, A.D. 161–80.

H   Lucius Verus. Died A.D. 169.

I   Juvenal, A.D. 60?–140? Satirical poet.

J   Ulpian (Domitius Ulpianus), died *c.* A.D. 228. Jurist.

K   Tertullian, A.D. 150?–230? Theologian.

L   *c.* 134. L. Julius Ursus Servianus, Hadrian's brother-in-law.

M, N   A.D. 193. Emperor Pertinax.

O   Constantine II, A.D. 312–40.

P   Theodosius I, A.D. 346?–95.

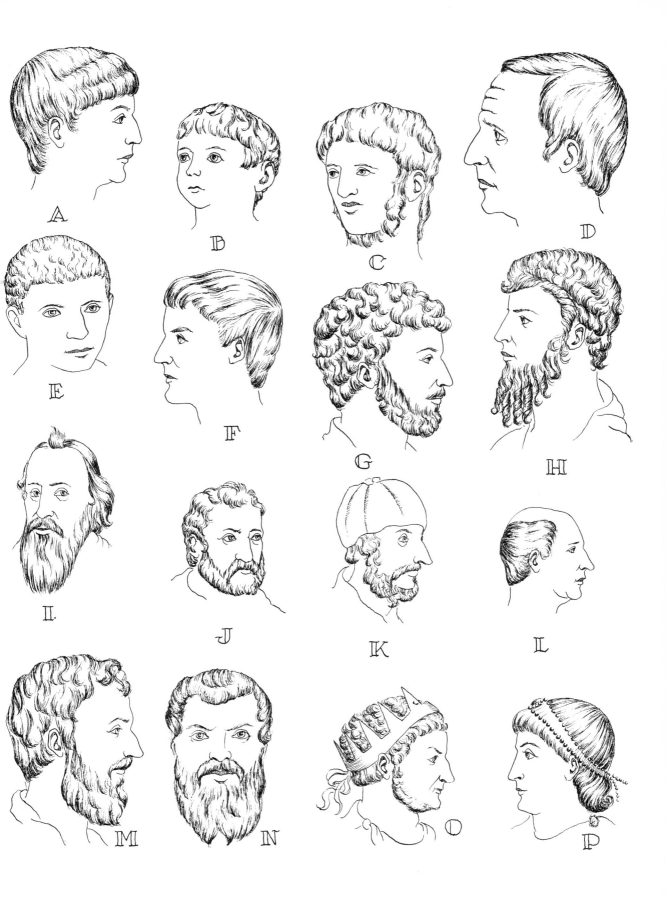

A B C D

E F G H

I. J K L

M N O P

PLATE 20 : ANCIENT ROMAN WOMEN 100 B.C.–A.D. 50

A   Date uncertain.

B   Dancing girl.

C   Dancing girl.

D   *c.* A.D. 1.

E   Minacia Pola. Wig. The centre parting, the full waves, the curls around the ears, and the escaping curls on the shoulders are all typical of the period. The hair was worn low in back, as shown in F below and in 21-B.

F, G   Early first century. Livia, 55? B.C.–A.D. 29. Typifies early Empire style (see also E above and 21-B).

H   Mid-first century B.C. Fulvia, wife of Marc Antony. Died 40 B.C. The puff at the forehead and the coil at the neck are typical of the fashion of the period. Sometimes the hair behind the front puff was braided and the braid carried over the top of the head and down to the coil on the neck. Braids were also worn around the head and over the head, as in L below.

I, J   Mid-first century B.C. Probably Octavia. The back hair was sometimes doubled into a coil hanging low on the neck, as in K below. The front hair in K is, however, of a slightly later period. The back hair might also be coiled without being braided. The hair was not elaborately waved or curled.

K   *c.* A.D. 30. This is a good example of the transition from the style of Fulvia (H above) to that of Livia (F, G). The puff has disappeared, and the hair is worn low on the neck. But the braid remains, and the hair is only slightly waved and not very full.

L   Probably first century A.D.

M   First century A.D.

N   Late first century B.C., or early first A.D. The fringe at the forehead is probably a development of the puff of the Fulvia style in H above. The hair is beginning to get a little fuller (see also Plate 21-A).

O   Late first century B.C., or early first A.D.

P   Late first century B.C., or early first A.D.

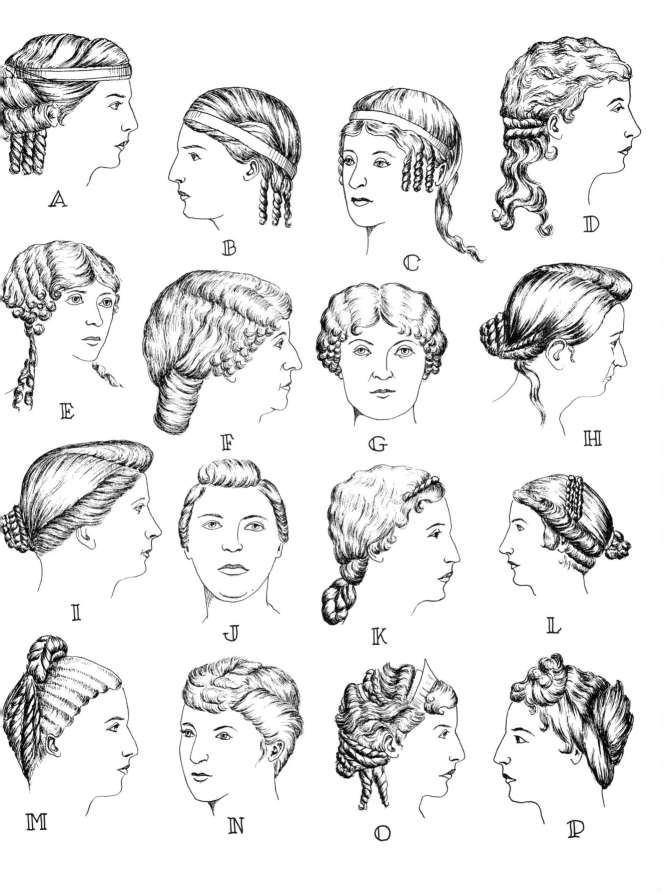

A

B

C

D

E

F

G

H

I

J

K

L

M

N

O

P

PLATE 21 : ANCIENT ROMAN WOMEN 20 B.C.–A.D. 260

A   *c.* 20 B.C. (see also Plate 20-N).

B   Early first century A.D. (see also Plate 20-K).

C   Late first century A.D.

D   Late first century A.D.

E   Possibly Valeria Messalina, notorious third wife of Claudius. Put to death in A.D. 48 for flagrant immorality. She had a number of wigs of different colours, partly for use as disguises.

F   Mid-first century A.D.

G   *c.* A.D. 80. Possibly Berenice, favourite of Titus.

H   *c.* A.D. 100. Plotina, wife of Trajan. This is her modification of the *orbis* style (see Plate 22-F-G, also I and J below). According to Palmerlee, 'the hair was still parted, brought forward, and supported on the wire frame, but it was no longer cut short. At the front, just over the forehead, the hair was evidently brought together in a knot. The ends then remaining were divided into two parts and wound around a narrow half circlet of metal which fitted on the forehead below the *orbis* and reached to the ears. If there were ends still left, they were curled and left hanging in front of the ears.'

I   *c.* A.D. 100. Marciana, sister of Trajan (see also Plate 22-J). A modification of the *orbis* (Plate 22-F-G).

J   Early second century. Style based on Plotina's modification of the *orbis* (see H above). The waved front hair was arranged over a wire frame.

K   Probably *c.* A.D. 140, period of Faustina the Elder (see Plates 22-K and 23-B).

L   Hairpins. They were of jet, bone, ivory, gold, or silver (see also Figure 13).

M   Late second century. It was fashionable in this period to comb the back hair forward and to show a definite separation from the front hair, which was in the form of waved bands.

N   *c.* A.D. 175. The two sections of hair were often separated by a braid, as they are here, or a twist of hair, as they are in P below, and the hair coiled loosely on the neck or arranged in coiled braids.

O   Second century.

P   *c.* A.D. 190. Empress Crispina, wife of Commodus (see M and N above).

Q   *c.* A.D. 215. Julia Cornelia Paula.

R   Third century.

S   Third century. Empress Cornelia Salonina, wife of Galienus.

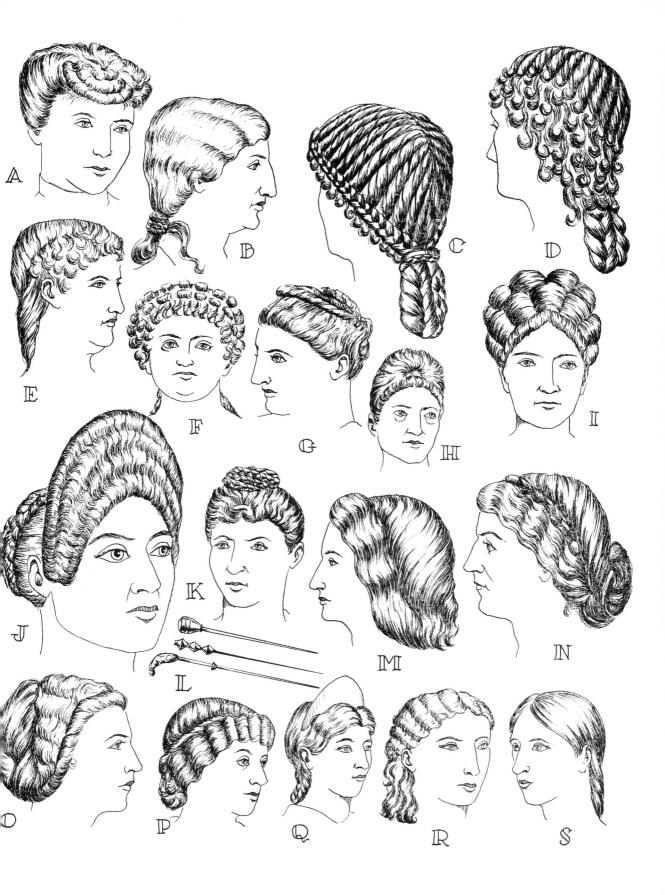

PLATE 22 : ANCIENT ROMAN WOMEN 50–120

A   *c.* A.D. 50.

B   *c.* A.D. 60. Octavia, wife of Nero. Wig.

C   *c.* A.D. 90. Domitia, wife of Emperor Domitian.

D   End of first century. (This is a modification of the *orbis* style in F and G below.)

E   Late first or early second century. A modification of the *orbis* (see F and G below).

F, G   Late first century. Style of Julia, daughter of Titus. *Orbis*. The curls are arranged on crescent-shaped wire frames. The back hair is divided into sections, braided, then curled. Sometimes the hair was coiled without braiding. (For modifications and variations see D, E, H, I, and J on this plate and 21-H-I-J.)

H   Early second century.

I   Probably *c.* A.D. 140 (see L and N below).

J   Early second century. Marciana, sister of Trajan (see also Plate 21-I).

K   Early second century. The front hair is wound around two metal bands to give it shape. Sometimes parts of the metal bands were allowed to show. It was customary to wind braids several times around the head, leaving the crown open.

L   Early second century. Wife of Trajan. Here also the ends of the hair are wound around a band. In this case there are three such bands instead of two, as in I above.

M   Young girl.

N   Mid-second century. Period of Faustina the Elder (23-B) and Antoninus Pius. According to Palmerlee, the hair at this time usually 'was parted, slightly waved, combed back, and braided into four, five, or six braids on each side at varying heights. These were brought upward and formed into a long, narrow coil, very high on the head. A band was often worn in front of this coil, while a lyre-shaped ornament, evidently formed of the hair, is sometimes seen.'

O   Second quarter of the second century. Hadrian period. Here the braids have spread over such a large area of the head that the diadem effect across the front has been crowded out.

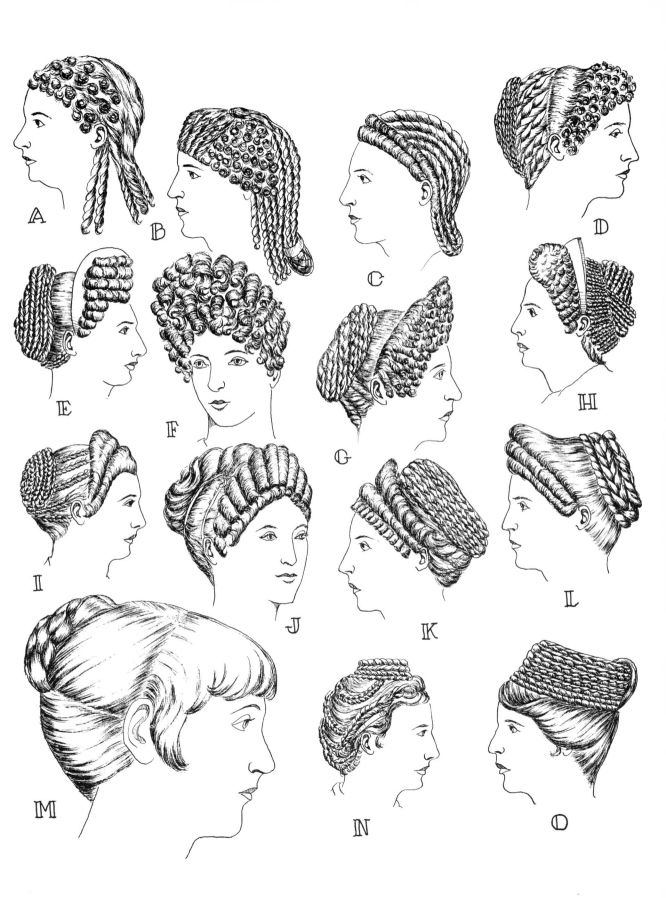

A

B

C

D

E

F

G

H

I

J

K

L

M

N

O

PLATE 23 : ANCIENT ROMAN WOMEN 50–120

A   Early second century. The very large crown of braids is typical of the Hadrian period and is a development of the smaller circlet which preceded it.

B   Second century. Faustina the Elder, 104?–41. Wife of Antoninus Pius. Typifies the hair style of her period.

C   *c.* A.D. 130. For other fashionable crown-of-braids head-dresses, see A, B, and D on this plate and Plate 22-N-O.

D   *c.* A.D. 140.

E   A.D. 195 (see J and K below).

F   Early third century (see J and K below).

G   Early third century. Julia Mamaea, mother of Alexander Severus.

H   Third century, probably second quarter.

I   Third century, probably second quarter.

J, K   Early third century. Julia Domna, wife of Septimus Severus. Typifies the padded hair style of her period. There were always massive braids or coils at the back of the head. Wigs were common. (See also E and F above and Plate 21-O.)

L   Third century.

M   Third century, second quarter. Orbiana, wife of Alexander Severus. The hair is less massive, and the coil at the back has shrunk. Notice also that the hair is lower in back. Later (O, P, Q, R below) it rose again.

N   Third century.

O   Third century. This is of a later period than Julia Domna (J and K above). Braids on top of and around the head (see also P, Q, and R below) once again assumed importance.

P   A.D. 313.

Q   Fourth century.

R   Fourth century.

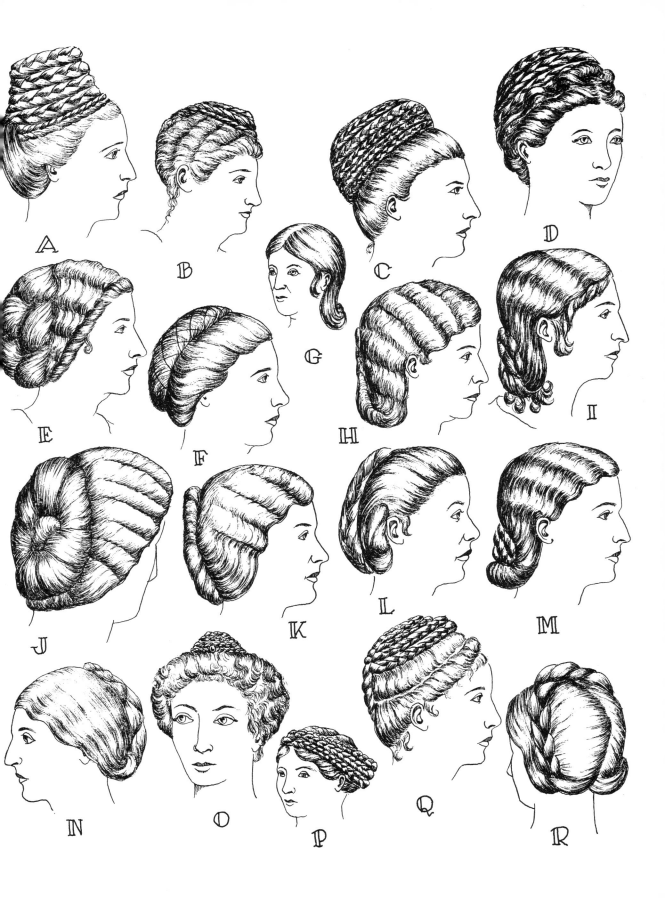

A

B

C

D

E

F

G

H

I

J

K

L

M

N

O

P

Q

R

5 · The Middle Ages

Hire yelwe heer was browdid in a tress
Behynde hire back a yerde long, I guess.
                                    CHAUCER

The period usually referred to as the Middle Ages extends roughly from the fall of the Roman Empire in 476 to the beginning of the fifteenth century in Italy and to the end of it in France and England. Unfortunately, our information about this long period, particularly the early years, is limited. Since the arts were not flourishing and printing had not been invented, most of the details of daily living, which we should like very much to have, are buried in the past. And the few which are available require considerable research by scholars of that particular period.

Many of the hair styles shown in the plates have been taken from sculpture, stained glass windows, mosaics, and carvings in stone, wood, or ivory. Allowing for limitations of the medium (particularly mosaics and stained glass), these sources give an acceptable picture of styles, though scholars have not always been able to pinpoint exact dates. But when we come to finding reasonable likenesses of famous people, we are in difficulty. Most of them that we have were not made by contemporary artists. In some cases they were, presumably, working from the most reliable sources available; in others one suspects they imagined the whole thing since the portraits they created contradict everything we know. There is no better example of this than engravings in the British Museum of the early kings of England. Some of them appear to be quite reasonable and were, in fact, taken directly from effigies on the tombs. Yet in one engraving King Henry I is depicted with long hair, a small moustache and a costume totally out of period. Others who are known to have been clean shaven are shown with moustaches or beards, frequently of a style fashionable when the engraving was made.

One must remember, however, that kings, along with other people, changed their hair styles and cut off their beards or let them grow, proof of which has often been lost. We do, however, have a striking example of such a change in Figure 38, Chapter 7, in which Ferdinand I of Germany is shown beardless and long-haired as a young man, then with beard and moustache and a totally different hair style at a later period. In the nineteenth century we find that the beard and moustache of Italy's Victor Emmanuel II (Figure 106, Chapter 11), as well as his hair style, changed markedly over the years. Some other examples can be found in the plates. In many instances, one can only accept artists' conceptions, based largely on imperfect contemporary descriptions which have come down to us.

THE BARBARIANS

The term is usually applied to any uncivilized peoples such as the early Goths, Saxons, and Gauls. Their single characteristic (which tended to distress the civilized peoples with whom they came into contact) was the tendency to wear very long moustaches and no beards. According to Strabo, the ancient inhabitants of Cornwall and the Scilly isles, a peaceable people and more civilized than some, wore 'their mustachios hanging down upon their breasts like wings'. We usually think of the barbarians with long, dirty, uncombed hair. The stereotype apparently holds good for certain tribes at certain times, but each tribe had its own customs and sometimes changed those customs on coming into contact with other races. In no case, apparently, were the hair and the beard neglected. They may not have been frequently washed and combed and oiled and perfumed, as they often were among more civilized peoples, but they were still a source of considerable pride.

According to Diodorus Siculus, the ancient Gauls 'frequently wash their hair with a lixivium made from chalk, turning it back from the forehead over the crown of the head and letting it fall down their necks. This gives them the appearance of satyrs and Pans. They indeed allow it to grow so thick that it scarce differs from a horse's mane. Some shave their beards; others make them grow in a modish way. The nobility [that is, chieftains] are shaved but wear moustaches, which hang down so as to cover their mouths, so that when they eat and drink, these brush their victuals or dip into their liquids.'

From 27 B.C. to A.D. 290 the Gaulish aristocracy are reported to have grown moustaches, whereas the rest of the nation wore pointed beards. The hair was a matter for great pride, and the Gauls are said to have sometimes dyed it bright red with goat's grease and ashes of beech timber. The Anglo-Saxons went a step further and coloured theirs, as Sparrow writes, 'a vivid green, a fine orange, and a deep, rich blue'.

Blue seems to have been the favourite, according to contemporary drawings, in which the hair is shown in various colours. But it has been suggested that after all, these were primitive people; and modern children, who go through a primitive stage in their first experience with drawing, have been known to colour hair blue or green or orange or anything else which happened to strike their fancy. There are also contemporary reports of blue-haired Saxons, but the question arises as to whether the writers saw the people or just the drawings or merely heard reports of the drawings.

It is known that the Germans reddened their hair with a preparation which was later introduced into Italy. They wore their hair long; and, according to Tacitus, short hair was a sign of ignominy. There were, however, many German tribes, and one cannot be sure which ones were meant. Plate 24-C and D show two striking hair styles which the *Encyclopédie Larousse* designates as coming from *Germanie*.

According to Sparrow, 'In 476 the Roman Empire of the West went down, and Clovis used its magnificent ruins as a foundation for the Merovingian dynasty. I

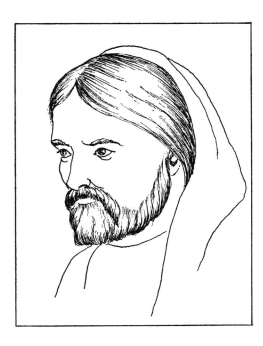

Fig. 14 : St Gregory of Tours (538–94)

remember a fine sketch in which some Frankish emigrants are seen entering the city of Lyons, A.D. 472. . . . They are tall men, fierce and strong, with no hair on their faces except a thin tuft of whiskers, through which they pass their rude combs incessantly. Each one has the back of his head shaven, while the hair in front, grown to its full length, is skilfully set up in a tall crest or topknot.' Mr Sparrow does not specify where he saw the sketch, when it was done, or how the artist was able to convey the impression of incessant combing. Sidonius Apollinaris, writing in the fifth century, gave a similar description of the Frankish hairdo, indicating that not all of the back hair was shaved:

'From the top of their red skulls descends their hair, knotted on the front and shaved in the nape of the neck. Their chins are shaven, and instead of a beard they have locks of hair arranged with the comb.' The locks of hair were their moustaches.

According to Gregory of Tours (Figure 14), it was for a long time the special prerogative of French royalty to wear long hair. Others were required to have their hair cut short as a sign of subservience. Hottoman says that 'to cut off the hair of a son of France under the first race of kings was to declare him excluded from the right of succeeding to the crown and his being reduced to the condition of a subject'. Sparrow suggests that 'to give them a flowing wig was to restore them to their former state. The King himself', he adds, 'had the finest beard and the longest ringlets: these were sometimes powdered with gold dust and ornamented with precious stones. When the King gave a single hair to anybody or let his beard be touched, his courtiers knew that he had just paid his most valued compliment, or else had brought happily to completion an important affair of state.'

As to the relative beardlessness, he goes on to say that the Franks 'were not always a shaven race. As their power increased and their social standing became

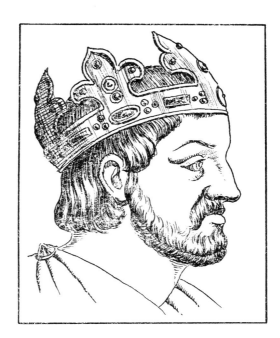

Fig. 15 : Pepin the Short (714–68),
King of the Franks

more and more marked by contrasts of wealth and poverty, the beard, like the hair, became a sign of liberty, of rank, and authority. At first the freemen left only a small tuft under the lower lip, but this little decoration grew and spread, till at last in the sixth and seventh centuries the slaves alone were beardless as well as bald.' The Germans in the sixth century were wearing long beards.

Fairholt reports that the Normans also shaved the back of the head and that after the Conquest both men and women wore their hair very long, the women's braided with silk and reaching nearly to the floor. And if their own hair wasn't long enough, they used false hair. The Normans were shaven in 1066 but later grew long beards. The Saxons wore beards, often carefully trimmed, and long hair, parted in the centre (25-S-U-W). The lower classes often cut the hair short.

The Gothic priests of Scandinavia shaved their heads except for a long tail which hung down from the crown, and they wore long beards (Figure 16). The Danish officers in England during the reign of Ethelred the Unready are said to have won the hearts of the ladies by the length and beauty of their hair, 'which they combed at least once a day'.

The Gauls are reported to have bleached their hair with lime water and worn it long and flowing like a horse's mane. The nobility shaved the beard but kept the moustache.

Very similar to the style of the Gothic priests is one of the Celtic styles, in which the temples, as well as the entire face, were shaved. The hair on top of the head was permitted to grow long and was drawn together in a *glib* or long lock, as shown in Figure 17. More common was the long, full hair and long moustaches with shaved chin, as illustrated in Plate 8-L, Chapter 2. The ancient Britons also wore the hair and moustaches long and shaved the chin.

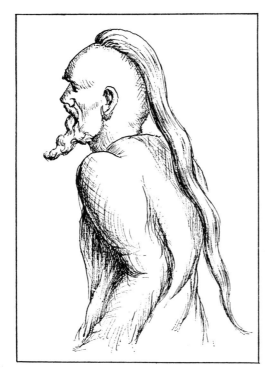

Fig. 16: *Drotte* or Gothic priest of Scandinavia

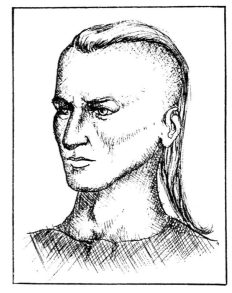

Fig. 17: Celtic warrior wearing his hair
in a *glib*

Perhaps the explanation for long hair among most of the barbaric tribes can be found in superstition. We have already mentioned the reluctance of primitive people to wash the hair for fear of giving offence to the protective spirit of the head. Sir James Frazer, writing on 'Taboo and the Perils of the Soul', points out that 'when the head was considered so sacred that it might not even be touched without grave offence, it is obvious that the cutting of the hair must have been a delicate and difficult operation. . . . There is first the danger of disturbing the spirit of the head, which may be injured in the process and may revenge itself upon the person who molests him. Secondly, there is the difficulty of disposing of the shorn locks. For the savage believes that the sympathetic connection which exists between himself and every part of his body continues to exist even after the physical connection has been broken and that therefore he will suffer from any harm that may befall the severed parts of his body, such as the clippings of his hair or the parings of his nails. Accordingly, he takes care that these severed portions of himself shall not be left in places where they might be exposed to accidental injury or fall into the hands of malicious persons who might work magic on them to his detriment or death. . . . The simplest way of evading the peril is not to cut the hair at all; and this is the expedient adopted when the risk is thought to be more than usually great. The Frankish kings were never allowed to crop their hair; from their childhood upwards they had to keep it unshorn. To poll

the long locks that floated on their shoulders would have been to renounce their
right to the throne.'

MEN: 500–1100 (Plates 24-26)

A great part of the history of hair during this period is written in the struggles of the
Church to regulate—both within the Church and outside—the length of hair and
beards. The Church has never looked kindly upon long hair for men, but the attitude toward beards has varied. St Wulstan, Bishop of Worcester, considered the wearing of long hair by men 'highly immoral, criminal, and beastly'. Other members of
the Church have agreed with him and expressed violent opinions on the subject.
But few have taken the matter into their own hands in quite the same way. It is said
that the bishop always carried a knife with him; and whenever a long-haired penitent
knelt to receive his blessing, the bishop would whip out his knife, cut off a handful of
hair, and throw it in the man's face. No doubt long-haired men began to think twice
before asking his blessing. Bishop Serlo in the twelfth century was slightly less precipitous, but then he was dealing with a king. However, we shall come to him
presently.

The shape of the tonsure (the shaved crown of a priest's head), Speight tells us,
'was the subject of long and violent debates between the English clergy on the one
hand and those of the Picts and Scots on the other. Amongst the former it was circular, whilst the Picts and Scots had it only semicircular. Not only, however, did the
Divines quarrel about the shape of the disfigurement, but some, resisting authority,
objected to it altogether.' The semicircular tonsure was known as the tonsure of
St John; whereas the completely circular one, which was preferred in Italy, Spain,
and Germany, was called the tonsure of St Peter.

According to an article in *All the Year Round*:

'In the reign of Oswie, the last of the Bretwaldas, who flourished toward the end
of the seventh century, a fierce contest arose between the See of Rome and the
Catholic church of England, Scotland, and Ireland, as to how the priests should
shave their heads and faces, or whether they should shave them at all. The British
priests held that shaving was superfluous; the Pope, however, maintained that the
use of razor was indispensable to salvation. The strife waxed warm; but, as things
seemed likely to go too far, Oswie, who feared interdict and excommunication,
convoked a meeting of ecclesiastics at Whitby, and there decreed: first, that priests
should shave all but a thin crown of hair off their heads; secondly, that they should
wear neither beard nor whiskers nor moustaches, upon pain of public penance. This
was peremptory, and the English priests gave in.

'Beards had come into fashion again for laymen long before this meeting at
Whitby. It is likely that Oswie himself wore a full-flowing beard, whiskers, and all

the appurtenances; but the Emperor Charlemagne, who ascended the French throne in 768, sported only a moustache; and for some reason or other, he had such an aversion to hairy faces that he not only required his courtiers to shave, but furthermore made it an express condition, when he gave the dukedom of Benevento to Grimoald, that the latter should oblige the Lombards to cut off their beards. Egbert of Wessex, the first king of all England, had spent a part of his youth at the court of Charlemagne; when he returned home to take possession of his throne, he brought with him a smooth face. The Danes, who, during this reign, infested England, were all bearded men. This was sufficient reason, had no other existed, for the Anglo-Saxons to shave: men in those days made it a point to be as unlike their enemies as possible.'

But by the middle of the ninth century the Roman Catholic priests were letting their beards grow and sometimes even neglecting to shave their heads. The Greek church was scandalized and unmoved by the arguments that the apostles had set a precedent in the wearing of beards. Wearing beards was specified as a major grievance in the edict of excommunication against Pope Nicholas in 856. But some centuries later the positions of the Greek church and the church of Rome were to be completely reversed with the Roman priests cleanly shaven and the Greeks happily bearded.

As for Charlemagne, evidently he later grew a beard, and there is also a possibility that still later he shaved it off.

The struggle between the bearded and the beardless continued throughout the Middle Ages and has erupted sporadically in one form or another ever since. A beard, when it is worn, becomes a cherished and sometimes a sacred possession. We have seen that Romans consecrated their first beards. The Moslems also kept every lost hair throughout their entire lives and had it buried with them. Pulling the beard was naturally not thought well of among the Moslems; and Reynolds points out that spitting on the beard, or even spitting on the ground and *saying* it was meant for the beard (which seems to show admirable restraint) was punishable by law.

In some countries merely touching another man's beard without permission was considered an insult; and shaving another man against his will was, not unreasonably, considered a very serious insult indeed—so serious, in fact, that it was punishable by precisely stipulated fines. It would appear that the forcible removal of other people's beards was a fairly popular pastime. There were also fines for pulling out hairs of the beard, usually reckoned at so much per hair. In some cases, during the early part of the Middle Ages, only the ruling classes were permitted to wear beards.

In the Ravenna mosaics (*c.* 547) there is a mixture of shaven faces and short beards. Justinian is among the clean shaven. However, in a Constantinople mosaic of the preceding decade he is shown bearded. Monks in the Middle Ages usually were bearded, and it is said that Constantine V, affronted by the opposition of the monks, set fire to some of their beards.

Of course, to say that a man was ever clean shaven in those days is somewhat misleading since even at the best there was usually some stubble left. And until soap

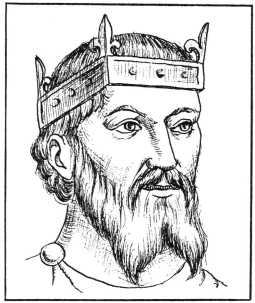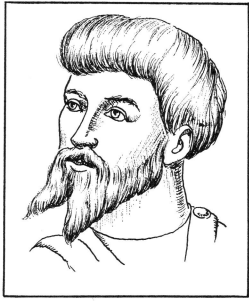

Fig. 18 : Two heads from a ninth-century British manuscript. The one on the left is an Anglo-
Saxon king

became generally available, daily shaving was almost unknown. Once a fortnight
seemed to be about the average. So even those who did not technically wear a beard
were well on their way toward one for most of the time. One is reminded of Chaucer's
lines from the *Merchant's Tale*:

> . . . he kisseth her full ofte;
> With thikke bristles on his beard unsofte,
> Like to the skin of houndfisch scharp as brere,
> (For he was schave al newe in his manere).

As a glance at the plates will show, the general tendency during the early part of
the Middle Ages was for hair to be of medium length, occasionally falling to the
shoulders or below. It was either combed out from the crown in all directions and
cut in bangs across the forehead, or parted in the centre. Beards were usually of
medium length, round or pointed. Long ones were often forked.

Stewart reports that 'in the eighth century it was the custom of people of quality
to have their children's hair cut the first time by persons they had a particular honour
and esteem for; who, in virtue of this ceremony, were respected as a sort of spiritual
parents or god-fathers to him; though this practice appears to have been more ancient,
in as much as we read that Constantine sent the pope the hair of his son Horacleus as
a token that he desired him to be his adopted father'.

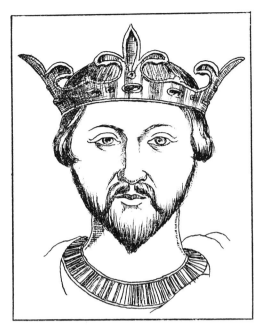

Fig. 19 : Henri I (1005?–60), King of France

In the ninth and tenth centuries (Plates 25 and 26) we find the hair generally short-er, especially among young men. The short bowl cut was to be popularized in even shorter form and without the beard by Henry V in the fifteenth century. Young men were frequently clean shaven, whereas older men wore beards. Otto I (crowned in 936) was bearded; but his son, Otto II, was not. The clergy usually shaved.

In Britain the conquering Danes were not without influence in setting the fashions. As Speight tells it, 'In the reign of those two very unsatisfactory Monarchs—Edgar, the Peaceable, and Ethelred, the Unready—there were Danish soldiers quartered upon the people of England who gave themselves high airs, and were probably looked upon as wells of the purest water. We can judge what they were from the old Danish poem, the death-song of Lodbroc, where we find a "lover of the lady beauteous in his locks". Royalty, too, did its duty as a leader of fashion, to some purpose, for we find that the locks of King Canute hung over his shoulders in rich profusion. At all events the young Danes were the beaux of the period, and particu-larly attentive to the dressing of their hair.'

During the eleventh century beards began to disappear, to some extent, in the western countries, and the Church did its best to make beardlessness complete. Still, a silver penny of 1065 shows Edward the Confessor with a fairly short pointed beard; one minted in 1066 portrays King Harold with a very short curly beard; and

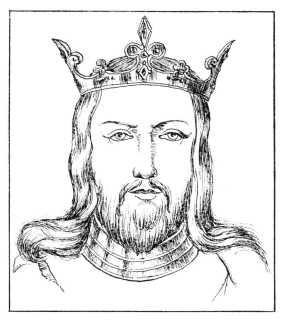

Fig. 20: Louis VII (le Jeune) (1120?–80), King of France

on yet another penny, dated 1068, William the Conqueror appears with a short, round beard. The hair was parted in the centre, if at all.

Despite the Church, long beards and long hair were revived late in the century; they were sometimes curled or crimped or even plaited. Plate 29-E shows a twelfth-century example of plaited hair.

'At this time', reports Fabian, the Chronicler, 'the Priests used bushed and braided heads, long-tailed gowns, and blasyn clothes shinying, and golden girdles, and rode with gilt spurs, using of divers other enormities.'

In 1073 Pope Gregory called a council at Gironne, from which an edict went out forbidding the clergy to wear beards. A few years later the Pope wrote to Ozroc, Podestà of Cagliary:

'We therefore order your bishop, our brother, to have his beard shaved, like all the Western clergy, who have preserved this custom ever since the commencement of the Christian faith: in consequence, we command you likewise to oblige all the clergy that are under your authority to be shaved, and to confiscate the property of those who shall refuse to obey, to the profit of the Church of Cagliary. Make use of severity, for fear lest this abuse should increase.'

The Archbishop of Rouen proclaimed that anyone wearing long hair or a beard should be excluded from the church both before and after death. This was officially enacted in 1096. In 1031 the Council of Limoges had decreed that the wearing of beards was optional. In France in 1094 the first known organization of barbers was formed.

MEN: TWELFTH CENTURY (Plates 27-29)

In 1102 a decree in Venice banned long beards; and on Christmas Day, 1105, the Bishop of Amiens refused to give communion to anyone wearing a beard. Clearly, beards were still being worn. Long forked ones were fashionable. The moustaches were often long and pointed and separated from the beard, which was taken great care of, often being covered with unguents and encased in a beard-bag overnight. Young men, however, were often beardless.

That the beard was highly regarded is clear from a charter made in 1121 and still in existence. It closes with this sentence: 'And that this writing may go down to posterity firm and stable like the oak, I have applied to my present seal three hairs of my beard.' The seal was then affixed with three hairs from the king's beard.

Early in the century the Templars, founded by nine French knights, wore long beards; and, defying the order of the original nine that heads should be cropped, many of the members also wore long hair.

Speight quotes an unidentified contemporary historian as relating that 'An event happened in the year 1129 which seemed very wonderful to our young gallants, who, forgetting that they were men, had transformed themselves into women by the length of their hair. A certain knight, who was very proud of his luxuriant hair, dreamed that a person suffocated him with its curls. As soon as he awoke from his sleep he cut his hair to a decent length. The report of this spread over all England, and almost all the knights reduced their hair to the proper standard. But this reformation was not of long continuance, for in less than a year all those who wished to appear fashionable returned to their former wickedness and contended with the ladies in length of hair. Those to whom nature had denied that ornament supplied the defect by art.'

The Church did not give up its campaign and, according to Reynolds, specified certain minimum requirements for cutting—namely, that part of the ear and the eyes should remain uncovered. One would not expect the latter requirement to cause any great hardship. Still, that which is never done is not forbidden.

In the Cistercian order of French monks, in about 1160, there was such a persistent rumour that Burchard, abbot of Bellevaux, had forbidden the lay brethren to wear beards that he felt compelled to refute the rumour in a treatise consisting of three books (now in the British Museum). The treatise, called the *Apologia de Barbis ad Conversos*, made clear that the abbot did not disapprove of beards so long as they were worn 'in a decent and orderly fashion and without vainglory'. He approached his subject from various points of view—theological, moral, monastic, social, and sanitary; and he designated the wearers of various types of beards as *pleniberbes*, *imberbes*, *rariberbes*, *eberbes*, *citiberbes*, *tardiberbes*, and *barbiflui*. He also provided the useful information that beards in heaven would be of a fixed and constant length and that in hell those who had sinned by the beard would be punished by the beard.

Bishop Serlo was particularly zealous in his denunciation of long hair and beards; and in 1105 when Henry I of England, convinced by the bishop of the evil of his hairy ways, agreed to being shorn and shaved, Serlo was prepared. He brought forth a pair of scissors from beneath his robes and did the job on the spot. The king's courtiers, naturally, followed his example. Wilton points out, however, that they

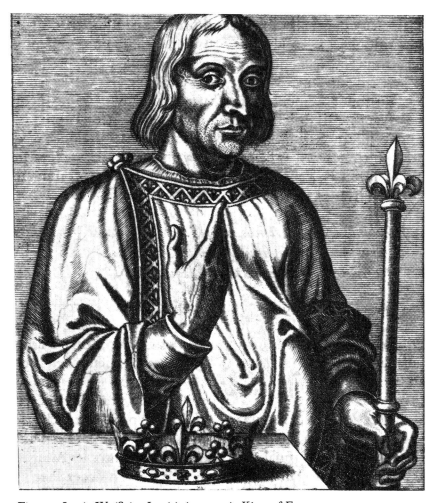

Fig. 21 : Louis IX (Saint Louis) (1214–70), King of France

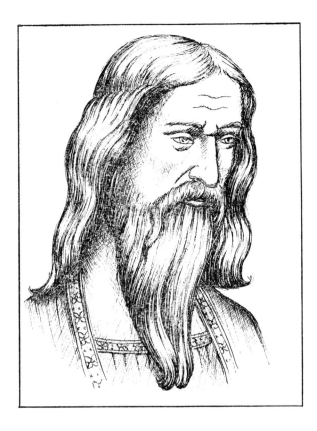

Fig. 22: Edward III, King of England 1327–77

appeared with long hair a few months after the Serlo incident and suggests that the explanation may lie in the use of wigs, which were mentioned in Stephen's reign.

In the middle of the twelfth century Louis VII, suffering, it is said, from pangs of conscience over the burning of 3500 refugees in the Vitry church, was persuaded by Peter Lombard, Bishop of Paris, that the best way to expiate his sin was to cut off his beard. Thus, submitting at last to the decree of 1096, he shaved his beard and cut his hair, much to the distress of his queen, Eleanor of Aquitaine, who, it seems, in lieu of a beard at home, found others further afield. The marriage was shortly dissolved; and she married the future Henry II of England, who received, along with his bride, the French provinces of Poitou and Guyenne. This was followed by three hundred years of bloody wars. The long-haired, bearded Louis is shown in Figure 20.

After the end of the twelfth century, beards and moustaches were not fashionable in France. During the twelfth and thirteenth centuries monks were required to shave twice a month in the winter and every ten days during the rest of the year. Protestants were to shave once a month. The penalty for failure to shave was bread and water for four consecutive Saturdays or (for the second offence) to be beaten with a scourge of cords.

In 1163 the Council of Tours forbade the clergy, who had been practising surgery, to draw blood; and as a result, the barbers took over most of the surgery.

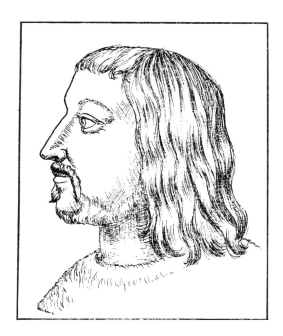

Fig. 23 : Jean II (le Bon), King of France.
Died in England 1364

MEN: THIRTEENTH CENTURY (Plates 29, 30)

Beards were not generally fashionable after the beginning of the thirteenth century, though they were still worn, especially by older men, as Plates 29 and 30 show. But they tended to be shorter than in the preceding century. England's Henry III wore a very short beard and hair of medium length, as did Edward I. Innocent III at the Council of Lateran in 1200 decreed that monks should not wear beards, but the order was not always obeyed. It was customary, as Reynolds points out, for St Augustine monks in Canterbury to shave each other. But it was decided in 1266 to hire professional barbers as a safety measure. Early in the century, according to Strutt, it was dangerous for a stranger to appear in Britain with a beard. In mid-century in France the Brotherhood of St Cosmos founded the first school for barber-surgeons.

Men curled their hair with crisping irons, as shown by the tight rolls on the forehead and at the neck. Sometimes they wore fillets. The hair was still worn with either a fringe on the forehead or a centre parting.

MEN: FOURTEENTH CENTURY (Plates 33-35)

The fourteenth century brought a return to long hair and beards—among the nobility at first, then gradually spreading to the general populace. In 1323, however, by a synodal statute of the Church of Orleans, clergymen were forbidden to wear long beards. Other councils made similar orders. Edward II was very proud of his beard and wore it carefully curled with drooping, curled moustaches. His long hair was also curled. Edward III (Figure 22) wore both his hair and his beard longer. Consequently, many long beards, as well as shorter ones, were seen. Plates 33-35 show some of the variations, 34-F and G being particularly interesting French styles. The French beards tended to be shorter than the English, and they disappeared sooner. The Church, notably in France, prohibited beards among the clergy but with evidently disappointing results since the prohibitions were frequently repeated. Finally (with resignation, one suspects), the Church forbade *long* beards.

In the middle of the fourteenth century false beards were much worn in Spain, and one man might have several colours and styles of beards to wear for various occasions. The ease with which one could disguise oneself led to various misdemeanours; and Peter, King of Aragon, was finally compelled to forbid the wearing of false beards.

The general availability of soap made shaving much easier; and by the end of the century, although long hair and beards were worn by older people, they were not really fashionable. The long-bearded Edward III was followed by Richard II, who wore a thin, drooping moustache and two tiny points of hair on the chin. The hair was also shorter. Others were clean shaven.

In 1308 the Worshipful Company of Barbours was founded in England, and in 1371 the barber-surgeons were organized in France.

WOMEN: 300–1100 (Plates 31, 32)

The early Byzantine hair styles were, in a sense, an extension of the Roman with an added Oriental richness and decorativeness. The hairdos were often very complex and built up over rolls and pads, bound with ribbons, and studded with jewels.

The early European hair styles, on the other hand, began very simply with the hair long and flowing and parted in the centre. A fillet or band was usually worn to help keep the hair in place. But even so, the long, flying hair proved to be impractical; and it was eventually divided into tresses and laced with ribbon into two double ropes, which could hang down the back but apparently were more often worn in front. Later, the hair was braided instead of being bound with ribbons, and the braids were arranged in a variety of ways, as shown on Plate 31.

As in all periods, women were frequently dissatisfied with their hair and found ways to change it. In Italy the monks complained about the use of secret ointments on the hair. One recipe which has been preserved instructed the lady to 'Take dried cauls from the Orient, grind them to a powder, and mix in equal proportions with the yolks of eggs that have been boiled, then mix them with wild honey. Rub on hair in evening, wrap head in kerchief, and wash in morning with olive oil, soap, and fresh water.' Having done this, the lady was required to sit in the sun all day.

Young girls wore their hair loose and flowing and usually bound it up after marriage. Unfortunately we know little of exact styles as the hair after marriage, during much of the Middle Ages, was covered.

WOMEN: TWELFTH CENTURY (Plates 31, 32)

In the second quarter of the twelfth century the hair was sometimes worn in very long plaits (even to below the knees), bound with ribbon as shown in Plates 31-L

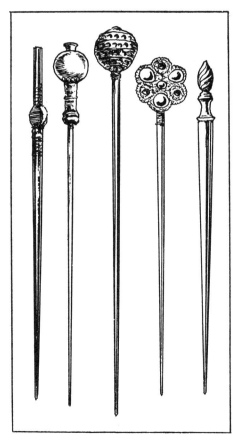

Fig.24 : Hairpins belonging to a Merovingian woman (*c*. seventh century)

and 32-I. Sometimes the ends were ornamented. When the natural hair was not long enough, false hair was added. In England this style was reserved for women of high rank. Often the back part of the hair was allowed to hang free, with only the sides being bound; and sometimes the hair was braided and not bound with ribbon. Later the braids were often wound around the head, or coiled into a chignon; but the hair in the latter part of the century was again concealed by a veil or often by a *mentonnière* or chin strap. Wigs were occasionally worn.

WOMEN: THIRTEENTH CENTURY (Plates 31, 32)

Hair was largely concealed until almost the end of the thirteenth century when a vogue for uncovered hair began. At this time also the hair was sometimes parted over the crown from ear to ear. But until such a time the hair was usually covered with a veil or a *mentonnière*, frequently combined with a *mortier* (a sort of hat, which was the forerunner of the modern academic mortar-board). Late in the century women began to roll the braids of hair on either side of the head over the ears. This style became quite popular in the following century. In the thirteenth century the braids were usually covered.

WOMEN: FOURTEENTH CENTURY (Plates 35, 36)

Braids were fashionable and were used in many ways, coils over the ears being particularly popular. Sometimes the coils were exposed, sometimes encased in crespines or crespinettes. Often the braids hung straight down instead of being coiled.

The hair was generally parted in the centre; and if the style required more, false hair was used. Sometimes cotton or wool was included for padding, feathers were worn, and hair dye was also used. The clergy, of course, were unhappy about this and made various threats, none of which seemed to have any effect.

In England, during the first half of the century, according to Cunnington, the hair was concealed except by children, unmarried girls, brides, and queens at their coronation, in which cases it was worn long and unconfined. It was also partially visible when worn with an open turban.

It was in this century (after 1320) that women began to pluck or shave the front hairline to move it farther up and back to give a higher and broader forehead. In the latter part of the century a Norman knight instructed his daughters: 'See that you pluck not away the hairs from your eyebrows, nor from your temples, nor from your foreheads, to make them appear higher than nature has ordained. Be careful

also not to wash the hair of your head in anything more costly than a plain lixivium.'
Perhaps the daughters obeyed, but other women went on plucking for another two
hundred years.

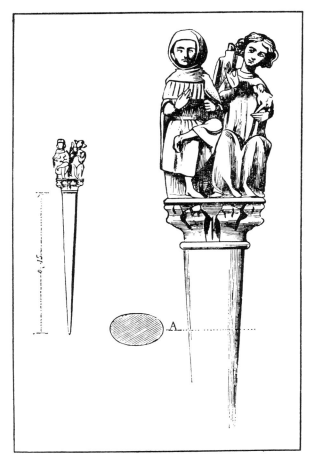

Fig. 25 : Fourteenth-century French hairpin of ivory.
From the *Dictionnaire Raisonné du Nobilier
Français*

PLATE 24 : ANCIENT AND MEDIEVAL MEN 300–550

A   Barbaric British chieftain.

B   Teutonic barbarian, perhaps Frankish (authenticity doubtful).

C, D   Goths or possibly early Franks. D is based on an obviously stylized drawing in the *Encyclopédie Larousse*.

E   *c.* A.D. 400, Roman.

F   *c.* A.D. 400, Roman.

G   *c.* A.D. 400, Roman.

H   Early fifth century, Roman.

I   Roman. Constantine I (the Great), 280?–337.

J   Mid-fifth century, Roman.

K   Mid-fifth century, Roman.

L   *c.* A.D. 450, Roman.

M   Fifth century, French.

N   Italian. St Ambrose, 339?–97. (From a mosaic in Milan completed a few years after his death.)

O   Fifth century.

P   Fifth century.

Q   Fifth century.

R   *c.* 547.

S   Sixth century, Gaul.

T   Sixth century, Gaul.

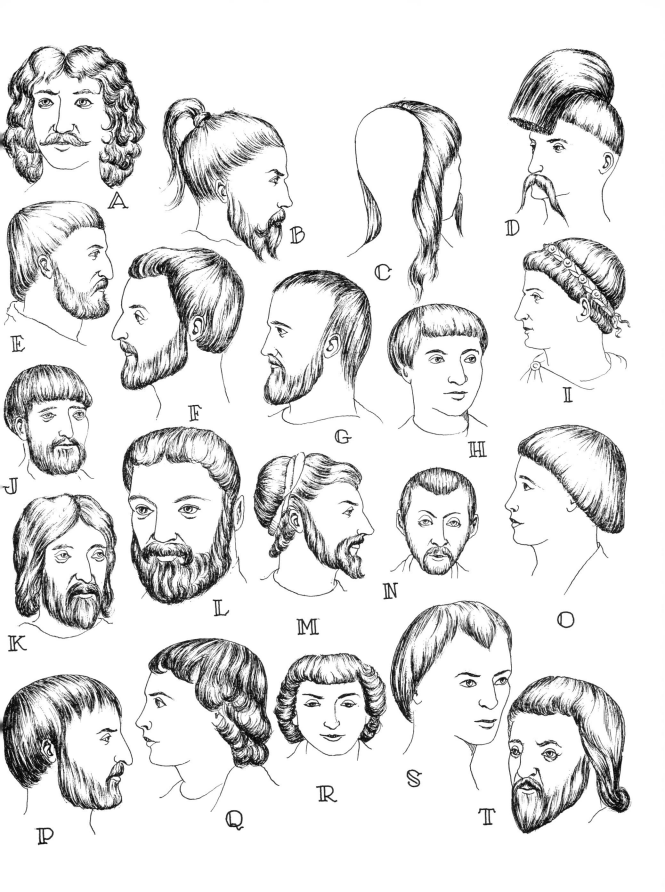

A
B
C
D
E
F
G
H
II
J
K
L
M
N
O
P
Q
R
S
T

PLATE 25 : MIDDLE AGES, MEN 500–1100

A   Sixth century. Note particularly the bands of hair combed forward on either side of the parting. These are typical of the period (see also 27-S, 28-G-S, and 29-D). Sometimes the centre band was not separated by a parting and was cut off short on the forehead, as in 26-A, 27-B-Q, and 30-C-O-Q. Another variation shows a short fringe below the parting, as in 26-R, 27-H, and 28-L.

B   *c.* 500, Byzantine.

C   Byzantine.

D   *c.* 500, Byzantine.

E   *c.* 547, Byzantine. A dignitary in the court of Justinian. Some of the members of the court were bearded; others were not. Although Justinian's hair style was much like this one, he was clean shaven. An earlier mosaic shows him bearded.

F   *c.* 547, Byzantine. Archbishop in the court of Justinian.

G   *c.* 675, Frankish.

H   *c.* 634. Short beards were usually either round (J, K, L) or pointed (D, P). Longer beards were frequently forked (Q, S, U, W). There are numerous additional examples on the following plates.

I   *c.* 634.

J   *c.* 634.

K   *c.* 640.

L   *c.* 705. Pope John VII.

M   *c.* 750.

N   *c.* 790. Offa, King of Mercia.

O   Ninth century. In this century and in the tenth, the hair was generally shorter than it had been. Although older men wore beards, younger ones were usually clean shaven.

P   *c.* 820.

Q   Ninth century, Byzantine.

R   *c.* 879.

S   *c.* 1000, Saxon.

T   Tenth century.

U   Late tenth century, Anglo-Saxon.

V   Egbert the Great—died 839. Anglo-Saxon king. (Portrait probably speculative.)

W   Eleventh century, British.

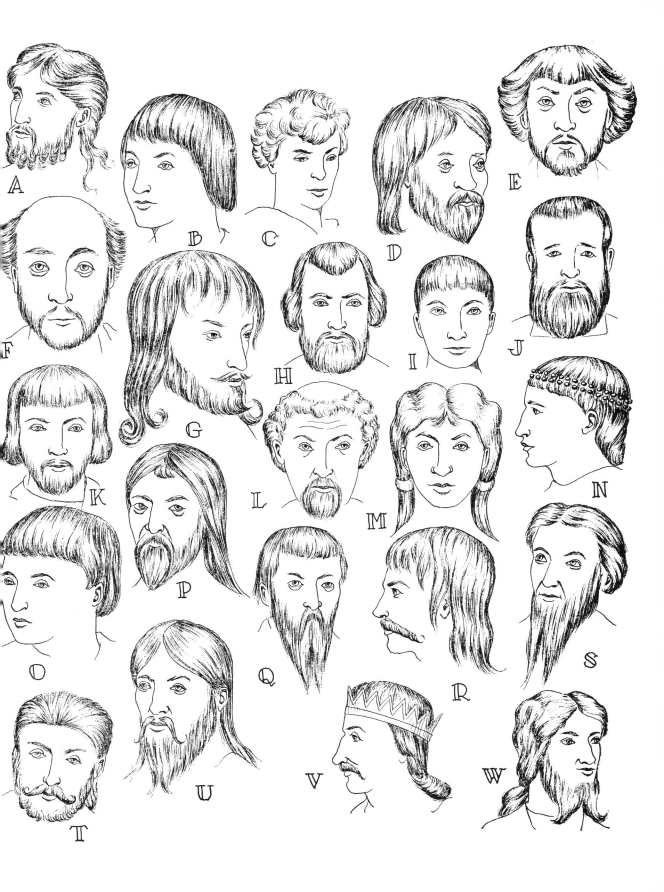

PLATE 26 : MIDDLE AGES, MEN 900–1100

A   *c.* 900, Constantinople.

B   Tenth century.

C   Tenth century.

D   French.

E   Tenth century.

F   Tenth century.

G   Late tenth century.

H   Late tenth century.

I   Late tenth century. This is a variation of the style shown in C above but is distinguished by its shortness at the back. In the fifteenth century it became still shorter.

J   Late tenth century.

K   Eleventh century. When a parting was used, it was always in the centre (see P, R, and T below).

L   German. Otto I (the Great), 912–73—crowned 936.

M   Pope Gregory VII, 1073–85—later canonized.

N   *c.* 1020.

O   *c.* 1050.

P   *c.* 1080, Norman.

Q   Eleventh century.

R   Late eleventh century. The slight fringe below the parting was common.

S   Late eleventh century.

T   Late eleventh century, Greek.

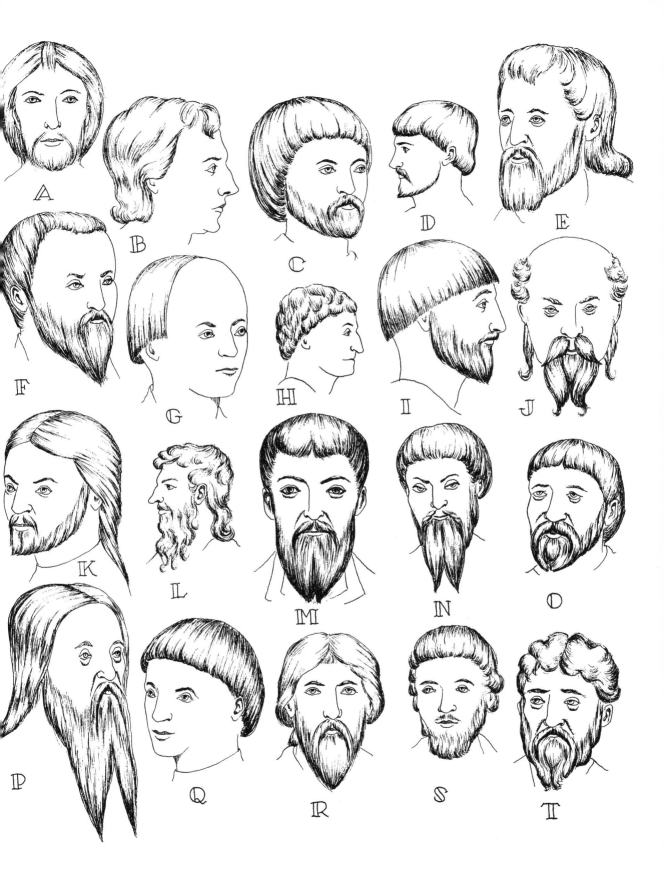

A B C D E

F G H I J

K L M N O

P Q R S T

PLATE 27 : TWELFTH-CENTURY MEN 1100–1150

A   *c.* 1100. The top hair was sometimes combed forward, as it is here, sometimes parted in the centre (C, H, N), or parted either side of a centre section, as shown in B, M, and Q. In S the centre section is divided into two parts. (Further twelfth-century examples can be found on Plates 28 and 29.)

B   *c.* 1100.

C   *c.* 1100.

D   *c.* 1100.

E   *c.* 1100.

F   French. Louis-le-jeune, 1120–80—reigned 1137–80. From a sixteenth-century manuscript (see also Figure 20).

G   1108, Russian. *Tonsure of St Peter.*

H   1108, Russian.

I   *c.* 1120, Roman empire.

J   Exact date uncertain. The hair is no doubt stylized.

K   Exact date uncertain.

L   Exact date uncertain.

M   1130–35. Although beards were commonly worn by older men, young men were usually beardless. The front hair was ordinarily combed forward and cut relatively short, but the back was sometimes left long, as it is here, or cut shorter, as in O and R below.

N   French.

O   Exact date uncertain.

P   Exact date uncertain.

Q   1130–35.

R   *c.* 1150, Italian.

S   Exact date uncertain.

T   Exact date uncertain.

U   *c.* 1150, Italian. Note that the hair radiates from a point on the natural hairline rather than at the crown. This was not an unusual style among the Italians and can be seen also on Plate 28-B-H.

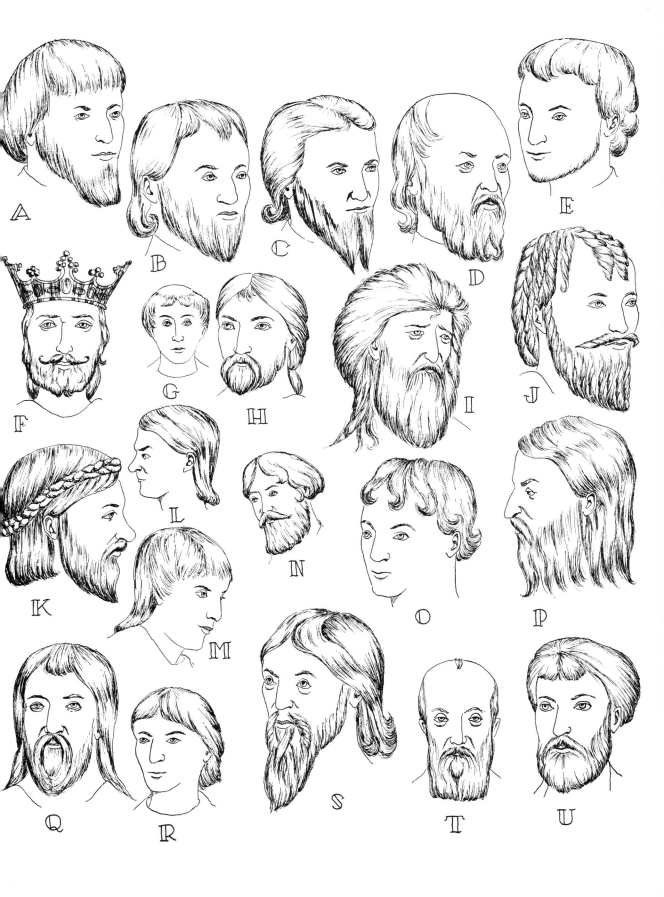

A

B

C

D

E

F

G

H

I

J

K

L

M

N

O

P

Q

R

S

T

U

PLATE 28 : TWELFTH-CENTURY MEN 1150–1200

A   King Stephen, 1105–54—reigned 1135–54. The drawing is based on an engraving in the British Museum. However, since the costume is not in period, clearly the engraving was not made from a contemporary portrait.

B   Italian. (Note similar hair style in H below and in 27-U.)

C   Exact date uncertain. Beards were sometimes worn without moustaches, but rarely was the reverse true.

D   Italian.

E   *c.* 1165.

F   French.

G   *c.* 1170.

H   *c.* 1180, Italian. (Note similar hair style in B above and in 27-U.)

I   *c.* 1180, Italian.

J   *c.* 1180, Italian.

K   *c.* 1180.

L   Italian.

M   Italian.

N   *c.* 1180.

O   Richard I, 1157–99—ruled 1189–99.

P   Exact date uncertain.

Q   Exact date uncertain.

R   Exact date uncertain.

S   Exact date uncertain.

T   Exact date uncertain.

U   St Thomas Aquinas, 1225–74. *Tonsure of St Peter,* the style preferred in Italy.

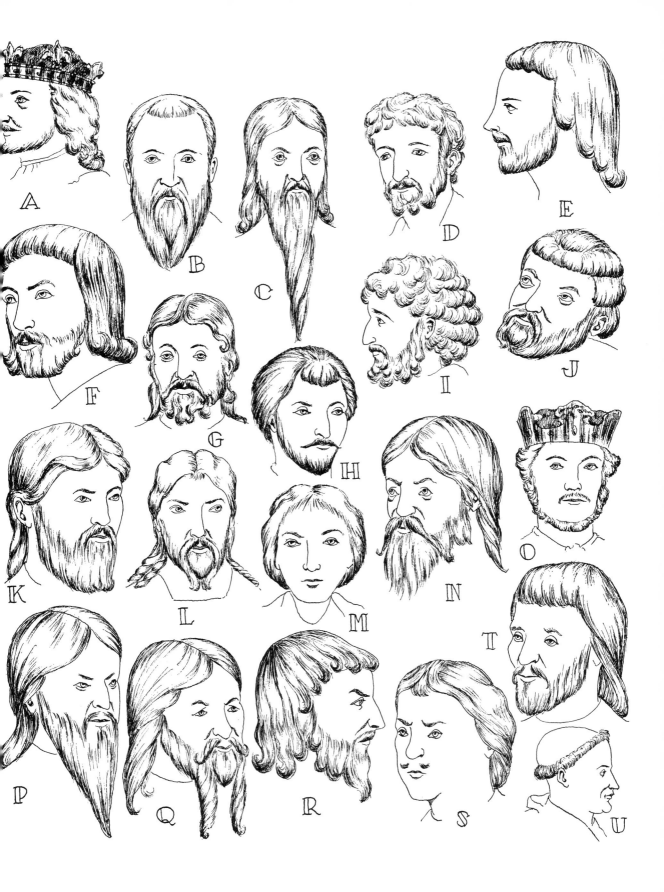

A

B

C

D

E

F

G

H

I

J

K

L

M

N

O

P

Q

R

S

T

U

PLATE 29 : MIDDLE AGES, MEN 1100–1275

A Early twelfth century, French. The long, pointed moustaches, separated from the beard, were fashionable at this time (see also C below).

B 1146. Pope Alexander. *Tonsure of St Peter.*

C *c.* 1130, French. Long hair and beards were fashionable, though younger men were often clean shaven.

D *c.* 1146, English. Long, forked beards were fashionable early in the century, despite objections by the Church.

E *c.* 1150, French. The hair was occasionally plaited in the eleventh century.

F *c.* 1150, Saxon.

G *c.* 1150, English.

H Henry III, 1207–72—King of England, 1216–72. From his tomb in Westminster Abbey, made in 1291.

I *c.* 1180.

J *c.* 1180.

K German. Supposedly a portrait of Frederick I, known as Frederick Barbarossa, 1122?–1190—crowned king of Germany in 1152 and emperor in 1155. The reliability of the portrait is uncertain (see O below).

L *c.* 1160, French.

M *c.* 1235, French.

N *c.* 1240, French. The forehead roll was made with a crisping iron.

O Frederick Barbarossa in his later years. Reliability of the portrait is uncertain (see K above).

P French. Louis VIII, 1187–1226—ruled 1223–26. The portrait is probably not contemporary.

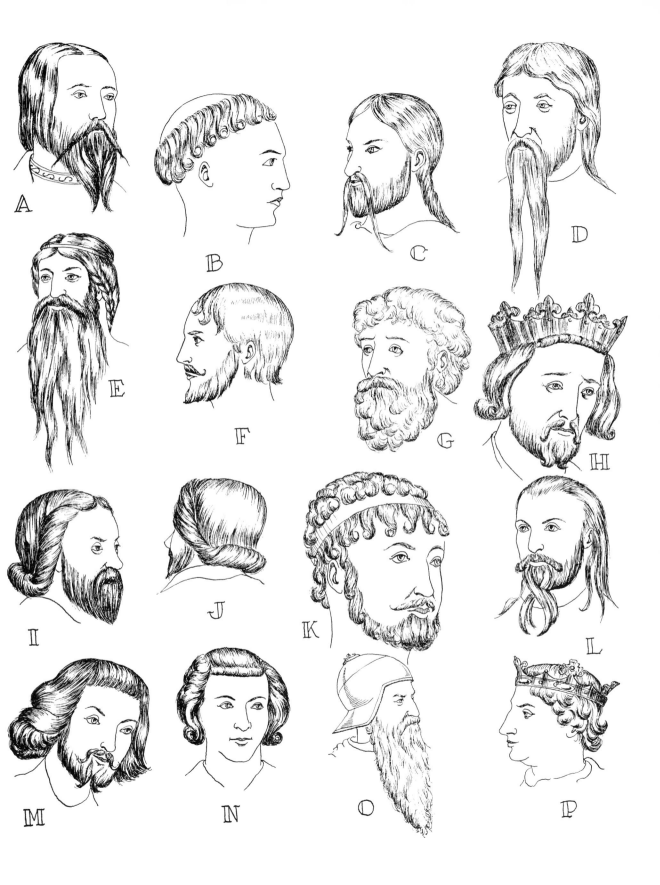

PLATE 30 : THIRTEENTH-CENTURY MEN 1200–1300

A   *c.* 1200.

B   *c.* 1215.

C   First quarter.

D   First quarter.

E   First quarter.

F   First quarter.

G   First quarter.

H   *c.* 1225. The tight forehead roll was made with a curling iron.

I   *c.* 1245.

J   Mid-century.

K   French. Louis IX (Saint Louis), 1214–70—ruled 1226–70.

L   Mid-century.

M   Mid-century, French

N   Mid-century.

O   Mid-century.

P   Mid-century.

Q   *c.* 1260.

R   King Edward I, 1239–1307—ruled 1272–1307. The portrait, from an engraving in the British Museum, is not contemporary. Another portrait (33-B), which appears to be more authentic, shows a slightly fuller beard and moustache and also obviously represents the king during his later years. It is possible that the beard varied from time to time.

S   Last quarter. The tight rolls of hair were made with a crisping iron.

T   Last quarter. The ends of the hair were curled with an iron.

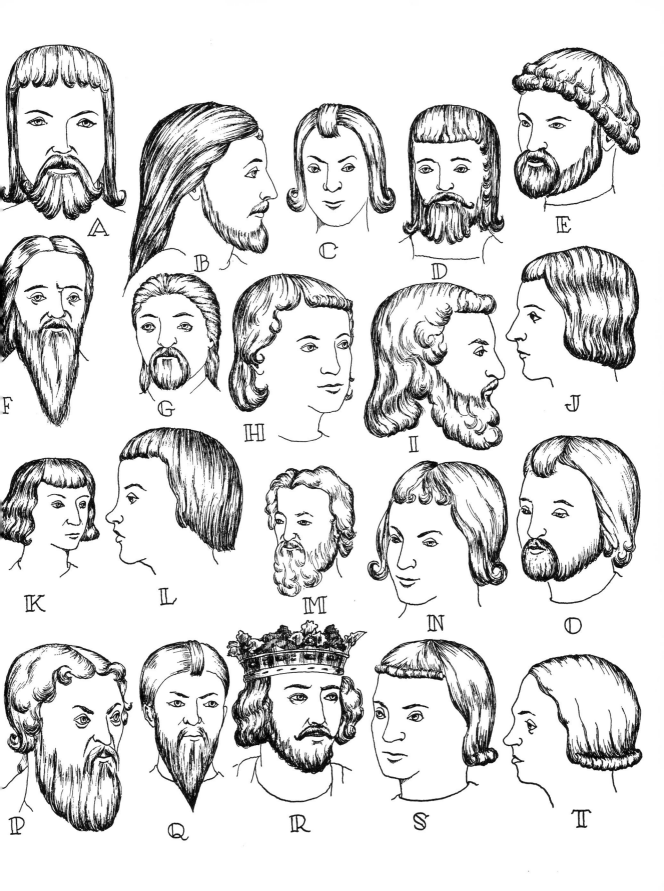

A

B

C

D

E

F

G

H

I

J

K

L

M

N

O

P

Q

R

S

T

PLATE 31 : MIDDLE AGES, WOMEN 300–1300

A   Third or fourth century, Italian princess.

B   *c.* 379, early Christian. Possibly Flacilla, first wife of Theodosius I.

C   Late fifth century.

D   *c.* 560, Byzantine.

E   Sixth century, Byzantine. The hair was built up over rolls and pads. Often it was studded with jewels (see also 32-B).

F   Sixth century, Byzantine.

G   Ninth century, French.

H   Tenth century, French.

I   Eleventh century, French (see also L and P below and 32-I).

J   *c.* 1108.

K   *c.* 1125.

L   *c.* 1140, French.

M   *c.* 1130, French.

N   Twelfth century, bourgeois French.

O   *c.* Twelfth century, German.

P   Twelfth century.

Q, R   Late thirteenth century. There was a vogue at this time for uncovered hair.

S   Twelfth century, French. Lady with chin cloth or *mentonnière*.

T   *c.* Twelfth-thirteenth century.

U   Thirteenth century, French. The *mortier* was here combined with the *mentonnière*, and the braids were wound around the head to form a very popular and fashionable style.

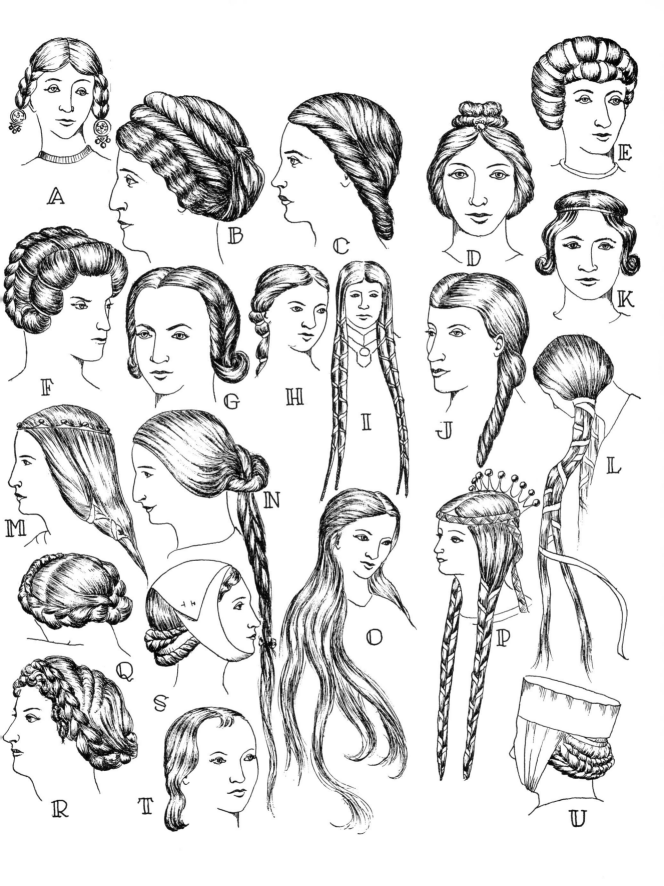

PLATE 32 : MIDDLE AGES, WOMEN 400–1300

A   Fourth or fifth century. Early Christian.

B   *c.* 400, Byzantine. Athenais Endocia, wife of Emperor Theodosius.

C   730, Polish. Queen Wanda.

D   Late eleventh century, Greek.

E   1083, French. Queen Mathilde.

F   *c.* 1100.

G   Mid-twelfth century, Italian.

H   Twelfth century, Spanish.

I   1180, French. Queen. The braids were worn very long and extended with artificial hair if necessary.

J   Late twelfth or early thirteenth century.

K   Thirteenth century, Italian (Florentine).

L   Thirteenth century, Italian. Young girl. It was customary for young girls to wear the hair loose and flowing before marriage.

M   Thirteenth century.

N   Thirteenth century, German.

O   Thirteenth century.

P   Thirteenth century.

Q   Late thirteenth century, Italian.

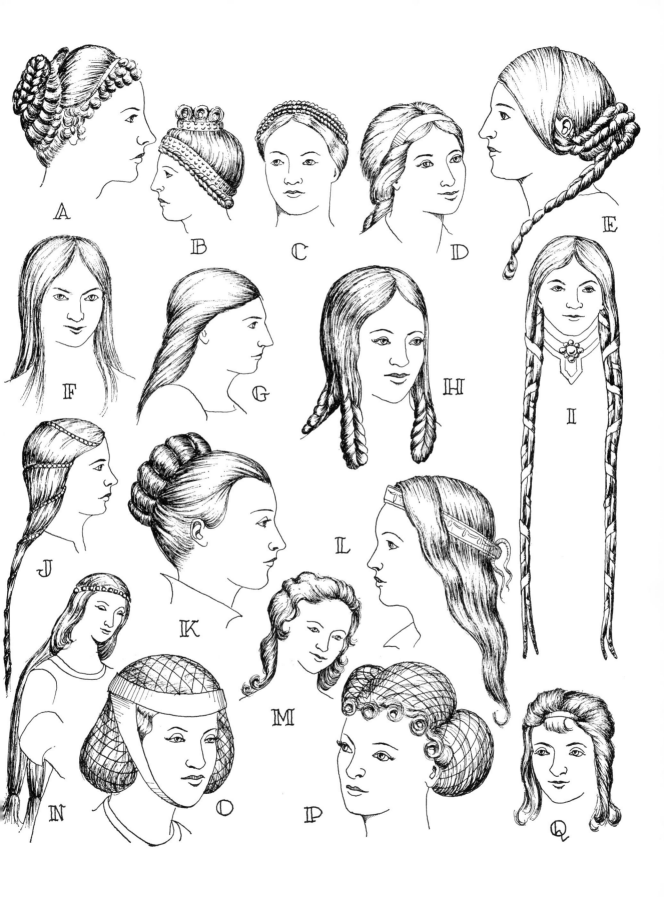

A

B

C

D

E

F

G

H

I

J

K

L

M

N

O

P

Q

PLATE 33 : FOURTEENTH-CENTURY MEN 1300–1350

A   First quarter.

B   King Edward I, 1239–1307—ruled 1272–1307. A late portrait and probably authentic (see also Plate 30-R).

C   First quarter.

D   Exact date uncertain.

E   King Edward II, 1284–1327—ruled 1307–27. His beard and moustache were always carefully curled.

F   *c.* 1320.

G   Second quarter.

H   Exact date uncertain.

I   First quarter, Italian.

J   First quarter, Italian. *Tonsure of St Peter.*

K   First quarter, Italian.

L   *c.* 1360, French.

M   Second quarter, Italian.

N   First quarter, Italian. *Tonsure of St Peter.*

O   *c.* 1340, Italian.

P   First quarter, Italian.

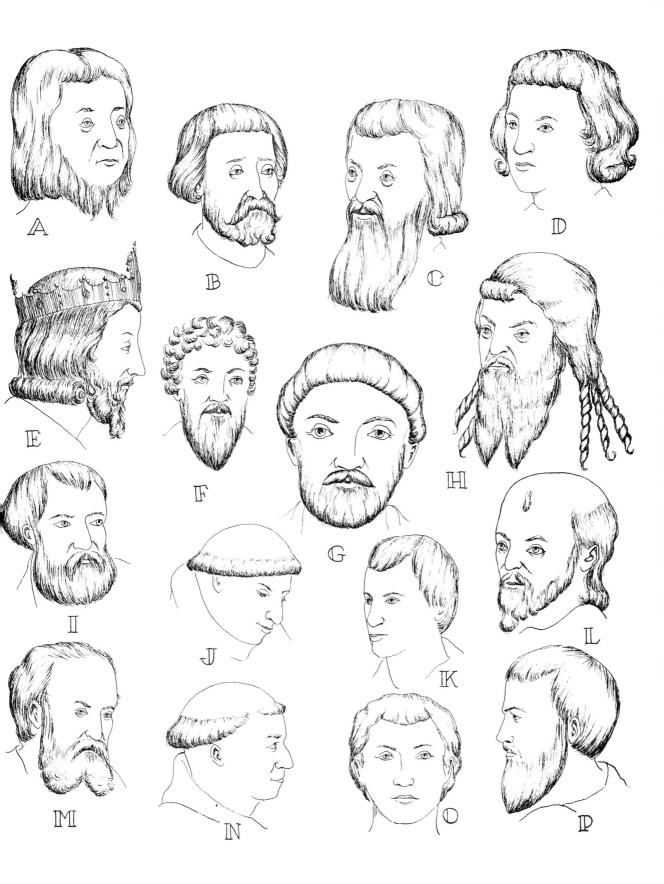

A

B

C

D

E

F

G

H

I

J

K

L

M

N

O

P

PLATE 34 : FOURTEENTH-CENTURY MEN 1350–1400

A   Charles V (the Wise), 1337–80. King of France, 1364–80.

B   King Edward III, 1312–77—ruled 1327–77. Some portraits show an even longer beard. A painting in the British Museum (not contemporary) shows the beard long, pointed, and wavy with long, turned-out moustaches. The hair is not visible. Reynolds refers to his long, forked beard, as shown here.

C   *c.* 1365, Italian.

D   Exact date uncertain.

E   *c.* 1370.

F   French.

G   Last quarter, French.

H   *c.* 1370, Italian. Long beards were not fashionable in the latter part of the century but were worn by older men.

I   *c.* 1370, Italian.

J   *c.* 1390.

K   Exact date uncertain.

L   English. Geoffrey Chaucer, *c.* 1340–1400.

M   Last quarter, Italian.

N   1396, Italian.

O   Richard II, 1367–1400—ruled 1377–99.

P   1380.

Q   *c.* 1390, Italian. Taddeo di Bartolo (from a self-portrait).

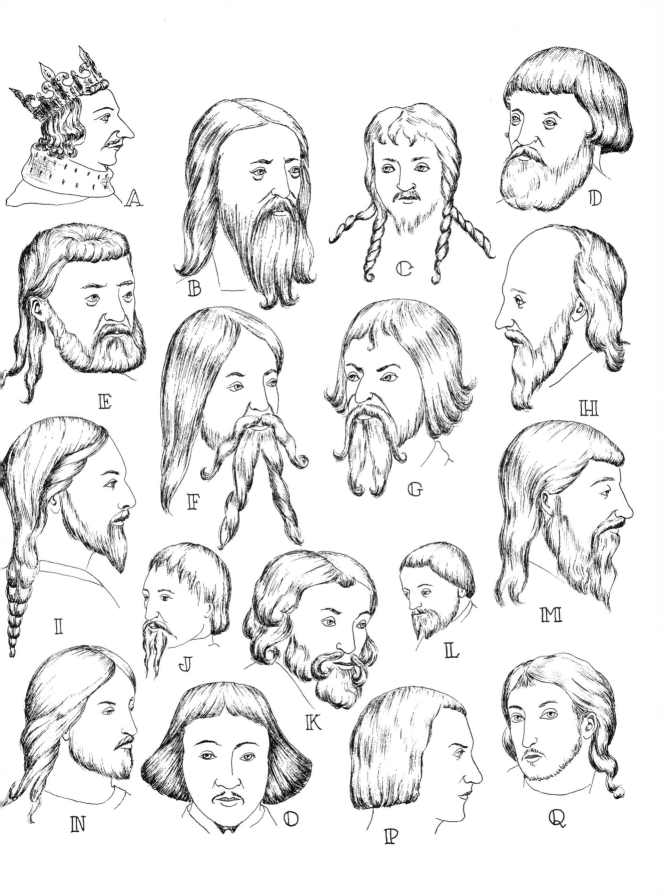

PLATE 35 : FOURTEENTH-CENTURY MEN AND WOMEN 1300–1400

A   Venetian magistrate, member of the Council of Ten.

B   *c.* 1303.

C   1357.

D   *c.* 1370.

E   *c.* 1376, French. Fashionable young man.

F   1390, French. Fashionable young man.

G   *c.* 1390, French. Fashionable young man.

H   *c.* 1380.

I   *c.* 1400, English.

J   *c.* 1310, French. Wearing a *gòrgière.*

K   *c.* 1330, French.

L   *c.* 1335.

M   *c.* 1340, French.

N   First quarter, French.

O   *c.* 1330. The braids originate at the parting, which extends down the back of the head to the nape of the neck. They are brought around the neck, up along the cheeks, and the ends are concealed beneath the front hair.

P   French.

Q   *c.* 1385, French.

R   French.

S   Last quarter, Italian.

T   *c.* 1360.

U   *c.* 1400, French.

V   Last quarter, French.

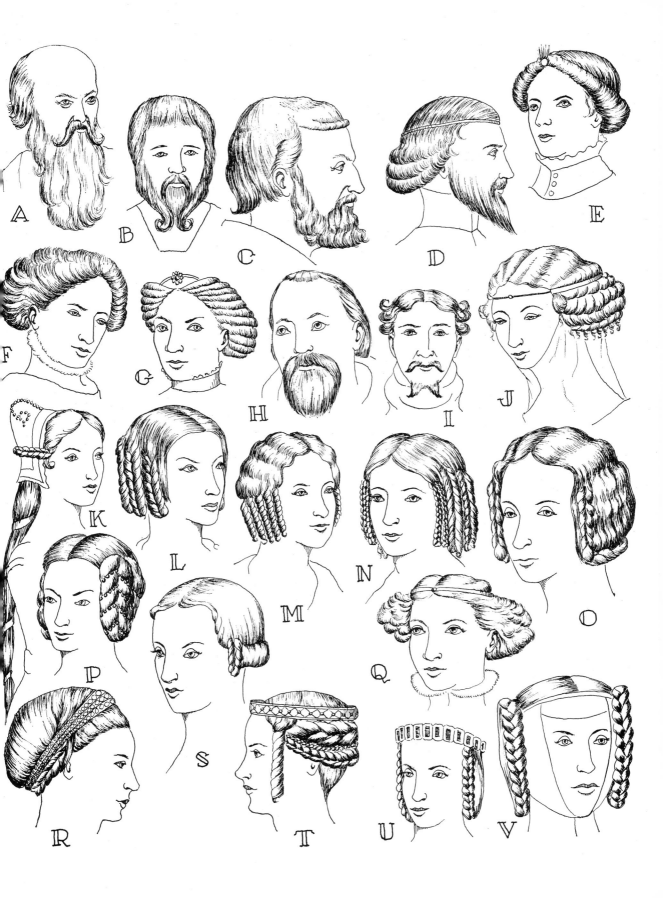

A

B

C

D

E

F

G

H

I

J

K

L

M

N

O

P

Q

R

S

T

U

V

PLATE 36 : FOURTEENTH-CENTURY WOMEN 1300–1400

A   First quarter, French.

B   *c.* 1305, Italian.

C   Exact date uncertain.

D   First quarter.

E   *c.* 1335, Italian.

F   *c.* 1350.

G   Italian (Florentine).

H   French. Laura de Noves, 1307–48.

I   First quarter, French.

J   Mid-century, German.

K   After 1320. It was in this century that women began plucking or shaving the hairline to give a higher forehead, as shown here.

L   Exact date uncertain.

M   1364, English.

N   Last quarter, Italian.

O   *c.* 1370, French.

Q   French.

P, R, S, T   Mid-century. Marie d'Espagne, wife of the Count of Alençon. P and T show the front and back views of the head-dress; R and S show steps in arranging the coiffure. (After Villermont)

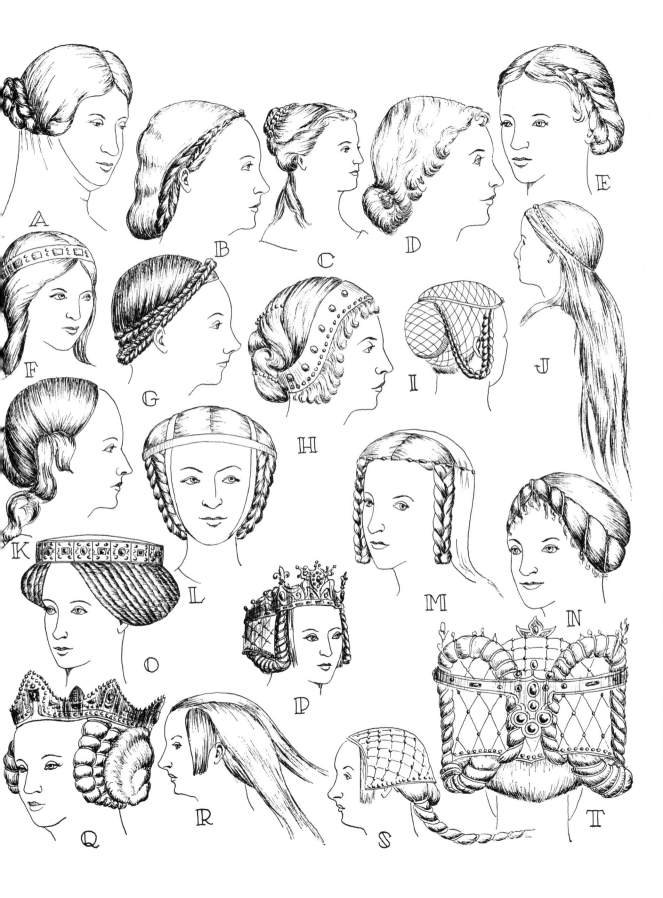

A

B

C

D

E

F

G

H

I

J

K

L

M

N

O

P

Q

R

S

T

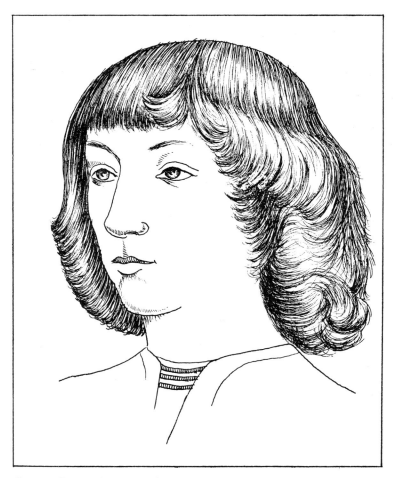

Fig. 26 : Duke of Cleves (fifteenth century)

6 · The Fifteenth Century

I love yt well to have syde here
Halfe a wote byneth myne ere
For ever more I stand in fere
That myne nek shold take cold.
I knyt up all the nyght,
And the day tyme komb yt downryght,
And then yt cryspeth, and shyneth as bryth
As any pyrled gold.

MEDWALL

Italy focuses our attention with its powerful and often brilliant families—the Sforzas, the Estes, the Gonzagas, and particularly the Medicis—and its remarkable painters, with Leonardo da Vinci overshadowing them all. The works of these painters are the source for most of our information about hair styles; and members of the famous families frequently sat for their portraits. These portraits are likely to prove to be the best source of current fashions; the religious paintings, though they show more or less contemporary hair styles, do not necessarily indicate the latest styles.

This is also the century of Gutenberg, who is generally credited with being the first European to print from movable type. This momentous event took place in 1436 or 1437. But probably not a great deal was being written about hair at the time; or if it was, it was not being printed by Herr Gutenberg and his colleagues, who had more important things on their minds. We shall have to wait until the printing press is at least a century old before we find the religious zealots assailing in print the wickedness of contemporary hair styles.

MEN (Plates 37-40)

Beards were not fashionable during the century and were almost never seen on young men. The plates, however, show a number of examples of beards worn by older men and important officials. Since they were a sign of age or dignity or importance, they tended to be fairly full or long or both. Sometimes they were rounded, sometimes pointed or forked. Since beards were not the fashion, we do not find the small, carefully trimmed and waxed, sometimes exotically or eccentrically shaped beards which appeared a century later.

According to William Barker, an eighteenth-century English hairdresser who tended to deal with the history of hair styles with, perhaps, more sweep than precision, 'A large flowing beard was esteemed the greatest mark of masculine beauty. If the beard naturally curled, they divided it into innumerable ringlets around the face. But if it was straight, they twisted it by means of small pieces of lead round the face and supported the weight by a chin cloth. In the morning, the first care was to dress the beard, which they parted in the middle of the chin, the curled beard resting on the cape of the under doublet. This continued to the latter end of Henry the VIIIth's reign, when the reformation having made some progress, the Protestants distinguished themselves from the Romish church party by a purity of manners and simplicity of dress, and the beards of the English, as well as their religion, underwent a considerable change.'

The most popular barber in Florence was Domenico di Giovanni Burchiello, whose shop was a favourite gathering place of poets, merchants, and intellectuals. Burchiello himself was quite a wit, and in 1480 a book of his topical verses was published.

An act passed in England in 1447, during the reign of Henry VI, decreed that 'no manner of man that will be taken for an Englishman shall have no beard above his mouth; that is to say, that he have no hairs on his upper lip so that the said lip be once at least shaven every fortnight or of equal growth with the nether lip; and if any man be found amongst the English contrary hereunto, that then it shall be lawful to

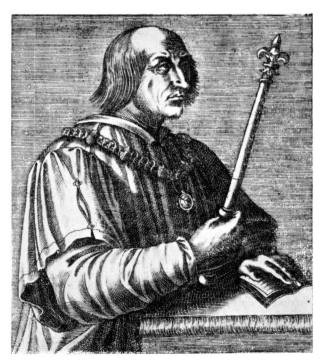

Fig. 27 : Louis XI (1423–83), King of France

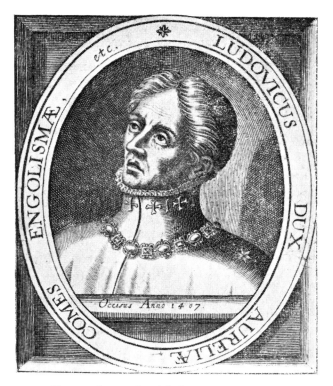

Fig. 28 : Louis, duc d'Orleans (1372–1407)

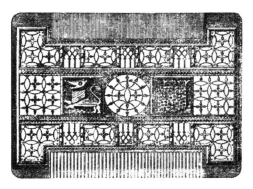

Fig. 29 : Fifteenth-century comb of carved wood

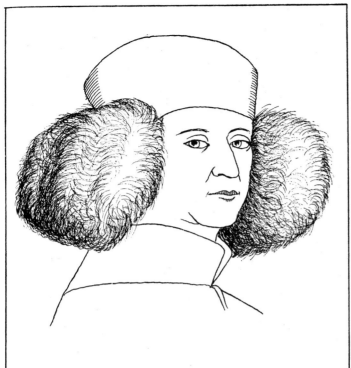

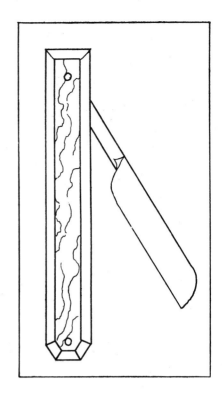

Fig. 30 : Late fifteenth-century Venetian hair style: a version of the *zazzera*

Fig. 31 : Fifteenth-century razor in wooden sheath

every man to take them and their goods as Irish enemies.' Plate 37-J shows a gentleman of the court of Henry VI with a very impressive beard below his mouth but no hairs above.

By an act passed during the reign of Edward IV certain Irishmen were required to 'wear beards after the English manner'. Most of the English, however, seem to have been clean-shaven at this time, though sometimes a slight beard was permitted on the chin. Reynolds reports that false beards were occasionally worn. In 1476 in France the Duke of Lorraine appeared at the funeral of the Duke of Burgundy wearing a false golden beard reaching to his waist.

Hair was short early in the century. The inverted bowl style of Henry V (Plate 38-F) was popular for about fifty years. For this cut, the hair was usually straight or curled under at the ends. However, Louis II (37-A), who died just as the bowl cut was coming into fashion, wore his hair longer and rather elaborately curled.

In the third quarter the hair was again allowed to grow below the ears and in the latter part of the century reached to the shoulders and below. Long bangs sometimes covered the entire forehead. Henry IV's hair was of medium length. Edward IV and Richard III both wore theirs almost shoulder length, and Henry VII permitted his to grow still longer. In France the long, flowing locks worn by Louis XI remained in style throughout the century. In 1461, when illness forced Duke Philip of Burgundy to have his hair shaved off, five hundred noblemen are said to have followed suit.

The hair was sometimes straight, sometimes curled or frizzed. If straight, the ends were usually turned under or sometimes up. One of the most popular Florentine hairdos late in the century was called the *ʒaʒʒera* (see Figure 30). It was simply a shoulder-length bob frizzed all over. From Italy it went to Paris and London, where it was appropriately called 'the Florentine cut'. There was clearly considerable freedom for individual choice in the wearing of the hair.

Sometimes wigs were worn by men of fashion, and the hair was dyed or bleached. Black and blond were both popular; red was not.

WOMEN (Plates 41-44)

Normally women covered their hair after marriage and wore it long and flowing before. However, a number of uncovered coiffures are available. Usually they followed the natural shape of the head and put considerable emphasis on braids, which were worn in various ways, as shown on Plate 41. Thick strands of hair might also be bound without being braided and be used to encircle the head (Figure 32).

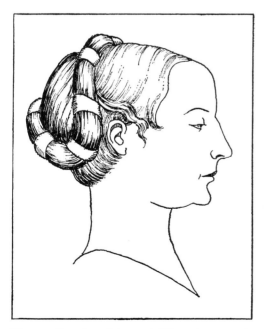

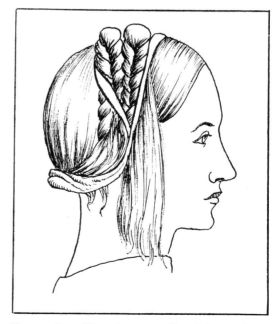

Fig. 32 : Beatrice of Aragon (fifteenth century)   Fig. 33 : Late fifteenth-century Dutch hair style

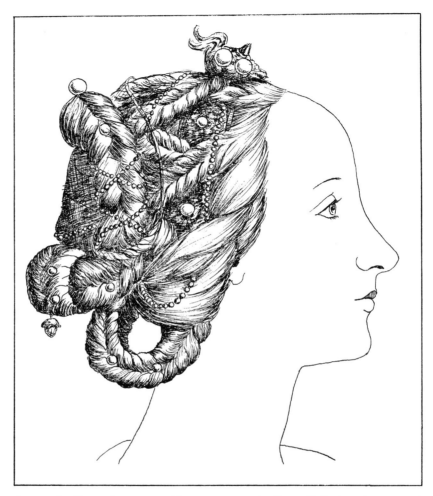

Fig. 34: La Bella Simonetta. From a painting by Piero di Cosimo (1462–1521)

Both styles were carry-overs from the fourteenth century. The hair was usually parted in the centre and worn straight or slightly waved. The Italian styles were more extreme (see Plate 42 especially) and were echoed in the 1960s.

The later styles are, in general, more complex and more highly decorative. The trend can be seen on Plate 44. In some cases, however, the hair itself is very simply done, and the decorative effect comes from the head-dress. All of these more complex hair styles are found in portraits of the nobility or in artists' conceptions of Venus, Aphrodite, and other mythical characters, executed in contemporary terms. They are not the styles of the common people.

A good deal of false hair was used, especially in Italy; and bleaches, dyes, curling irons, and wigs (sometimes made of silk floss instead of hair) were used. In the latter part of the century wigs from Italy were imported into France. Some women sat in the moonlight to beautify their hair. Blonde hair was popular in Italy; and in Venice, according to Child, various dyes and bleaches were used to achieve a variety of tones —brilliant, smoky, golden, tawny, honey, or a combination of them. Again, these were not for the common people.

The custom of plucking the front hair and eyebrows continued throughout the century, though some later portraits show hair which clearly was not plucked. And women did not hesitate to pluck stray hairs in public.

Although general patterns do show up (such as the centre parting and the extensive use of braids), the styles show a good deal of individuality, and there seems to have been no overpowering compulsion to adopt whatever style Battista Sforza or Cicilia Gonzaga might be wearing at the moment.

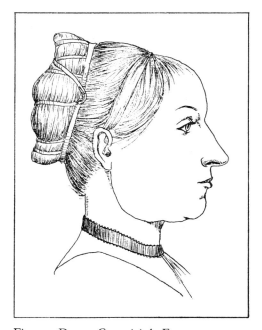

Fig. 35 : Donna Canonici da Ferrara. 1477

PLATE 37 : FIFTEENTH-CENTURY MEN 1400–1500

A   Louis II, Duc d'Anjou, Comte de Provence, 1377–1417.

B   *c.* 1400, French.

C   Italian (Florentine). Tommaso Guidi, known as Masaccio, 1401–28?

D   English. Sir John Oldcastle, died 1417. (Portrait may not be authentic.) Leader of the Lollards, friend of Henry V. Hanged and burned for heresy. Originally Shakespeare's Falstaff was called Sir John Oldcastle, but apparently only the name and a few other details, such as his friendship for Prince Hal, resembled the original.

E   Swiss courier. Presumably the hair is stylized.

F   Mid-century. French king. Beards were not fashionable, but long ones were sometimes worn by dignitaries as a symbol of their importance and to set them apart.

G   *c.* 1440, French.

H   1445.

I   1448. Alfonso V (the Magnanimous), 1396–1458. King of Aragon and Sicily, 1416–58 and of Naples, 1443–58.

J   English. Gentleman of the court of Henry VI, who reigned 1422–61. Henry himself was not bearded.

K   Last quarter. Young Italian gentleman.

L   Italian. Cardinal Mezzarota.

M   Third quarter, Italian (Florentine).

N   1472, German. Hardly a fashionable style.

O   German.

P   Theodorus Gaza, 1398?–1478. Greek scholar, taught and wrote in Italy.

Q   *c.* 1480.

R   Johann Fust, *c.* 1400–66. German printer, partner of Gutenberg. Later, with Peter Schoffer, first to print in colours. Issued first dated book in 1457. (See Plate 38-I for similar beard.)

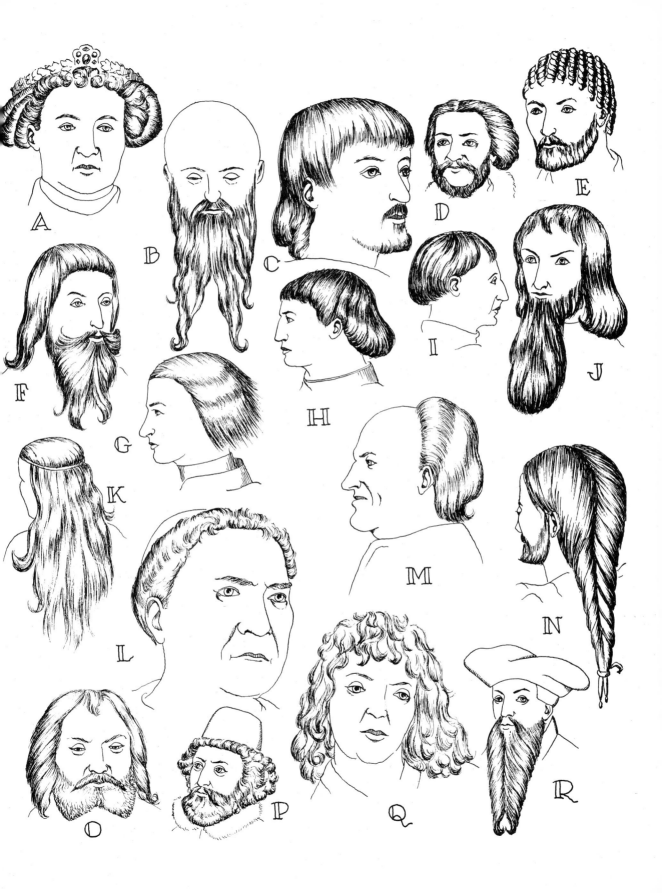

A

B

C

D

E

F

G

H

I

J

K

L

M

N

O

P

Q

R

PLATE 38 : FIFTEENTH-CENTURY MEN 1400–1470

A   1412. This style remained fashionable until about 1460 and was still worn somewhat later.

B   Probably mid-century. (From a wood carving in the Louvre.)

C   1416. The pointed or forked beard without side-whiskers was worn at the beginning of the century but in 1416 was disappearing.

D   First quarter.

E   First quarter. Very old-fashioned.

F   Henry V, 1387–1422. Reigned 1413–22. This was the fashionable and popular hair style during the first half of the century. Frequently the ends were curled under, as in A and B above.

G   Probably c. 1400.

H   Henry of Portugal, 1394–1460, known as Henry the Navigator. The moustache is unusual and would probably not have been worn in England or France.

I   Mid-century, probably French or German. Not fashionable. (Note a similar beard on Johann Fust, Plate 37-R.)

J   1438. This, also, was very old-fashioned.

K   1451, French.

L   Carthusian monk. Notice the fashionable hair and the unfashionable beard.

M   Charles VII, 1403–61. In 1429 Joan of Arc had him crowned king at Rheims.

N   c. 1470. This is an early example of the newest fashion, with forehead fringe and long hair to shoulders.

O   King Henry IV, 1366–1413—reigned 1399–1413. The portrait is taken from his tomb in Canterbury and is not entirely in accord with a painting in the National Portrait Gallery. The moustache is similar in both; but in the painting the beard, though equally short, extends further along the jaw. In neither case is much of the hair visible.

P   Mid-century. Unfashionable length.

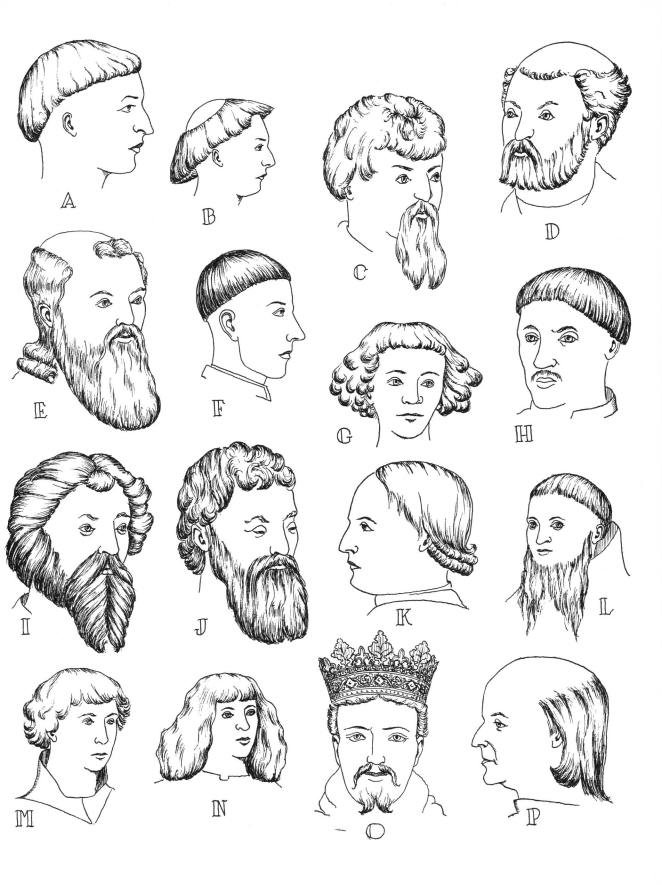

A   B   C   D

E   F   G   H

I   J   K   L

M   N   O   P

PLATE 39 : FIFTEENTH-CENTURY MEN 1470–1490

A   *c.* 1477, Italian. Federigo da Montefeltro, Duke of Urbino. The portrait was painted when his son, Guidobaldo, was about five. The drawing here is reversed. As a result of a jousting accident, his nose was broken and he lost his right eye. Consequently, only his left profile was painted. (His wife, Battista, is shown in Plate 44-N and Guidobaldo's wife in Plate 43-L.)

B   *c.* 1470.

C   Third quarter, Italian. Development of the earlier bowl crop, in which the hair was permitted to grow longer. Later it became still longer (see G below).

D   Last quarter.

E   1476, Italian (Venetian).

F   *c.* 1470, Italian (Florentine). Fashionable young man.

G   Italian. Probably wig.

H   *c.* 1470, German. Fashionable young man.

I   First half.

J   Lorenzo de' Medici, 1449–92 (for later portrait see Plate 40-H).

K   Last quarter, Italian.

L   1489, German. Hans Waldman.

M   Matthias Corvinus, 1443?–90. King of Hungary, 1458–90.

N   1480.

O   1480, French.

P   1486, Italian. Fashionable young man.

Q   Last quarter, Flemish.

R   Giuliano de' Medici, 1453–78.

S   German.

T   1488.

U   Piero de' Medici, 1471–1503.

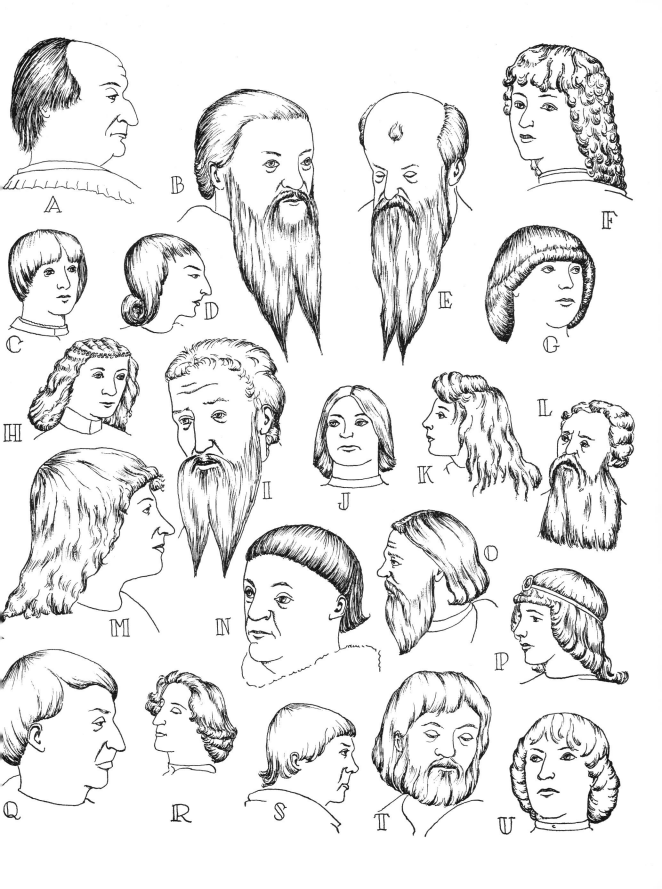

A

B

C

D

E

F

G

H

I

J

K

L

M

N

O

P

Q

R

S

T

U

PLATE 40 : FIFTEENTH-CENTURY MEN 1490–1500

A   Giovanni Pico della Mirandola, 1463–94. Brilliant Italian humanist. Fashionable hair style.

B   Flemish.

C   Italian.

D   *c.* 1490. The hair style was not fashionable at so late a date, and the beard was very unfashionable.

E   Last quarter, Italian (Milanese). Fashionable young man.

F   *c.* 1490. Very unfashionable.

G   Italian. Note the bangs turned up rather than under, as was more common (see also K below).

H   1491, Italian. Lorenzo de' Medici (for earlier portrait see Plate 39-J).

I   *c.* 1490.

J   *c.* 1490. Long bangs were fashionable in the last decade.

K   1491, Italian. Hair length is very conservative, but the long bangs are fashionable.

L   German. Fashionable style.

M   *c.* 1490, probably French.

N   Ferdinand V, 1452–1516. King of Spain (see Plate 41-Q for Isabella).

O   French.

P   *c.* 1495, German. Fashionable style.

Q   Possibly Flemish.

R   1492.

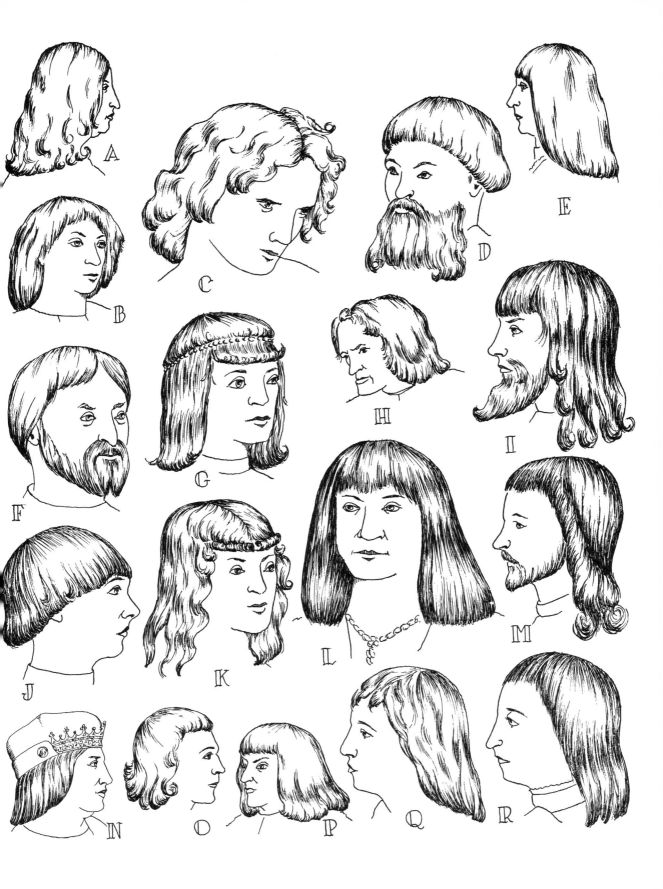

PLATE 41 : FIFTEENTH-CENTURY WOMEN 1400–1500

A   *c.* 1400, probably Italian.

B   Last quarter (before 1491), German.

C   *c.* 1500, Italian.

D   *c.* 1500, Italian.

E   Last quarter, German.

F   *c.* 1440, French. Jeanne de Saveuse, wife of Charles d'Artois.

G   Last quarter, German.

H   First half, French.

I   Second quarter, Italian. From a sketch by Pisanello for *St George and the Princess.* In the sketch the bindings are of rolls of hair, as shown. In the finished painting, however, they are of a dark material in strong contrast to the blonde hair (for other Pisanello hair styles see P below and Plate 42-E-F-G).

J   Noble Italian lady. Back hair is probably false.

K   Mid-century or third quarter, French.

L   Italian.

M   *c.* 1400, German.

N   French.

O   Italian.

P   Second quarter, Italian. Princess d'Este (see I above).

Q   Isabella I, Queen of Castile, 1451–1504 (for portrait of King Ferdinand, see Plate 40-N).

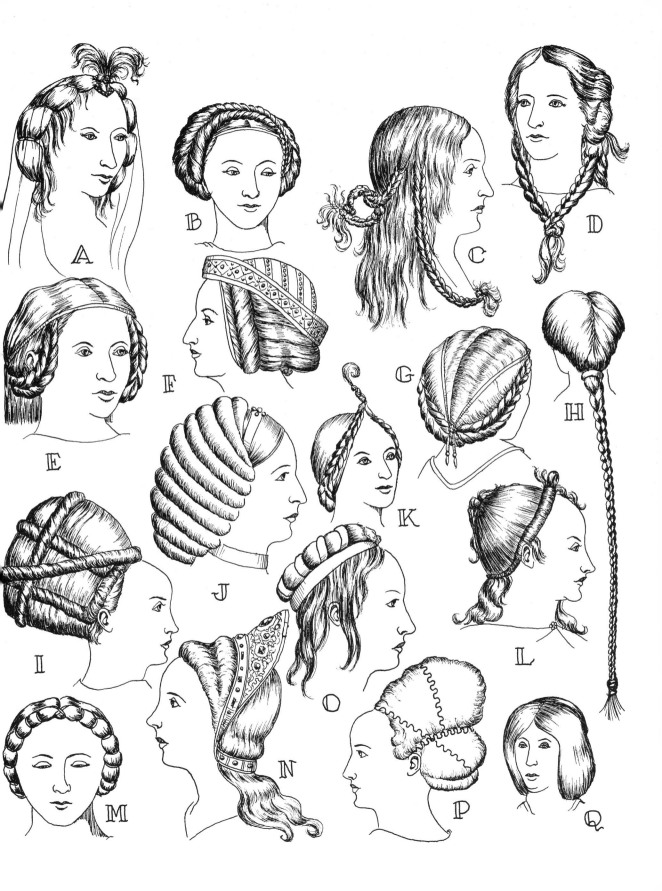

A

B

C

D

E

F

G

H

I

J

K

L

M

N

O

P

Q

Plate 42 : Fifteenth-Century Women 1400–1470

A First half, Italian (Florentine).

B 1436.

C 1450, Flemish.

D Third quarter, Italian (Florentine).

E, F Probably second quarter, Italian. From paintings by Pisanello (see also Plate 41-I-P).

G 1447, Italian. Cicilia Gonzaga (see also Plate 41-I-P).

H German.

I 1465, Alsatian.

J *c.* 1470, German.

K Mid-century, Italian (Venetian).

L Last quarter.

M *c.* 1500, French. Ste Marie-Madeleine. (From a wood sculpture in the Musée de Cluny.)

N German.

O First half, Italian.

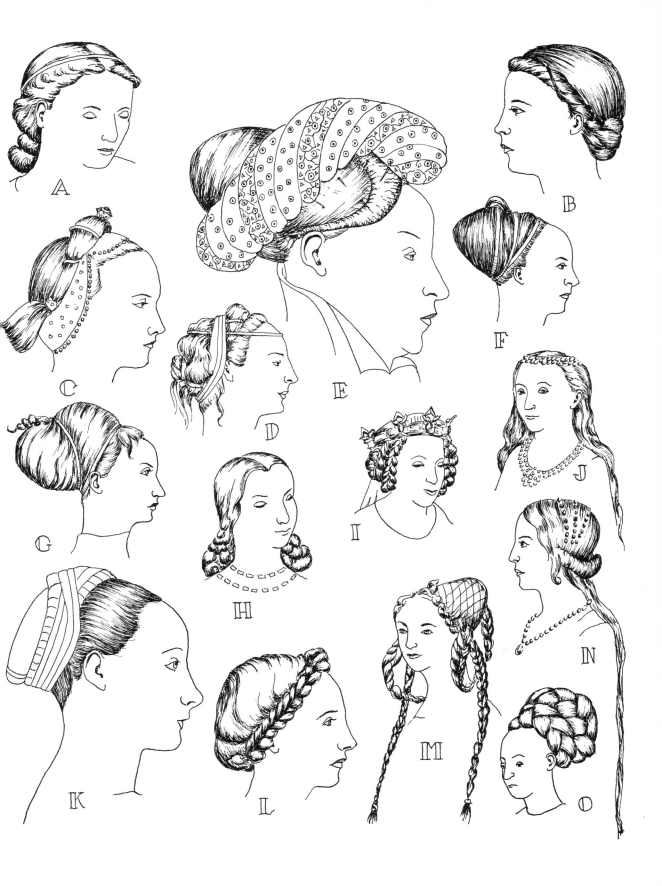

A

B

C

D

E

F

G

H

I

J

K

L

M

N

O

PLATE 43 : FIFTEENTH-CENTURY WOMEN 1470–1500

A Italian.

B Italian (Perugia).

C Last quarter.

D Last quarter.

E 1476, Italian.

F Italian.

G *c.* 1500, Italian. Isabella d'Este, 1474–1539, wife of Francesco Gonzaga.

H 1480, French. Marie de Bourgogne.

I *c.* 1480–90, German.

J 1492, Italian (Venetian). Worn only by fashionable upper-class ladies.

K Italian.

L 1495, Italian. Elisabetta Gonzaga, wife of Guidobaldo da Montefeltro, son of the Duke of Urbino (Plate 39-A).

M French.

N Italian.

O Last quarter.

P Italian.

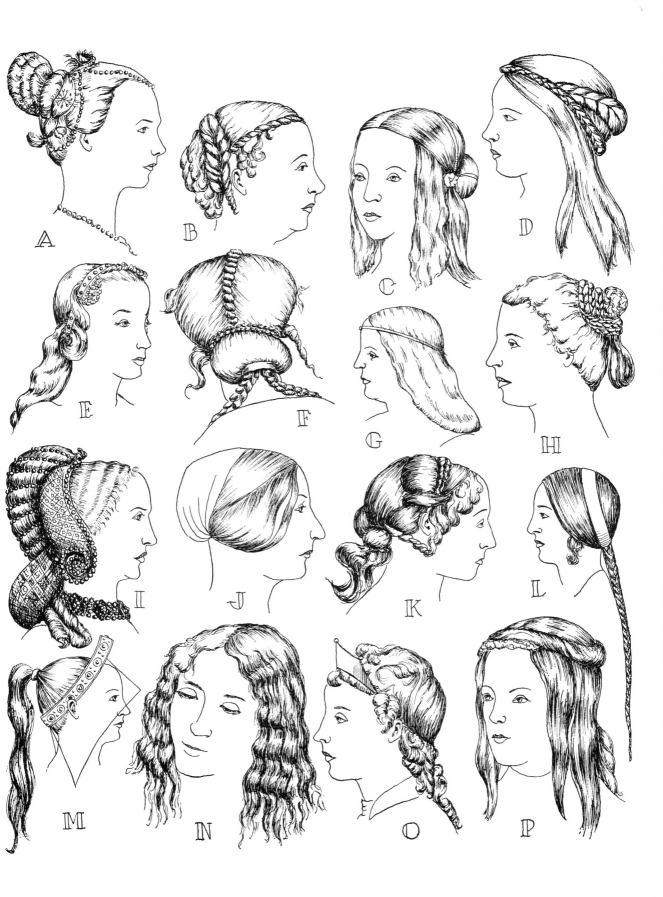

A B C D
E F G H
I J K L
M N O P

PLATE 44 : FIFTEENTH-CENTURY WOMEN 1470–1500

A   1488, Italian. Fashionable lady.

B   Last quarter, Italian (Milanese). Clarice Pusterla.

C   Last quarter, Italian.

D   Last quarter, Italian.

E   Italian. Probably Bianca, daughter of Ludovico Sforza.

F   Last quarter, Italian (Florentine). Fashionable.

G   *c.* 1470, German.

H   Italian.

I   *c.* 1480, Italian.

J   Italian. Fashionable.

K   Bianca Maria Sforza, daughter of Francesco I, second consort of Maximilian I.

L   Italian.

M   1490, Italian (Florentine). Fashionable.

N   Probably 1472, Italian. Battista Sforza, second wife of Federigo da Montefeltro, Duke of Urbino (Plate 39-A). Died in 1472, giving birth to her only son, Guidobaldo. The hair is parted in the centre, continuing down the back and drawn into two sections, one for each side. These are each bound with ribbon and about 6 inches of the ends left hanging loose. The hair is then formed into a coil over each ear and tied and secured with a brooch. The curls in front of the coil are made with an iron on short hair in front of the ears. The veil in back conceals the bareness of the back of the head. The jewel attached to the ribbon which goes over the top of the head was probably secured in place before the coil was made. The very fine line following the jaw is a delicate silk cord, probably for the purpose of securing the ribbon and the jewel. The hair in the painting is light reddish gold in colour.

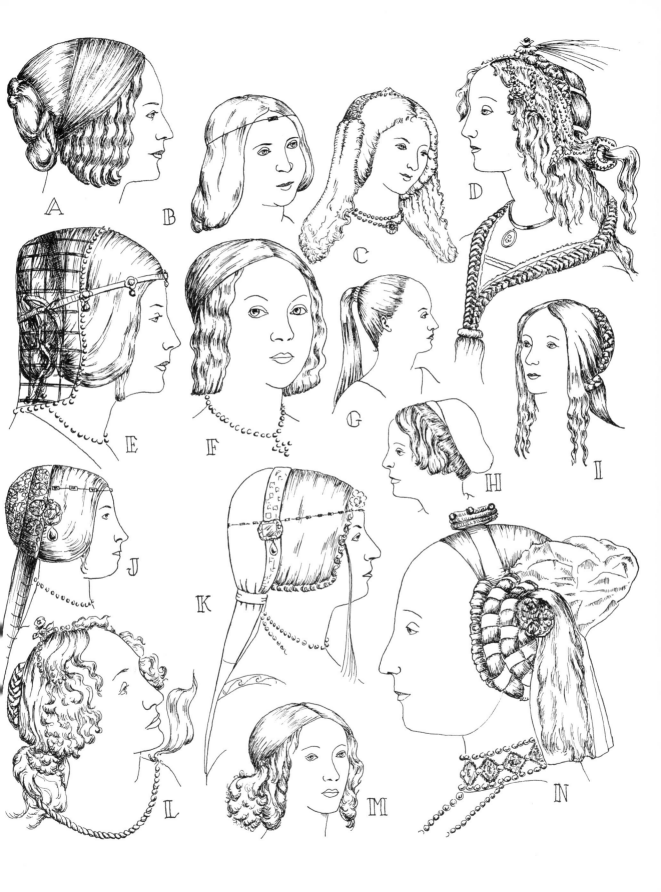

A

B

C

D

E

F

G

H

I

J

K

L

M

N

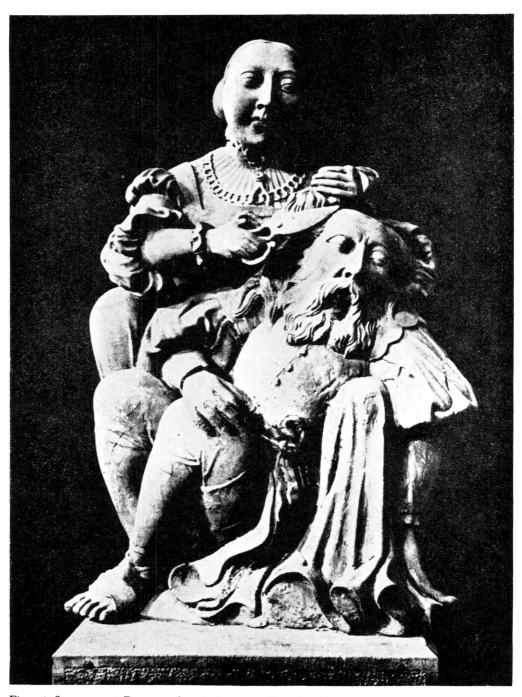

Fig. 36: SAMSON AND DELILAH. Sixteenth-century French sculpture

7 · The Sixteenth Century

Sir, will you have your worship's hair
cut after the Italian manner, short and
round, and then frounst with the
curling-yrons, to make it looke like
a halfe moone in a mist?

ROBERT GREENE

This is the age of Henry VIII, Elizabeth I, and Francis I; and all of them, not surprisingly, had a profound effect on the hair styles of the period.

MEN'S HAIR (Plates 45-51)

At the beginning of the century the long bob with bangs was fashionable. Wigs were worn when the natural hair was inadequate. We know, for example, that in December 1529 the royal treasury paid out twenty shillings 'for a perwyke for Sexton, the king's fool'. The *perwyke* was also known, at various times, as *peruique*, *perruque*, *perewake*, *periwinkle*, *perriwigge*, *periwigge*, and *periwig*.

In the 1520s there occurred in France an event, quite insignificant in itself, which sent Frenchmen, and therefore a good part of the Western world, to their barbers. As usual in such cases, there are various and conflicting versions of the story, but the end result in all cases is the same. According to Dulaure, one winter evening in 1521 when the court was at Remorantin, Francis and several of his favourites, all being in a playful mood and using snowballs in lieu of cannon balls, stormed the house of the Count Montgomery in the rue de la Pierre. As the invaders closed in, the Count or one of his guests hurled a flaming torch, striking the king on the head. The wound was serious enough to require cutting the hair short, and of course the king's courtiers very wisely adopted a similar style.

Plate 45-P, taken from a bust in the Louvre, shows Francis before the accident, whereas 47-J shows him with his post-accident coiffure.

Henry VIII, when he ascended the throne, wore his hair at what was then a fashionable length. But being favourably impressed by the new French style, he decided he wished not only to wear it himself, but to see it worn by others; and instead of waiting for his courtiers to follow his example, he made sure his wishes would be complied with by issuing an edict. According to Stow's *Annals*, in 1535 'the King commanded all about his Court to poll their heads, and to give them example, he caused his own head to be polled, and from thenceforth his beard to be notted and no more shaven'.

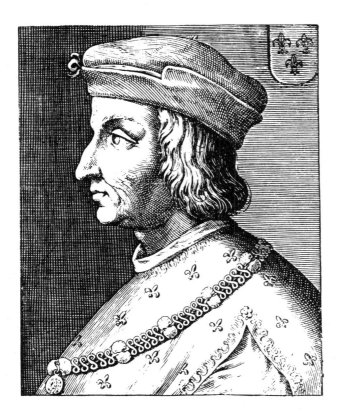

Fig. 37 : Louis XII (1462–1515),
King of France

With Francis and Henry both advocating short hair, the long-hair faction had no chance; and until very nearly the end of the century hair remained short. At first it was usually brushed forward from the crown when it was long enough to be brushed at all. In the latter part of the century the hair was a little longer and was brushed up stiffly away from the forehead rather than forward over it. The portrait of the duc de Guise (Plate 49-O) is the best example of the style. In the eighties the hair, still fairly short, was often curled all over.

In the nineties the peak of the short-hair period was past; and men of fashion were beginning to let the hair grow, even to the extent of wearing lovelocks, a French innovation which will be discussed at some length in the next chapter.

Robert Greene, in his *Quip for an Upstart Courtier* of 1592, has the barber ask: 'Sir, will you have your worship's hair cut after the Italian manner, short and round, and then frounst with the curling-yrons, to make it looke like a halfe moone in a mist? Or like a Spanyard, long at the eares, and curled like the two endes of an olde cast perriwig? Or will you be Frenchefied, with a love-locke downe to your shoulders, wherein you may weare your mistris' favour?' This was the year Greene died 'of a surfeit taken at pickeld herrings and Rhenish wine, as witnesseth Thomas Nash, who was at the fatall banquet'.

Clearly the hair was growing longer in 1597 when Hall wrote: 'When as thine oyled locks smooth platted fall, shining like varnish'd pictures on a wall'. It was the beginning of two hundred years of long hair, both real and false, for men.

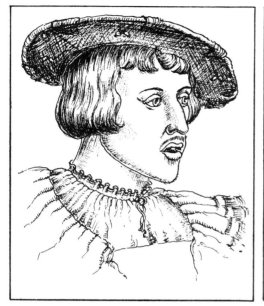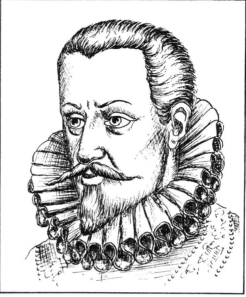

Fig. 38: Emperor Ferdinand I (1503–64), in 1531 and in mid-century

BEARDS (Plates 45-51)

It is the beards which provide the colour and most of the interest in the sixteenth-century treatment of hair. Men usually like to have a reasonable display of hair somewhere on the head. It may be the hair or it may be the beard. They seldom want both long hair and long beards at the same time, and they are rarely contented for very long with short hair and no beards. Therefore, when the hair came off, the beards were allowed to grow. Henry encouraged this and set no limits on size or style.

There were occasional beards early in the century, including the extraordinarily impressive German one shown on Plate 45-I and the equally impressive Italian one on Plate 48-B; but they were not fashionable and were not usually worn by young men. However, it is interesting to note that at Rouen in 1508 and again in 1513 men were forbidden to wear false beards. And had they not been wearing them, they would presumably not have been forbidden to do so, certainly not twice in five years.

Apparently the urge for beards was asserting itself and needed only the encouragement of two influential kings. Probably one would have been enough. But wherever there is a beard faction, there is usually somewhere an anti-beard faction. And as late as 1542 members of Lincoln's Inn were not allowed to dine in the hall when wearing a beard. In 1550 this was specified as meaning any beard over a fortnight's growth.

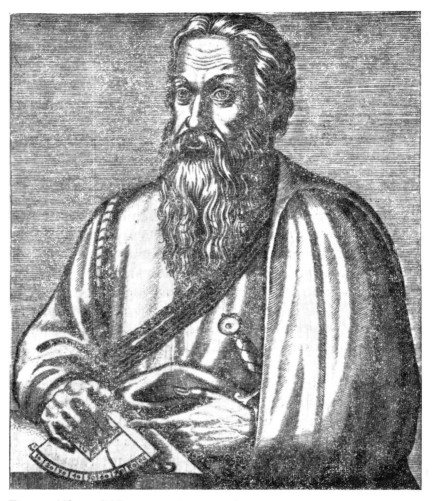

Fig. 39 : Alfonso d'Albuquerque (1453–1515)

In 1553 there was an order to the effect that members wearing a beard must pay twelve pence per meal and that any who were not shaven would be put out of commons. It was not until 1560 that the powers who made the rules gave up the fight and repealed all previous orders on the subject.

For once the clergy seemed to be in step with the laity (or vice versa), and beards were worn by everybody. However, in some circles the wearing of the beard still seemed to pose an awkward problem. Dr John Doran mentions the rather perplexing Jesuit casuists 'who wrote on the lawfulness of beards, and who most lucidly proved, under three heads—first, that we are bound to shave the beard; second, that we are bound to let it grow; third, that we may do either the one or the other'.

In 1535 in France the so-called Edict of Beards forbade anyone to appear in the hall of justice with a long beard. There are several cases on record of litigants who were refused justice until they had shaved off their beards. In 1561 the Sorbonne forbade its clerks to wear them.

In some countries the emphasis was on style, and neatly trimmed beards were worn; but in others, where quantity counted for more than style, there are records of some rather astonishing growths. Bulwer, tripping over his own syntax, is critical of the Germans, who, he says, 'affect a prolix Beerd, insomuch as some of them have been seen to have their Beerds so long that they would reach unto their feet, which they have worne trussed up in their Bosomes'.

Reynolds mentions Andreas Eberhard Rauber von Talberg who 'went habitually on foot, the better to display his beard'. It is said to have been long enough to reach to the ground, back up to his belt, and around his staff. Reynolds estimates that the beard must have been eight or nine feet in length.

Equally impressive but considerably less fortunate was the famous beard of Hans Steiniger (or Johann Staininger), a burgermeister in Braunau, Austria. His beard also was rather longer than he was and required tucking up. But on September 28, 1567, he evidently neglected to tuck it up; and on ascending the staircase to the council chamber, he tripped over the beard, fell down the stairs, and was killed. The 8 ft. 9 in. beard is reportedly still on display in the museum in Braunau.

Fig. 40 : Old man, German. 1514

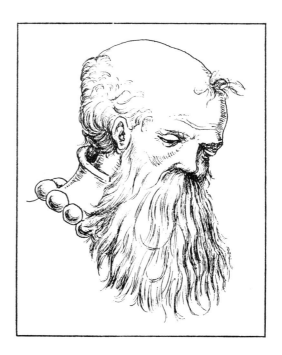

The enormously long beards probably required little but washing and combing. But the shorter, precisely cut beards worn by the fashion-conscious were curled, powdered, starched, waxed, perfumed, and often dyed, red being a fashionable colour. Ben Jonson in *Silent Woman* has the barber remark: 'I have fitted my divine and canonist, dyed their beards and all.' And as Brophy points out, 'Bottom was not thinking only of fake hair from the theatre wardrobe when he offered to play the part of Pyramus in "either your straw-colour beard, your orange-tawny beard, your purple in-grain beard, or your French-crown colour beard, your perfect yellow".'

Barker says that: 'The Puritans were divided as to the fashion of their beards, some of them wearing no whiskers at all, yet suffering the hair to grow from the chin very long. They cut the points square, so that the beard was not much unlike a pantile, as Butler, the author of Hudibras, very humorously describes it.'

Compiling an index to beard styles would undoubtedly prove to be an interesting and perhaps useful task for an antiquarian; but since the purpose of this work is to make it possible to reproduce the beards rather than to name them, I shall not try to provide any definitive listing, a task at which a number of other writers have already failed. Very likely it is impossible. There are many contemporary references to beards, some naming them, some describing them, but often in such vague or confusing terms that we cannot be sure exactly what was meant.

A case in point is the *spade beard*, which is assumed by many modern writers (and some, including Repton, not so modern) to be more or less rectangular, like a spade for digging. And this seems at first glance to be supported by the *Ballad of the Beard*, which will be quoted more fully in the next chapter:

> The soldier's beard doth march in, shear'd
> In figure like a spade,
> With which he'll make his enemies quake,
> And think their graves are made.

But all spades for digging are not rectangular. In fact, Randle Holme in his *Academy of Armoury* (1688) shows two 'turf spades' with very sharp points, one of them being shaped almost exactly like the lower part of the spade in a deck of playing cards.

Reginald Reynolds, in his witty and scholarly book entitled simply and informatively *Beards*, points out that in *Piers Penilesse* the spade beard is described as *sharp* and undoubtedly resembles the spade on a playing card. The broadness of the beard, which is mentioned several times, probably refers to the top of the beard, not the bottom.

One thing is certain, and that is that the style was particularly popular with the military. And an examination of a large number of prints and paintings featuring soldiers reveals a number of broad, pointed beards and very few broad, square-cut beards. So we shall call a spade a spade and have done with it. (For examples see Plates 49-R and 50-B.)

The clergyman William Harrison in his *Description of England* supplies us with descriptions of several beard styles after having said that he isn't going to:

'I will saie nothing of our heads, which sometimes are polled, sometimes curled, or suffered to grow at length like women's lockes, manie times cut off above or under the ears, round as by a wooden dish. Neither will I meddle with our varieties of beards, of which some are shaven from the chin like those of Turks, not a few cut short like to the beard of the Marques Otto, some made round like a rubbing-brush, others with a *pique devant*, (oh! fine fashion!) or now and then suffered to grow long, the barbers being growen to be so cunning in this behalfe as the tailors. And therefore if a man have a leane and streight face a Marques Otto's cut will make it broad and large; if it be platter like, a long slender beard will make it seem the narrower; if he be wesell-beeked, then much heare left on the cheekes will make the owner looke big like a bowdled hen, and so grim as a goose, if Cornelis of Chelmeresford saie true. Manie old men do weare no beards at all.'

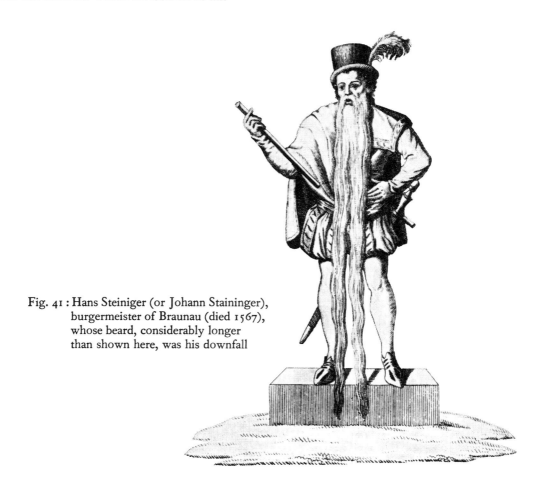

Fig. 41 : Hans Steiniger (or Johann Staininger), burgermeister of Braunau (died 1567), whose beard, considerably longer than shown here, was his downfall

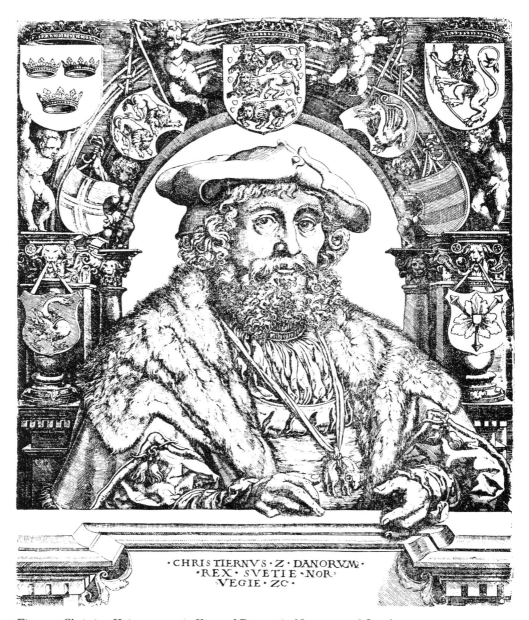

·CHRISTIERNVS·Z·DANORVM·
·REX·SVETIE·NOR·
VEGIE·ZC·

Fig. 42 : Christian II (1481–1559), King of Denmark, Norway, and Sweden

The 'beard of the Marques Otto', Reynolds points out, is a corruption of the French *marquisotte*. Later writers usually refer to the *marquisette*, meaning any very small beard cut close to the face. (See Plates 47-T and 50-A-M.)

The *pique devant* mentioned above was perhaps the most popular of all the styles. There are a number of illustrations in the plates, that of the duc de Guise, Plate 49-O, being especially noteworthy. The moustache varied, but the beard was always pointed, always neatly trimmed. If it bulged out and became rather broad before coming to a point (Lord Burghley's, 49-R), then it was a *spade*. Reynolds prefers not to distinguish between the *stiletto* and the *pique devant* (and, for that matter, between the *bodkin* and the *Pisa*); but if one were to make a distinction, it would seem that the extremely sharp beard shown in Plate 50-J might well be called a *stiletto*.

The pointed beard, whatever you wish to call it, stayed in fashion throughout the century; and in 1591 Lyly, in his *Midas*, has Motto ask:

'How, sir, will you be trimmed? Will you have your beard like a spade or a bodkin? A pent-house on your upper lip, or an alley on your chin? A low curl on your head like a Bull, or dangling locke like a Spaniell? Your Mustachios sharpe at the ends like shoemakers' awles, or hanging downe to your mouth like Goates' flakes? Your love-lockes wreathed with a silken twist, or shaggie to fall on your shoulders?'

The following year, in Greene's *Quip for an Upstart Courtier*, we find this reference to the barber:

Fig. 43 : Henri II (1519–59), King of France

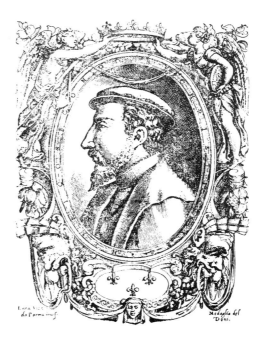

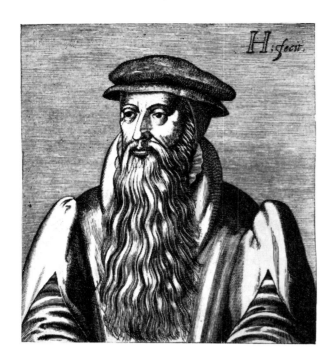

Fig. 44 : John Knox (1505?–72), Scottish religious reformer, wearing a *cathedral* beard

'He descends as low as his beard and asketh whether he please to be shaven or no, whether he will have his peak cut shorte and sharpe, amiable like an *inamorato* or broade pendant, like a spade, to be terrible like a warrior and a soldado; whether he will have his *crates* cut lowe like a juniper bush, or his *suberches* taken away with a rasor; if it be his pleasure to have his *appendices* primde or his *mouchaces* fostred, to turn about his eares like the branches of a vine or cut downe to the lip with the Italian lashe, to make him look like a halfe faced bauby in bras. These quaint tearms, barber, you greet Master Velvet-Breeches withal, and at every word, a snap with your sissars and a cringe with your knee; whereas, when you come to poore Cloth-Breeches, you either cutte his beard at your owne pleasure, or else, in disdaine, aske him if he will be trim'd with Christ's cut, round like the halfe of a Holland cheese.'

Beard styles listed by Stubbes in 1583 included the French, Spanish, Dutch, Italian, new, old, bravado, mean, gentlemen's, common, court, and country.

The *cathedral* beard, taking its name from its popularity with some churchmen, was a long, full beard, square cut or rounded, never pointed or forked, broader at the bottom than at the top (see Plates 47-E-R and 49-F). This was not a fashionable beard but was, like many beards, associated with a particular profession. The *sugar-loaf* beard was also long and rounded but was wider at the top than at the bottom (Plate 48-I-P).

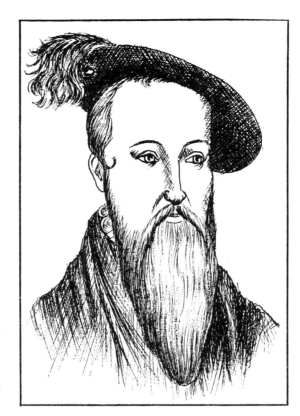

Fig. 45 : Thomas, Lord Seymour of
Sudeley (1508?–49), wearing
a *sugar-loaf* beard

The *forked* beard was quite frequently found. The *swallow-tail* is a variation, the term usually being used for forked beards in which the fork is rather widely spread (Plate 48-R).

The *fantail* beard, which was introduced during the reign of Henri IV, is described by Sparrow as 'a thing three inches long, in the shape of a fan, rounded, and set off with two long stiff whiskers, cat like in appearance. At night the fan-beard had a wadded bag to sleep in, and for the good reason that the scented wax with which the beard was coloured and stiffened took some time to manipulate, and was easily cracked.' Any beard requiring this much care would not have been worn by the working class.

Finally, there was the simple *square-cut* beard (Plate 50-D), which could be of various lengths, and the *round* beard (Plate 45-E), which was in some instances, when the name seemed appropriate, called a *bush* beard or simply a *bush* (Plate 45-I).

It is hardly surprising, in view of the importance attached to facial hair and the necessity for keeping it well trimmed and shaped, that barbers, and especially the king's barbers, should have been considered of sufficient importance that the names of two of them—Thomas Vicary and John Pen—have come down to us. Regulations for their conduct were carefully laid down:

'It is also ordeyned that the King's Barbour shalle daylie by the King's upriseinge be readdye and attendant in the King's Pryvie Chamber, there having in reddyness his water Basons, knyves, combes, scissours and such other stuffe as to his Roome

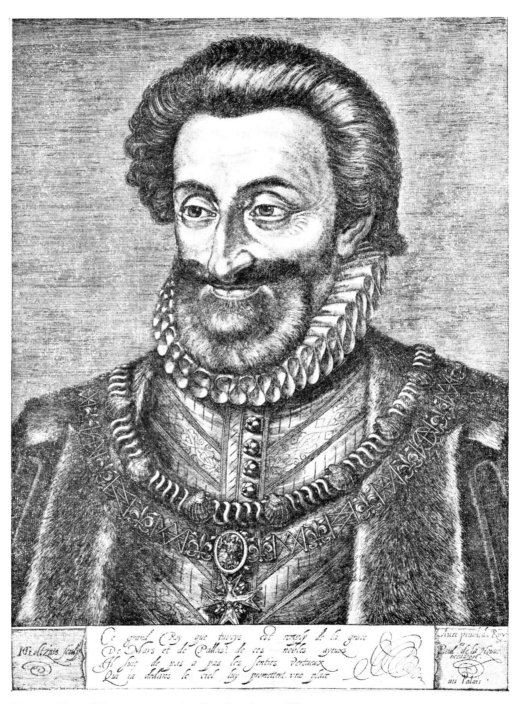

Fig. 46: Henri IV (1553–1610), first Bourbon king of France

doth appertaine for trymminge and dressinge of the King's heade and bearde, and that said Barbour take a speciall regard to the pure and clean keepinge of his own p'son and apparrell, usinge himself alwayse honestlye in his conversationne without resortinge to the companye of vile personnes or of misguided women, in avoydinge such danger as by that means he might doe unto the King's most royall person.'

Lesser men had their hair and beards trimmed in the public barbers' shops, popular gathering places which served as a sort of clearing house for local gossip. Musical instruments were usually provided for those who cared to play them. There were, however, certain strict regulations, conspicuously posted, for the customers' behaviour. Forfeits were to be paid for handling the razors, talking of cutting throats, calling hair powder flour, and meddling with anything on the shop board.

WOMEN'S HAIR (Plates 51-54)

In the early years there was a continuation of the fifteenth-century style, the hair being frequently concealed, especially by married women. When it was exposed, it was usually straight and combed smoothly from a centre parting, the long ends formed into braids, twists, curls, rolls, or chignons or a combination of all of them, and frequently interwoven with ribbons. Sometimes the hair hung loose; sometimes it was partially covered. Plates 52 and 53 show some of the many possible variations in treatment. The more or less stable elements of the early coiffure were the centre parting and the straight, smooth hair conforming to the natural shape of the head. What was done with the hair falling below the ears varied considerably.

After about 1540 in England, earlier in France and Italy, the hair was sometimes waved or curled among fashionable women; but the centre parting was maintained. Instead of smooth, flat hair at the temples, there tended to be a fluffing out or frizzing. In 1548 we find a reference to 'the heare of woman that is layde over hir forehead', and we are informed that 'gentlewomen do call them their rolles'. Among the lower classes the centre parting and braids were common. In 1545 the first metal hairpins were used in England.

The most notable development came after mid-century, when the hair began to be turned up and back over pads to give it fullness. Sixteenth-century Dutch portraits even show little girls (of the upper class) wearing the style. It reached its greatest peak during the last quarter of the century, when the hair was sometimes dressed over wire frames instead of pads to give it height in front (see Plates 52 and 54). Jewels were often worn in the hair during this period.

Wigs became fashionable in the latter part of the century; and, as Godey's expressed it some centuries later, 'the making of them furnished employment for decayed gentlewomen'. According to Doran, there is no evidence that English women wore wigs until the second half of the century. Queen Elizabeth, who had a large collection of wigs, favoured tightly curled hair, whereas Mary of Scotland, who is believed to have had an even larger collection, preferred the winged or horned style with smooth hair. Marguerite de Valois is said to have kept blond pages to provide hair for her wigs. Catherine de' Medici, who helped to popularize the wearing of wigs, paid, according to existing records, five sous to a woman for her daughter's hair.

In Venice fake hair was kept in place with a gum pomade, and hair was sometimes powdered. In 1593 even nuns were said to have been seen on the streets of Paris frizzed and powdered. English ladies of the court also powdered or dyed their hair yellow to match Elizabeth's natural hair colour. Black hair was not fashionable. Dyeing and bleaching hair were commonly practised among fashionable women, the bleaching especially among the Italians, who greatly admired blonde hair.

Writing in 1589, Cesare Vecellio described the elaborate arrangements for the process:

'The houses of Venice are commonly crowned with little constructions in wood, resembling a turret without a roof. On the ground these lodges or boxes are formed of masonry, floored like what are called terazzi at Florence and Naples, and covered with a cement of sand and lime to protect them from the rain. It is in these that the Venetian women may be seen as often, and indeed oftener, than in their chambers. It is there that with their heads exposed to the full ardor of the sun during whole days, they strain every nerve to augment their charms, as if they needed it, as if the constant use of so many methods known to all did not expose their natural beauty to pass for no better than artificial. During the hours when the sun darts its most vertical and scorching rays they repair to these boxes and condemn themselves to broil in them unattended. Seated there they keep on wetting their hair with a sponge dipped in some elixir of youth, prepared with their own hands or purchased. They moisten their hair afresh as fast as it is dried by the sun, and it is by the unceasing renewal of this operation that they become what you see them—blondes. When engaged in it they throw over their ordinary dress a *peignoir* or dressing gown of the finest white silk, which they call a *schia-ronetto*. They wear on their heads a straw hat without a crown, so that the hair drawn through the opening may be spread upon the borders; this hat, doing double duty as a drying-line for the hair and a parasol to protect the neck and face, was called a *solana*. In winter, or when the sun faded, they wetted and dried their hair before a fire.'

In her *Memoirs and Essays* Mrs Jameson mentions having seen 'a curious old Venetian print which represents this process. A lady is seated on the roof or balcony of her house, wearing a sort of broad-brimmed hat without a crown; the long hair is drawn over these wide brims and spread out in the sunshine, while the face is completely shaded. How they contrived to escape a brain fever or a *coup de soleil* is a wonder; and truly of all the multifarious freaks of fashion and vanity, I know nothing more strange than this.' The curious old Venetian print referred to was made by Vecellio and is reproduced in Figure 48.

Venetian ladies did *not* always escape the unpleasant consequences of too much sitting in the sun. Bulwer records in some detail (and with a certain relish, one suspects) the case of one unfortunate lady:

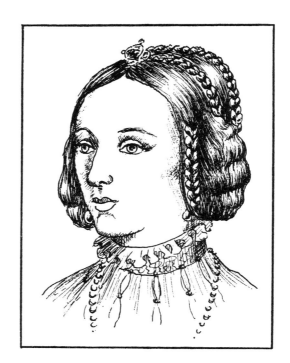

Fig. 47: Isabella of Portugal, wife of
Charles V (Emperor 1519–56)

'The Women of old time did most love yellow Haire, and it is found that they
introduced this colour by safron and by long sitting daily in the Sun, who instead
of Safron sometimes used medicated Sulphur. . . . The Venetian Women at this day,
and the Paduan, and those of Verona, and other parts of Italy practice the same
vanitie, and receive the same recompence for their affectation, there being in all these
Cities, open and manifest examples of those who have undergone a kinde of Martyr-
dome, to render their Haire yellow. Schenkius relates unto us the History of a cer-
taine Noble Gentlewoman, about sixteen or seventeen yeares of age, that would
expose her bare Head to the fervent heat of the Sun daily for some houres, that shee
might purchase yellow and long Haire, by anointing them with a certain unguent;
and although she obtained the effect of her desires, yet withall, shee procured to her
selfe a violent Head ach, and bled almost every day abundantly through the Nose;
and on a time being desirous to stop the Blood by the pressing of her Nostrils, not
farr from her right Eye toward her Temple, through a pore, as it were by a hole
made with a needles point, the Blood burst out abundantly, and taking away her
fingers, againe caused it to run through her Nose; and at that very time shee was
diseased by the obstruction of her courses. Another Maid also by using this same
Art, became almost blind with sore Eyes.'

Mixtures of alum, black sulphur, and honey were sometimes used for bleaching.
Even as early as 1562 Dr Marinello of Moderna, writing in the *Light of Apothicaries
and Treasure of Heroborists*, a 'Treatise upon the Adornment of Women', cautioned
strongly against hair dyes:

'Permit me to remind you honored and honorable ladies that the application
of so many colors to your hair may strike a chill into the head like the shock of a

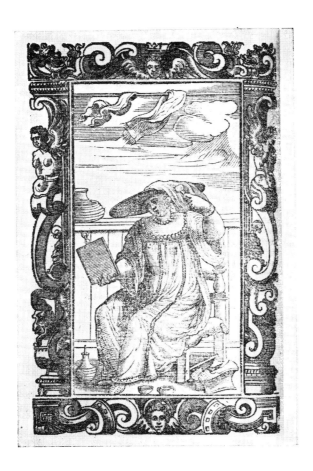

Fig. 48 : Woman bleaching her hair
in sixteenth-century Venice

shower-bath, that it affects and penetrates, and what is worse, may entail divers grave maladies and infirmities; therefore, I should advise you to take all possible precautions. . . . We frequently see the hair affected in its essentials, or at its roots grow weak and fall off and the complexion destroyed through the use of so many injurious liquids and decoctions.' Working-class women were, of course, spared all this.

As always when women are passing through a cycle of extravagance and distortion in their hair styling, they are subjected oftentimes to quite vehement criticism (almost exclusively from men), to which they pay absolutely no attention. But it gives the complainers something to complain about, and it frequently provides posterity with an enlightening description of the hair styles of the period.

Phillip Stubbes, a complainer, fortunately included women's hair styles in *The Anatomie of Abuses*, which was first published in 1583. It was apparently a great success, for the third edition, from which the following quotation is taken, was published two years later. It should, perhaps, be pointed out that Stubbes was not without staunch supporters, one of whom took the trouble to compose some verses to the glory of Phillip Stubbes, which Mr Stubbes thoughtfully included at the beginning of his volume:

If mortall man maie challenge praise
    For anything doen in this life;
Then may our Stubbes, at all assaies,
    Injoy the same withouten strife.

Not onely for his godly zeale,
    And Christian life accordinglie;
But also for his book in sale
    Here present now before thine eye.

Herein the abuses of these daies,
    As in a glass thou maiest beholde;
Oh, buy it then, heare what he saies,
    And give him thankes an hundred folde.

But let our Stubbes speak for himself:

'Then followeth the trimming and tricking of their heades, in laying out their haire to the shewe, whiche of force must be curled, frisled, and crisped, laid out (a World to see!) on wreathes and borders, from one eare to an other. And least it should fall down, it is under propped with forks, wiers, and I cannot tell what, like grim sterne monsters, rather than chaste Christian matrons. Then, on the edges of their boulstered haire (for it standeth crested rounde about their frontiers, and

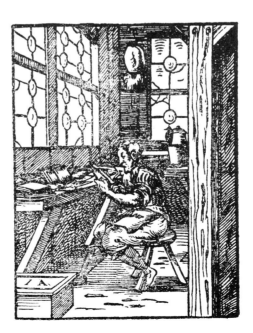

Fig. 49 : Workshop of a sixteenth-century
      comb-maker

hanging over their faces like *pendices* or vailes, with glasse windowes on every side)
there is laied great wreathes of gold and silver, curiously wrought, and cunningly
applied to the temples of their heades. And for feare of lacking any thing to set
forthe their pride withall, at their haire, thus wreathed and creasted, are hanged
bugles (I dare not say babels), ouches, rynges, gold, silver, glasses and suche other
childishe gewgawes, and foolish trinkets besides, whiche, for that they be innumerable, and I unskillfull in women's tearmes, I cannot easily expresse. . . . If curling and
laying out their owne naturall haire were all (which is impious, and at no hande
lawfull, being, as it is, an ensigne of pride, and the standerd of wantonnesse to all
that behold it), it were the lesse matter; but thei are not simplie content with their
owne haire, but buye other haire, either of horses, mares, or any other straunge
beastes, dying it of what colour they list themselves. And if there be any poore
women (as now and then, we see, God doth bless them with beautie as well as the
riche) that hath faire haire, these nice dames will not rest till they have bought it, or
if any children have faire haire, they will entice them into a secret place, and for a
penie or two they will cut off their haire, as I heard that one did in the citie of
London of late, who, meeting a little childe with very faire haire, inveigled her into
a house, promised her a penie, and so cutte off her haire; and upon the other side,

Fig. 50: THE SIN OF PRIDE. 1570

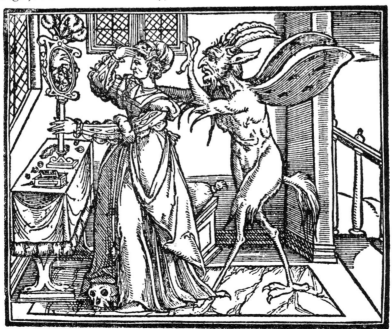

if any have haire of her own naturall growing, whiche is not faire ynough, then will they dye it in divers colours, almost chaunging the substaunce into accidentes by their devilish, and more then thrise cursed devyses. So where as their haire was geven them as a signe of subjection, and therefore they were commaunded to cherish the same, now have they made it an ornament of pride, and destruction to themselves for ever, excepte they repent.'

Of course they did not repent but continued in their wicked ways right into the seventeenth century.

Plate 45 : Sixteenth-Century Men 1500–1525

A   French. Louis XII, 1462–1515. Succeeded Charles VIII in 1498.

B   1501, German.

C   1500, German. Albrecht Dürer, 1471–1528. (From a self-portrait.) (For later portrait see Plate 46-T.)

D   1515, German.

E   1500, German. *Round* or *bush* beard.

F   Polish. Nicolas Copernicus, 1473–1543.

G   German.

H   Italian. Giuliano de' Medici, Count of Nemours, 1478–1516.

I   1510, German. Unusually large *round* or *bush* beard.

J   *c.* 1505, probably French.

K   Italian.

L   1520, German. Martin Luther, 1483–1546 (for later period see Plate 47-L).

M   Pope Julius II, 1443–1513. He was followed by Leo X, who was not bearded.

N   Young German prince.

O   *c.* 1525, Dutch.

P   Francis I, 1494–1547. King of France, 1515–47 (for later portrait see Plate 47-J).

Q   1514, German.

R   1510–20, Flemish. *Swallow-tail* beard.

S   Probably French.

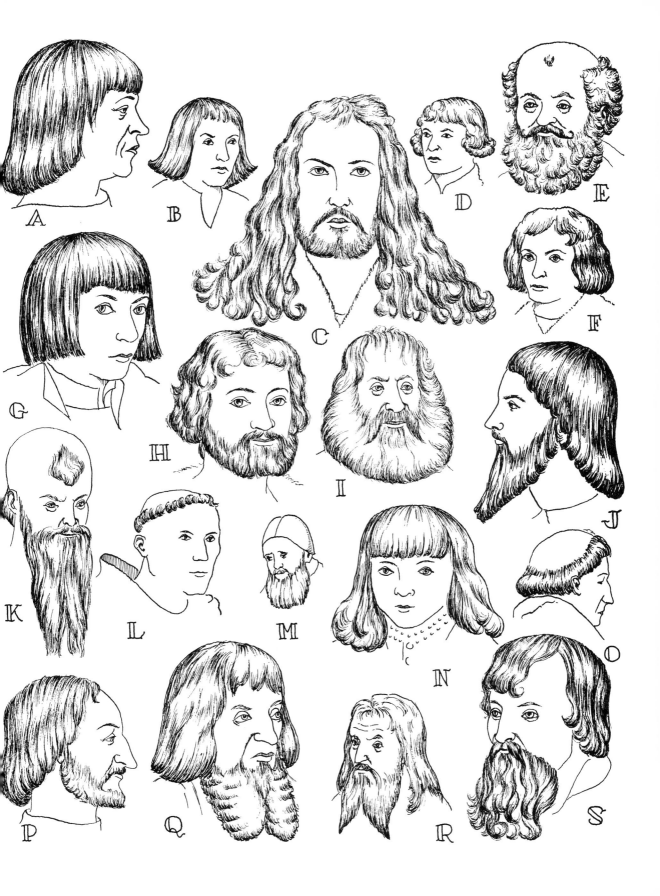

A

B

C

D

E

F

G

H

I

J

K

L

M

N

O

P

Q

R

S

PLATE 46 : SIXTEENTH-CENTURY MEN 1520–1530

A   1520, German. Hieronymus Holzschuher.

B   1528, Italian.

C   Italian.

D   Dutch.

E   1524, German. Wilibald Pirkheimer.

F   Italian boy.

G   German.

H   Exact date uncertain.

I   *c.* 1525, German. The long locks in front of the ears are not uncommon in German portraits of this period. When the hair is crisp and very curly, they give the impression of very long sideburns.

J   German.

K   German.

L   1530, Martin Luther's father (for portraits of Luther see Plates 45-L and 47-L).

M   German.

N   *c.* 1525, Swiss.

O   German.

P   1522, German. Frederick III, 1463–1525.

Q   Charles V, 1500–58. Emperor, 1519–58; King of Spain (as Charles I), 1516–56.

R   French. Robert de Montal.

S   1522, German.

T   1527, German. Albrecht Dürer, 1471–1528 (for earlier portrait see Plate 45-C).

U   1526, German. Philipp Melanchthon, 1497–1560. Scholar and humanist (see also Plate 47-T).

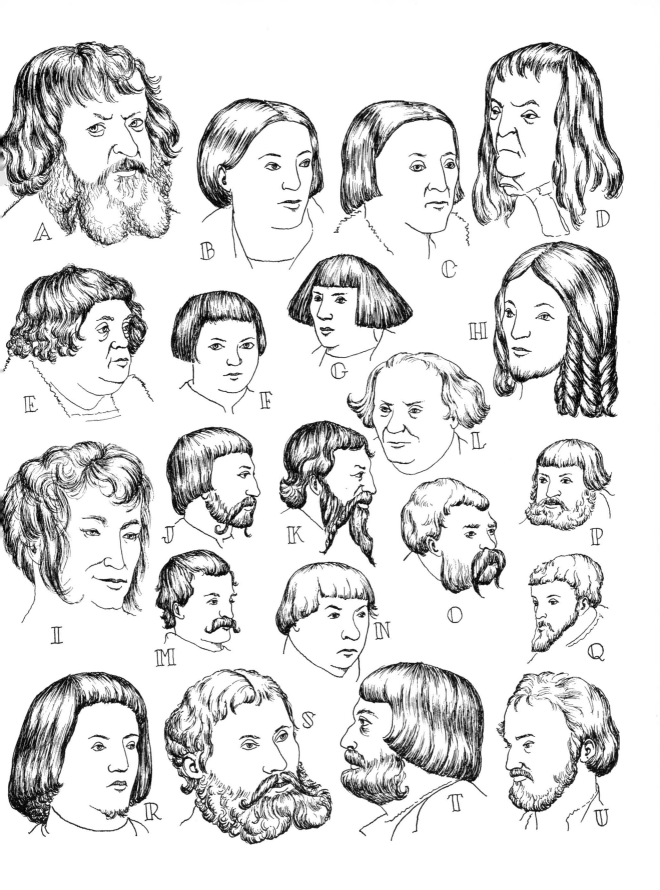

PLATE 47 : SIXTEENTH-CENTURY MEN 1520–1550

A   French. John Calvin, 1509–64. Protestant theologian (for other portraits see Plates 48-I and 49-N). *Forked* beard.

B   Johannes Sturm.

C   *c.* 1525, Swiss. Rudolf Coolin. Teacher.

D   1543, probably Dutch.

E   German. Johannes Oekolampadius, 1482–1531. Reformer and associate of Zwingli. *Cathedral* beard.

F   1535, German. Count Ulrich von Württemberg.

G   Italian. Michelangelo, 1475–1564.

H   1529, German. Philipp Künstler, age 7.

I   Mid-century, English.

J   Francis I, 1494–1547. King of France, 1515–47 (for earlier portrait see Plate 45-P).

K   1534, German. Duke George of Saxony.

L   German. Martin Luther, 1483–1546 (for earlier portrait see Plate 45-L).

M   Mid-century, Italian.

N   Henry VIII, 1491–1547. King of England, 1509–47 (see also Plate 51-E).

O   *c.* 1524, Swiss. *Swallow-tail* beard.

P   German. Long *forked* beard.

Q   English. Sebastian Cabot, 1483?–1557? *Forked* beard.

R   French. *Cathedral* beard.

S   1547–50.

T   German. Philipp Melanchthon, 1497–1560. *Marquisette* beard (see also Plate 46-U).

U   1540.

V   1530, German.

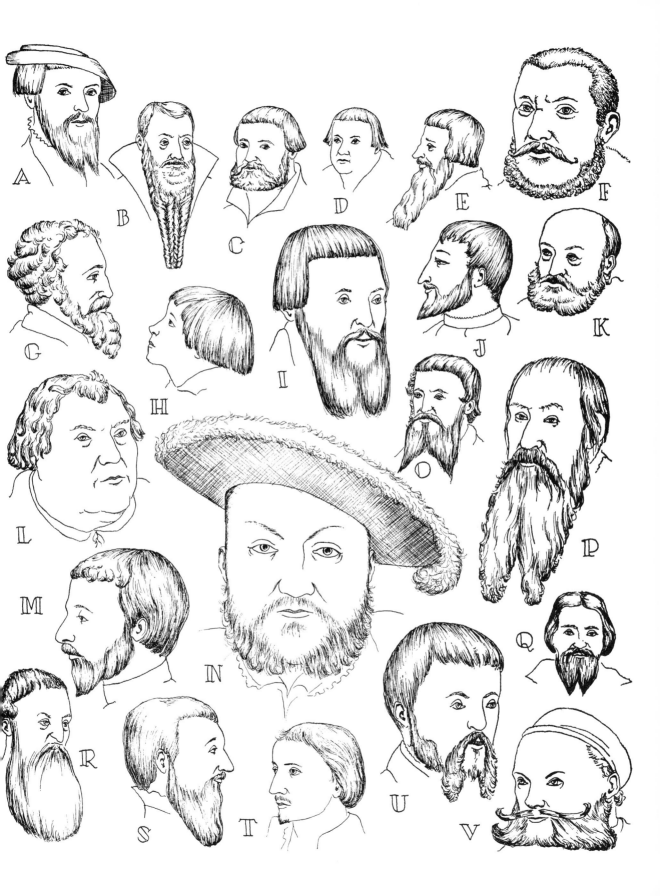

PLATE 48 : SIXTEENTH-CENTURY MEN 1520–1600

A *c.* 1525, French.

B *c.* 1520, Italian.

C 1531, German.

D 1531, German.

E Second quarter, Italian.

F *c.* 1559, English. William Parr.

G Third quarter, Italian. *Bush* beard.

H Mid-century French. Long *forked* beard.

I French. John Calvin, 1509–64 (for other portraits see Plates 47-A and 49-N). *Sugar-loaf* beard.

J Third quarter, Italian.

K Third quarter, Italian.

L Third quarter, Italian.

M Third quarter, English. *Forked* beard.

N Third quarter, Italian.

O Last quarter, Italian. Long *forked* beard.

P Last quarter, English. *Sugar-loaf* beard. Style worn by Lord Seymour of Sudley.

Q 1587. *Pique devant* beard with inverted moustache.

R 1596, English. *Swallow-tail* beard.

S English. Beard of George Clifford, Earl of Cumberland.

T *c.* 1594, Italian. Small *bush* beard.

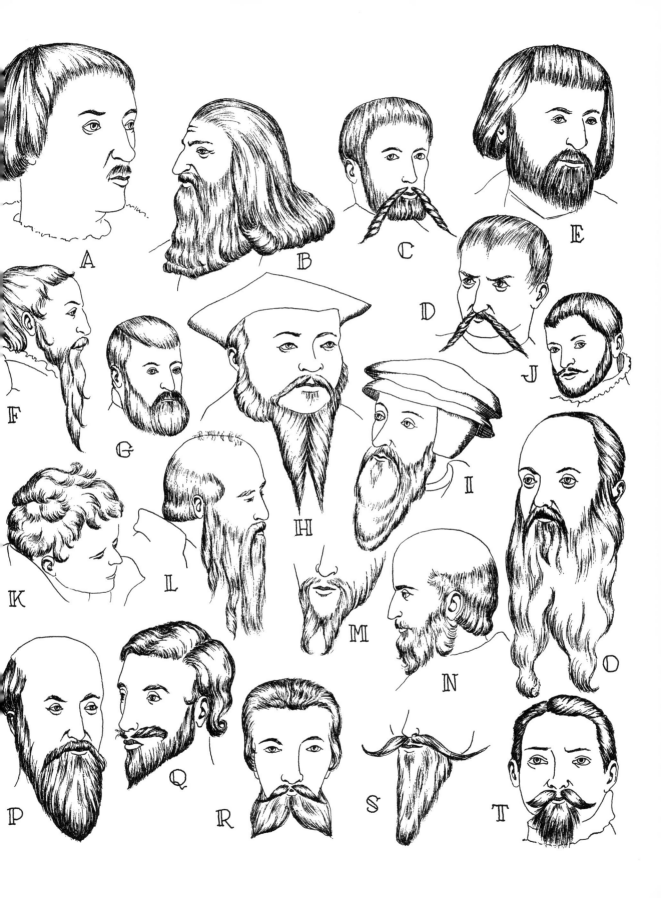

PLATE 49 : SIXTEENTH-CENTURY MEN 1540–1580

A   Italian. Cosimo I de' Medici, 1519–74. Duke of Florence.

B   1555.

C   German.

D   Spanish. Michael Servetus (Miguel Serveto), 1511–53. Theologian and physician. *Pique devant* beard.

E   1550, German. Lukas Cranach the Elder, 1472–1553. Long *forked* beard. (From a self-portrait.)

F   1550, English. Reginald Pole, 1500–58. Archbishop of Canterbury, 1556–58. *Cathedral* beard.

G   Italian. Jacopo Sansovino, 1486–1570. Sculptor and architect. *Forked* beard.

H   *c.* 1560.

I   1555.

J   French. Henri II, 1519–59. King, 1547–59.

K   Edward VI, 1537–53.

L   Flemish. Andreas Vesalius, 1514–64. Anatomist.

M   French.

N   French. John Calvin, 1509–64 (for other portraits see Plates 47-A and 48-I).

O   French. Henri de Lorraine, duc de Guise, 1550–88. *Pique devant* beard with inverted moustache.

P   German. Martin Bucer, 1491–1551. Reformer.

Q   French. Charles IX, 1550–74. Reigned 1560–74. *Pique devant* beard.

R   English. William Cecil, Lord Burghley, 1520–98. *Spade* beard.

S   Scottish.

T   Venetian.

U   Spanish. Philip II, 1527–98. *Pique devant* beard.

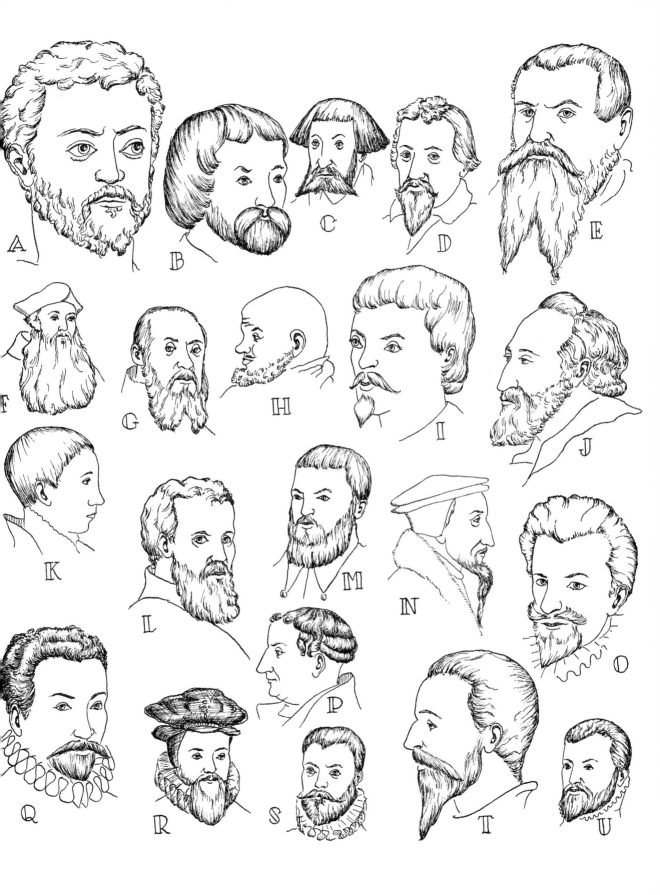

PLATE 50 : SIXTEENTH-CENTURY MEN 1575–1600

A   Italian. *Marquisette* beard.

B   1580, Spanish. Don Alvardo de Bazan. Admiral. *Spade* beard.

C   English. William Shakespeare, 1564–1616. Small *forked* beard. There are no authenti-
cated contemporary portraits of Shakespeare. This one is an idealized composite of
several (see Plate 55-P in the next chapter for a portrait done a few years after his
death).

D   1597, English. *Square-cut* beard.

E   1580–85, Flemish. *Pique devant* beard.

F   1577. *Marquisette* beard.

G   English. Edmund Spenser, *c.* 1552–99.

H   English. Sir Walter Raleigh, 1552?–1618. *Pique devant* beard.

I   *c.* 1595, Dutch. *Forked* beard.

J   1581–82. *Stiletto* beard.

K   1583.

L   1599, English. Sir Henry Neville.

M   1580–85, Flemish. *Marquisette* beard.

N   1599.

O   English. Robert Dudley, Earl of Leicester, 1532–88.

P   *c.* 1575, Scottish.

Q   French. Henri IV, 1553–1610.

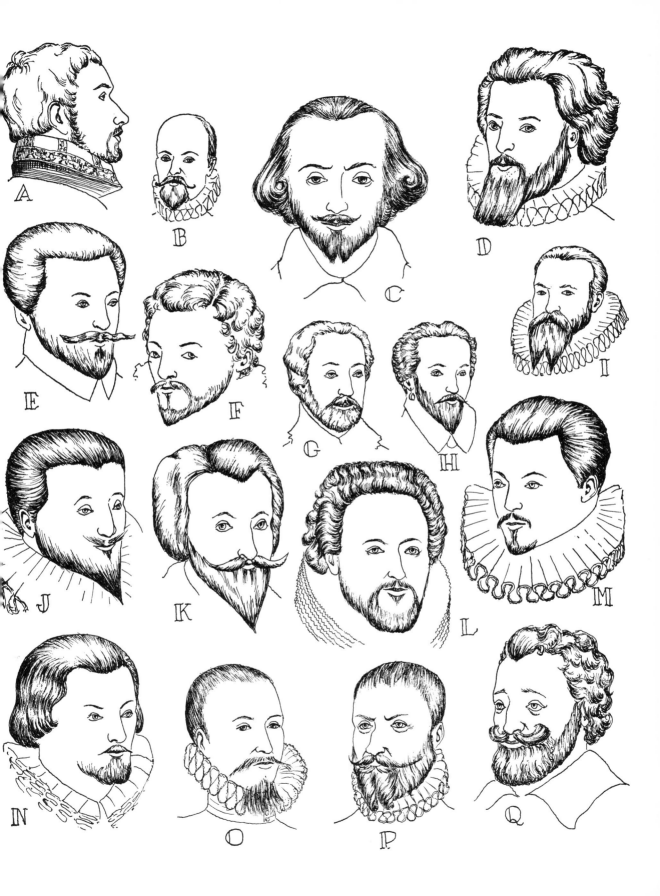

A

B

C

D

E

F

G

H

I

J

K

L

M

N

O

P

Q

PLATE 51 : SIXTEENTH-CENTURY MEN AND WOMEN 1500–1600

MEN:

A   Franz von Sickingen, 1481–1523. German knight.

B   English. Edward Courtney, Earl of Devonshire, died 1536.

C   Italian. Pietro Bembo, 1470–1547. Poet.

D   Sigismund I, 1467–1548. King of Poland, 1506–48.

E   1545. Henry VIII, 1491–1547. King of England, 1509–47 (see also Plate 47-N).

F   French. Henri II, 1519–59. King, 1547–59 (see also Figure 43).

G   Gustavus I, 1496–1560. King of Sweden, 1523–60.

H   Italian. Matteo Bandello, 1480?–1562? Writer.

I   Italian. Girolamo Frescobaldo, 1538–1644. Organist, singer, composer.

J   1581.

K   Flemish. Abraham Ortelius, 1527–98. Geographer.

L   Beard of J. Stumppius.

M   Flemish. Gerardus Meractor (Gerhard Kremer), 1512–94. Geographer.

N   Cornelius Vandun, 1483–1577. Soldier with King Henry, Yeoman of the Guard and usher to King Henry, King Edward, Queen Mary, and Queen Elizabeth.

WOMEN:

O   First quarter, Italian.

P   Mid-century, French.

Q   Mid-century, French.

R   Mid-century, French.

S   c. 1597, Italian (see also Plate 54-R-S-T-U).

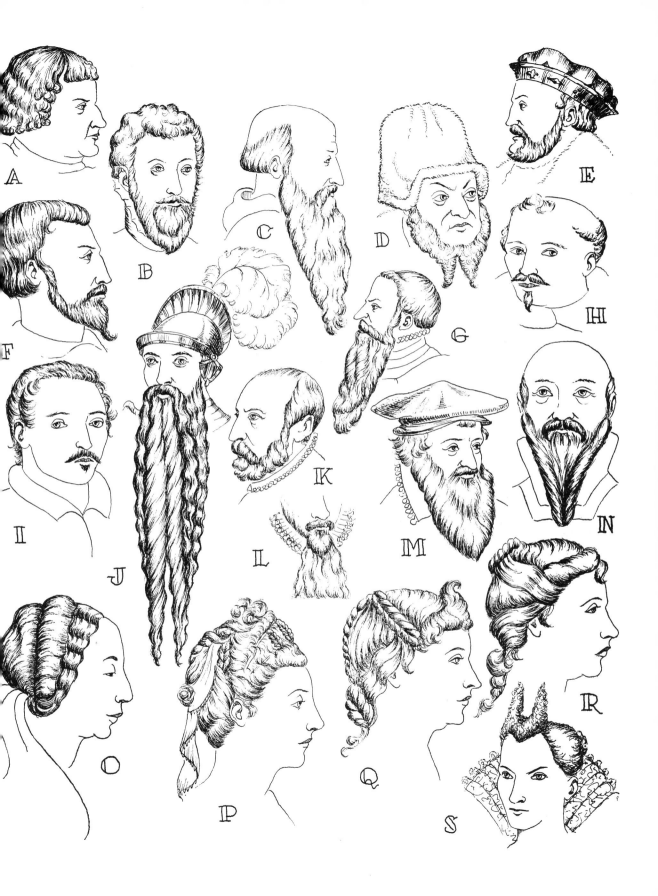

A

B

C

D

E

F

G

H

I

J

K

L

M

N

O

P

Q

R

S

PLATE 52 : SIXTEENTH-CENTURY WOMEN 1500–1600

A   *c.* 1500, Italian.

B   *c.* 1500.

C   *c.* 1512, Italian.

D   Italian.

E   *c.* 1515, Italian.

F   *c.* 1530. Style of Eleanor of Austria.

G   Second quarter, French.

H   Before 1545.

I   *c.* 1550, French.

J   *c.* 1550, Italian.

K   *c.* 1560, probably English.

L   Last half, Italian.

M   *c.* 1575, French. Hair dressed over pads.

N   Last quarter, French. Hair dressed over wire frames (see also R and S below and Plate 54-N-O; extreme Italian versions are shown in 51-S and 54-R-S-T-U).

O   Mid-century, French.

P   Last quarter, French. Marie Touchet, duchesse d'Entraques. Hair dressed over pads or a wire frame.

Q   Last quarter, French. Probably a wig.

R   *c.* 1595, French. Wig.

S   Marguerite de Valois, 1553–1615. Queen of France and Navarre, wife of Henri IV. Wig.

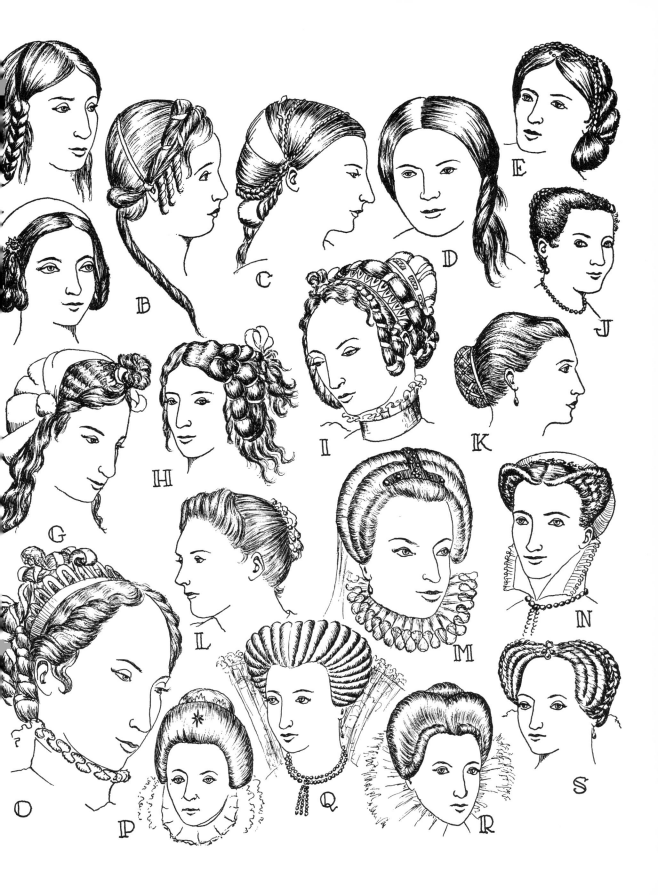

PLATE 53 : SIXTEENTH-CENTURY WOMEN 1500–1550

A   Early.

B   1520, Italian.

C   1510–20, Flemish.

D   1500–10.

E   Early, possibly French.

F   Early, French.

G   Italian. Lucrezia Borgia, 1480–1519.

H   Before 1520, Italian.

I   French. Marguerite d'Angoulême, Queen of Navarre, 1492–1549, sister of Francis I, author of the *Heptameron*. The style seems more typical of a slightly later period, and it is entirely possible that the sculpture from which this drawing was made was not contemporary and is not a reliable indication of the queen's actual hair style.

J   1543. Mary I, 1516–58. Queen of England, 1553–58.

K   Italian, probably mid-century.

L   Italian.

M   1525.

N   *c.* 1530–40, French.

O   Very early, Italian (possibly late fifteenth century).

P   Very early, Italian (possibly late fifteenth century).

Q   1529, German. Luther's wife.

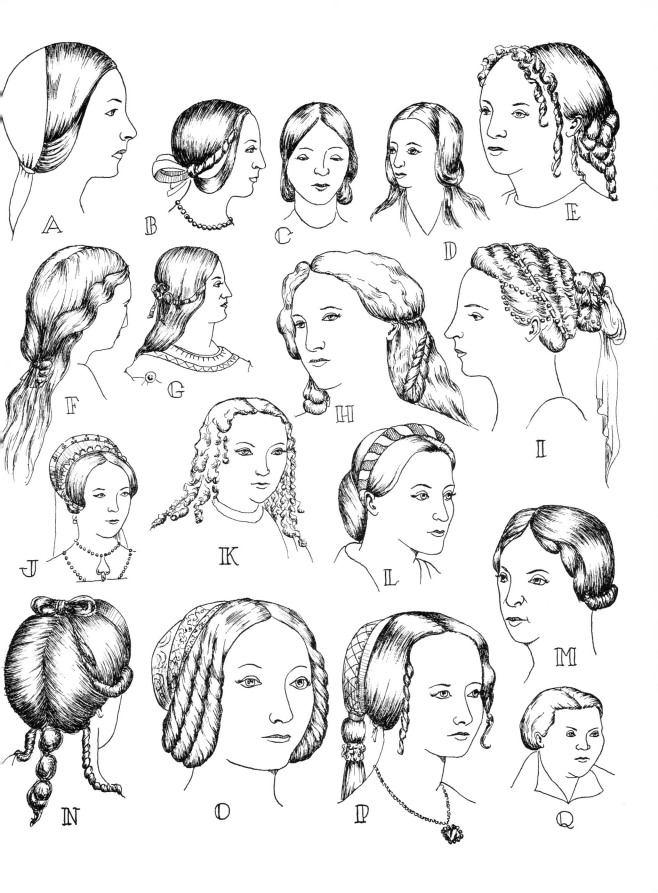

A B C D E

F G H I

J K L M

N O P Q

PLATE 54 : SIXTEENTH-CENTURY WOMEN 1550–1600

A   Elizabeth I, 1533–1603. Queen of England, 1558–1603 (see M below for later period).

B   1560.

C   Mid-century.

D   German peasant.

E   German peasant.

F   Probably French.

G   German.

H   German peasant.

I   Mid-century, Italian.

J   Italian. Duchess Renata of Ferrara.

K   Mid-century, probably French.

L   1560.

M   Elizabeth I. Wig (see A above for earlier period).

N   1579, French. Hair dressed over pads or a wire frame.

O   English. Hair dressed over pads (see similar styles on Plate 52).

P   German. Hair dressed over pads.

Q   *c.* 1570.

R   1597, Italian. Hair dressed over a wire frame.

S   1597, Italian. This was also worn with a cone-shaped head-dress similar to the one in U below but more like a fifteenth-century hennin and not a part of the actual coiffure.

T   *c.* 1597, Italian. Horns of hair dressed over a wire frame.

U   1597, Italian. The same treatment of the front hair was also used without the cone-shaped arrangement at the back, as shown in Plate 51-S. Hair dressed over wire frames.

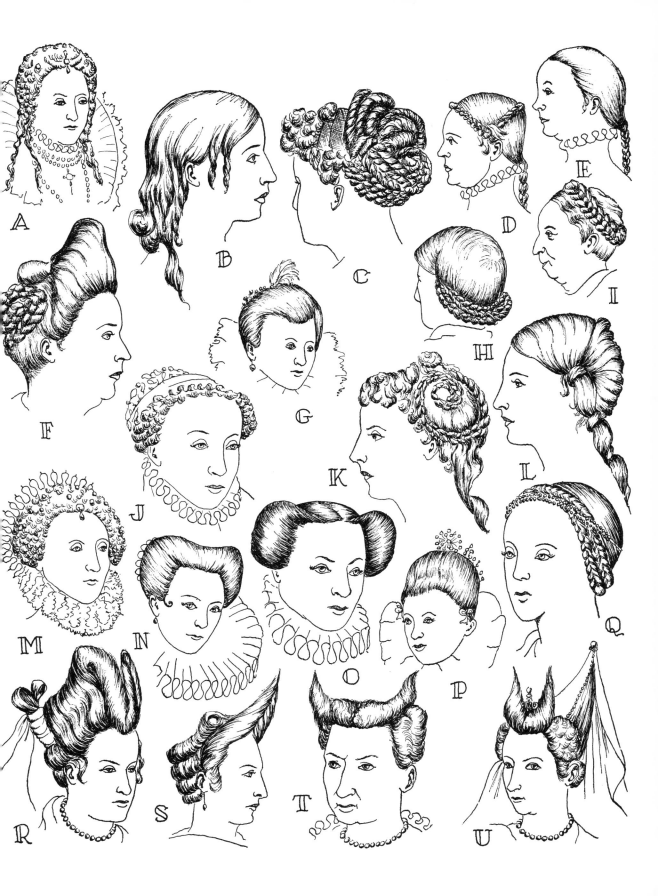

A

B

C

D

E

F

G

H

I

J

K

L

M

N

O

P

Q

R

S

T

U

8 · The Seventeenth Century

Take the Oyles of White Henbane and
Fenugreek Seed, and with them mix
a little Gum Arabick, and over a
gentle Fire make it into a flowing or
soft Ointment, and anoint your Hair
with it before you turn it up, and it
will be Curiously Curled.
The Ladies Dictionary

The seventeenth century was one of dramatic change for men, whereas for women the innovations were less startling. It saw the end of beards and men's widespread use of wigs for the first time since the days of the ancient Egyptians. Fashionable women's coiffures were high at the beginning of the century, high at the end, and low, though sometimes unnaturally wide, in between.

BEARDS

It was Henry VIII who had dictated the short hair and allowed freedom of choice of beards. But Henry was gone and the beards were going. And the hair at the turn of the century was just beginning to be a little longer. Although some of the older men still kept their long beards, the younger ones tended to trim theirs smaller. This did not, however, diminish their importance. Great care was taken of the beard, which was arranged with the help of a small beard brush and comb and kept in shape with perfumed wax. It was also dyed when necessary.

John Bulwer, in his *Anthropometamorphosis*, better known as *The Artificial Changeling*, first published in 1650, expressed his opinion on the dyeing of beards:

'Nor is the Art of falsifying the naturall hue of the beard wholly unknown to this more civilized part of the world; especially to old Leachers, who knowing grey haires in the Beard to be a manifest signe of a decay of the generative faculty, and an approaching impotency incident to Age, vainely endeavour to obliterate the naturall signification thereof. For there are some grown so foolish . . . who being now grown old, decrepid, and unable for any kind of use or exercise, and this their weaknesse being notorious, and well known to all the worlde, and this their rotten building ready to fall; yet are they willing to deceive themselves, and every body else, (if they could) contrary to all truth and reason, by dying the haires of their beardes and heads, as if any man were so ignorant, and did not know that there are none of these changeable coloured beards, but at every motion of the Sun, and every cast of the eye they present a different colour, and never a one perfect, much like unto those in the necks of Doves and Pigeons: for in every haire of these old Coxcombs you shall meet with three divers and sundry colours; white at the roots, yellow in the middle, and black at the point, like unto one of your Parrats feathers.'

In *Pylades and Corinna* (1731), which records the life of Mrs Elizabeth Thomas, there is a reference to her grandfather, Mr Richard Shute: 'He was very nice in the mode of that age, his valet being some hours every morning in starching his beard and curling his whiskers during which time a gentleman whom he maintained as a companion always read to him upon some useful subject.'

Davies, in *Scourge of Folly*, writes:

> Crispus doth spend his time in labour sore
> To bring his beard in fashion if he could:
> Quils, irons, and instruments he hath good store,
> To fashion it and make it fashion hold.

There were a number of fashionable styles, some of which were described in the famous *Ballad of the Beard*, mentioned in the preceding chapter:

> Now a beard is a thing that commands in a king,
>   Be his sceptre ne'er so fair;
> When the beard bears the sway, the people obey,
>   And are subject to a hair.
>
> .   .   .   .   .
>
> Now of beards there be such a company,
>   And fashions such a throng,
> That it is very hard to handle a beard
>   Tho' it be never so long.
>
> The Roman T in its bravery
>   Doth first itself disclose,
> But so high it turns that oft it burns
>   With the flames of a torrid nose.
>
> The stiletto beard, oh! it makes me afeard,
>   It is so sharp beneath,
> For he that doth place a dagger in's face,
>   What wears he in his sheath?
>
> But methinks I do itch to go thro' stitch,
>   The needle-beard to amend,
> Which without any wrong, I may call too long.
>   For a man can see no end.

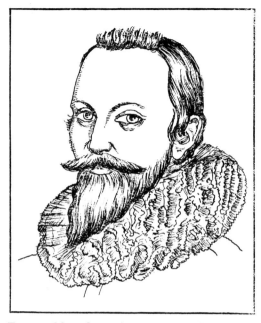

Fig. 51 : Marc Garrard (1561–1635). From an
engraving by Wenceslaus Hollar

> The soldier's beard doth march in, shear'd
>   In figure like a spade,
> With which he'll make his enemies quake,
>   And think their graves are made.
>
> But, oh! let us tarry, for the beard of King Harry
>   That grows about the chin,
> With his bushy pride, a grove on each side,
>   And a champion-ground between.

The *Roman T* or *hammer cut* is shown in Plate 59-U in a drawing based on Repton and is probably the most authentic example of the style. It seems to tally well with the description in the ballad.

In *The Queen of Corinth* (1618) Fletcher and Massinger speak of a 'beard, Which now he puts i' th' posture of a T, The Roman T; your T beard is in Fashion'. In the following year in Henry Hutton's *Follies' Anatomie* these lines appeared:

> With what grace, bold, actor like he speaks,
> Having his beard precisely cut i' the peake.
> How neat's mouchatoes do at a distance stand,
> Lest they disturbe his lips or saffron band:

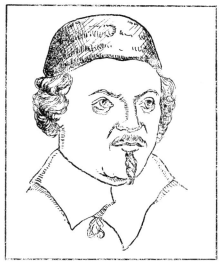 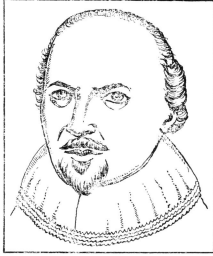

Fig. 52, 53 : John Taylor, the 'Water Poet' (died 1653), as shown in the Bodleian portrait and the Granger portrait

> How expert he's; with what attentive care
> Doth he in method place each straggling haire.

The description refers to the *pique devant*, which appears a number of times in the plates and which we have discussed in the preceding chapter. Plate 55-M and Q perhaps provide as good examples as any. Plate 55-R would probably also be called a *pique devant*, though the moustaches certainly do not 'at a distance stand'.

Randle Holme refers to the *pick-a-devant* (an anglicization which is frequently used) as ending 'in a point under the chin and on the higher lip, chin, and cheeks'. Whether or not the term was used for a pointed beard which was confined to the chin, with the cheeks shaved, is uncertain.

The *needle* beard mentioned in the ballad and illustrated in Plate 58-I was long, thin, and sharply pointed. The *stiletto* beard referred to any very sharply pointed beard, such as the one in Plate 55-N. The *spade* beard has been discussed at some length in the preceding chapter.

The inverted moustache (Plate 56-M) was still being worn; and in *Cynthia's Revels* (1601) Mercury says to the barber, 'Come invert my mustachio'. But fashions change; and in *Time's Metamorphosis* (1608) we find the line, 'Why dost thou weare this beard? . . . 'Tis cleane gone out of fashion'.

Fashion decreed that the beard should go, but the moustache outlived it by some years. The Latin countries put more emphasis on the moustache than the northern ones, and the very long (Plate 57-K) or oddly-shaped (Plate 57-G) moustaches are quite often found to be Spanish.

The difficulty in matching names and shapes of beards has already been mentioned. Perhaps we would do well to stick with John Taylor in his *Superbiae Flagellum* or *The Whip of Pride*, in which for the most part he contents himself with describing a large number of beards in rather general terms. Repton says that Taylor himself wore a *screw* beard, which is not mentioned in the poem; and the Bodleian portrait does show him with such a beard (Figure 52). However, the 1630 portrait in Granger, whom Repton used as a source for some of his beards, shows Taylor with an entirely different beard (Figure 53). This is the portrait which was used in the collection of his complete works.

But whatever beard Taylor wore himself, his recital of contemporary styles has proved invaluable:

> Now a few lines to paper I will put,
> Of men's Beards' strange and variable cut;
> In which there's some doe take as vaine a Pride,
> As almost in all other things beside.
> Some are reap'd most substantial, like a brush,
> Which makes a nat'rall wit knowne by the bush;
> (And in my time of some men I have heard,
> Whose wisedome have been only wealth and beard);
> Many of these the proverbe well doth fit,
> Which sayes—Bush naturall, more haire then wit.
> Some seeme as they were starched stiffe and fine,
> Like to the bristles of some angry swine;
> And some (to let their Loves desire on edge),
> Are cut and prun'd like to a quickset hedge.
> Some like a spade, some like a forke, some square,
> Some round, some mow'd like stubble, some starke bare,
> Some sharpe, stiletto fashion, dagger-like,
> That may with whispering a man's eyes outpike:
> Some with the hammer cut, or Romane T,
> Their beards extravagant reform'd must be,
> Some with the quadrate, some triangle fashion,
> Some circular, some ovall in translation,
> Some perpendicular in longitude,
> Some like a thicket for their crassitude,
> That heights, depths, bredths, triforme, square, ovall, round,
> And rules Geometricall in beards are found,
> Besides the upper lips strange variation,
> Corrected from mutation to mutation;

As 'twere from tithing unto tithing sent,
Pride gives to *pride* continual punishment,
Some (spite their teeth) like thatch'd eaves downward grows,
And some grow upwards in despite their nose;
Some their moustaches of such length do keep,
That very well they may a manger sweep,
Which in beer, ale, or wine they drinking plunge,
And suck the liquor up as 'twere a sponge.
But 'tis a sloven's beastly pride, I think,
To wash his beard where other men must drink.
And some (because they will not rob the cup)
Their upper chops like pot hooks are turned up.
The barbers thus (like tailors) still must be
Acquainted with each cut's varietie.

And yet not many years later, in 1657, a man named Foscari was denounced as a boor for wearing a beard and cutting his hair.

The trimming of the beard, whatever the style, was usually left to the professional barber-surgeon. In the time of Elizabeth I and James I the apprentice barbers were sometimes restive, no doubt with good reason, and became difficult to handle; and after having been punished by one of their superiors, they would sometimes waylay him in the street and beat him up. To forestall this, a coat, popularly known as a 'bulbeggar', was devised. This coat, according to Sidney Young, 'was a garment somewhat like a sack with apertures for the eyes and arms, which was put over the head and body of the person appointed to flog an unruly apprentice, who was thereby prevented from identifying his castigator'. There is on the records of the Worshipful Company of Barber-Surgeons for 1607 an entry reading: 'Item bought a pece of Blacke buckaram to make Coote for correction of Appr. . . . 16 shillings'.

Sometimes, it would seem, merely showing the bulbeggar was sufficient to achieve the desired effect:

'This daye the weife of Saloman Carr made complaint against her apprentice George Tether formerly bound to Jeffery Baskerville deceased and he had the bulbeggar showed him, whoe upon his humble submission to his M^{ris} was spared in hoape of his better service to her hereafter.'

But clearly bulbeggars were not always sufficient, for the records abound in notations about apprentices being brought into court on the complaints of their masters or mistresses. The following entry is for November 14, 1615:

'In the complaynt made by the Servant of William Corbett against his M^r wch beinge examyned at this Court It is aparyant that the boy hath very stubburnlie & naughtielie behaved himself unto his Mr Whereupon it is this daie ordered that the boy shall goe home agayne wth his M^r & behave himselfe more honestlie than formerlie he hath done wch the boy promiseth to doe.'

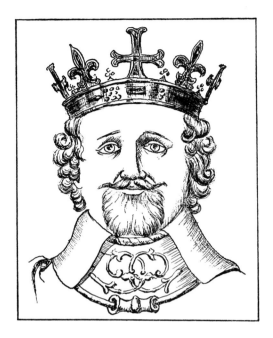

Fig. 54 : James I, King of England 1603–25

On February 18, 1616, the year of Shakespeare's death, the court dealt with an even naughtier apprentice:

'In the complaint made by M^ris Wooten against her app'ntice Thomas Hill for his neclect of service & for pleaing at dice & whoring It is therefore ordered that the boy be corrected.'

Occasionally the tables were turned, as in this entry for the same day:

'In the complaint made by David Richardson against his M^r ffletcher for lack of vittualls It is ordered that ffletcher shall take the boy home & kepe him as an app'ntice ought to be kept.'

A memorandum for August 9, 1647, suggests that by mid-century things hadn't changed very much:

'Mr. Heydon complayneing to this Court of his apprentice here present in Court ffor his evill and stubborne Behavior towards him and frequent absences out of his service in Day time and in late hours at night The said apprentice being in court to answer to the same did rudely and most irreverently behave himselfe toward his said M^r and the whole Court, in sawcy language and behaviour, useing several Oathes protesting that he will not serve his M^r whatever shall come of it This Court did therefore cause the Haire of the said apprentice (being undecently long) to be cut shorter.'

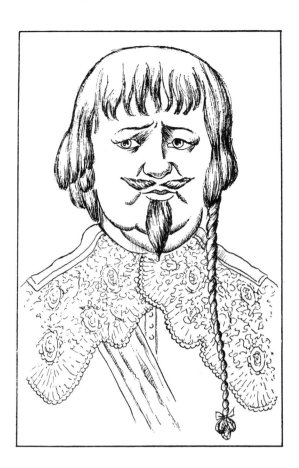

Fig. 55 : Christian IV (1577–1648),
King of Denmark

MEN: EARLY YEARS (Plates 55-59, 62)

The accession of James I in 1603 and of Louis XIII in 1610 undoubtedly added considerable impetus to the fashion of long hair. Louis, being very young, had long, beautiful curls and no beard, and James had a decided preference for long hair.

When one's own hair would not grow fast enough or thickly enough, false hair was sometimes added. The fashion of wearing wigs started in France fairly early in the century but did not gain great popularity until later. It was Louis XIII who was responsible. Since he was losing his hair, he started in 1624 to wear a wig; and when the king wore a wig, wigs were worn. It was not until much later that the whole process began to get out of hand. The fashion did not become general in England until the time of Charles II. Stewart points out (in *Plocacosmos*) that 'at first it was reckoned a scandal for young people to wear them, by reason the loss of their hair, at that age, was attributed to a disease, the very name of which is a reproach; but at length the mode prevailed over the scruple, and all ages and conditions wore them; foregoing without any necessity, the conveniences of their natural hair.'

In 1634 the General Court of Massachusetts passed a law which forbade long hair 'if uncomely or prejudicial to the common good', and the boys at Harvard were not 'permitted to wear Long Haire, Locks, Foretops, Curlings, Crispings, Partings, or Powdering of Ye Haire'.

Although beards were growing somewhat smaller, they were far from disappearing and, it appears, were a matter of some pride to the owners, as beards always have been. But Louis XIII was not a beard fancier and wore only a tiny one himself. If it had been anything else that he did not fancy, it would probably have disappeared promptly from his court. But getting a man to part with his beard, as we have seen, requires some fairly drastic action. The personal pleasure of the king was obviously not enough. So one day in 1628 when he could think of nothing better to do, Louis decided it would be amusing to shave his courtiers' beards. This he did, leaving only the moustache and a tiny pointed tuft on the chin. This, then, became the new style. The moustaches continued to be carefully curled and put up at night.

LOVELOCKS

One of the most curious and inexplicable fashions of the seventeenth century was the lovelock, a single lock of hair, much longer than the others, hanging down over one shoulder, usually the left. Sometimes it was curled (Plate 60-J), sometimes not (Plate 59-P); and occasionally it had a bow or a rosette at the end (Figure 55).

The style was introduced in France by one of its elegant leaders of fashion, Honoré d'Albert, maréchal de France, seigneur de Cadenet, who wore one on each side. Others later wore as many as six. The lock came to be called a *cadenette* in his honour, and still later it was called a *moustache* when worn by either men or women.

The fashion (and it was confined to the fashionable) was mentioned as early as 1592 by Greene in *Quip for an Upstart Courtier*, quoted in the preceding chapter. In 1613 Rich noted in *Opinion Deified* that 'Some by wearing a longe locke that hangs dangling by his ears do think that lousie commodity to be esteemed'. Burton in *Anatomie of Melancholie*, published in 1621, was equally disapproving: ''Tis the common humour of all suitors to trick up themselves to be prodigal in apparel . . . neat combed and curled, with powdered hair, with long love-lock, a flower in his ear, perfumed gloves, ring scarves, feathers, points.' And in 1628 we find Rowlands complaining in *Earth's Vanity Flye It* that 'Your gallant is no man unless his haire be of the woman's fashion, dangling and waving over his shoulders.'

More curious than the fashion itself and its durability is the offence it evidently gave to a great number of people and the vehemence with which they denounced it.

In 1628, the year Louis XIII took to barbering, there was published in London an extraordinary book by William Prynne entitled *The Vnlouelinesse, of Loue-lockes, or A summarie Discovrse, proouing: The wearing, and nourishing of a Locke, or Loue-locke, to be altogether vnseemely, and vnlawfull vnto Christians.* (It is hoped that scholars will not seriously object to the exchanging of the u's and v's henceforth.)

The sixty-three pages of the book, containing more invective than logic, is addressed 'to the Christian Reader' and begins straightforwardly:

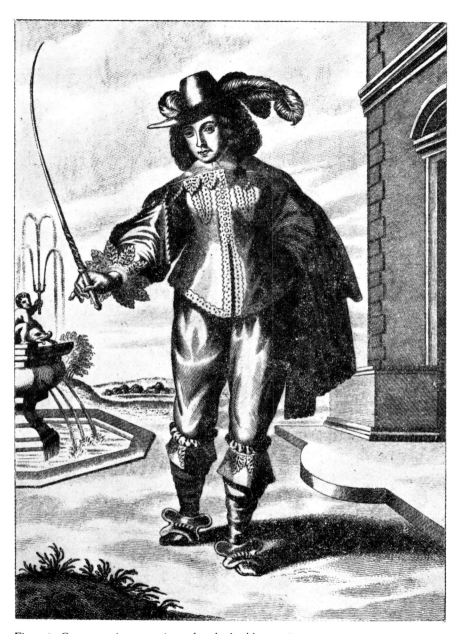

Fig. 56 : German prince wearing a lovelock. About 1650

'I here present unto thy view and censure a rough and brief discourse, whose subject, though it bee but course and vile, consisting of Effeminate, Proud, Lascivious, Exorbitant, and Fantastique *Haires*, or *Lockes*, or *Love-lockes* (as they stile them), which every Barbar may correct and regulate; yet the consequence of it may be great and profitable in these Degenerous, Unnaturall, and Unmanly times; wherein as sundry of our Mannish, Impudent, and Inconstant female sexe, are Hermophradited, and transformed into men; not onely in their immodest, shamelesse, and audacious carriage (which is now the very manners and courtship of the times), but even in the unnaturall Tonsure, and odious, if not whorish Cutting and Crisping of their Haire, their Naturall vaile, their Feminine glory, and the very badge and character of their subjection both to God and Man; so divers of our masculine and more noble race are wholy degenerated and metamorphosed into women; not in Manners, Gestures, Recreations, Diet, and Apparell only; but likewise in the Womanish, Sinfull, and Unmanly, Crisping, Curling, Frouncing, Powdring, and nourishing of their Lockes and Hairie excrements, in which they place their corporall Excellencies and chiefest Glory. . . . Alas, may I not truely say of too to many, who would be deemed not onely English-men, but Devout and faithfull Christians: that the Barber is their Chaplaine; his Shop, their Chappell, their God? that they bestow more cost, more thoughts, more time and paines upon their Hairie Lockes and Bushes from day to day then on their peerelesse and immortall Soules? that they consult more seriously and frequently with the Glasse and Combe then with the Scriptures? that they conferre more often with their *Barbers* about their Hairie Excrements then with their *Ministers* about the meanes and matter of their owne Salvation? Are not most of our young Nobilitie and Gentrie, yea, the Elder too, under the Barbers hands from day to day? Are they not in dayly thraldome and perpetuall bondage to their curling Irons, which are as so many chaines and fetters to their Heads, on which they leave their Stampe and Impresse? Good God, may I not truely say of our Gentrie and Nation, as Seneca once did of his: that they are now so vaine and idle that they hold a Counsell about every Haire, sometimes Combing it backe, another time frouncing and spreading it abroad; a third time Combing it all before, in which, if the Barber be any thing remisse, they will grow exceedingly angry, as if they were trimming of the men themselves; doe they not rage excessively if any Haire bee but cut to short, if it lye not to their liking and fall not readily into its rings and circles? Would they not rather have the Common-wealth disturbed than their Haire disordered? doe they not sit all day betweene the Combe and the Glasse? are they not more sollicitous of the neatnesse of their Haire, then of their safetie? and more desirous to be neate and spruce then Honest? Is it not now held the accomplished Gallantrie of our youth to Frizle their Haire like women and to become Womanish, not only in exilitie of Voyce, tendernesse of Body, levitie of Apparell, wantonnesse of Pace and Gesture, but even in the very length and Culture of their Lockes and Haire? Are not many now of late degenerated into *Virginians, Frenchmen, Ruffians,* nay, *Women,* in their Crisped-Lockes and Haire? have they not violated the Grave and Ancient Cut and

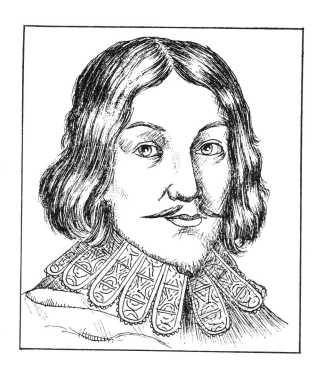

Fig. 57 : Bernhard (1604–39), Duke of Sachs-Weimar

decent Tonsure of their Ancestors; and broken the very ordinance and Law of God and Nature by their Womanish, Embroidered, Coloured, False, Excessive Haire and Love-Lockes? . . . Did ever any Saints of God, that wee can heare or read of, weare a Locke? or Frizle, Powder, Frounce, Adorne, or Decke their Haire?'

This gives a good indication of the tone of the book, which expands on the theme with remarkably little variation. In summary, one may say that Mr Prynne considered lovelocks and the wearing of them to be Unlovely, Sinfull, Unlawfull, Effeminate, Vainglorious, Evil, Odious, Immodest, Indecent, Lascivious, Wanton, Fantastique, Disolute, Singular, Incendiary, Ruffianly, Graceless, Whorish, Ungodly, Horred, Strange, Outlandish, Impudent, Pernicious, Offensive, Ridiculous, Foolish, Childish, Unchristian, Hatefull, Exorbitant, Contemptible, Sloathfull, Unmanly, Depraving, Vaine, and Unseemly. Prynne was twenty-eight when the book was published. It had no effect on the wearing of lovelocks.

THE LOATHSOMNESSE OF LONG HAIRE

During the middle years of the century the fashion, except in the French court, where wigs were worn, was for long, curled, natural hair at least to the shoulders. Whereas the beard, or what remained of it, was usually carefully waxed, the hair was worn in studied disarray, the curls irregular and the top often short and combed forward or perhaps parted and brushed casually to one side, seldom brushed back from the forehead, as it had been earlier. And the controversial lovelocks continued in fashion.

But this style was by no means universally accepted. In England the Cavaliers wore their hair very long, wearing wigs when necessary, whereas the Puritans defiantly cropped their hair short and thus came to be known as Roundheads. Once again hair was mixed up with politics.

But it wasn't entirely a political matter. The long, curled, perfumed, and sometimes powdered hair was just as distasteful to a great many people as the lovelocks and was considered foppish by those who did not follow the fashion. In 1640 a verse called *On Monsieur Powder-wig* appeared:

> Oh, doe but marke yon crisped sir, you meete!
> How like a pageant he doth walk the street!
> See how his perfumed head is powder'd o'er!
> 'Twould stink else, for it wanted salt before!

In the following year we find the opposition expressing itself in a song called *The Character of a Roundhead*, which began:

> What creature's this, with his short hairs,
> His little head and huge long ears,
> That this new faith hath founded?
> The Puritans were never such,
> The Saints themselves had ne'er so much—
> Oh! such a knave's a Roundhead!

Those who were inclined to blame the devil for anything of which they disapproved, wasted no time in pointing out long hair as a flagrant example of his handiwork. The following poem appeared in 1655:

> At the devill's shopps you buy
> A dresse of powdered hayre,
> On which your feathers flaunt and fly;
> But I'de wish you have a care,
> Lest Lucifer's selfe, who is not prouder,
> Do one day dresse your haire with a powder.

One of the blame-the-devil group, Thomas Hall, B.D., Pastor of Kingsnorton, who was terribly cross about the whole thing, broke into print in 1653 with a volume twice the length of Prynne's entitled *Comarum, The Loathsomnesse of Long Haire: or, A Treatise Wherein you have the Question stated, many Arguments against it produc'd, and the most materiall Arguments for it refell'd and answer'd, with the concurrent judgement of Divines both old and new against it. With an appendix against Painting, Spots, Naked Breasts, &c.* The book, we are informed, was 'printed by J. G. for Nathaniel Webb and William Grantham at the signe of the Bear in S. Pauls church-yard near the little North door'.

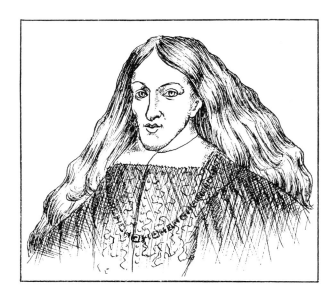

Fig. 58 : Charles II (1661–1700),
King of Spain

Although Hall's language may be slightly more restrained than Prynne's, his opinions are equally strong; and all those who disagree with him are automatically labelled as ruffians. He begins his treatise with relative calm:

'Amongst other vices, I observe that Pride is very predominant in this licentious age; Pride in Heart, Pride in Habit, Pride in Long haire; Pride in the Clergy, Pride in Professors, &c. Had it raigned only in the under foot I had been silent; but when I saw Gods owne people by profession, yea, and many Ministers (who should be patterns of Gravity and Modesty to their Inferiours) to be tainted, appearing like Ruffians in the Pulpit, I could no longer forbeare; especially considering how few have appeared against this sin, either in the Pulpit or the Presse. Master Pryn is the onely man that I know who hath appeared (in our language) in a set Treatise against it; and yet his bent is principally against Love-locks: I shall give one clip nearer, & will see what may be said against the long-locks especially of Ministers and Professors, who have of late exuded in this kind: they draw neerer unto God, and so their sins are more displeasing unto him, and should be more grievous unto us.'

Hall's thesis is *That it is unlawfull for any man ordinarily to weare Long Haire*, and he proposes to enlarge upon his thesis by first explaining the terms, then setting forth 'Arguments drawn from the Word of God, &c.' and then finally to 'answer all the cavills (of any weight) which are made against it'.

This naturally leads us to the question, *when may wee say that a man's Haire is too long?* The Reverend Hall is ready with the answer:

'1. The Haire of a Mans Head is too long when tis an impediment to him and hinders him in the workes of his calling; therefore such men as are faine to get

Strings or fillets to tie up their Haire that it fall not in their eyes when they worke, offend in excessive Long-Haire. Even the Stoicks should say that tis time to cut our Haire when it is a burden to us or hinders us in our Callings.

'2. 'Tis excessive when it is so long that it covers the eyes, the cheeks, the countenance, &c. God hath ordeined those parts to be visible, for the face is a special glass wherein the glory & Image of God (in respect of the body) doth shine forth and appeare, and therefore may not be hidden with long haire, since the haire of the head is ordeined by God for the covering of the head, and not the face.

'3. When it is so long that it lyes on the back and shoulders; the haire of mans head is given to man for a cover to his head and not to his back and body, which apparell must cover.

'4. When it is scandoulous and offensive, when it is so long that the godly are thereby grieved, the weak offended, and the wicked hardened.

'5. When it is contrary to the civil and laudable custome of those civiliz'd Nations which we live in; for when the customes of a Nation are good and agreeable to the role of God's word, we are bound to observe them. Now the known commendable custome of our horde (all the reigne of Queen Elizabeth, King James, and the beginning of the late King's reigne) was short haire: 'Tis true indeed, *de facto*, that of late in these licentious times (where so many amongst us change both their Practice and their Principles) some have brought up the fashion of long haire; but *quo jure*, what Law of God or Man command them so to do I know not; and that you may see I am not singular, you shall have the judgement of Mr. Perkins, a man famous in his generation for his piety and experience in the ways of God. *The Wearing of long haire in the younger sort* (saith he) *is an abuse of it; it began (indeed) amongst the aged, but now it is become a trick of youth and is the badge of a proud heart. . . . If it be said, to weare long haire is our English fashion: I answere, it is not our ancient English fashion, but indeed it is a forraigne trick and therefore as unlawfull as forraign attire, which God condemnes. Our ancient English fashion (except it were amonst the aged) was to weare short haire; and in every country the most ancient and grave fashion ought to be followed, &c.* Thus he.

'Lastly, as no man weare his owne hair excessively long, so he may not weare the long haire of another, be it of a man, a woman, or it may be of some harlot, who is now in Hell, lamenting there the abuse of that excrement. These Periwigs of false-coloured haire (which begin to be rife, even amongst Schollars in the Universities) are utterly unlawfull, and are condemned by Christ himselfe, Mat. 5. 36. *No man can make one haire white or black*: but wee have those in our dayes that can do both; by powdering their haire, they can make that white which was black, (the powder forgets the dust); others by Periwigs and false haire, can make themselves black or white. Even what please themselves; what is this but to correct God's handywork, and in the pride of their heart to think they can make themselves better than God hath made them, and can correct his creation?'

Further on, in his detailed arguments, one finds this instructive passage:

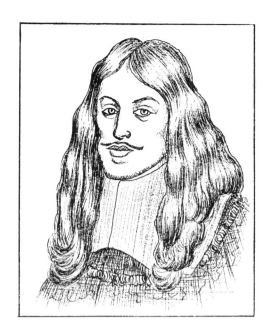

Fig. 59 : Emperor Leopold I (1640–1705)

'It is clear that long haire is one of the sinfull customes and fashion of the wicked men of the world. This will appeare if we look abroad into the remote parts of the world, we shall there see that long haire was, and still is, the guise and fashion of the most barbarous, idolatrous, heathenish Nations that know not God but worshippe the Devill, as the Virginians in America, to whom the Devill appeares in the shape of a Virginian, with a long black lock on the left side hanging downe neere to the feete, whom the Virginians imitate in this Divellish Guise.'

He quotes an unidentified divine ('famous for his Piety and Paines in the Ministry') as saying that it is 'the duty of Christians not onely to sacrifice their eyes and eares, but also their heads to God, in a sober and modest wearing of their haire, which the Apostle (by the testimony of Nature itselfe) commendeth to us, viz. that men weare short haire, because 'tis a shame for them to have long haire'. This concludes his sixth argument.

There are echoes of Prynne when he states categorically that 'where one wicked man weare short haire, there is a thousand weare long'. His description of the various methods of wearing the hair is of some interest:

'How strangely do men cut their haire—some all before, some all behind, some long round about, their crowns being cut short like cootes or popish priests and friars; some have long lockes in their eares, as if they had four eares, or were prick-eared; some have a little long locke onely before, hanging down to their noses, like the taile of a weasell; every man being made a foole at the barbers pleasure, or making a foole of the barber for having to make him such a foole.'

As for beards, Hall informs us that 'long haire is . . . a shame and a dishonour to a man, but so is not a long Beard. The Scripture no where condemns a long Beard, but it oft condemns long haire. A decent growth of the Beard is a signe of Manhood and given by God to distinguish the Male from the Female sex. . . . God would have his people to preserve their Beards and enjoynes them not to shave the corners of their Beards, as the Heathen did. Levit. 19. 27. they must not deforme and disfigure their faces by shaving off the haire of their beards. The Council of Carthage at which S. Austin himselfe was present, made his Canon, *Comam nec nutriant sacerdotes, nec barbam radant.* Let not Ministers weare longe haire, nor shave their beards.'

The translation, however, is somewhat in question, as is the existence of the Council. According to the Catholic Encyclopedia, the canon reads, '*Clericus nec comam nutriat nec barbam*'—a priest shall not nourish his hair nor his beard. But the precise wording of the Latin became a sort of *cause célèbre* in the Church, the opposing side claiming that it should read, '*Clericus nec comam nutriat nec barbam radat*'. In other words, 'a priest shall not nourish his hair nor shave his beard'. One suspects that the wording of the canon accepted depended largely on whether or not one wished to wear a beard. The Reverend Hall clearly did.

The good Reverend includes in his book several verses which he feels support his point of view:

> Good Ramus pardon me, for I
> Have always lov'd Trichotomy,
> But now I doe affect it more
> By far, than ever I did before.
> How many doe I daily see
> Given up to Muliebritie!
> A female head to a male face
> Is marryed now in every place,
> And some doe make, so vain they are,
> A Galaxias in their haire.
> Now sure Trichotomy it is
> Can banish these sad vanities.

Another is entitled 'To the Long-Hair'd Gallante of these Times':

> Go Gallants to the Barbers, go.
> Bid them your hairy Bushes mow.
> God in a Bush did once appeare,
> But there is nothing of him here.
> Here's that he deeply hates: beside,
> That execcrable sin of Pride;
> Here also is that Felony. . . .

Later in the same poem (it's rather a long one) there is a reference to 'Plica', which is described in a footnote by Reverend Hall, with what seems to be a certain gleeful relish, as 'a most loathsome and horrible disease in the haire, unheard of in former times; bred by moderne luxury & excess. It seizeth specially upon women; and by reason of a viscous venomous humour glues together (as it were) the haire of the head with a prodigious ugly implication and intanglement; sometimes taking the forme of a great snake, sometimes of many little serpents, full of nastiness, vermin, and nay some smell; and that which is most to be admired, and never eye saw before, pricked with a needle they yeild bloody drops. And at the first spreading of this dreadful disease in Poland, all that cut off this horrible and snaky haire, lost their eyes, or the humor falling downe upon other parts of the body turned them extremely.'

It is said that his book was a great success and enjoyed considerable popularity for a number of years. It was followed by the longest hair in history, most of it false.

The Coming of Wigs

As we have pointed out, wigs were introduced in France early in the century. When Louis XIV ascended the throne in 1643, he had unusually long, thick, luxuriant hair, of which he was very proud (see Plate 62-H for Louis at sixteen). But this had no lasting effect on the wearing of wigs since the courtiers' heads were shaved and the wigs were necessary in order to maintain the style set by the king. But eventually the king's hair thinned, whereas the courtiers' wigs grew in size and elegance. In order not to be outshone, the king at last (when he was thirty-five) reluctantly began to add false hair to his own. Eventually he agreed to have his head shaved, which was done daily thereafter, and to wear a wig. He is said to have employed forty wig-makers.

By 1665 wig-making was so well established that the wig-makers in France banded together in a guild. Although wigs were worn in England, the fashion did not really become established until the Restoration. Charles II began to wear a wig when his naturally black hair started to grey. And since the king had black hair, black hair was popular. Later brown and blond hair were fashionable. Horsehair and goat hair were used for wigs as well as human hair.

As a sign of the times it is interesting to note that by 1660 wigs were beginning to appear tentatively on a few of the more courageous and independent abbots in Britain. But when the Abbé de la Rivière (later Bishop of Langres) tried the same thing in France (he was not entirely without followers) the clergy was outraged. Dr John Doran writes:

'Nor was this feeling confined to the Romish church in France. The Reformed Church was fully as hostile against the new and detested fashion. Bordeaux was in a state of insurrection, for no other reason than that the Calvinist pastor there had refused to admit any of his flock in wigs to the sacrament. And when Reviers, Protestant Professor of Theology at Leyden, wrote his *Libertas, Christiana circa ilsum capillitii Defensa* in behalf of perukes, the ultraorthodox in both churches turned to gore him. The Romanists asked, what could be expected from a Protestant but rank heresy? and the Protestants disowned a brother who defended a fashion which had originated with a Romanist.'

Although certain of the clergy began to wear wigs, the controversy did not abate, especially in France. And Dr Doran goes on to say that 'No primitively-minded prelate would license a curé who professed neutrality on the matter of wigs. The wearers of these were often turned out of their benefices; but then they were welcomed in other dioceses, by bishops who were heterodoxly given to the mundane comfort of wiggery. Terrible scenes took place in vestries between wigged priests ready to repair to the altar, and their brethren or superiors who sought to prevent them. Chapters suspended such priests from place and profit; Parliaments broke the decree of suspension, and Chapters renewed the interdict. Decree was abolished by counter-decree, and the whole church was rent in twain by the contending parties.'

James Stewart, writing on the history of the peruke, reports that 'the cardinal Grimaldi, in 1684, and the bishop of Louvar, in 1688, prohibited the use of the peruke to the clergy, without a dispensation and necessity. M. Thurs has a treatise expressly to prove the peruke indecent in an ecclesiastic and directly contrary to the decrees and canons of councils; a priests head, embellished with artificial hair, curiously adjusted, he esteems a monster in the church; nor can he conceive anything so scandalous as an abbot with a horrid countenance, heightened with a jolly peruke.'

In England Charles II forbade the clergy to wear wigs. Tillotson, believed to be the first English clergyman to wear a wig, recalled in one of his sermons the time, not far gone, when 'the wearing of the hair below the ears was looked upon as a sin of the first magnitude; and when ministers generally, whatever their text was, did either find or make occasion to reprove the great sin of long hair; and if they saw anyone in the congregation guilty in that kind, they would point him out particularly and let fly at him with great zeal'.

But despite intramural squabbling in the church and the censure of most of the clergy, the wearing of wigs by men was the fashion and was to remain the fashion for another 130 years.

On March 8, 1663, Samuel Pepys wrote in his diary: 'At Mr Jervas's, my old barber. I did try two or three borders and periwigs, meaning to wear one; and yet I have no stomach for it; but that the pains of keeping my hair clean is so great. He trimmed me, and at last I parted; but my mind was almost altered from my first purpose, from the trouble which I foresee will be in wearing them also.'

In October he took his wife to the periwig-maker's, and she approved the wig he had had made. But he was less approving of her experiments with her hair; and on May 13, 1664, he wrote: 'This day my wife began to wear light-colored locks, quite white almost, which, though it made her look very pretty, yet, not being natural, vexes me, that I will not have her wear them'.

One might suppose that naturalness being the criterion, he had given up the idea of wearing a periwig, but no such thing. On November 3, 1663, he had written in his diary: 'Home, and by-and-bye comes Chapman, the periwigg-maker, and upon

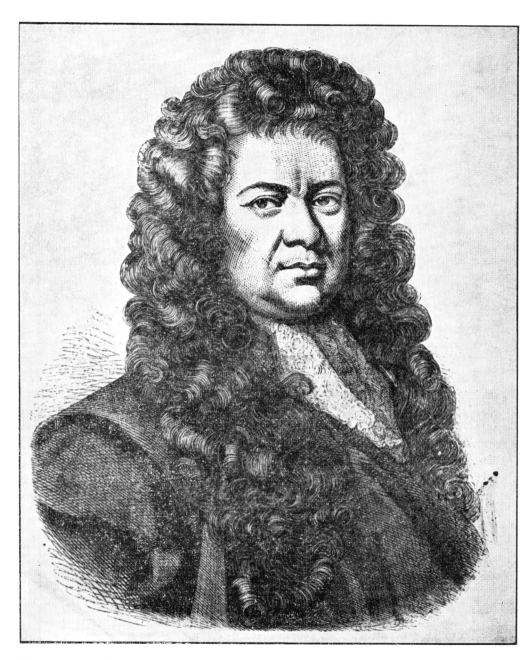

Fig. 60 : Samuel Pepys (1633–1703) wearing his periwig

my liking it (the wig), without more ado I went up, and then he cut off my haire, which went a little to my heart at present to part with it; but it being over, and my periwigg on, I paid him £3; and away went he with my own haire to make up another of; and I, by-and-bye, went abroad, after I had caused all my maids to look upon it, and they concluded it do become me, though Jane was mightily troubled for my parting with my own haire, and so was Besse.'

On November 8th he went to church 'where I found that my coming in a peri-wigg did not prove so strange as I was afraid it would, for I thought that all the church would presently have cast their eyes upon me, but I find no such things'.

In 1665, while his wig was being repaired, he wrote that 'this day, after I had suffered my own hayre to grow long, in order to wearing it, I find the convenience of periwigs is so great that I have cut off all short again and will keep to periwigs'.

In September of the same year he notes: 'Up, and put on my coloured silk suit, very fine, and my new periwig, bought a good while since, but durst not wear, because the plague was in Westminster when I bought it; and it is a wonder what will be the fashion, after the plague is done, as to periwigs, for nobody will dare to buy any hayre for fear of the infection, that it had been cut off the heads of people dead of the plague'.

In 1667 he spent £4 10s for a fine periwig—'mighty fine; indeed too fine, I thought, for me'. But two days later he recorded that he had been to church 'and, with my mourning, very handsome; and new periwig made a great show'.

But the plague notwithstanding, periwigs remained the fashion; and by 1669 Pepys was taking them more for granted:

'Having made myself a velvet cloak, two new cloth skirts, black, plain both, a new shag gown trimmed with gold buttons and twist, with a new hat, and silk tops for my legs, and many other things; being resolved hence forward to go like myself. And also two periwigs, one whereof cost me £3 and the other 40s. I have worn neither yet but will begin next week, God willing. . . . Up and put on a new summer black bombazin suit; and being come now to an agreement with my barber to keep my perriwig in good order at 20s a year, I am like to go very spruce, more than I used to do.'

Evidently others than Samuel Pepys found the periwig more convenient and more desirable than the natural hair. In 1673 in *The Dutch Lover* we find the line: 'Do you remember, Sir, how you were wont to go at home, when instead of a Periwig, you wore a slink, greasy Hair of your own?' Convenient or not, it was fashionable. In *The Man of Mode* (1676) Medley, speaking of Sir Fopling Flutter, says: 'He was yesterday at the Play, with a pair of Gloves up to his Elbows, and a Periwig more exactly Curl'd than a Ladies head newly dress'd for a Ball'.

The fashions in wigs changed slightly from year to year. In 1678 *Le Mercure Galant* described two wigs, half frizzed and half curled, not so long as the preceding year, and also cavalier wigs with a large curl falling from the knot. Some of the most famous perruquiers had their own individual style which was easily identifiable.

Various terms were used to refer to wigs. James Stewart, writing a century later, explained that 'The term peruke, or perriwig, was anciently used for a long head of natural hair; such, particularly, as there was care taken in the adjusting and trimming of. Menage derives the word, by a long detour, from the Latin *pilus*, hair; the several stages of its passages, according to the critic, are *pilus, pelus, pelutus, pelutuus, pelutiac, perutica, perruca, perruque.* . . . Peruke is now used for a set of false or borrowed hair, curled, buckled, and sowed together on a frame, or caul; anciently called cappilamentum, or a false peruke.'

Randle Holme describes the various types of wigs in use, first explaining that 'a Peruque or Perawicke . . . is a counterfeit Hair which Men wear instead of their own, a thing much used in our days by the generality of Men, contrary to our forefathers, who got Estates, loved their Wives, and wore their own Hair; but in these days there is no such things'. Having made his own position in the matter clear, he lists the 'Sorts of Perawicks' (references in square brackets are the author's):

'A BORDER OF HAIR is only Locks to cover the ears and Neck, and is fixed to a Cap, having no head of hair. [You will recall that Pepys tried on "two or three borders and periwigs".]

A SHORT BOBB, a HEAD OF HAIR, is a Wig that hath short Locks and a hairy Crown.

A LONG PERAWICK with SIDE HAIR and a POLE LOCK behind, which some term a Wig with a Suffloplin or with a Dildo. [See Plate 58-U.]

A CAMPAIGN WIG hath Knots or Bobs (or a Dildo on each side) with a Curled Forehead. A TRAVELLING WIG. [See Plate 58-O.]

A GRAFTED WIG is a Perawick with a turn on the top of the head, in imitation of a Mans hairy Crown,'

Holme then lists the various terms used in curling hair:

'A CURLED HAIR is when a Lock of hair turns round and round in it self.

A CRISPED HAIR is when it lyeth in a kind of Wave.

A FRISE or FRISSED HAIR is when the hair is full of small Crispings and when one hair will not sort or fall into order with another, but stand bunching out; yet some are more flying, others more close. [Plate 58-A.]

A CURLE and FRISE is when the hair is neither Curle nor Frise, but both, or between both.

A SNAKE CURLE is when the Locks turn round many times and hang down, as the Dildo or Pole lock doth. [Plate 61-L.]

A DRAKE or DRAKE TAIL CURL, when the ends of the hair only turn up, and all the rest hangs smooth. [Plate 60-G.]

An OPEN CURLE is when it turns round and wide in all the ends.

An HIGH CURLE is between both, and so keeps Curle.'

This is followed by a list of the 'Parts of a Perawick':

'The BOTTOM LOCKS are the side locks that hang down on the shoulders and back. [Plate 61-G.]

The SIDE LOCKS are those as cover and keep warm the ears and neck, being a degree shorter than the former. [Plate 61-F and others.]

The CROWN is that hair as compasseth about, to make the turn of the crown of the head. [Plate 61-F.]

The FORETOP is that as makes the forepart of the head.

The FULL FRONT is the frisled and curled hair of the topping or forehead, the Brow hair.' [Plate 61-F.]

The various terms used by the periwig makers are, perhaps, too technical to be of interest here; but we may note in passing that in weaving, a few hairs drawn out of the hank were known as a *hatch*, a *catch*, a *draft* or a *thought* of hair.

The periwigs spelled the end of the beard. There were some who hung on to a pencil-line moustache long after taking up the periwig (Plate 61-L); but in general, as the size of the wig increased, what remained of the facial hair shrank until it vanished completely. When Louis XIV shaved off his moustache in 1680, that was the final blow; and civilians, for the most part, remained shaven until the nineteenth century.

In Russia, where the French fashions were not so eagerly followed, beards hung on longer, especially among the common people; but in 1698 Peter the Great decided they had hung on long enough. In order to get rid of them, he imposed a beard tax—a hundred roubles (about sixteen pounds or forty-five dollars) for noblemen, gentlemen, merchants of St Petersburg, etc., sixty roubles for tradesmen and servants of noblemen, thirty roubles for residents of Moscow, and for peasants, two duqui (about threepence or three cents). Tax collectors were stationed at the gates of each town to collect the tax; and when it was paid, the bearded recipient received a copper disc which showed that he had paid the tax, and this became his beard licence for one year.

The wearing of wigs, of course, caused even more attention to be focused on the hair than had been the case before. According to John Bulwer, who might have been referring either to natural hair or to wigs:

'Our Gallants' wittie noddles are put into such a pure witty trim, the dislocations of every Haire so exactly set, the whole bush so curiously candied, and (what is most prodigious) the natural jet of some of them so exalted into a perfect azure, that their familiar Friends have much adoe to own their faces: for by their powdered heads you would make them to be Mealmen.'

With the long hair, both natural and artificial, combs took on considerable importance, and it was considered not only proper but fashionable to comb the hair in public with large combs. It was a nicety to be cultivated, like taking snuff. In 1663 in the stage directions of Killigrew's *Parson's Wedding*, a group of fashionable gentlemen are instructed to 'comb their heads and talk'.

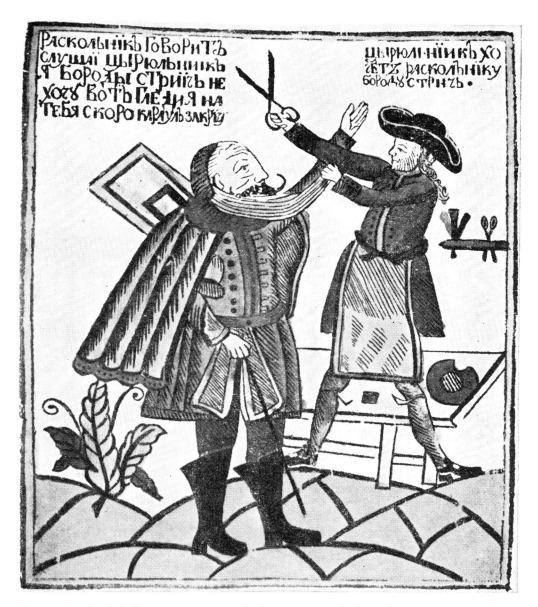

Fig. 61 : Russian folk illustration depicting the forcible removal of beards by the order of Peter the Great. From *Russian Folk Illustrations*, St Petersburg, 1881

Thirteen years later, in *The Wrangling Lovers*, these lines appeared:

> How we rejoic'd to see 'em in our pit!
> What difference we thought there was
> Betwixt a Country Gallant and a wit,
> When you did order Perriwig with comb,
> They only us'd four fingers and a thumb.

Chambers Journal in 1860 pointed out that 'combing the wig in Charles II's time was just what twirling the moustaches is now; it served when conversation slackened from a lack of ideas—it was a mask for insolence, and was used by intrigue for a signal. When fashionable idlers met to promenade at Fox Hall or at the Spring Gardens, to part cheesecakes, and drink toasts in Rhenish—there the idlers met and combed their black or white wigs with combs which they kept in cases in their pocket with their snuff-boxes. Gentlemen stayed at the door of a drawing-room to comb their wigs, just as they do now to adjust their ties; even the lover sighed and combed, and combed and sighed alternately. The pit of a theatre was a great place for combing, and Dreyden shews us the wits rising in a mass when an unknown beauty in a mask appeared, and beginning to gracefully comb their wigs that so well set off their nut-brown faces. You could tell a country novice, we read, by his rustic habit of combing his wig with his fingers.'

Beard combs are mentioned in Heywood's *The English Traveller* in 1533. Randle Holme, mine of technical information, goes into some detail about the combs currently in use. He first lists the 'Sorts of Combs' (references in square brackets are the author's):

'The HORSE or Mane comb, a strong wood comb with a thick back.
The WISKE COMB, have teeth on one side, and are wide and slender.
The BACK TOOTH COMB, having teeth but on one side.
The BEARD COMB, a small sort of comb, almost 4 square.
The DOUBLE COMB, two combs one clasped into the other.
The MERKIN COMB.
The PERUWICK COMB, haveing teeth on both sides, one side wider than the other.'

Then he explains 'Of what combs are generally made':

'WOOD COMBS, made of light and close wood as black thorn.
BOX COMBS, made of Box tree.
HORN COMBS, made of oxe and cows horns.
IVORY COMBS, made of elephants teeth.
BONE COMBS, made of the shank bones of Horses and other large beests.
TORTOIS COMBS, made of the sea and land Tortois shell; the counterfeit combs of this sort are Horn stained with Tortois shell colours.
COCUS COMBS, made of cocus wood.

LEAD COMBS, used by such as have red hair, to make it of another color.' [Red hair at the time was not in fashion.]

Periwigs were of various types. The earlier ones in England can be seen in portraits of Charles II (Plates 58-L, 61-L). The curls were usually irregular and tumbling about the shoulders. Many of the new wigs were smaller, less pretentious, and more like natural hair. The earlier French wigs were not so full (Plate 61-F-G) and might have the top hair combed forward or parted. Plate 61-H shows a German wig of this general type with a moustache far larger than was worn in either France or England.

Then came the periwigs, still very large but with more regular curls (Plate 61-M), and finally the enormous wigs familiar on portraits of Louis XIV (Plate 61-N), parted in the centre, with the hair rising very high on either side of the parting and falling far below the shoulders. Variations can be seen on Plate 61. Plate 67 in Chapter 9 shows additional wigs worn at the turn of the century.

Those who could afford it often had more than one wig—a large one for dress and a smaller one for at home or sport or informal occasions. Louis XIV had a number of wigs—a relatively short one for rising, another for mass, another for after dinner, another for supper, still another for the hunt, etc. And these were all donned ceremoniously. It is said, however, that during his lifetime nobody but his barber ever saw the king without a wig.

The tying of the ends of the periwig, which became popular in the eighteenth century, had its origin late in the seventeenth and can be seen in the portrait of Bibbiena (Plate 61-I).

The hair was still scented and sometimes dyed; and powder made of orris, nutmeg, etc., was worn on both natural hair and wigs. In 1698 a French author in *Memoires et Observations en Angleterre* remarked, when describing the English, that 'their perruques and their habits were charged with powder like millers, and their faces daubed with snuff'.

Late in the century the wife of Racine wrote in a letter to her son, on his becoming Secretary to the Embassy in Holland, where wigs were in fashion: 'Your father deeply regrets the necessity which you say you are under of wearing a wig. He leaves the decision to the Ambassador. When your father is in better health he will order M. Marguery to make you such a one as you require. Madame la Comtesse de Gramont is very sorry for you that you should lose the attraction which your hair gave.'

The wearing of wigs, though widespread, was not so universal as it was to become in the eighteenth century. The large wigs, which were extremely expensive and considered a major investment, were often willed with other valuables to one's heirs. As *Chambers Journal* points out, 'Wigs came as a broad mark to distinguish rich and poor; and though beginning only at the price of £2 or £3, they soon rose to £50, and were indeed a formidable class barrier'.

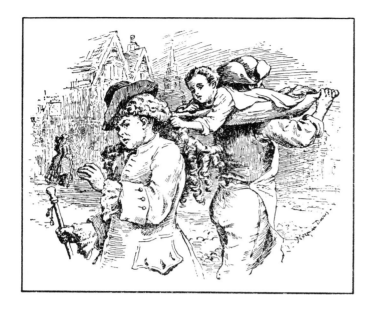

Fig. 62 : Stealing a wig in seventeenth-century England. From Andrews's *At the Sign of the Barber's Pole*

In *The Weekly Comedy*, 1690, we find Snarl asking Brim: 'How many bad women do you think have laid their heads together to complete that mane of yours? . . . It makes you look, in my mind, like an Essex calf peeping out of thicket of brambles, for I can scarce see any part of your face but your mouth for periwig.' And Brim answers: 'As slight as you make of my wig, sir, I would have you know, sir, it cost me fifty guineas; and if I was to tell you how it was made, I am sure you would think it was worth the money.'

A contemporary satirist, taking a jaundiced look at a fashionably bewigged gentleman, referred to his face as 'a small pimple in the midst of a vast sea of hair'.

Speight suggests that 'When we hear of a wig costing as much as thirty to forty guineas, we must not be surprised to hear of many an ingenious theft. A small dog in a butcher's tray poised on the shoulders of a tall man could frequently get through a large amount of business in this way. The wig was adroitly twitched off, and whilst the astonished and dismantled owner looked round for it in vain, the tray-bearer made off, an accomplice impeding the wigless victim under the pretence of assisting him.' Small boys were used for the same purpose and in the same way, as illustrated in Figure 62.

Many who wished to be fashionable but could not afford a periwig wore their own hair to look as much as possible like a wig. Tradesmen often wore their natural hair cut much shorter than the fashion, and of course labourers wore their own. In 1698 in Ned Ward's *The London Spy* there was a reference to 'A couple of airy youths who by their cropped hair, stone buckles in their shoes, broad gold hat bands, and no swords I took to be merchants' sons or the apprentices of topping tradesmen'.

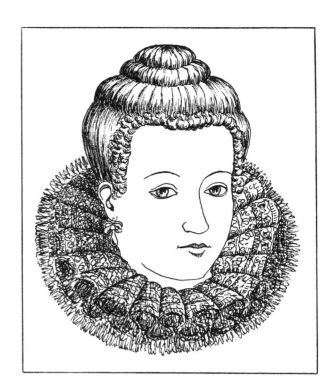

Fig. 63 : Marie de Médici, Queen of France,
second wife of Henri IV, in 1601

We have one final, rather grumpy comment on periwigs from a work published in 1694: 'And, to speak plainly, Forty, or Threescore pound a year for Periwigs, and Ten to a poor Chaplain to say Grace to him that adores Hair, is sufficient demonstration of the Weakness of the Brains they Keep Warm'.

WOMEN: 1600–1645 (Plates 62, 63, 66)

Wigs were still fashionable for women at the beginning of the century. The hair of the wigs was curled by rolling it over heated *bilboquets* or *roulettes*. When wigs were not worn, the hair was usually dressed high over rolls or pads or a wire frame and sometimes frizzed or curled. The back hair was usually in a flat bun covered with a net or caul. Coloured hair powders (such as blonde or reddish) were sometimes used. The high head-dresses were not really fashionable after about 1615.

Then the hair was lowered and the emphasis moved to the back; and until late in the century the dressing of the back of the head remained much the same—usually a kind of large, round chignon made of braids or twisted rolls or puffs. But this was subject to endless variations, a number of which are shown on Plate 63. The chignons were sometimes plain but were frequently decorated with ribbons and bows or even feathers. Plate 63-M shows the popular French *bourrelet*, a crescent-shaped pad concealing the hair around the chignon.

Among the fashionable there was usually a fringe across the forehead and frizzed or slightly curled hair at the temples; among women of the middle and lower classes,

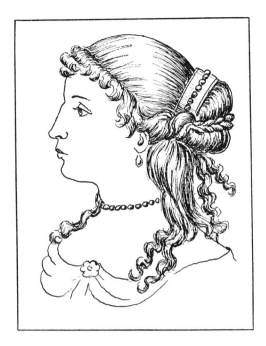

Fig. 64 : Marie Thérèse (1638–83), daughter of Philip IV of Spain and wife of Louis XIV

this often took the form of wisps of loose hair around the face. Variations can be seen on Plate 63. The spaniel ears in G are typical. These were called *bouffons*. In France a single curl called a *cadenette* (see discussion under 'Lovelocks') was sometimes allowed to hang down on either or both sides, usually ending in a rosette or a bow called a *gallant* (Plate 63-T).

Then the side hair began to grow longer and more important; and as it did, the coil or bun at the back tended to grow larger. The fringe was sometimes carefully curled and plastered down on the forehead, and sometimes (after 1640) it disappeared completely.

Patches, which were essential to the fashionable lady, were to be had in a variety of shapes, and their positioning often had a great significance. A patch close to the eye was called *la passionée*, one beside the mouth, *la baiseuse*, on the cheek, *la galante*, etc. In 1637 Beaumont and Fletcher found occasion to mention them in *The Elder Brother*: 'Your black patches you wear variously, some cut like stars, some in half moons, some in lozenges'.

WOMEN: 1645–1670 (Plates 62, 64-66)

In mid-century the side curls of the lady of fashion began to take more definite form and to be wired to stand out away from the face, as in 64-C. This encouraged the use of false hair, and in Marston's *Mountebank's Masque* we find the line, 'A great

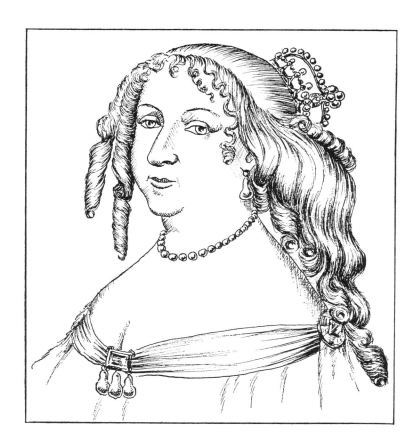

Fig. 65 : Marie-Jeanne-Baptiste,
Duchess of Savoy,
in 1666

lady should not wear her own hair; for that's as meane as a coate of her own spinning'. Later the curls receded and were worn closer to the face (Plate 64-O).

The curious Spanish hair styles of the period may at first glance seem unrelated to those of other countries. But they really follow the general pattern of hair of medium length in a low, extremely wide coiffure. The hair was usually waved or frizzed all over, and the top and side hair was not separated. Nor was there any fringe. Plate 64-J shows a simpler, perhaps earlier version. Compare it with the still earlier Italian style shown in Plate 63-D.

Masks were worn out of doors to preserve the complexion and sometimes indoors as well. Patches were still being worn in profusion. In 1650, in *The Artificial Changeling*, Bulwer says, 'Our ladies have lately entertained a vaine custom of spotting their faces out of an affectation of a mole, to set off their beauty, such as Venus had; and it is well if one black patch will serve to make their faces remarkable, for some fill their visages full of them, varied into all manner of shapes and figures'. Eight years later, in *Wit Restored*, there appeared a few lines on the subject:

> Their faces are besmear'd and pierc'd
>   With severall sorts of patches,
> As if some cats their skins had flead
>   With scarres, half moons, and notches.

WOMEN: 1670–1700 (Plates 62, 65, 66)

In 1671 there appeared in Paris a new style created by Martin and called the *hurlu-berlu* (Plate 65-I). When Madame de Sévigné saw it being worn by Madame de Never, she wrote to her daughter (on 18 March) that it was the most ridiculous thing she could imagine; and she advised the daughter not to change her own style, which her maid had learned to do so well. In another letter, written on the first of April, she confessed to being 'diverted' by the new coiffure. Three days later, having seen it on the duchesse de Sully and the comtesse de Guiches, she advised her daughter to adopt it immediately since it was obviously the mode for her face. She not only promised to do the coiffure on a doll and send it so that her daughter might see for herself, but she added that her present coiffure (which on 18 March had been so becoming) was simply impossible and that the *hurluberlu*, though ridiculous on older women, was just the thing to set off her beauty. The style became extremely popular among the fashion-conscious in both France and England.

Then, in about 1680, came the *fontange*. Starting out as a few curls with ribbons or bows, as shown in Plate 65-L, it developed into a high and elaborate structure of curls (Plate 66-O), often combined with a sort of cap of starched linen and lace worn forward on the head. Whether this entire structure was referred to as a *fontange* or only the lace and linen decoration is disputed. In any case, there were other terms used for the curls and their foundation, as we shall see presently.

The story of the origin of the *fontange* is frequently told and seldom with the same details. According to Leloire's version, Marie de Scoraille de Roussilhe (duchesse de Fontanges), maid of honour to Madame and mistress to the king, was accompanying the king on a hunting party when her hair came down. She took off a garter and put it around her head. The king was enchanted, and, so it is said, all of the ladies of the court immediately adopted the style. Unfortunately, Marie died in 1681 at the age of twenty, but the *fontange* (perhaps also unfortunately) lived on for a good many years. In its later form the king came to dislike it intensely but seemed powerless to do anything about it until one day he publicly admired the simple coiffure of a visiting Englishwoman, Lady Sandwich, whereupon the elaborate French constructions are said to have come down overnight. But that was not until the early eighteenth century.

The high pile of curls was frequently false, and this false hair was called a *tour*. Sometimes the term was translated as *tower*; but it appears that usually the French word was used, as in Wycherly's *The Plain Dealer* (1696): 'Is not this Tour too brown? . . . This Tour must come more forward, Madam, to hide the wrinkles at the corners of your eyes.' Or, in George Etherege's *The Man of Mode, or, Sir Fopling Flutter*, published in 1676, Medley says: 'I have plaid with her now at least a dozen times, till she'as worn out all Her fine Complexion, and her Tour wou'd keep in Curl no longer'.

The hair was dressed over a wire foundation known as a *commode* (see Plates

66-O and 78-A-B-D). In order to make the coiffure, the hair was parted from one ear to the other and the back hair tied between the crown and the neck, then formed into a chignon. The front hair was parted in the centre and formed into a high torsade of curls. False curls on pins were often used, as well as pearl or jewelled pins for decoration.

But the *tours* and *palisades* and *commodes* are only the beginning. John Evelyn (Plate 60-Q), who wrote prolifically on an astonishing variety of subjects, published in 1690 a satiric piece in rhymed couplets called *Mundus Muliebris: or, The Ladies Dressing Room Unlock'd and Her Toilette Spread*. The piece, actually written by Evelyn's nineteen-year-old daughter, covers the entire toilette. The following are those couplets referring to the hair:

> A saphire bodkin for the hair
> Or sparkling facet diamond there.
> *Calembus* combs in *pulvil* case
> To set and trim the hair and face:
> And that the cheeks may both agree,
> Plumpers to fill the cavity.
> The *settee*, *cupee*, place aright,
> *Frelange, fontange,* favorite;
> *Monte la haute,* and *palisade,*
> *Sorti, flandan* (great helps to trade),
> *Bourgoigne, jardine, cornett,*
> *Frilal* next upper panier set,
> Round which it does our ladies please
> To spread the hood called rayonnés;
> Behind the noddle every baggage
> Wears bundle *choux*, in English cabbage;
> Nor *cruches* she, nor *confidents*,
> Nor *passages*, nor *bergers* wants;
> And when this grace Nature denies,
> An artificial *tour* supplies;
> All which with *meurtriers* unite,
> And *creve coeurs* silly fops to smite,
> Or take in toil at park or play,
> Nor holy Church is safe, they say,
> Where decent veil was wont to hide
> The modest sex religious pride;
> Lest these yet prove too great a load,
> 'Tis all comprised in the *commode*;
> Pins tipt with diamond point and head,
> By which the curls are fastened,

> In radiant firmament set-out,
> And over all the hood *sur-tout*;
> Thus face that erst near head was plac'd.
> Imagine now about the wast,
> For *tour* on *tour*, and tire on tire.
> Like steeple Bow, or Grantham spire
> Or Septizonium, once at Rome,
> (But does not half so well become
> Fair ladies head), you here behold
> Beauty by tyrant mode controll'd.

The references, though intriguing, are not so enlightening as they might be. Evelyn (or his daughter) apparently anticipated this and appended *The Fop-Diction-ary, Compiled for the Use of the Fair Sex*. Again, here are those definitions which apply to the hair:

COMMODE. A frame of wire, cover'd with silk, on which the whole head-attire is adjusted at once upon a but or property of wood carved to the breasts, like that which perruque-makers set upon their stalls.

CONFIDANTS. Smaller curles near the eares.

CREVE-COEURS. Heart-breakers, the two small curl'd locks at the nape of the neck.

CRUCHES. Certain smaller curles, placed on the forehead.

FAVORITES. Locks dangling on the temples.

FIRMAMENT. Diamonds, or other precious stones heading the pins, which they stick in the tour and hair, like stars.

FONT-ANGE. The top-knot, so call'd from Mademoiselle de Fontange, one of the French Kings mistresses, who first wore it.

MEURTRIERS. Murderers; a certain knot in the hair which ties and unites the curls.

PALISADE. A wire sustaining the hair next to the dutchess, or first knot.

PASSAGERE. A curl'd lock next to the temples.

SEPTIZONIUM. A very high tower in Rome, built by the Emperor Severus, of seven ranks of pillars, set one upon the other, and diminishing to the top, like the ladies new dress for their heads, which was the mode among the Roman dame, and is exactly described by Juvenal in his 6th Satyr:

> Such rows of curles press'd on each other lye,
> She builds her head so many stories high,
> That look on her before, and you would swear
> Hector's tall wife Andromache she were,
> Behind a pigmy.

TOUR. An artificial dress of hair on the forehead, &c.

The tour was so common at the time that a more informative definition probably seemed quite superfluous. But common as it was, it was not the easiest thing in the world to manage. The following contemporary description gives an idea of some of the difficulties inherent in wearing a commode or a tour:

'And now her ladyship brandishes the combs, and the powders raise clouds in the apartment. She trims up the commode, she places it ten times, unplaces it as often, without being so fortunate as to hit upon the critical point; she models it to all systems, but is pleased with none, for you must know that some ladies fancy a vertical, others an horizontal position, others dress by the northern latitude, and others lower its point 45 degrees.'

And even when the commode was finally placed to the lady's satisfaction, it had a disconcerting tendency to slip rakishly on some heads. It is reported that there was some sentiment in favour of flattening the heads of female babies a bit so that when they grew up, the commode would stay properly anchored.

In addition to his other lists relating to hair, Randle Holme has one entitled 'The Several ways Women wear Hair about their Face.' These are the several ways:

In LOCKS, when the hair lyeth on each side the Cheeks.

In CURLES, when the hair swells or puffeth out from the Cheeks.

In FALLS or FLATS, when the hair hangs loose down about the shoulders, having nothing to tie it up.

In SHADES, when it lieth plain and streight on each side the forehead.

In CROSS SHADES, when it lieth cross the Forehead, with a Silk Thread in the middle of it.

In a SHORT FILLET or CURL, when it lieth so all the breadth of the forehead from one side to the other.

In a TOPPING or FORE-LOCK, when a Lock is laid from the foretop to the Crown of the head, as little children that have long hair are usually dressed.

In TAURES, when the hair on the forehead is curled and standeth out.

In BULL HEADS, when the said curled forehead is much larger than the Taure.

THE LADIES DICTIONARY

In 1694 there was published in London 'A Work Never Attempted before in English' and entitled *The Ladies Dictionary; Being a General Entertainment for the Fair-Sex*. Under the heading of *Hair, how to cause it neatly to Curl*, it is pointed out that 'Hair twining in curious Curls is very graceful and modish to the Ladies, but especially to the other Sex, whose Faces if any thing comely, it sets off to a wonder, and these kind of Curls were once so taking with the Fair Sex, though now reduced much shorter, that none were thought Paragons for Beauty, save those whose graceful Locks did reach the Breasts and make Spectators think those soft tempting ivory Globes of Venus were upheld by the friendly aid of their Crispy twirls. . . .

'Hair, if you would have it curiously to Curl, must be first washed and cleansed well; that done, take oak-galls to the number of twenty, two ounces of Maiden-hair, boil them well stamped in a small quantity of Water and Salt, till the Water be boiled to the Consistence of Honey, work them well together, and then at sundry times for two days anoint the Hair with it, and on the third day cleanse it in this Bath, *viz*. Take Beet-Leaves and Fern-Roots, of each a handful, bruise them in two quarters of water, till a third part of the Water be consumed, then taking it off, put in a little piece of Gum-arabick, and use it cool; after which on Twirling Irons turn up your Hair, in what Curls or Ringlets you please, and it will continue so a long while; but finding it begin to fall and grow Limber, it must be renewed: or for want of the former Receipt, take the Oyles of White Henbane and Fenugreek Seed, and with them mix a little Gum-Arabick, and over a gentle Fire make it into a flowing or soft Ointment, and anoint your Hair with it before you turn it up, and it will be Curiously Curled.'

This is followed by instructions for taking the curl out of curly hair and the bush out of bushy hair and then an entry which reads:

'*Hair, how to make it of any Colour*: Hair of a yellow or shining golden Colour was in highest esteem among the Ancients, the Poets rarely delineating any excellent Beauty without appropriating that to her as a singular Ornament; yet since the time of the Danes, it has been (in spite to those cruel invaders, who turned up almost all the Women they came near) loaded with Obloquies, and is held as a sign of lustful Constitution; for it is a Fancy generally received that the Locks can never sparkle with Golden Flames without, unless there lodges some cherished heat of that kind within; but indeed though black is now in Vogue amongst the most celebrated Beauties, yet in this as in all other Colours, Peoples Minds and Fancy vary; some are for the Curious flaxen, others for the Light Brown, and so what best suits their Humours.' This is all very enlightening but might well prove disappointing to any lady dissatisfied with the unfashionable colour of her hair and wanting desperately to know 'how to make it of any Colour'.

However, if black was the colour she had in mind, she was in luck, for there follows another entry:

'*Hair, Grey or otherwise, to make it black*. Hair to render it black, take the Bark of an Oak Root, the Green Husks of Walnuts, three ounces of each, the deepest and oldest Red-Wine a Pint, boil them, bruised and well mixed to the Consumption of half a Pint, strain out the juice, and adde of the Oyl of Myrtle a pound and a half, set them six days in the Sun in a Leaden Mortar, stirring them well, and the anointing the Hair, it will turn any Coloured Hair as black as Jet in often doing.' There are no further instructions for colouring the hair.

There are, however, instructions for doing a number of other things to the hair; and they seem well worth a digression. The first entry has to do with *Scurf and Dandriff how to cleanse the Head of it*: First one must purge the body 'with some convenient Medicine; after that, wash the Head or other parts affected with lye thus made, *viz*. Take the Ashes of the Roots of Beets and Coldworts, make a Lixivium with them, wherein boil Lupins and Beans a sufficient quantity, then strain the decoction, and add a sixth part of Honey. When the Head has been well washed with this, dry it well, and rub it hard with a Coarse warm Cloth, then take this Unguent and anoint it, *viz*. bitter Almonds lightly heated in an oven or Stove, and old Walnuts, each six Ounces, two drams of the Honey of Squills, two Ounces of the dregs of old Wine, Sulphur half an Ounce, Vitriol two drams, make it into an Unguent for your use with red Wax. Having not these Ingredients, take Oyl, Rue, one Ounce, Sope an Ounce, Salt finely beaten half an Ounce, work them together into a Mass, and anoint the Head, *&c*. after washed with the following Compound decoction, *viz*. Boil Beets, Fenugreek, Briony-Roots, Bean-Meal, each a good handful in a Gallon of Spring Water, till it be consumed, then take it off, and when it is cool use it three or four days successively, and your Expectation will be satisfied.'

The next instructions come under the intriguing heading, *Hair, how to fasten, and keep it from falling off*:

'Have in a readiness or procure Myrtle leaves, the Bark of a Pine-tree, and Maidenhair, of each half a handful, bruise them well together, and add to these a double quantity of pounded Labdanum, put them into a sufficient quantity of White-wine to steep them well, then add an Ounce of the Oyl of Radish-seed; and being sufficiently steeped, strain out the Liquid part, and anoint your Head, or any place where the Hair is defective, going to Bed, and have next Morning in readiness a Bath to wash your head in, made of Sorrel, Maiden-hair, Myrabolans and Emblick; these are to be boiled in water, and a little pounded Myrrh added, and in a few times using it will fasten your Hair extreamly; or for want of these take Willow-leaves, Plantane, Roch Allum, and Hyssop, of each a moderate proportionable quantity, boyl them in Water, and add some Powder of Myrrh and Tutty. Hair is secured this way by the Golden Water drawn from Honey in a Glass Still; or take the roots of Vervine, together with the Leaves, stamp them well, and put them into Oyl of Green Grapes, and set them in the Sun ten days, then strain out the moist part and anoint your Hair with it, as you see occasion; or for want of any of the former, take Juniper-berries, Nigella-Seeds, Wormwood, Labdanum and Vervine, each a like quantity, bind them well, bruited in a linen Cloath, and Macerate them five days in Oyl, and it will not only by anointing fasten the Hair, but make it grow comely.'

But there were more treasures. And had the men not been wearing wigs, they might have dipped into the book for this one:

'*Hair, wanting, how to make it grow on a Bald Place, &c*. However, Ladies, if some disasters have trod too hard on your Heads, and kill'd those pleasant Plants that were used to flourish there; you may again by the following helps, attire with their Native Beauty and repair all former ruins and render it more fair and lovely than nature before had planted it. Indeed the Hair is a very great Ornament and where it is wanting in its proper Places, it throws a kind of an Eclipse over the Face of Beauty; to recover it then take Fern Roots, burn them to ashes, mingle with them

Linseed Oyl and bruised Almonds, Bran of Wheat, and half an ounce of Mastick Powder, spread them well tempered together upon a piece of fine Leather, and lay it as a Plaister to the place where the Hair is wanting, and in three or four times applying, and washing with Rose-water and Butter of Orange-flowers, the Hair will appear and grow up very full, decently, and in order.' An alternative recipe containing 'Oyl of Roses and a little Deers Suet' is then suggested. If neither of these appealed to the reader, there was a third which must have seemed a godsend to any ladies whose medicine chests were overstocked with Housleek Juice and Oyl of Mugwort. The resulting ointment would, they were advised, give to the hair 'a lighter Colour and more curious than before'.

Finally, there is a recipe for taking hair away:

Take 'Auripigmentum an ounce and a half, quick lime four ounces, Florentine Irish Roots an ounce, Sulphur, Nitre, of each half an ounce; these must be laid in a Quart of Lye made of Beanstalks, and being well mixed and temper'd, boil them in a glaz'd Pot, till putting in a Feather, you will find all the shag come off the Stalk then add half an ounce of Oyl of Mirrh, or any Fragrant Oyl, and well mixing all, anoint the part of the Body from which the Hair is to be taken, it not being a place that is sore, and you will in a short time find the effect.' The reader, it is only fair to add, was warned to have some Oyl of Roses handy to 'cool and Mollifie the Heat'. There was an alternative recipe calling for Orpiment, quick lime, henbane, fleawort seeds, sublimate gum, and a scruple of opium, but it also required a soothing oil to allay the after effects. If by any chance the lady didn't want the hair to come back, there was still another recipe requiring, among other things, emmetts' eggs and the blood of a frog.

And on this eminently practical note we come to the end of the seventeenth century.

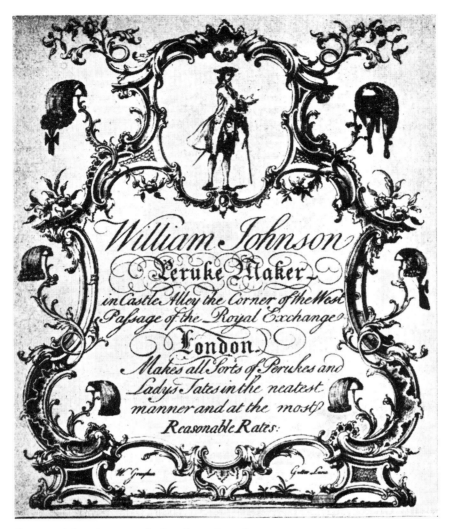

Fig. 66 : Advertisement of a London wig-maker

PLATE 55 : SEVENTEENTH-CENTURY MEN 1600–1620

A   *c.* 1610, English. *Square cut* beard.

B   1600.

C   *c.* 1600, English. Robert Devereux, Earl of Essex, 1566–1601. The portrait in the National Portrait Gallery, London, painted in 1597, shows a somewhat larger and bushier beard.

D   *c.* 1600, French.

E   Italian. Galileo Galilei, 1564–1642.

F   Goldzius, died 1616.

G   1604, English.

H   1604, Spanish. *Goat* beard.

I   1604, Austrian. *Spade* beard.

J   1604. *Stiletto* beard.

K   German. Johannes Kepler, 1571–1630.

L   1604, Spanish.

M   Dutch. *Pique devant* beard.

N   *c.* 1615, English. *Stiletto* beard.

O   *c.* 1600, Italian. Rutilio Manetti, painter. Randle Holme would no doubt call this a *mouse-eaten* beard.

P   English. William Shakespeare, 1564–1616. From an engraving by Martin Droeshout in 1623 (see also Plate 58-A).

Q   *c.* 1620, possibly French. *Pique devant.*

R   1614, German. *Pique devant.*

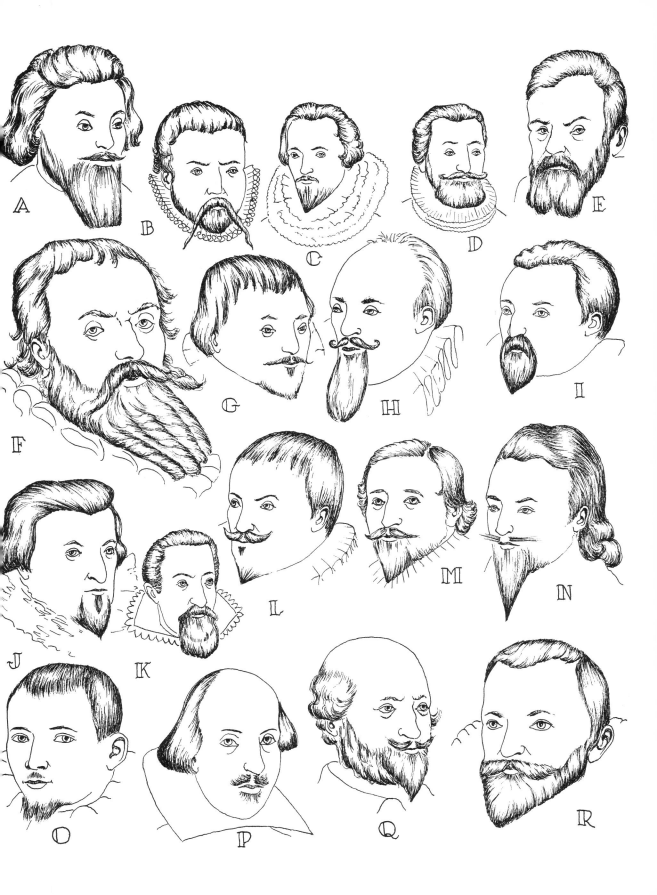

A

B

C

D

E

F

G

H

I

J

K

L

M

N

O

P

Q

R

PLATE 56 : SEVENTEENTH-CENTURY MEN 1620–1650

A   1628. Spanish peasant.

B   1628. Spanish peasant.

C   1628. Spanish peasant.

D   *c.* 1630, Dutch. Crispin Van de Passe the Younger. *Square cut* beard.

E   1624, Italian. Giovanni Battista Marino. Poet. *Bodkin.*

F   Cardinal Richelieu, 1585–1642. *Stiletto* beard.

G   Swedish. King Gustavus Adolphus, 1594–1632—reigned 1611–32. *Stiletto* beard.

H   Flemish. Sir Anthony Van Dyck, 1599–1641 (see K below and Plate 58-D). *Stiletto* beard, later called a *Van Dyck* or *Vandyke.*

I   Paulus Moreelse, 1571–1638. Painter.

J   1635. Daniel Mytens, painter.

K   *c.* 1640, Flemish. Sir Anthony Van Dyck. From a self-portrait (see H above and Plate 58-D).

L   *c.* 1640, English.

M   *c.* 1630, French. *Bodkin.*

N   Bavarian. Gottfried Heinrich, 1594–1632. Imperialist general in the Thirty Years War. *Stiletto* beard.

O   French. Pierre Corneille, 1606–84.

P   Italian. Sassoferrato (Giovanni Battista Salvi), 1609–85. Painter. *Bodkin.*

Q   Italian. Giovanni Lorenzo Bernini, 1598–1680. Sculptor and architect. *Hammer cut* beard.

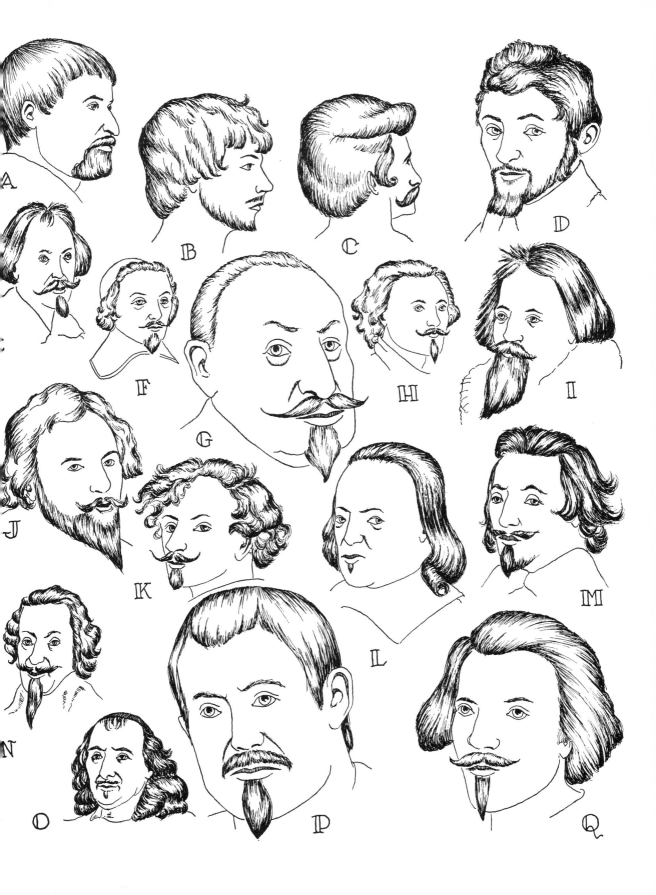

A

B

C

D

E

F

G

H

I

J

K

L

M

N

O

P

Q

PLATE 57 : SEVENTEENTH-CENTURY MEN 1610–1685

A   Christian IV, King of Denmark and Norway, 1577–1648. Notice the small braid in front of the ear. The fashion of wearing a single pearl ear-ring was started by Henri de Lorraine, duc d'Harcourt, who subsequently became known as '*le Cadet à la perle*'.

B   *c.* 1615.

C   English. Thomas Howard, Earl of Arundel, 1586–1646. (Other portraits show some variation in the beard.)

D   *c.* 1630, Dutch. *Stiletto* beard.

E   Spanish. Velasquez, 1599–1660. *Stiletto* beard.

F   *c.* 1635.

G   Ferdinand III, King of Hungary and Bohemia, 1608–57.

H   1632, Spanish. Charles of Austria, son of Philip III, 1607–32.

I   Dutch. Gerard van Honthorst, 1590–1656. Painter. *Lovelock*.

J   Italian. Cardinal Leopold de' Medici.

K   *c.* 1635, Spanish.

L   1677, French.

M   English. John Dryden, 1631–1700. (Another portrait in the National Portrait Gallery shows Dryden wearing a full-bottom wig.)

N   *c.* 1675, Italian painter.

O   1685, English. Sir Godfrey Kneller, 1646–1723. (From a self-portrait.)

P   1683. Nathanial Dilgerus. Beards had long been out of fashion and were seen only occasionally on the elderly or on individual or eccentric types.

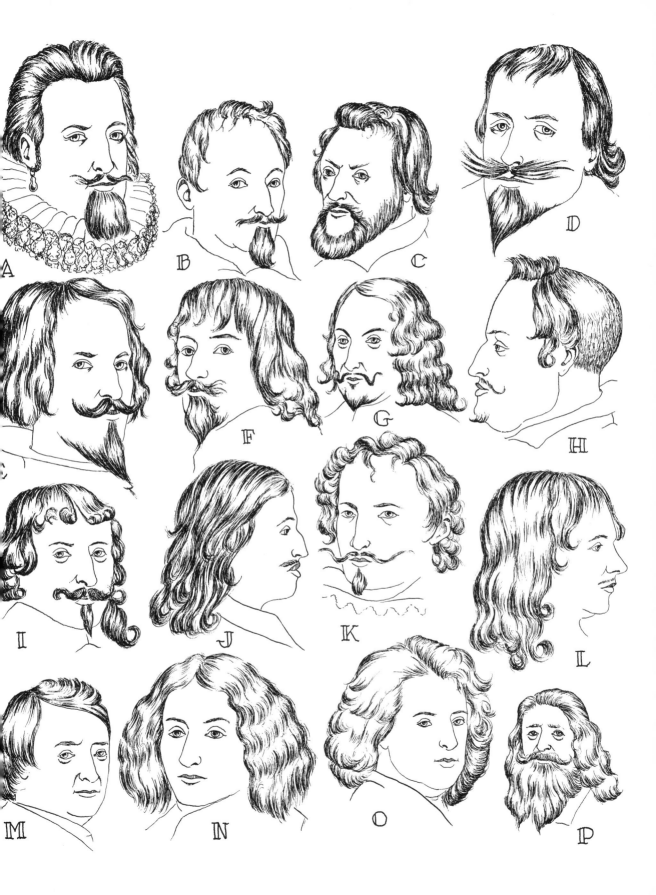

A

B

C

D

E

F

G

H

I

J

K

L

M

N

O

P

PLATE 58 : SEVENTEENTH-CENTURY MEN 1610–1690

A   William Shakespeare, 1564–1616. (The drawing is based on the Chandos portrait).

B   English. James I, 1566–1625—reigned 1603–25.

C   1626, English. Charles I, 1600–49—reigned 1625–49 (see also F below).

D   Anthony Van Dyck, 1599–1641. *Stiletto* beard (see also 56-H-K).

E   1645, English. Oliver Cromwell, 1599–1658.

F   1649, English. Charles I (see C above).

G   Italian. Evangelista Torricelli, 1608–47. *Stiletto* beard.

H   Captain John Smith, 1579–1631. English adventurer. *Round* beard.

I   English. John Endicott, 1589–1665. Governor of Massachusetts colony. *Needle* beard.

J   French. François Mansart, 1598–1666. Architect.

K   German. Otto von Guericke, 1602–86. Natural philosopher.

L   1660, English. Charles II (for later portrait see Plate 61-L).

M   Italian. Luca Giordano, 1632–1705. Painter.

N   English. John Dryden, 1631–1700. Poet, dramatist, critic.

O   1688, English. *Campaign* or *Travelling wig.*

P   French. Le Grand Dauphin, son of Louis XIV.

Q   1688, English. *Crisping* or *curling irons* for men's hair.

R   1660, Dutch. Cornelius de Graef.

S   *Curling pipe*, around which false hair was rolled while boiling or baking.

T   *Periwig thimble.*

U   'A *Peruque* or *Perawick* (or a long Perawick with a Pole Lock). This is the Sign or cognizance of the Perawick Maker. This is by Artists called a long Curled Wig, with a Suffloplin or with a Dildo or Pole-lock.' (*Academy of Armoury*, 1688.)

V   '*Beard cisers*' with 'short nippers and larg handles' (*Academy of Armoury*).

W   1688, English. *Curling stick.*

X   Beard of Erasmus Schmidt, 1560–1637. *Swallow-tail.*

Y   1648. Beard of H. Everhard Cratz. *Pique devant.* (Repton calls this a *stiletto* or *bodkin.*)

Z   Beard of Christian IV of Denmark, according to Repton.

AA   Beard of Francis à Domia. *Spade.*

BB   Beard of an Italian painter. *Pique devant.* (Repton calls this a *bodkin* or *stiletto*, but the designation is questionable.)

CC   1625. Beard of an Italian painter. *Pencil.*

DD   Beard of N. Vigelius de Dreisa.

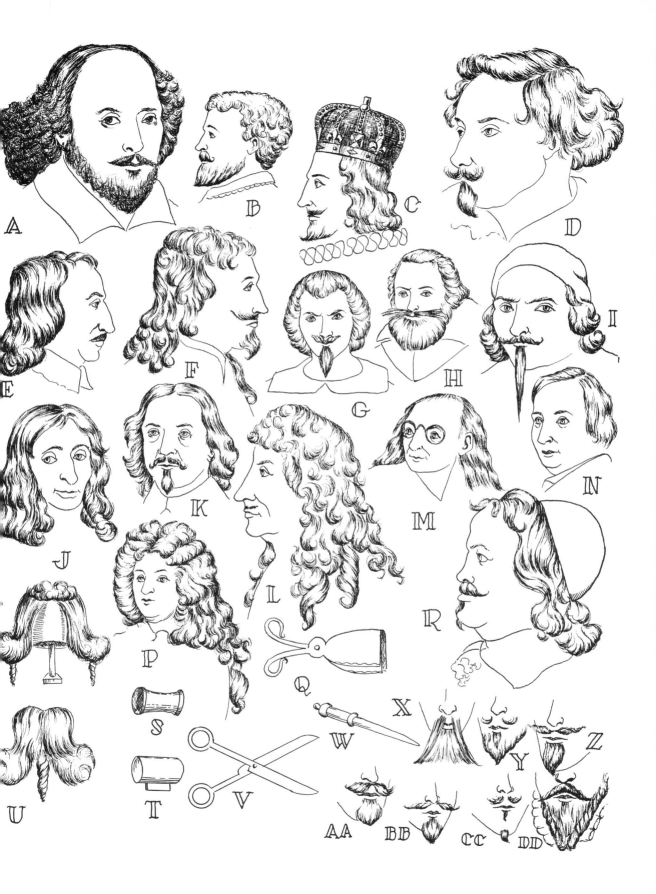

PLATE 59 : SEVENTEENTH-CENTURY MEN 1614–1670

A   1617, Dutch.

B   *c.* 1617, Dutch.

C   *c.* 1621. Beggar.

D   1617, Dutch.

E   1614, Italian. Francesco de' Medici, brother of the Grand Duke.

F   1627, French. Jacques Callot, 1592–1635. Engraver and etcher. (Callot's work is the source of a number of hair styles on these plates.)

G   1624, English. Court of James I.

H   1624, English. Court of James I.

I   1640, Spanish. Gaspar de Guzman, conde de Olivares, 1587–1645.

J   English. *Screw* beard. (After Repton.)

K   Italian. Mask of Pantaloon with false beard and moustache.

L   1633, French. Fashionable gentleman with *lovelock.*

M   Dutch beggar.

N   *c.* 1635. Dutch peasant.

O   Dutch. Willem Burchgraeff. (From a portrait by Rembrandt.)

P   1649, English. Cavalier with lovelock.

Q   1649. Beard of David Gloxen.

R   1645, English. Fop with two lovelocks.

S   Date uncertain. (After Repton.)

T   1653. Dutch peasant.

U   1649. Beard of N. G. Raigersperg. (After Repton.) *Hammer-cut* or *Roman-T* beard.

V   1653, Dutch. *Square-cut* beard.

W   1669, Dutch.

X   French. Claude Ballin. Parisian goldsmith.

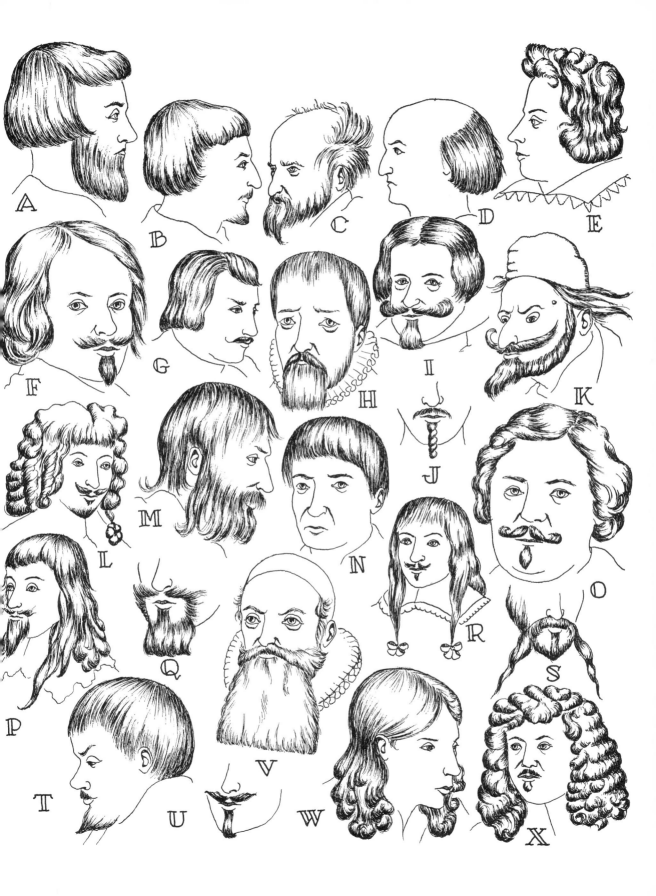

PLATE 60 : SEVENTEENTH-CENTURY MEN 1640–1670

A   1649, Dutch.

B   *c.* 1650, Spanish. *Bodkin.*

C   *c.* 1645. Fabritius. (From a self-portrait.)

D   1647.

E   Spanish. Philip IV, 1605–65 (see Plate 59-I for the beard of the Duke of Olivares, who dominated Philip's reign).

F   1651. French painter.

G   1649, Dutch. Pieter de Hooch. (From a self-portrait.)

H   *c.* 1645. Dutch painter.

I   *c.* 1650. Dutch painter.

J   *c.* 1650. French nobleman.

K   *c.* 1640.

L   1652. Cardinal Mazarin, 1602–61. *Bodkin* with *inverted* moustache.

M   Henri de la Tour d'Auvergne, vicomte de Turenne, 1611–75—Marshal of France.

N   1650, French. Nicolas Poussin, 1594–1665. (From a self-portrait.)

O   Dutch.

P   *c.* 1650, French. Molière, 1622–73.

Q   *c.* 1650, English. John Evelyn, 1620–1706.

R   *c.* 1658, French. Sébastien Bourdon. (From a self-portrait.)

S   1662, Dutch.

T   1668, French.

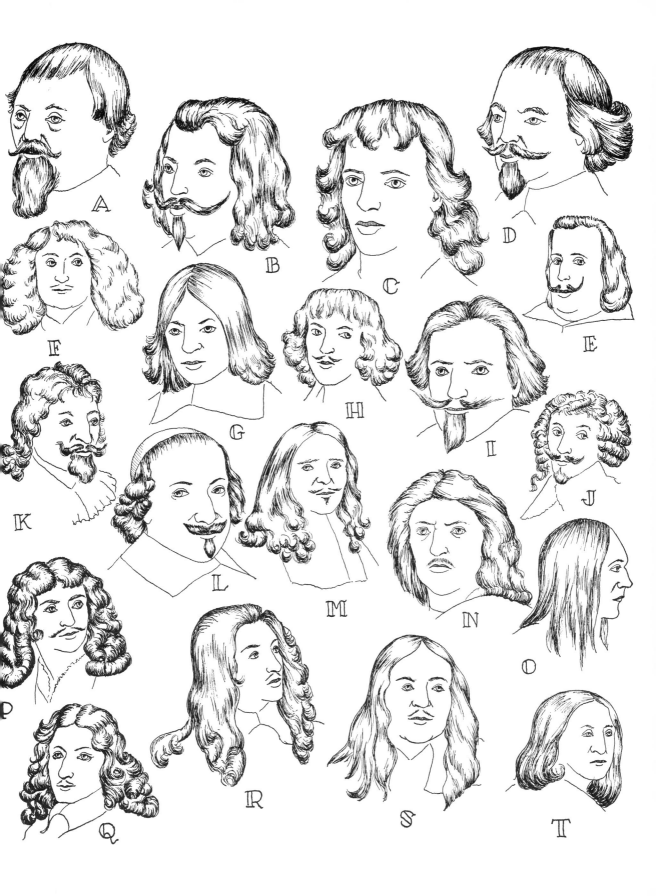

PLATE 61 : SEVENTEENTH-CENTURY MEN 1650–1700

A   *c.* 1670, Dutch. Adriaen van de Velde, 1636?–72. (From a self-portrait.)

B   1674. Italian painter.

C   1670, English.

D   *c.* 1690, Dutch.

E   *c.* 1665, French. Real and false hair.

F   *c.* 1650, French.

G   *c.* 1650, French.

H   1682, German. The full moustache would not have been worn in France or England at this time.

I   Italian. Bibbiena (Francesco Galli), 1659–1739. Wig.

J   *c.* 1685. English painter.

K   *c.* 1690. Spanish painter.

L   English. Charles II, 1630–85—reigned 1660–85 (for earlier portrait see Plate 58-L).

M   French. Michel Le Tellier, marquis de Louvois. Minister of War under Louis XIV. Wig.

N   French. Louis XIV, 1638–1715—reigned 1643–1715. Wig.

O   English. Daniel Defoe, 1660–1731. Wig.

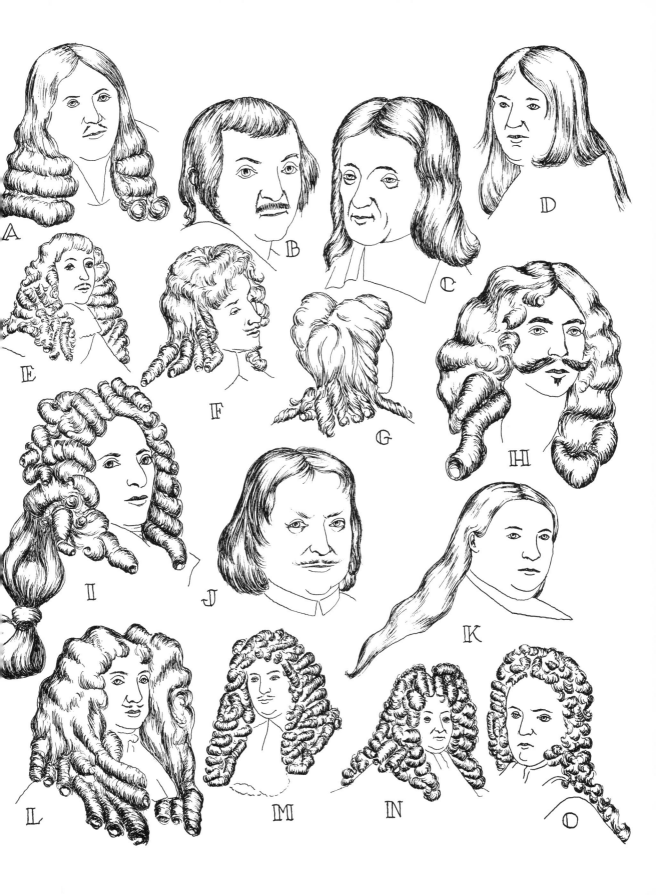

A

B

C

D

E

F

G

H

I

J

K

L

M

N

O

PLATE 62 : SEVENTEENTH-CENTURY MEN AND WOMEN, 1600–1680

MEN:

A   1619, English. Henry Percy, Earl of Northumberland—died 1632.

B   1632, English. William Lee—'Memorable for his numerous progeny'.

C   English. John Lamotte, 1577–1655—'Citizen of London'. *Bush* beard.

D   English. William Slater, D.D.

E   1635. Sir William Brog. Colonel of Scots troops. *Square-cut* beard.

F   German. Jacob Bobart, 1598–1679.

G   English. Sir Thomas Browne, M.D., 1606–82.

H   1654, French. Louis XIV at age 16.

I   1635, English. Richard Brome. Poet. *Screw* beard with inverted moustaches.

WOMEN:

J   1620, English. Susanne Temple.

K   1603, English. Lady Anne Clifford.

L   Third quarter, English.

M   Dutch.

N   Anne, Duchess of Albemarle.

O   Dutch. Maria van Reygersbergh.

P   1660, Dutch. Catherina Horft.

Q   English. Ann Hyde, Duchess of York.

R   *c.* 1680, English.

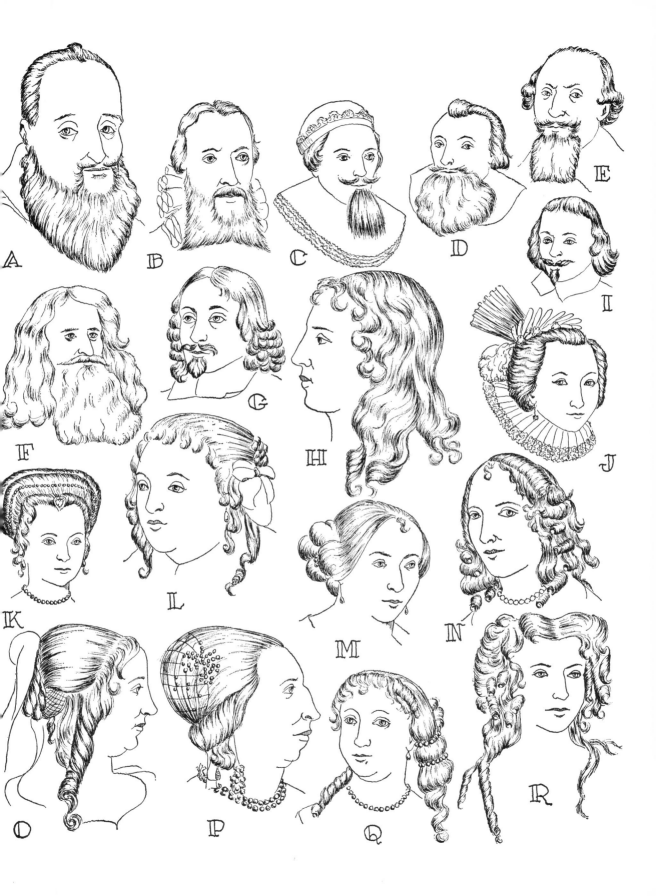

A

B

C

D

E

F

G

H

I

J

K

L

M

N

O

P

Q

R

PLATE 63 : SEVENTEENTH-CENTURY WOMEN 1600–1645

A   1610, French. Wig (see also Plate 66-A-B).

B   1615, probably Spanish. A simplified version of the head-dress shown in Plate 66-E. Wig.

C   Marie de Médici, 1573–1642. Wig.

D   *c.* 1630, Italian.

E   French or Italian. Peasant girl.

F   *c.* 1630, Dutch. Hélène Fourment, wife of Peter Paul Rubens.

G   *c.* 1630, French.

H, I   *c.* 1630, German.

J   1635, English.

K   *c.* 1640, Dutch.

L   *c.* 1630, French.

M   *c.* 1635, French.

N   *c.* 1635, French.

O   *c.* 1640, Dutch.

P   1640, French.

Q   1640, French.

R   *c.* 1645, Dutch.

S   1645, French middle-class.

T   1643, French.

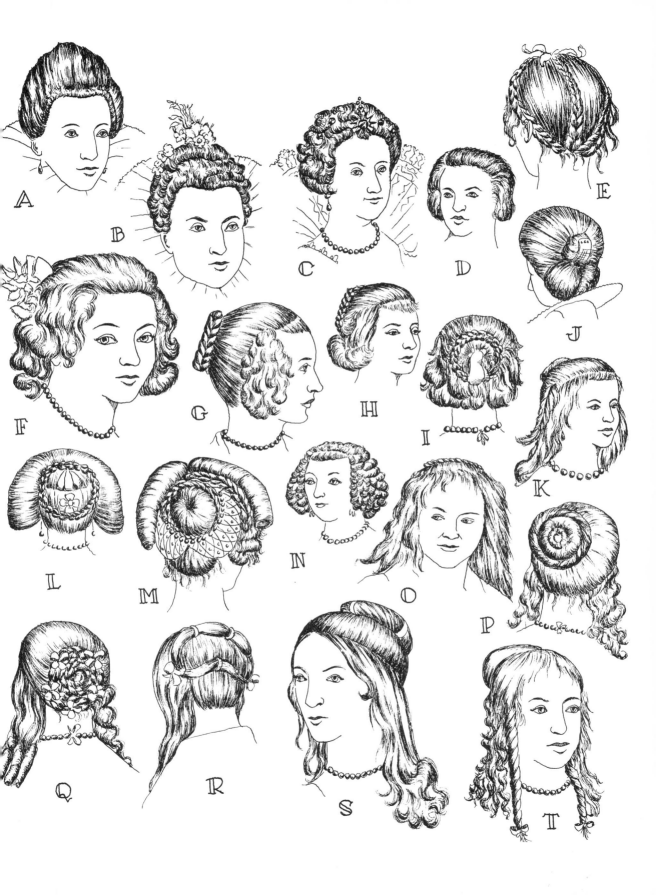

A

B

C

D

E

F

G

H

I

J

K

L

M

N

O

P

Q

R

S

T

PLATE 64 : SEVENTEENTH-CENTURY WOMEN 1645–1660

A   1647, French.

B   French. Anne Geneviève, duchesse de Longueville, 1619–79. Celebrated beauty and politician.

C   French. Anne of Austria, 1601–66. Queen of France, mother of Louis XIV (see later portrait, O below).

D   French. Marie de Rohan-Montbazon, duchesse de Chevreuse, 1600–79. Intimate of Anne of Austria, conspired against Richelieu.

E   *c.* 1650, Italian.

F   *c.* 1645, Flemish.

G   *c.* 1650.

H   *c.* 1645.

I   *c.* 1650, Flemish.

J   *c.* 1650, Spanish.

K   1650s. Infanta Maria Theresa. Hair crimped and arranged over wire frame.

L   *c.* 1650, Dutch.

M   *c.* 1650, Spanish.

N   *c.* 1660, Dutch.

O   French. Anne of Austria (see C above for earlier portrait).

P   *c.* 1660, Portuguese.

Q   *c.* 1660.

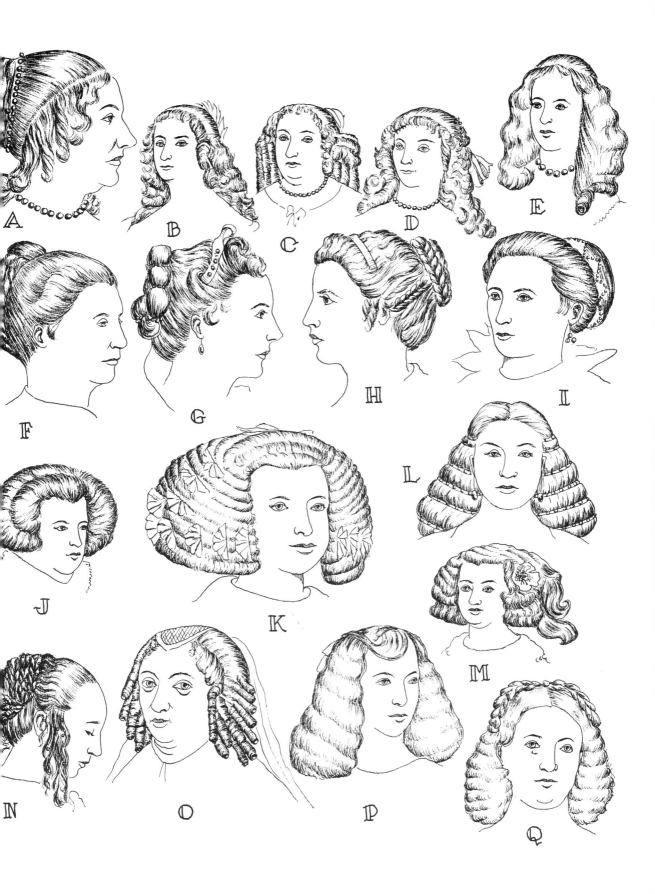

A

B

C

D

E

F

G

H

I

J

K

L

M

N

O

P

Q

PLATE 65 : SEVENTEENTH-CENTURY WOMEN 1660–1700

A   1665, French. Side curls are wired to stand out.

B   Louise de la Vallière, 1644–1710. Became mistress of Louis XIV in 1661, made a duchess in 1667.

C   French. Head-dress *en serpenteux*.

D   Dutch.

E   Dutch.

F   Dutch maidservant.

G   English. Nell Gwynn, 1650–87. Actress and mistress of Charles II after 1669 (see K below).

H   French. Duchesse de Monpensier.

I   1671, French. *Hurluberlu* style. Created in 1671 in Paris by Martin.

J   1680, English. *Hurluberlu.*

K   English. Nell Gwynn (see G above).

L   1680s, French. Early *fontange* (see later development, Plate 66-O and Plate 78 in Chapter 10).

M   1680, French. *À la bergère* style.

N   1680s, Spanish.

O   1688, French. Early *fontange* (see L above).

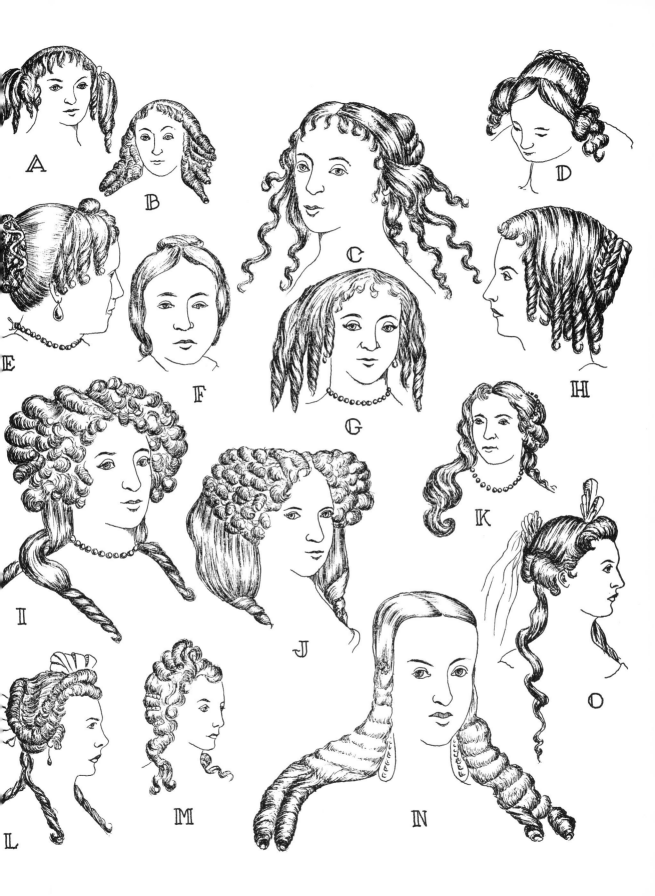

A

B

C

D

E

F

G

H

I

J

K

L

M

N

O

PLATE 66 : SEVENTEENTH-CENTURY WOMEN 1600–1700

A   *c.* 1600, French. Probably natural hair dressed over pads (see also Plate 63-A).

B   1600, French. Court of Henri IV.

C   *c.* 1610, French. Probably wig.

D   1615, French. Probably wig.

E   1615, Spanish. Probably wig.

F   Nobility of Lorraine.

G   German.

H   1628, Dutch.

I   *c.* 1633, French.

J   1635.

K   1645. Mistress Tracy, first wife of Wenceslaus Hollar.

L   Elizabeth of Bohemia, 1596–1662.

M   *c.* 1650. French duchess.

N   1680s, French. An early *fontange* (see also Plate 65-L-O).

O   1690s, French. *Fontange* with *tour*, decorated with jewelled pins.

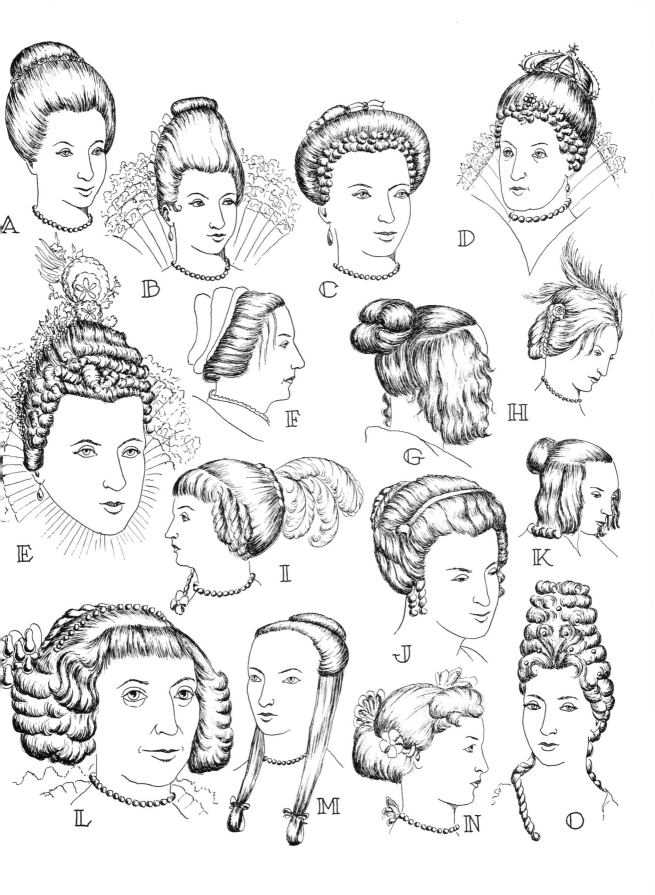

A

B

C

D

E

F

G

H

I

J

K

L

M

N

O

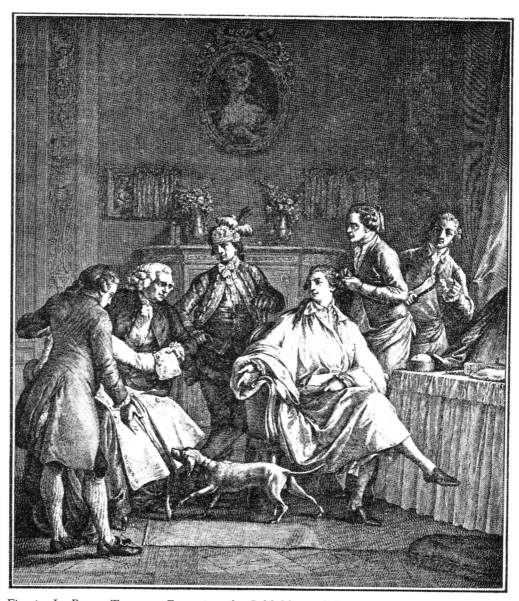

Fig. 67 : La Petite Toilette. Engraving after J. M. Moreau le jeune, c. 1779

9 · The Eighteenth Century—Men

Who, in this enlightened age, would put
the least confidence in a physician
who wears his own hair?

JACQUES DULAURE

This was the century of wigs for men. And though they could not match those fashionable at the end of the preceding century in sheer overpowering bulk, they more than made up for it in variety. It was not that the styles changed rapidly but that once they were introduced, they stayed, along with all of the other styles which had been introduced. Some of them, it is true, reached a point at which they were no longer considered fashionable, but they continued to be worn by men of certain ages or certain professions. Never before had men had such a wide choice of hair styles—styles which could be changed as quickly and as often as one wished, depending on the number of wigs one could afford.

THE EARLY YEARS

Beards were not worn throughout the century except in very special cases, and the barbers were kept busy shaving. The story is told (with endless variations) of an officer (sometimes a gentleman), with a face 'richly carbuncled with the rubies of red wine' who entered a barber's shop to be shaved. Placing his sword on the table, he said menacingly to the barber, 'Examine my features, sir; if you shave me without bleeding, there is a guinea for your expertness; but, mind the alternative, if one drop of blood be drawn, I will run you through the body!' The barber was unwilling to accept the challenge, but his more wily apprentice volunteered. Upon completion of the operation with no blood drawn, the soldier said to the boy, 'Here is your guinea, my brave fellow, but first tell me how you dared to risk your life when your master would not?'

'Oh,' answered the apprentice lightly, 'it was no risk at all, sir, because if I had drawn blood, I should have seen it first, and I would have cut your throat!'

In view of the opportunities afforded to barbers for misusing their tools, it is very much to their credit that they evidently maintained the confidence of most of their patrons. There were some unsettling rumours about barbers in Paris who were able to provide bodies at any time for those who required them; and Procter mentions the infamous assassin-perruquier, who supplied fresh corpses to a *pâtisserie* in the rue de la Harpe, which became famous for its savoury *pâtés*. 'The conspiracy was discovered through the agency of a faithful dog that refused to quit the street without its master. After the trial and execution of the two confederates, their shops were raised [*sic*], a memorial pillar erected upon the site, and a decree issued that bearded men are never more to be there shaven, nor are savoury patties to be again compounded on that spot.'

Nor was this sort of activity confined to the Left Bank. Procter also tells of a barber named Joseph Orcher, who lived in the Faubourg St Antoine and regularly shaved the Marquis de Courzi at his residence. One day he arrived there just as a tenant farmer was leaving, after having paid his yearly rent. A thousand gold louis were still lying on the table. Succumbing at last to the overwhelming temptation, Orcher dispatched the marquis with his razor and fled to Calais with the thousand louis. Twenty-nine years later, one year short of the statute of limitations, he returned to Paris, where he was recognized and guillotined.

It was customary in the days of the dentist-barber-surgeons for them to indicate their multiple profession by appropriate window displays. One of these is described by Gay in *A Goat Without a Beard*:

> His pole with pewter basin hung;
> Black rotten teeth in order strung;
> Ranged cups, that in the window stood,
> Lined with red rags, to look like blood;
> Did well his threefold trade explain:
> Who shaved, drew teeth and breathed a vein.

The red and white stripes on the barber's pole were originally meant to represent bandages. The bowl represented the shaving basin, and the pole itself was an enlarged version of the one provided for the customer to hold on to in order to keep his hands steady.

At the beginning of the century the full-bottom wig was still in favour. Even as late as 1697, in Vanbrugh's *The Relapse*, we find Mr Foretop, the wig-maker, proudly presenting Lord Foppington with his new wig, assuring him that it is 'so long & full of hair, it may serve you for a Hat and Cloak in all weathers'. When Lord Foppington complains that the wig is too skimpy—'not nine hairs of a side', Foretop moans: 'Oh Lord! Oh Lord! Oh Lord! Why, as God shall judge me, your Honour's side-face is reduc'd to the tip of your nose.'

Lord Foppington replies: 'My Side-Face may be in an Eclipse for aught I know; but I'm sure, my Full-Face is like the Full-Moon.' Upon being assured that the broadest place in his face is not two inches in diameter, Foppington retorts that that is two inches too much and adds that 'a Perriwig to a man shou'd be like a Mask to a Woman: nothing shou'd be seen but his Eyes'.

But the Lord Foppingtons were in a dwindling minority; and during the first twenty years of the century, the wig declined in both height and length. In 1721 the Society of Friends in Hampton, Massachusetts, proclaimed that 'the wearing of extravagant wigges is altogether antagonistic to truth'. Very early in the century new styles began creeping in (see Plate 67); and after the second or third decade, the full-bottom wig was out of fashion but continued to be worn by older conservative men and especially in certain professions. In the legal profession it persists to the present writing and shows no signs of giving up.

With the ponderous full-bottom out of the way, the road was clear for the leaders of fashion and the peruke makers; and they wasted no time. In May 1739 the following perruquier's advertisement appeared in *The Kentish Post or Canterbury News Letter*:

'All sorts of Perukes, curiously made, after the best Manner, viz. Tye Wigs, Clergymens Bobs and Long Bobs, with a handsome Feather Crown in the manner of a Tye-Crown, after the newest fashion and never yet made use of in Canterbury. Also Bag-Wigs, Spencers, Tuck-up Wigs, and Naturals, all drawn with a handsome Topee done in such a manner as scarcely to be perceived from one's own Hair. All made of the best of Hair by William Hilles at the Rose in St. George's, Canterbury. Where may be had fine Bottle Pale Beer at 6d. per Bottle, drank in the House, or 5s. per Dozen delivered out of the House, the Bottles to be exchanged or paid for at the Delivery.'

But even earlier than that—in 1724—Joseph Pickeaver, a Dublin wig-maker, who had formerly lived at the Black Lyon in Copper-alley and was now to be found 'under Tom's Coffee House, where all gentlemen may be furnished with all sorts of perukes', was prepared to supply 'full bottom tyes, full bobs, ministers' bobs, naturalls, half naturalls, Grecian flyes, curley roys, airy levants, qu perukes, and bag wigges'.

In March 1762 there appeared in the *London Chronicle* a brief article on 'The History of Male Fashions', subtitled 'Upon Wigs'. The article provides not only a peek at the attitude toward wigs in general but rather pungent descriptions of a few of the more popular styles:

'Elaborately have both ancients and moderns expressed themselves concerning the Brain, the Pineal Gland, Ideas, and Cogitations, by which the Head, or the Animal Spirits of the Head, properly trammel'd, might pace in good order.

'But the only persons who can properly be of benefit to Heads are Periwig-makers, and Doctor Monro, Physician to Moorfields Hospital.

'Wigs are as essential to every person's head as lace is to their clothes; and although understanding may be deficient in the wearer, as well as money, yet people dress'd out look pretty; and very fine Gentlemen, thus embellished, represent those pots upon Apothecaries shelves, which are much ornamented but always stand empty.

'Behold a Barber's Block unadorned: can we conceive any higher idea of it than that of a bruiser just preparing to set to? Indeed, with a foliage round its temples, it might serve in an auction room for the Bust of a Caesar; and provided it was properly worm-eaten, would be bid for accordingly. But of that hereafter, our business now is to show the consequence of Wigs.

Imprimis

'The 'Prentice Minor-bob, or Hair-cap; this is always short in the neck, to show the stone stock-buckle, and nicely stroaked from the face, to discover seven-eights of the ears; and every Smart we meet, so headed, seems, like Tristram Shandy, to have been skaiting against the wind; and his hair, by the sharpness of the motion, shorn from his face.

'Next the Citizen's Sunday buckle, or bob-major; this is a first rate, bearing several tiers of curls, disposed in upper, middle, and lower order.

'Then the Apothecary's bush, in which the hat seems sinking like a stone into a snow heap.

'The Physical and Chirurgical ties, carry much consequence in their fore-tops, and the depending knots face fore and aft the shoulders with secundem artem dignity.

'The scratch, or the Blood's skull-covering, is combed over the forehead untoupeed, to imitate a head of hair, because those gentlemen love to have everything natural about them.

'The Jehu's jemmy, or white and all-white, in little curls, like a fine fleece on a lamb's back, we should say something upon, were in not for fear of offending some gentlemen of great riches, who love to look like coachmen.'

This is to say nothing of the *Spencer*, the *Adonis*, the *cauliflower*, the *Tyburn scratch*, the *caxon*, the *brigadier*, and many others.

It seems clear that the best way out of the maze of wig styles (there are more than two hundred illustrated in this chapter, and there could be many more) is to approach the century analytically rather than chronologically, by first examining the hair itself, then the wig and its various parts and the forms they assumed.

Wigs and Hair

Since the custom of wearing wigs was well established in the seventeenth century, there was no striking change involved in its continuance, even, it would seem, to the stealing of them in the street. According to John Gay:

> Nor is the wig with safety worn;
> High on the shoulder, in a basket born,
> Lurkes the small boy, whose hand to rapine bred,
> Plucks off the curling honors of thy head.

Even the method hadn't changed very much. (See Figure 62, Chapter 8.)

An even more drastic method was brought to the attention of the public in the *Weekly Journal* of March 30, 1717. It seems that wig thieves were robbing gentlemen by cutting through the backs of the hackney coaches in which they were riding, snatching their wigs, and making off with them into the night. 'So a gentleman was served last Sunday in Tooley Street and another but last Tuesday in Fenchurch Street, wherefore this may serve as a caution to gentlemen or gentlewomen that ride

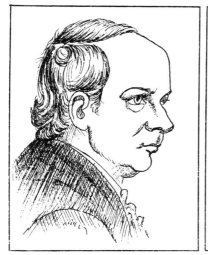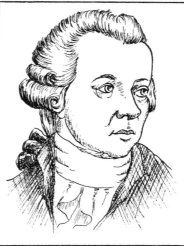

Fig. 68 : Oliver Goldsmith (1728–74) with and without his wig

single in the night-time, to sit on the fore seat, which will prevent that way of robbing.'

A century later, when they were no longer in fashion, the wigs which the thieves went to such trouble to steal could be bought for sixpence apiece in street markets by reaching sight unseen into a barrel and taking whichever wig one happened to come up with. If the first try was not successful, one could dip in as often as one liked for sixpence a dip. Often the wigs were used as dustmops or polishing cloths. But that ignominious end was a long time in coming.

Since the full-bottom wigs which were fashionable at the beginning of the century had obviously gone about as far as they could go in size and weight, to say nothing of expense, a drastic change was called for. No doubt the death of Louis XIV and the accession of the young Louis XV with his beautiful natural hair was the final stroke which put an end to the full-bottom wig as a fashionable style in France and thus throughout the Western world. It was, of course, the opportune moment for a change to natural hair. However, with the upper classes being accustomed to wigs as a status symbol, with the wig-makers becoming well established, along with the source of supply of hair, and with the heads beneath the wigs neatly shaved, the path seemed to lead not back to natural hair, but to a different type of wig.

This had one inevitable consequence. As wigs became less pretentious and less expensive (in 1700 a fine wig sold for as much as £140), they were taken up by the middle classes and even the lower classes so that eventually nearly every man who could afford a wig (with the exception of an occasional eccentric) wore one. And often if he couldn't afford one, he dressed his own hair to look like a wig.

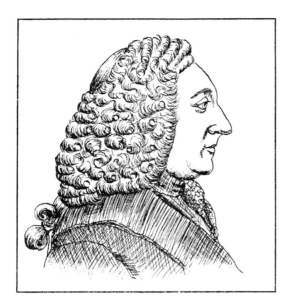

Fig. 69 : Lord Chesterfield (1694–1773)

Still, there were holdouts, even among the upper classes. In 1748 bewigged Lord Chesterfield (Figure 69) wrote in a letter to his son:

'I can by no means agree to your cutting off your hair. I am very sure that your head-aches cannot proceed from thence, and as for the pimples upon your head, they are only owing to the heat of the season, and consequently will not last long. But your own hair is at your age such an ornament, and a wig, however well made, such a disguise, that I will on no account whatsoever have you cut off your hair. Nature did not give it to you for nothing, still less to cause you the head-ache. Mr. Elliot's hair grew so ill and bushy that he was in the right to cut it off. But you have not the same reason.'

Even the children in upper class families wore wigs for dress. But for those who did not Stewart suggested the following:

'First, every morning thoroughly wash the child's neck with cold water, especially behind the ears: and let it be well dried with a coarse cloth. Rub the head well till it smokes; this promotes circulation and dissolves all secretions and stagnations in the head. Afterwards, comb the hair with a large comb; then take about the bigness of a large nut of sweet pomatum, put it in the palm of your left hand, and with the points of your right fingers rub it well into the pores of the head all over; after which, let it be pretty well combed with a small comb, but not too much. This will sweeten the head, take all scurf from the roots of the hair, and nourish it exceedingly, always remembering that the hair be cut regularly every new moon, and that by an experienced hand.'

According to an article in *All the Year Round*, 'The price of a common wig was one guinea; a journeyman usually treated himself to a new one once a year; and it was a frequent clause in an apprentice's indentures that his master should provide him with "one good and sufficient wig yearly during the term of his apprenticeship"'.

Perhaps the spread of wigs to the lower classes in England was not entirely spontaneous. At any rate, it seems that England, anticipating a demand for wigs, had bought up all available hair; but the demand was disappointing and it was necessary to create a demand. Peter Pindar relates his version of the story in verse:

> A hair-brain'd animal from head unknown,
> Yet born and educated near the throne,
> Dropp'd down—(so will'd the dread decree of fate)
> With legs wide-sprawling, on king George's plate.
> The wily Pitt, who soon perceiv'd, no doubt,
> What this new incident might bring about,
> Assured his sovereign that such vermin fed,
> Not on a royal, but a plebeian head;
> And straight advis'd, that every cook and page,
> And servants all, of every sex and age,
> Should shave their heads as smooth as barbers' blocks,
> And all wear wigs of artificial locks.
>
> Ye Gods! What horror seiz'd the varsal band,
> At this despotic, absolute command!
> From garret to the cellar, all turn pale,
> And sadly their devoted locks bewail;
> But no expostulations could prevail,
> Here stood the barber—there the threat'ning jail;
> So all resign'd their heads to fashion's priest,
> And of two evils, wisely chose the least.
>
> As Pitt foresaw, this courtly fashion spread,
> And every loyal subject shaved his head;
> Throughout the island the contagion flew,
> And even cross'd the British channel too;
> The inconstant French of every sex and age,
> Soon cropp'd their hair, and wigs were all the rage.
> O power and greatness! what unstable things!
> Those wigs, which once were worn alone by kings,
> Whence they derived their air of awful state,
> Now decorated every plebeian pate.
> The French, alas! were then compell'd to wear
> Those made in England of the cheapest hair;
> This proved the death of genius and of taste,
> And nobles scorn'd a fashion so bebas'd.

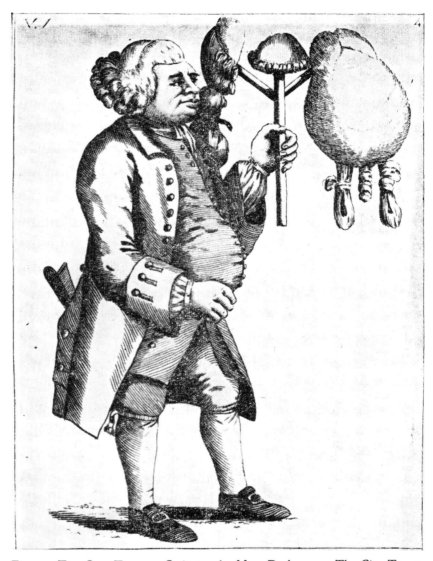

Fig. 70 : THE CITY TONSOR. Caricature by Mary Darly, 1771. The City Tonsor is wearing a major bob and carrying on the stand a cadogan, a minor bob, and a physical tie

Nobody, of course, was happier than the wig-makers, who, during the reign of Louis XIV, became well established as a guild separate from the barber-surgeons. In the 1760s, however, they had a bad scare when there seemed to be evidence of a return to natural hair. Even George III, when he ascended the throne in 1760, wore his own hair powdered and arranged to look as much like a wig as possible. Later he wore an inelegant brown wig without powder, a style referred to thereafter as a 'brown George'.

In 1765 in London the peruke-makers petitioned the king to require by law that all adult citizens wear wigs. It is reported, however, that some of the petitioners were not wearing wigs at the time; and this can hardly have helped their cause. Furthermore, a sly petition purporting to be from the guild of wooden leg makers, which humbly requested His Majesty to wear a wooden leg in order to make them fashionable, probably didn't help either. The petition was denied. In spite of their failure with the king, however, the return to natural hair proved to be premature; and the wig-makers had work for another twenty-five years.

Wigs, even when widely worn, were still the subject of satire. There was a certain police official in Brighton whose wig was immortalized in a bit of doggerel considerably more popular than the man himself:

> Of all the wigs in Brighton town,
> The black, the grey, the red, the brown,
> So firmly glued upon the crown,
> There's none like Johnny Townsend's.

> Its silken hair and flaxen hue,
> It is a scratch and not a queue;
> Whene'er it pops upon the view,
> 'Tis surely Johnny Townsend's!

And over the door of an English barber's shop one might find a sign bearing a picture of David weeping over the dead Absalom and under it the lines:

> Oh, Absalom! Oh, Absalom!
> Oh, Absalom! my son,
> If thou hadst worn a periwig,
> Thou hadst not been undone!

The verse was equally popular in France, where it is said to have originated:

> Passans, contemplez la douleur
> D'Absalom pendu par la nuque;
> Il eut évité ce malheur
> S'il avait porté perruque!

Finally, in the *London Magazine* for 1753 there appeared a satirical piece purporting to be an advertisement for a French periwig maker, which is worth quoting at some length:

'Monsieur de la Papillotte, merchant perriwig-maker, hair-cutter and frisseur, educated under the celebrated artist the Sieur Lattoupe at Paris, now begs leave to advertise you, that being animated by the rising taste of the gentry of this kingdom, he is resolved to abandon his native country, in order to settle in Dublin. . . . His innate modesty would fain cast a veil over his accomplishments, but justice constrains him to publish them for the benefit of mankind and the good of the publick; which obliges him to inform you that he fabricates all kinds of perriwigs for churchmen, lawyers, physicians, military, mercantile, and country gentlemen in a most new, exquisite, curious and extraordinary taste: As for example, to ecclesiastical perriwigs he gives a certain demure air; he confers on the tye-wigs of the law an appearance of great sagacity and deep penetration; on those of the faculty of physick, he casts a solemnity and gravity that seem equal to the profoundest knowledge. His military smarts are mounted in a curious manner, quite unknown to every workman but himself; he throws them into what he calls the animating buckle, which gives the wearer a most warlike fierceness. He has likewise invented a species of major or brigadier for the better sort of citizen and tradesmen, which, by adding a tail to them, that may be taken off and put on at pleasure, may serve extremely well, when they either do duty in the militia or intend to ride the franchises. He also flatters himself upon hitting the taste of the Irish country gentlemen and fox hunters, by his short cut bobs of nine hairs on a side.

'For the gentlemen of the beau monde whose taste and talents lie in dress, he prepares perriwigs frized in the following taste and fashion, all of which are now worn at Paris, viz. *en ailes de pigeon, à la comette, à la choux fleure, à l'oiseau royale, en escalier, en échelle, en brosse, en dos de sanglier, à la temple, à la rhinoceros, en pâte de loup garroté, à la Saxe, à la dragone, en rose, en béquille, en négligé, à la chancallier, à face coupée, en long, en boucle demi naturelle, en chaines, à la bordage, en boucle detachée, à la Janseniste, en point, en escargot, en grain d'épinards, en cul d'artichaut,* &c. &c.

'For young gentlemen of the law, who are not troubled with much practice, he has invented a perriwig, the legs of which may be put into a smart bag during the vacation, and which in term time may be restored to its pristine form. He intends to keep from two to three hundred of this sort always in readiness to hire out occasionally.

'He also makes white woollen bobs, which fit as close as night-caps, very proper to be worn by young persons of distinction, either when they chuse to mount the coach box, or walk in a morning like their footmen in dishabille with an oaken club in their hands. For such as love to save their cash, he will have perriwigs made of calves tails, which he engages will last a long time; this kind (as there is but very little profit to be had by them) he only makes to oblige the fathers of such young sparks who honour him with their custom.

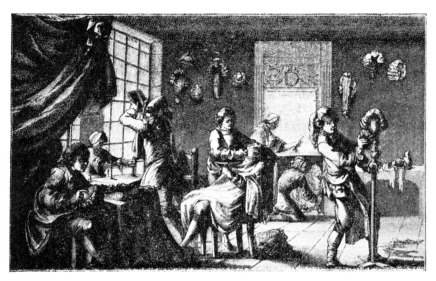

Fig. 71 : Eighteenth-century barber's and wig-maker's shop.
Engraving after Cochin

'He assures the publick that there are but few conditions in life who may not reap a sensible benefit by his labours, as many of his customers have experienced, having by the diversity of his perriwigs contributed greatly to advance the affairs and interest of the wearers; for all the world must allow that it is necessary to have a man's head put into a proper order for business, to have any affair terminate happily.

'He dresses, cuts, curls, and frisses hair in the most elegant taste, either for ladies or gentlemen; and to prevent loss of time at the toilette (a consequence the Irish gentry may at first complain of, but which custom will render in a short time as familiar as in France, where they give up the whole morning to so necessary a duty) he has by long standing and labour discovered and invented a commodious machine, called the night basket, by which ladies and gentlemen may have their heads dressed while they divert themselves at cards without loss of time. This basket being constructed on mathematical principles, is fitted on the inside with several iron points covered with velvet, that attract the hair (it being first oiled and powdered with loadstone dust) and frisses it into the form of the inside of the basket, which is moulded into the tete du mouton, and all other most fashionable shapes now in vogue. The said points preserve the buckles in an admirable symmetry, and the velvet, being dipped in a soporiferous liquor, contributes greatly to comfort the brain and bring on sleep, provided the wearer has not had an ill run at cards.

'He has an admirable secret to colour all kinds of hair on the head and give any tint the wearer pleases; and this he performs without the use of lead combs, mercury or any outward application whatsoever; for as all naturalists allow the hair to be only certain tubes which take their colour according to the quality of the juice with which they are nourished, he has invented a syringe, with which he injects the hair with a liquor of the colour the person chuses to have, or that which may happen to be most in the mode. This method being dear is little used in France, the people of that nation, though they love to shine, love to do it at a cheap rate; on the contrary, the generosity of the Irish, and their contempt of money is well known; the fame thereof has spread to Paris, so that the artist flatters himself his noble designs will meet with the countenance and protection of a people celebrated for their attachment to the beaux arts. This liquor is perfectly innocent and might be a means of conveying several supplies to the internal organs of sensation; but he leaves this as a hint to be prosecuted by the gentlemen of the faculty; and though he boasts himself a barber-surgeon of the honourable fraternity of St. Cone at Paris, he does not mean to encroach on the upper branch of a profession he has only the honour of being an understrapper of.'

Unfortunately, some of these satires on contemporary customs are so subtle in their exaggeration and the fact and fiction so skilfully interspersed that occasionally later writers have accepted them verbatim and have listed as historical fact that which was invented purely for purposes of satire. In fact, little more than a century later the method of hair dyeing described above was reported quite seriously as one of the curiosities of eighteenth-century life.

The hair of the wig was treated in three different ways—it was curled, frizzed, or left more or less straight. It was seldom really waved. Most wig styles called for two of these treatments in combination, sometimes all three.

Curled Hair. The full-bottom wig, as we have noted before, was a mass of cascading curls, which were eventually confined to the back of the wig when used at all. But smaller spiral curls, soft, loose curls, or stiff roll curls, either alone or in tiers, were used throughout the century (see Plate 72).

Pipes or *roulettes* were used in curling wigs. According to Redfern, 'these were of pipe-clay and were heated over a stove, and when the pipes were sufficiently hot they were used on the wigs in the same way as curling-tongs are now employed. The various sizes range from the small pipe for the upper part of the wig to the enormous roulette which formed the larger curls at the lower end of it.' (See Plate 58-S.)

The natural hair was often curled by means of *papillottes* or curl papers, as shown in Plate 68-M. This might be done by either oneself or one's valet.

Frizzed Hair. Whenever a bushy effect was desired, as it frequently was, the hair was *frizzed* or *frizzled*, terms used to refer to very small tight curls or crimped hair which could be combed out into a bush (Plate 68-A, for example). This was sometimes fashionable, sometimes not; but it was worn in one form or another throughout the century. It was usually combined with straight hair (Plate 68-I) and sometimes with both straight hair and curls (Plate 76-G).

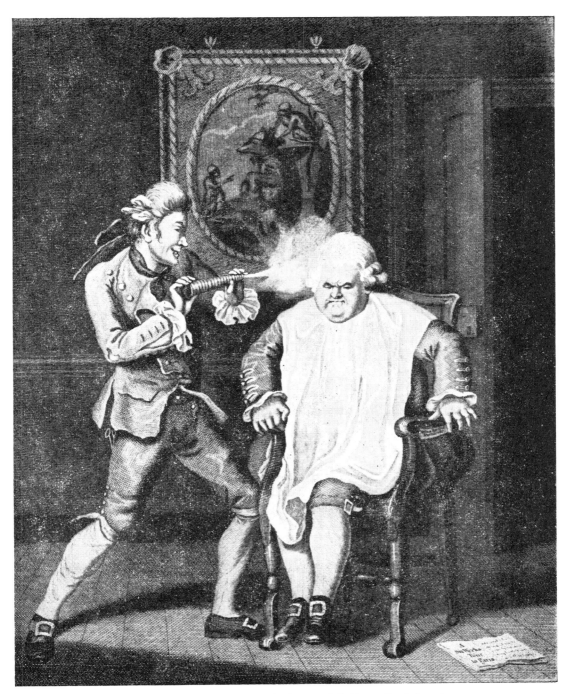

Fig. 72 : THE ENGLISHMAN IN PARIS. Powdering the hair with bellows. English caricature, 1770

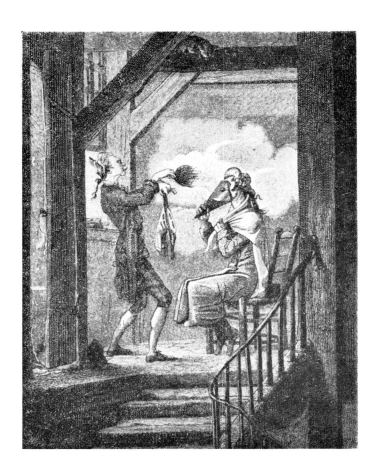

Fig. 73 : LA TOILETTE. Engraving after Carle Vernet, late eighteenth century. A gentleman holding a face cone is being powdered by his valet.

All of this frizzing and curling came in for its share of criticism, for those who are in fashion are always criticized by those who are out. In the December 1772 issue of *Gentleman's Magazine* a disgruntled correspondent submitted the following verse:

> To describe, in its dressing, the taste of the time,
> (To answer your purpose, and fill up my rhime)
> Your choice must be made, for a figure exemplar,
> Of a captain, a cit, maccaroni, or templar.
> Let his figure be slender, and lounging, and slim,
> Confoundedly formal, and awkwardly trim.
> Hang a hat on his head, let it squint fiercely down,
> And be cut, slash'd, and scollop'd, and par'd to the crown.
> Behind this strange head a thick queue you must tye on,
> Like a constable's bludgeon, or tail of a lion;
> And before, when you try to embellish his hair,
> Let your fingers be quick, and your powder be fair;
> Be-friz it, and paste it, and cut it, and curl it,
> Now slope it in ranges, in rollers now furl it.
> For the head of a fribble or beau (without doubt)
> Having nothing within, should have something without. . . .

Straight Hair. Nearly all wig styles contained some straight hair with the notable exceptions of the full-bottom and the unfashionable *cut wig*, which, when curled all over, was sometimes referred to as a *cauliflower wig* for obvious reasons (Plate 69-CC). Even in the styles which show no straight hair from the front (Plate 68-A), there is straight hair at the crown, as in Plate 68-C.

Few wigs were composed entirely of uncurled hair, and those which were or which came close to it (Plate 72-B) were never fashionable. Natural hair (also unfashionable until late in the century, except briefly in the sixties) might be worn uncurled; but there was often a slight natural wave.

Length of the Hair. The long full-bottom wigs became shorter in the third decade. In fact, after that, hair generally tended to be shorter, though one must distinguish between the body of the hair and the queue. Wigs without queues were seldom much more than shoulder length, with the exception of those full-bottoms which remained. However, queues were often quite long, though late in the century they were shortened considerably. At the end of the century rather short hair was in fashion.

Colour of the Hair. Even before the beginning of the century powder had been used sporadically to change the colour of the hair. About 1703 a plain white powder is believed to have been used for the first time. About 1714 bleaching was tried, but it was not successful; and for the greater part of the century powdering was commonplace. No house of any consequence built during the period was without at least one wig closet, where the powdering was done. Those who lacked powdering facilities of their own sent their wigs by messenger to the wig-maker or, if necessary, went themselves.

Wigs could be powdered by one's valet (or the wig-maker) without one's being involved in the mess at all; but if the natural hair was to be powdered or if one's own front hair was to be blended into the wig, that involved a rather special technique. Since the powder was blown on with special bellows (Figure 72), and as there was no really practical way of confining the powder to the hair, it was necessary to devise some means of keeping the powder off the man during this process. This was done by means of a cape or apron and a face mask, two versions of which are shown in Plate 69-R (see also Figure 73). The mask was held in front of his own face by the man being powdered, while the servant operated the bellows. The powder might be blown directly towards the hair, or it might be blown upward and allowed to float down. Either way it was undoubtedly all encompassing.

The effect of freshly powdered hair was both striking and becoming; but unfortunately, all of the powder did not stay on the hair. Gay prudently advised his readers on meeting a coxcomb to pass 'with caution by, lest from his shoulders clouds of powder fly'. In the National Gallery of Art in Stockholm there is a portrait of George Washington by A. U. Wertmüler clearly showing a fine dusting of powder on the shoulders.

The powder was encouraged to stick to the hair by first plastering it with grease or pomatum; but even though that proved a deterrent to the production of clouds of powder drifting in one's wake, it hardly prevented anything touching the hair from being rather the worse for the encounter.

Various substances were used for powdering, wheat flour being the first. It was calculated that in the time of George II, every soldier used a pound of flour a week on his hair. But in about 1715 riots in Caen, resulting from the fact that badly needed flour for bread was being used by aristocrats to put on their heads, encouraged a search for substitutes. One of these was a powder made from a soft white earth, accidentally discovered and developed by John Schnorr, a German ironmaster. Another was a mixture of starch and plaster of paris. There is a record of fifty-one English barbers being fined twenty pounds for possessing powder not made of starch. Later another forty-nine were arrested and fined for the same infraction of the law.

Early hair powder was usually either white or grey, sometimes black or brown, very occasionally blond. Later it was tinted in various colours—pink, blue, and lavender—and strongly scented. Cunnington quotes the diary of John Crosier for May 1782: 'Much aversion as people in general have to red hair, the appearance thereof was so much admired that it became the fashion, for all the Beaus, and Bells wore red powder'. But this was unusual. In the *Monthly Magazine* of 1806 Fox is described as having 'his red-heeled shoes and his blue hair powder'. Though tinted powders were popular with the dandies, the average man stuck with the white and the grey.

The use of powder declined somewhat during the latter years of the century, and the Revolution saw the end of it in France. In England the end came when a law was enacted by Pitt's government requiring anyone using hair powder, no matter how little, to purchase a licence at one guinea per year. It is reported that revenue the first year amounted to £210,136. But that was not to continue for long. The opposition, who called the licence purchasers 'guinea-pigs', was led by several prominent Whigs, including the Duke of Bedford. In a meeting at Woburn Abbey, they cut off their pigtails (presumably they were no longer wearing wigs) and vowed to use no more powder. *Sic transit gloria mundi.*

There were interesting and curious exemptions specified in the Act, among them, according to William Redfern, 'the Royal family and their servants, clergymen not possessing an income of a hundred pounds a year, subalterns in the army and officers in the navy, under the rank of masters and commanders . . . and in families all daughters except the two eldest were also exempted'.

Materials Used. Better wigs were always made of human hair, most of which was imported, although it is recorded that in 1700 a young English countrywoman received fifty pounds for her hair, at the rate of three pounds per ounce. Hair from the northern countries was preferred, and Stewart tells us in his *Plocacosmos* that 'the merit of good hair consists in its being well fed and neither too coarse nor too slender; the bigness rendering it less susceptible of the artificial curl and disposing it rather to frizzle, and the smallness making its curl of too short duration. Its length should be about 30 inches; the more it falls short of this, the less value it bears. There is no certain price for hair; but it is sold from 5 shillings to £5 per ounce, according to its quality. The scarceness of grey and white hairs have put the dealers in that commodity upon the method of reducing other colors to this. This is done by spreading the hair to bleach on the grass, like linen, after first washing it out in a lixivious water; this lye, with the force of the sun and air, brings the hair to so perfect a whiteness that the most experienced person may be deceived therein. . . . Hair made perfectly clean and moistened with the solution of silver in aqua fortis, exposing it to the sun, in order to hasten the appearance and deepen the colour, will be changed from a red, grey, or other disagreeable color, to a brown or deep black.'

For cheaper wigs animal hair was sometimes used. Perhaps the most curious substitution was that of feathers, used largely for the foretop. Thus, one finds references to 'feather-top' wigs, which were used a good deal for outdoor activities and, it seems, by parsons. One peruke-maker's advertisement reads, 'Very durable wigs, not to be hurt at least by wet, made of the single feathers in mallards tails'. Another advertisement, in January 1761, offers 'Gentlemen's perukes for sporting made of drakes' tails'. English weather being what it is, the feather tops were no doubt quite practical.

It was reported in May 1750, in the *Ipswich Journal*, that 'a certain peruke maker has distanced all his brethren by a new invention of making a wig of copper wire which will resist all weathers and last for ever'. But apparently the invention did not sweep the country.

Our investigation of the actual dressing of the hair, which was done by the local peruke-maker if one did not have a valet skilled in the art, can probably best be accomplished by dividing the hair into three areas—the foretop, the temples, and the back.

FORETOP

The term was used to refer to the front part of the hair or the wig immediately above the forehead.

The full-bottom wigs of the seventeenth century were usually parted in the centre; and the centre parting was maintained, though not universally, into the beginning of the eighteenth century. But it was little seen after 1730. When a parting was used, however, it was invariably in the centre.

Usually the foretop of the wig was built up slightly, as in Plate 67-N, or considerably, as in 68-A. The reason for this may have been partly that men were accustomed to the high foretops of the full-bottom wigs; but surely it was also governed by the fact that the construction of wigs at that time did not make possible a natural hairline, and the clumsiness of the hairline became less apparent when the front hair was worked forward and then combed up and back.

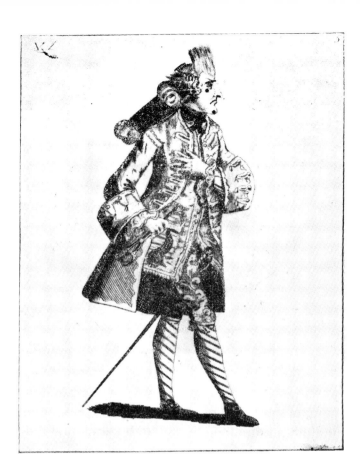

Fig. 74 : Monʳ Le Frizuer (sic). Caricature by Mary Darly, 1771, showing a Macaroni hairdresser with his high toupee and enormous club behind

Sometimes, in order to make a more natural hairline and to simplify the construction and lower the cost of a wig, the natural front hair was combed over the front edge of the wig and blended into the hair of the wig. ('I suffered my hair to grow long enough to comb back over the foretop of my wig, which, when I sallied forth to my evening amusement, I changed to a queue.') If the wig was powdered, the blending caused no problem. Eventually the partial wigs, specifically designed to be worn with natural front hair, became quite small, being attached below the crown and serving only to provide a queue. The drawing of John Adams in Plate 77-P is taken from an unusual and rare etching which clearly shows the rather unconvincing join between the real hair and the false.

As it developed in importance, the foretop of the natural hair or of the wig came to be known as the *toupee*. The meaning of the term has since changed slightly; but whenever it is used in this chapter, it will refer to the raised or extended foretop, whether natural or artificial.

During the century the toupee gradually became increasingly important, sometimes shooting dramatically upward, as in the 1770s (Plate 72-L), but always creeping slowly back toward the crown (72-N), past the crown (72-K), and down toward the neck (76-E) and eventually almost enveloping the head, leaving nothing but a tail behind (77-F).

The dramatic development of the seventies was brought about in England directly by the Macaronis, a group of elegant young men who had spent some time in Italy and had brought back new ideas with them. Plate 72-J shows a typical Macaroni style. The highly exaggerated toupee was built up on wire frames or cushions of wool or felt. Even the children were affected by the style, as shown in Plate 73-M. As early as the sixties, however, before the Macaronis became influential, the toupee was being brushed up over pads. The Macaronis merely gave it a little extra push.

The toupee was soon lowered and resumed its backward move, forming itself into a modified horseshoe shape when viewed from the rear (Plate 73-S). This was called a *grècque*, the French word, as so often happened, being adopted.

From the mid-eighties to the mid-nineties the toupee, in addition to extending farther back and being lower, was often wider and frequently bushy and slightly wavy or frizzled rather than smooth. We can see the style in the familiar likeness of George Washington (Plate 74-Q), Mozart (Plate 76-M), Robespierre (76-S), and Lafayette (Plate 77-F).

In some styles of wigs the foretop was composed of a brush of short hair. This took two forms—*la coque*, which was brushed straight up, as shown in Figure 77-A-B-E-G-H, and *l'étoile*, which was curled toward the centre, as in Figure 77-C-D.

At the end of the century the toupee as such tended to disappear as the hair of the foretop was combed forward (Plate 75-T). Although this was not the first time in the century this had been done, it was the first time it had been really fashionable. Sometimes the foretop of a wig, especially the scratch wig, was brought forward in order to give a more natural hairline, as in Plate 71-A. In the latter part of the century (about 1785–95) the toupee, which obviously had come to encompass a good deal more than the foretop, could not really be separated from the hair at the temples, which will be our next consideration.

SIDES

With the passing of the full-bottom, this area began to take on an individuality of its own. When the bulk of the hair began to be drawn to the back and tied, side sections were left hanging in front of the ears. The French called them *ailes de pigeon*. The term was sometimes used in English, sometimes translated simply as *pigeon's wings* or *pigeon wings* or occasionally as *wings*. The origin of the term is not hard to understand (Plate 68-H is a good example); however, it came to be applied to any similar arrangement of the side hair even when the resemblance to the wings of a pigeon was more remote. Hogarth seems to have used the term to refer to all side hair, as, for example, in all five orders of periwigs (Figure 76). But pigeon wings, in the original sense of the term, with the hair hanging loose or frizzed or lightly curled, went out of style about 1740, though they continued to be seen and were

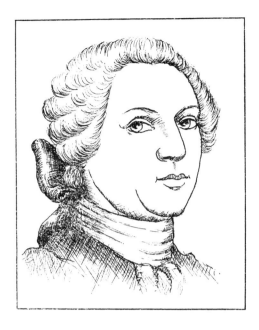

Fig. 75 : Louis XV (1710–74), King of France

revived to some extent late in the century. They were largely replaced by from one to five stiff, horizontal roll curls (Plate 76-E, for example). These were called *buckles*, a corruption of the French *boucles*. A wig with such side curls might be called a *buckled* wig. Sometimes these side curls became *puffs*, rolled over a foundation of frizzed hair (Plate 77-D). When the natural hair was worn, it was done up in curl papers to make the buckles (see Plate 68-M).

The size, length, number, and placement of the curls varied considerably, as can be seen from the various plates. Stewart says, 'A full dress is five curls, which when wore, fills up the side of the head considerably more by which means there is less top or feather'. At the end of the century there was a fashion for a single roll curl, usually not large, extending around the head from ear to ear (Plate 76-S).

BACK OF THE HEAD

The greatest variation of all is found in the treatment of the back part of the wig or the hair, and it is from the style of this part that the wig usually takes its name—bob, tie, bag, cadogan, etc.

Wigs can be divided into two general categories—those with queues and those without. Both were worn throughout the greater part of the century, and those who could afford to often had both types for different occasions, the wig with queue being the dressier of the two. Both types were fairly long in the beginning and became shorter later on. And both types were sometimes powdered, sometimes not. A powdered wig was considered more formal than one of natural colour.

WIGS WITHOUT QUEUES

The first and most obvious of these is the well established *full-bottom*, a carry-over from the seventeenth century.

Full-bottom Wig. In 1700 the style was at its peak and ready to go into a decline. The long, high-peaked wig (Plate 67-A) began to shrink, as we can see in the sketch of Handel (Plate 67-P). There the wig is not only greatly reduced but also powdered. George II (Plate 67-Q) retains more curls than Handel, but the body of the wig is less voluminous. The curious Italian wig shown in Plate 67-I hardly deserves to be called a full-bottom at all.

Along with the shrinking came various modifications, such as the *square wig*. The version on Plate 67 is from Diderot's *Encyclopedia*, and that on Plate 68-C is Hogarth's so-called *Lexonic wig* from his satiric five orders of periwigs (Figure 76). Another version of the full-bottom is called by Hogarth the *Aldermanic* because it was worn by aldermen; the *Parsonic*, so called for the obvious reason, seems to hover between being a full-bottom and a bob.

Knotted Wig. This is an outgrowth of the full-bottom wig, which cannot have been particularly comfortable at any time and was certainly hot in summer. The ends were sometimes knotted together on either side for comfort, and a very durable style was born. Although the central portion in back was sometimes knotted, it more frequently ended in a spiral curl like that on the square wig. Hogarth calls this curl a *necklock*, whereas Randle Holme refers to it variously as a *pole lock*, a *suffloplin*, or a *dildo*. Diderot's version is shown on Plate 69 and Hogarth's in Figure 76. Much fuller and higher bushy knotted wigs can be found in Plates 67-M and 70-A. These were also known as *campaign wigs* or sometimes as *travelling wigs*, and they were very popular, especially with older men. The knots were allowed to fall where they might. The bushy knotted wig was also called a *physical tie*. ('The Physical and Chirurgical ties carry much consequence in their fore-tops, and the depending knots face fore and aft the shoulders with secundem artem dignity.')

Bob Wig. This is a comprehensive term including what appears at first glance to be a variety of styles. And many of the modifications were indicated in popular names of the wig—*long bob*, *short bob*, *'prentice minor bob*, *physical bob*, *bob major*, *full dress bob*, *scratch bob*, *full bob*, *clergymen's bob*, etc. Some of these are identified along with the drawings. In the eighteenth century the term *bob* applied only to men since there was no occasion to apply it to women. In the mid-twentieth century it was defined in Webster's dictionary as 'a woman's or girl's short haircut'. The essential characteristic of the bob in either case was that the hair was cut off more or less evenly all around. The short bobs (Plate 71-J) were cut high enough to expose the neck, whereas the long bobs (Plate 72-A) covered the neck and might be shoulder length.

Early in the century the bob was often parted in the centre, but in the thirties or after it was more likely to be brushed straight back. Usually there was either a bush of frizzed hair, a single roll curl, or a tier of roll curls, sometimes smooth and even, sometimes broken, from ear to ear around the back. Plate 72-C shows a very bushy bob, usually designated as a *physical bob*, a term used to refer to any very full, bushy bob. This one seems to answer perfectly to the description referred to earlier, 'the Apothecary's bush, in which the hat seems sinking like a stone into a snow heap'.

Scratch Wig. This was a small undress wig, which was especially popular with the lower classes because it was relatively inexpensive. The term, like so many others, covers a variety of styles, and the final effect depended a good deal on how it was worn. It could be dressed to become a 'natty scratch' or it could hang limp and look fairly disreputable. It deserves special attention because it was often used as a partial wig, comparable to the *fall* later used for theatrical purposes. It could be worn with the natural front hair combed into it, combining the advantages of a natural hairline and a smaller, lighter, less expensive wig. Sometimes the front hair of the scratch was combed down over the forehead to give a more natural effect. This would have to be done if one had only a scratch to wear and no front hair to blend into it.

Plate 69-G is probably a *scratch bob* (in other words, a partial bob). Drawing O on the same plate could be natural hair but is probably a scratch. V shows rather clearly how the scratch is combined with natural hair, in this case by a man who doesn't much care how he looks. A, C, and I on Plate 71 show scratches with the front hair combed forward, and B shows a scratch merely set on the head like a cap with no attempt to make it look presentable or to blend it with the natural hair. The best example of a scratch wig is probably that of Denis Diderot, shown in Plate 73-AA.

An article in *Leisure Hour* in the late nineteenth century takes a definite stand on the scratch wig:

'We suppose it will be admitted that the last age of the wig is, after all, the most contemptible in point of fashion—the scratch-wig—the lineal descendant, however, of that which has, for want of any better designation, been called by a writer in the *Quarterly* the George-the-Fourthian Peruke. Lest we should seem irreverent, we may quote this high conservative authority, who speaks of it as "an upstart sham among wigs, hideous, artificial, and gentish looking; its painful little curls haunt us. We scarcely ever see that type now in its full original horror, but bad is the best; it seems at first thought very odd that barbers cannot make a decent imitation of a head of hair." From this descended, we say, the scratch-wig, whose highest ambition consists in being like the natural hair; its aim is to make age look youthful, and to give to the baldness of Cicero and Caesar the beauty, if not of flowing locks, the reverse of the prophetic condemnation in the adornment of well-set hair.'

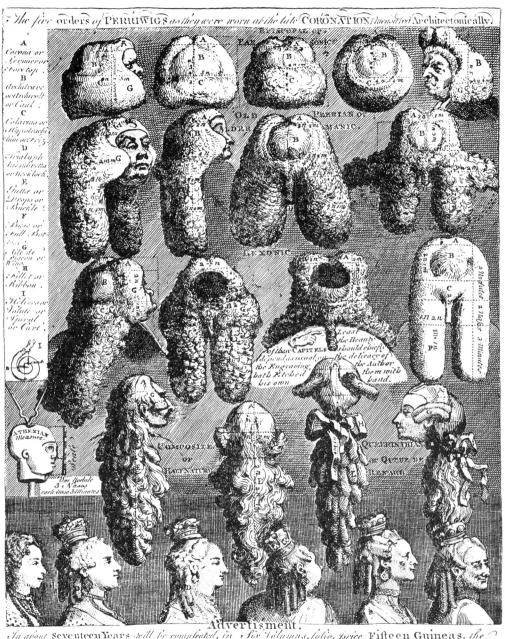

Fig. 76 : THE FIVE ORDERS OF PERRIWIGS by William Hogarth, 1761

It would seem from this that the term may also have applied, especially later, to any small wig used to represent the natural hair and to conceal baldness—in other words, what has since come to be called a toupee. Perhaps it was some such small wig that Cowper was referring to in a letter to his cousin, Lady Hesketh, when he wrote:

'As for me, I am a very smart youth of my years; I am not, indeed, grown grey so much as I am grown bald. No matter; there was more hair in the world than ever had the honour to belong to me. Accordingly, I have found just enough to curl a little at my ears, and to intertwine with a little of my own that still hangs behind. I appear, if you see me in the afternoon, to have a very decent head-dress, not easily distinguished from my natural growth, which, being worn with a small bag and a black ribbon about my neck, continues to me the charms of my youth, even on the verge of old age.'

Cut Wig. This is a small, fairly short-haired wig worn largely by coachmen, riders, artisans, etc. It might be curled all over (Plate 69-CC), a style favoured by coachmen; or it might be straight. The cut wig shown in Plate 76-F is about halfway between. Possibly it was once curled and now has lost most of the curl. The fleecy white Jehu's jemmy, previously described as a favourite among 'gentlemen of great riches, who love to look like coachmen', would be a curled and powdered cut wig.

WIGS WITH QUEUES

In the earliest years of the century wigs with queues, first worn for convenience by the military, were not considered fashionable and were worn mostly when travelling or when engaging in some physical activity for which they were more practical than the large full-bottom wigs. But after their modest beginning, they became fashionable in about 1740 and retained their supremacy in one form or another until the very last years of the century.

There was a variety of queues. The *Irish Quarterly Review* gives a partial list:

'There was the thick braid of hair hanging down between the shoulders; the smaller tail, tightly bound up with black ribbon; the loosely-tied tail; the tail of the courtier, with a bag attached to it; the short medical tail; the gentleman's tail, and military tails of all kinds—the most whimsical of which was that invented in the time of the Duke of York, which, looking like a small riding-whip and hanging between the shoulders, was supposed to ward off the cut of a sabre; but which caused so much pain and inconvenience when fastened to the hair, that officers frequently attached theirs to their caps or helmets; and a row of tails might be seen hanging up in the hall, while their owners were at dinner, rejoicing in their freedom.'

Tie Wig. Just as the knotted wig was evolved to keep the hair under control, so was the tie (or tye) wig. In this case the hair was kept even tidier by pulling it all to the rear, tying it together, and letting the curls fall freely down the back. In the early tie wigs, however, the ears frequently remained covered; in the later ones they were

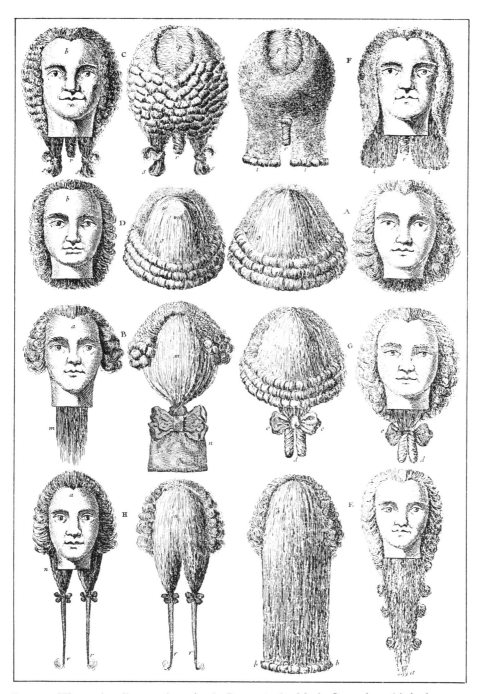

Fig. 77 : Wig styles illustrated in *Art du Perruquier* by M. de Garsault, published 1767

more likely to be exposed. In Hogarth's *foxtail wig* we see all of the curls at the back securely tied by a great deal of ribbon. Plate 69-J shows a very simple tie with the hair hanging straight instead of curled. G and H on Plate 75 show much later and more elegant ties, the one with quite a wide ribbon; and 69-A shows the *solitaire*, the long ends of the bow (always black) being brought around the neck and tied in front—the origin of the bow tie. More examples of the solitaire, which was considered very dressy, will be found with other styles of queue wig. The early tie wig had a centre parting; later ones usually did not. Plate 76-A, representing rather a late style, shows a tie with the hair combed forward from the crown; 71-U shows another late tie with as much ribbon as hair in the queue.

In a letter written in 1745, Horace Walpole said of Lord Sandwich, 'I could have no hope of getting at his ear for he has put on such a first-rate tie wig that nothing without the lungs of a boatswain can even think to penetrate the thickness of the curls'.

Writing in the 1780s, hairdresser William Barker expressed the opinion that 'Tye wigs, of all others, seem most becoming and graceful, more especially since the late alteration they have undergone. Formerly tye wigs, which have been worn by judges and counsellors ever since the reign of Charles II, entirely covered the ear, intimating perhaps the propriety of avoiding law suits, as in many instances Justice may be said to be deaf as well as blind.'

Bag Wig. In the very early days of the tie wig it was customary for soldiers to encase their queues in black bags with draw strings as a matter of convenience. Eventually the practice became fashionable, and after about 1730 bag wigs were seen increasingly. They were usually of black silk or taffeta, tied with a drawstring and decorated with a matching stiff bow or rosette. Plate 73-Q, R, and W show the front and back view of Diderot's bag wig with its rosette. The size shown there is the normal size in comparison to the size of the wig. The early ones were square, of medium size, and stuffed to appear full of hair; later they became narrower, longer, and flatter. In the 1770s there was a fashion for very large bags (Plate 77-A). The bow took various shapes. Sometimes we see the bag wig combined with a solitaire.

The bag could be combined with almost any style for the body of the wig or for the natural hair if it was long enough. James Stewart in his instructions on hairdressing said that 'if the hair is worn in a bag behind, you must tie it in the smallest twist or club you can, to keep the bag on, the bag to be put on after powdering'.

Once the bag wig was established among civilians and accepted by fashionable men, it maintained its position as a dress wig until very nearly the end of the century. The dressiness depended on the care with which the wig itself was dressed and the smartness and crispness of the bag and the bow.

In 1772 George Washington wore his natural brown hair, unpowdered. During the Revolution he wore powdered hair and the queue in a black silk bag, which was sometimes tied with a narrow ribbon, sometimes with a broad bow or even a wide bow with a pinked edge. Later he occasionally 'wore it pinned with a brooch set with a single diamond, to match the knee buckles he wore in 1793 at his second inauguration when he appeared in black velvet and powdered hair'.

Ramillies Wig. This was a wig with a long braided tail (Plate 73-Y), usually having two bows. Late in the century (particularly in the 1790s), the braided queue was sometimes looped up and secured with a comb below the crown (Plate 77-J). This was especially popular with the military. The name was in honour of the battle of Ramillies in 1706, in which the English defeated the French.

Pigtail Wig. This was an extremely durable style, considered smart but not dressy, and was very popular with the military. The queues were tightly bound with black, often with a few hairs sticking out at the end. The early pigtails tended to be fairly long, but late in the century they became much shorter. Their width varied from thick to very slender; they could be worn with or without a small bow at the top; and sometimes, more frequently in France than in England, there were two tails (see Plate 75-L and Figure 78.)

Although early military pigtails were made of the natural hair, later ones were often of black leather or, in the British army, whalebone (for officers) or metal wire (for the men) bound with black ribbon. Tufts of real hair frequently protruded from the ends. British sailors sometimes smeared their pigtails with tar. Early military pigtails were as much as two feet long. Usually, except among some of the officers, they were part of or attached to the natural hair rather than being part of a wig.

Cadogan or Club Wig. The cadogan, named after the Earl of Cadogan, did not appear until the 1760s; but after that it became extremely popular and lasted almost until the end of the century. The hair of the queue hung down straight, broad, and flat and then was doubled up on itself and tied around the middle, usually just below the neck (see Plate 72-O). The size of the club varied but was at its largest in the early seventies when the Macaronis balanced their enormously high toupees with huge cadogans or clubs. This, naturally, provided plenty of material for satirists. We can see examples in the Darly caricatures in Figures 74 and 78. There is also a cadogan on the wig stand in Figure 70.

There were even songs about the Macaronis. One of them was called simply *The Macaroni*:

> Ye belles and beaux of London town,
>   Come listen to my ditty;
> The Muse in prancing up and down
>   Has found out something pretty.
> With little hat and hair dress'd high,
>   And whip to ride a pony;
> If you but take a right survey,
>   Denotes a Macaroni

Along the street to see them walk,
  With tail of monstrous size, sir,
You'll often hear the grave ones talk,
  And wish their sons were wiser.
With consequence they strut and grin,
  And fool away their money;
Advice they care for not a pin,—
  Ay,—that's a Macaroni!

With boots and spurs and jockey-cap,
  And breeches like a sack, O;
Like curs sometimes they'll bite and snap,
  And give their whip a smack, O.
When this you see, then think of me,
  My name is Merry Crony;
I'll swear the figure that you see
  Is called a Macaroni.

Five pounds of hair they wear behind,
  The ladies to delight, O;
Their senses give unto the wind,
  To make themselves a fright, O.
This fashion who does e'er pursue,
  I think a simple-tony;
For he's a fool, say what you will,
  Who is a Macaroni.

Major and Brigadier Wigs. There has been considerable confusion about this terminology. It was thought at one time that the major had one tail and the brigadier two, but contemporary references to a two-tailed major have made it clear that this was not so. So far as we know, they were the same thing. The term *brigadière* was used by the French and *major* (and to a somewhat lesser extent *brigadier*) by the English. Plate 73-U is the French brigadier wig shown in Diderot's *Encyclopedia*. It is a dress bob with the queue added. There was always a bow or a rosette and always two spiral curls.

Quite different in appearance was the English major (Plate 71-L), in which the two curls and a small bow were attached directly to the underside of the wig. The fact that one was a bushy bob and the other a buckled bob adds to the contrast, but this has nothing to do with the general classification.

In Plate 71-G we see the back view of a long, bushy bob with a single tail. Although this was less common than the double tail, it may also have been called a *major*. Since one eighteenth-century gentleman left scribbled notes indicating that

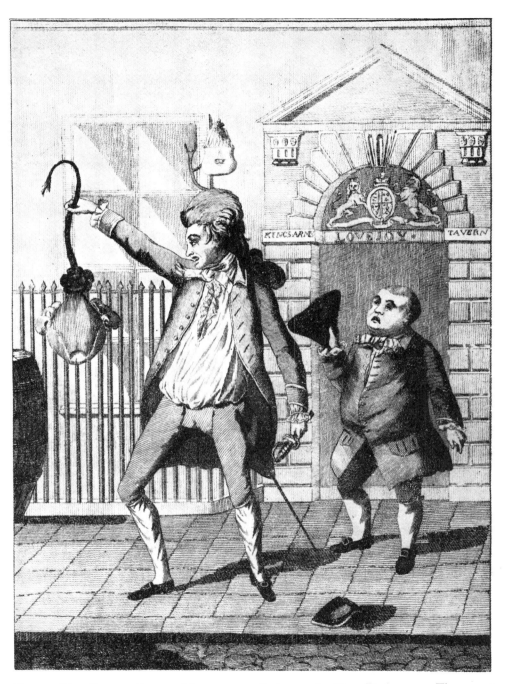

Fig. 78 : THE COVENT GARDEN MACARONIES. Caricature by Mary Darly, 1771. The young
Macaroni, registering mock distaste for his companion's old-fashioned pigtail, appears
to be on the point of cutting it off

he considered the one-tailed wig a *major* and the two-tailed, a *brigadier*, it's entirely possible that it started out that way and that subsequently the terms became interchangeable with careless usage. But even though the two-tailed wig was called a *major*, the one-tailed was presumably not called a *brigadier*. Plate 76-P shows a German version of the one-tailed major. Both the major and the brigadier were primarily military wigs but were also worn by civilians.

Men with a practical turn of mind sometimes made one wig do for two by turning a *bob* into a *major* with the addition of a tail or two. In the July 18, 1754, issue of the *Connoisseur*, an essay complaining about the 'Vanity of People Making an Appearance above their Circumstances' refers patronizingly to 'a man of this cast who has but one coat; but by now and then turning the cuffs and changing the cape, it passes for two. He uses the same artifice with his peruke, which is naturally a kind of flowing bob; but by the occasional addition of two tails, it sometimes appears as a Major.' A glance at Plate 71-L will show how easily this could be done.

Spencer Wig. There is still further confusion about the Spencer, shown in Plate 72-H. It was frequently mentioned by contemporary writers, who considered it a fashionable wig, although none of them ever bothered to describe it. Hogarth, however, in his *Analysis of Beauty*, refers specifically to the wig illustrated as a *Spencer*. Although Cunnington, who lists the Spencer as 'not identified', calls this wig a *major*, there seems to be no reason to discredit Hogarth in the matter, particularly since this wig is quite different from wigs we know to have been called *majors*.

Natural Wigs. This is a general term covering those wigs which were made to look like natural hair or in which the hair was allowed to hang loose without being tied up or frizzed or excessively curled. Hogarth refers to Plate 68-E as a *half-natural*.

Related to these is the *peruke naissante* or *à l'enfant* (Plate 75-D), little worn in England but fashionable in France late in the century. A more formal version is shown in Diderot's *Encyclopedia*, published about 1770 (see Plate 73-O-P).

TO EACH HIS OWN

One of the most curious aspects of eighteenth-century men's hair, apart from the almost universal use of wigs, is the identification of certain styles with certain professions. Normally, the leaders of fashion set the style, which gradually gains acceptance among the middle and lower classes. That, in turn, makes it necessary for the leaders to develop new styles if they have not already done so. This also happened in the eighteenth century; but at the same time there were professional groups who, on the whole, stuck to their conventional wigs, though there were fashion-followers in every group.

James Stewart, writing in 1782, said that 'As the perukes became more common, their shape and forms altered. Hence we hear of the clerical, the physical, and the tie peruke for the man of the law, the brigadier or major for the army and navy; as also the tremendous fox-ear or cluster of temple curls with a pig-tail behind.

'The merchant, the man of business and of letters were distinguished by the grave full-bottom, or more moderate tie, neatly curled; the tradesman by the snug bob or natty scratch, the country gentleman by the natural fly and hunting peruke.

'All conditions of men were distinguished by the cut of the wig, and none more so than the coachman who wore his, as there does some to this day, in imitation of the curled hair of a water dog.' The latter we have already noted on Plate 69-CC.

There is a contemporary listing of special wigs in Colman's Prologue to Garrick's *High Life Above Stairs*:

> Fashion, in everything, bears sovereign sway,
> And words and periwigs have both their day;
> Each have their purlieus, too, — are modish each
> In stated districts, wigs as well as speech.
> The Tyburn scratch, thick club, and Temple-tie,
> The parson's feather-top, frizzed broad and high,
> The coachman's cauliflower, built tier on tiers,
> Differ not more from bags and brigadiers,
> Than great St. George's or St. James's styles
> From the broad dialect of broad St. Giles.

In 1786 Jacques Dulaure, referring to the French fashions, wrote:

'A tradesman . . . to appear as he ought, should have his head shaved and wear a round wig; physicians and surgeons too should do the same. Who, in this enlightened age, would put the least confidence in a physician who wears his own hair, were it the finest in the world? A wig, certainly, can't give him science, but it gives him the appearance, and that is everything nowadays.' There is a footnote to this: 'Strip a physician of his wig, gold headed cane, ruffles, and diamond ring; what will he have left?'

In the *Connoisseur* for April 24, 1755, a mode of behaviour and dress is described as being 'as improper as a physician would seem ridiculous prescribing in a bag-wig, or a serjeant pleading in the Court of Common Pleas in his own hair instead of a night-cap periwig'.

As to the men of fashion, they abandoned the full-bottom and went on to the knotted wig, the tie, the bag (which proved extremely durable), the club, etc. These have all been discussed under their respective headings.

Fashion is always a popular and legitimate target for the satirist, and the eighteenth century provided a plethora of material. In 1753, when the bag wig was in fashion, the following verse appeared in the *London Magazine*:

> Take a creature that nature has form'd without brains,
> Whose skull nought but nonsense and sonnets contains;

With a mind where conceit with folly's ally'd,
Set off by assurance and unmeaning pride;
With commonplace jests for to tickel the ear
With mirth, where no wisdom could ever appear;
That to the defenceless can strut and look brave,
Although he to cowardice shews he's a slave.
And now for to dress up my beau with a grace,
Let a well frizzled wig be set off from his face;
With a bag quite in taste, from Paris just come,
That was made and ty'd up by Monsieur Frisson;
With powder quite grey, then his head is complete;
If dress'd in the fashion, no matter for wit. . . .

In the fall of 1754 the editors of *Connoisseur* described the ultra-fashionable men of the time:

'They have their toilettes, too, as well as the ladies, set out with washes, perfumes, and cosmetics, and will spend the whole morning in scenting their linen, dressing their hair, and arching their eyebrows. Their heads (as well as the ladies') have undergone various mutations and have worn as many different kinds of wigs as the block at their barber's. About fifty years ago they buried their heads in a bunch of hair; and the beaux (as Swift says) "lay hid beneath the penthouse of a full-bottomed perriwig". But as they then shewed nothing but the nose, mouth, and eyes, the fine gentlemen of our time not only oblige us with their full faces, but have drawn back the side curls quite to the tip of the ear.'

This description, of course, brought letters from the readers; and one of these, from a Mr W. Manly, was published the following April. Mr Manly closes his letter by saying:

'I am ashamed to tell you that we are indebted to Spanish Wool for many of our masculine ruddy complexions. A pretty fellow lacquers his pale face with as many varnishes as a fine lady. . . . I fear it will be found, upon examination, that most of our pretty fellows who lay on Carmine are painting a rotten post.'

The young editors, who went under the collective name of Mr Town, took the opportunity for further comment:

'The male beauty has his washes, perfumes, and cosmetics and takes as much pains to set a gloss on his complexion as the footman in japanning his shoes. He has his dressing-room and (which is still more ridiculous) his Toilet too, at which he sits as many hours repairing his battered countenance as a decayed toast dressing for a birth-night.'

The collective Mr Town then describes a visit to a young gentleman's dressing-room:

'I could not but observe a number of boxes of different sizes, which were all of them Japan, and lay regularly disposed on the table. I had the curiosity to examine the contents of several: in one I found lip-salve, in another a roll of pig-tail, and in another the ladies black sticking plaister; but the last which I opened very much surprised me, as I saw nothing in it but a number of little pills. I likewise remarked, on one part of the table, a tooth-brush and sponge, with a pot of Delescot's opiate; and on the other side, water for the eyes. In the middle stood a bottle of Eau de Luce and a roll of perfumed pomatum. Almond pastes, powder puffs, hair combs, brushes, nippers, and the like, made up the rest of this fantastic equipage. But among many other whimsies, I could not conceive for what use a very small ivory comb could be designed, till the valet informed me that it was a comb for the eyebrows.'

In 1770, Ellis Pratt, a hairdresser, wrote under the name of E. P. Philocosm a long poem called *The Art of Dressing the Hair*, one of the rare poetical tributes to men's hair. Although it is too long to quote in its entirety, parts of it seem worth including here:

> With various Art the tortur'd Curls to place,
> Confirm their Structure, and dispose with Grace;
> The Puff to manage with exactest Care,
> And pour the Snow-white Show'r on ev'ry Hair,
> I teach; embolden'd by the Muses' Aid
> To leave the shaving for the tuneful Trade.

> Oh *Phoebus*! Patron of the Sons of Song,
> God of the quacking and the fiddling Throng;
> Let my low Shop be with thy Presence blest,
> And all thy Raptures struggle in my Breast!
> What tho' untaught by Art thy Ringlets twine,
> No engines scorch, or Papillotes confine;
> What tho', unshorn, the Honours of thy Head
> In wild Luxuriance down thy Shoulders spread,
> Nor Bag hath dar'd enclose, or Ribbon tye,
> Nor borrow'd Locks their friendly Help supply;
> What tho' no Bristles thy smooth Chin conceal,
> But Down eternal, innocent of Steel;
> Let not in vain an honest Barber sue,
> Tho' ne'er the Labours of his Hand you knew;
> But like my Razor make my Lines appear,
> Smooth, tho not dull; and sharp, tho' not severe.
> And since these Hands, on many an empty Pate
> Ne'er form'd by Nature for dispensing Fate
> Oft have been taught the mighty Bush to lay,
> Which gave the Bearer Privilege to stay;
> Who without Learning had obtained Degrees,
> By stealing Theses, and by paying Fees:

Teach me what Unguents will the Loss repair,
When falling Tresses leave the Temples bare;
What styptic Juices will Assistance lend,
Relax'd and weaken'd if the Curls depend.

.   .   .   .   .

See the *Frisseur* disclose his ample Store,
And all his Implements of Toil explore!
The various *Comb* to various Cares applied,
Now to compose the Ringlets, now divide;
Pomatum with undying Odours frought,
Wool from Siluria's sable Fleeces brought;
The glowing *Forceps*, the confining *Pins*,
With Skill he ranges, and the Work begins.
While his quick Hand in weaves the crisped Hair,
A Mirror in your snow-white Fingers bear;
From Curl to Curl the happy Progress trace,
Exhaust his Art, and labour ev'ry Grace.

Let pointed Wires each waving Hair restrain
When eddying Whirlwinds sweep the dusty Plain,
Hapless that Youth, who, when the Tempest flies,
Unarm'd each rushing Hurricane defies!
In vain on Barbers or on God he calls,
The ringlets yield, the beauteous structure falls.
Nor less, when soft-descending Show'rs prevail,
Dread the moist influence of the Southern Gale:
Oft will its tepid Breath the Curls unbend,
While dropping Dews from ev'ry Spire depend.
Yours be the Care to watch, with cautious Eye,
When threat'ning Clouds portend a Tempest nigh.
Mark the Papilio-Race; the little Elves,
As gay, as soft, as silken as yourselves,
To vernal Suns their painted Wings unfold,
But shun the driving Blast and wint'ry Cold.

.   .   .   .   .

Your gentle Limbs on downy sofas throw,
And bid secure each happy moment flow,
Not unimprov'd: in secret Conclave mix;
The Laws of Dress, the Change of Fashions fix.
If pondr'ous *Clubs* shall from behind depend,
Or *Queues* in formidable Length descend;

If high the double Curl shall rise in Air,
Shoot up aloft, and leave the Temples bare;
Or in one Circle of Extensive Fold,
Belles shall admire your graceful Tresses roll'd.
Exert your Eloquence, display your Taste,
In Praise of *Wash-balls*, or of *Almond Paste*:
What *Dentifrice* a lasting White bestows,
What healing *Lip-Salve* emulates the Rose.

.   .   .   .   .   .

So may no Chance the latent Wires disclose,
Or your false Locks to titt'ring Belles expose!
So may your Tresses the Attack sustain
Of ruffling Tempests, or of moist'ning Rain;
And ev'ry Curl in lasting Order stand,
Unmov'd, and faithful to the Artists' Hand!

This just preceded the formation in 1772 of the Macaroni Club, which we have already mentioned briefly in connection with foretops and cadogans. The sight of the very elegant Macaronis in the streets of London very shortly brought forth the following comment in *Town and Country*:

'They make a most ridiculous figure with hats of an inch in the brim, that do not cover but lie upon the head, with about two pounds of fictitious hair, formed into what is called a club, hanging down their shoulders as white as a baker's sack. . . . Sir William Lofty approves of the ludicrous scheme of raising the tops of chairs and coaches that the ladies heads may not be discomposed; and yet with his foretop (which is full six inches high) there is never a chair or coach in town that can carry him without he stoops; Billy Mushroom swears that Lady Bridget's head has not been combed these four months, and yet two of his hair-dressers have refused dressing him unless he cleans his head.'

Although the wig shown in Plate 72-J is the original Macaroni style which was the subject for derision by all except those who chose to follow it, the name came to be associated with any display of elegance in fashion, particularly any fashion not sanctioned by long usage. It rather connoted affectation in dress, which presumably included the adoption of any new fashion. Thus, Plate 71-M was considered a Macaroni style even without the huge club.

But any disturbing elegance in English styles could hardly be compared to that of the French ones. The extraordinary bag wig called *en medallion*, shown in Plate 75-E, is described in the July 1777 issue of *The Lady's Magazine*. (In the same issue are to be found instructive articles on the 'Pernicious Consequences of Gaming' and an 'Account of the Most Romantic Parts of North Wales'.) The hair style, which is designated as the latest fashion in England, is, of course, a French import:

'The toupee is something like that à la maréchalle, only higher and more separated on the crown, and quite divided and upright on the back part of the head, so that

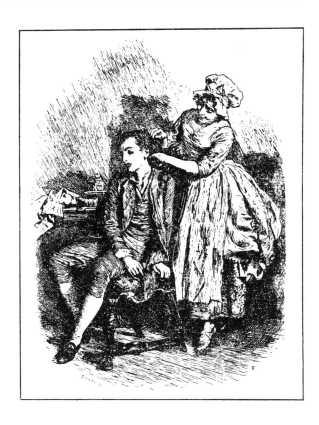

Fig. 79 : Denis's Valet. Young man having his hair dressed by a serving girl. Illustration from *Denis Duval* by William Makepeace Thackeray

each side forms a regular round, in imitation of a medal, with one large curl under it. From under the curls a three breast-plated queue descends loosely on each side, the ends of which are tied up with the rest of the hair into the bag. The bag is also in form of a large medal, though something oval, trimmed all around with a ribbon in small puffs, imitating the circumscription in medals. In the middle is a large rose, also ornamented with small puffs. The bag is tied to the hair with a large knot, on each side of which the bows and streamers are left flying.' The illustration accompanying the article (and it is the source of the one on Plate 75) showed no rose in the centre. So either the writer let her imagination get the better of her, or the artist, frought with disbelief, refused to put it in.

But the roses and high toupees and braids and bags were having their final fling before disappearing in the Revolution.

RETURN TO NATURAL HAIR

James Stewart, writing of wigs in 1783, said that 'now, indeed, they are much left off, as the hair of late years has been worn more generally than in the last age'. The first step in discarding the wig was to dress the natural hair to look like a wig. In his extensive treatise on hairdressing, Stewart goes into great detail concerning all aspects of the subject. His directions for dressing a woman's hair are quoted at length in the next chapter. He suggests that the procedure for gentlemen is much the same but adds a number of informative comments:

'The top is the brush, or feathered part, which bends backwards like that of the ladies. The sides is that which is done into curls, buckles, and ringlets, and takes, when more than one row of curls is wore, about 2 inches of the front hair, from the top of the ear upwards; the rest of each side all belong to the top and is drest as a vergette, or feather, or brush. The first row of curls slants regularly from the peak of the temple, passing over the top of the ear, pointing to the tail behind, seldom less than 6 inches of a regular slant, the feather, or brush, above the curls, in regular declension. A full dress is 5 curls, which, when wore, fills up the side of the head considerably more, by which means there is less top or feather. They are placed like 5 small tubes, or short joints of the smallest flute. The first one very small and short, not above an inch long. The two second in a line below the first, as if only broke rather larger in the curls, and at least about 2 inches long to spread backwards, and come more forward. The two under ones still larger in a line, as if just broke also, each about 3 inches long, to reach still further back, and the front one to come forward, the back one slanting downwards, as the front points upwards, the latter being rather from the head, while the former lies close to the head. In common dress, the 3 top curls are taken away, and the feather or brush supplies their place.'

As for curling, Stewart says that 'it is certain gentlemen's hair cannot be curled and dressed in perfection without putting it in papers'. He therefore recommends 'that every young gentleman's hair should be put in papers as carefully as the ladies, but not twisted or craped in curling this hair; therefore you are to proceed in every shape as you did when you curled the ladies hair, only with this difference, you must make more curls, or papers, the hair being shorter, else it will not have a curl strong enough'. He later adds that 'Most gentlemen, for four or five months in the year, have their hair in a brush, within half an inch of their scull, which must naturally strengthen it much, and effectually counteract any bad consequence from the toupee irons. When, therefore, gentlemen's hair is turned, or toupeed, it is done in regular rows exactly as the ladies has been directed. . . . If the gentleman wears a false tail, you are to shove it in the middle of the tail, when the hair covers it on all sides; you are then to press the hair exceeding tight down with your hands, and in order that it may tie well, the gentleman must fall his head between his shoulders. . . . As the head is thus held, you must have the lace in your right hand and the hair grasped hard by your left, when you must proceed to tie it very firm, full 5 inches from the head to make it hang well. . . . If queued, the ribbon is slantingly rolled round the hair till you come within 2 inches of the ends of the hair, when you reverse the rolling of the ribbon, slanting it back to the top, tying the ends you have in your hand with that you left at the top in a handsome bow; if clubbed, the hair is frizzed on the inside, then wound round your fingers in a large bow, which the ribbon completes by tying in the middle. If twisted, divide in two . . . then double

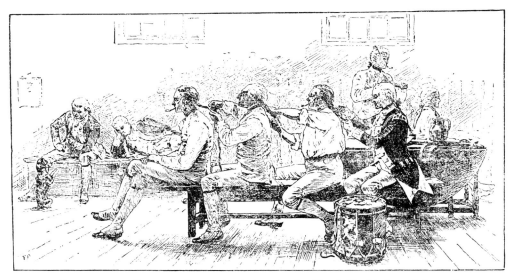

Fig. 80 : Pᴇᴛᴀɪʟs ᴀɴᴅ Pᴏᴡᴅᴇʀ. Pen and ink drawing by Frank Dodd, late eighteenth century

it up about 6 or 7 inches in length, and tie it with the ribbon round the middle. The length of the ribbon depends on the length of the hair; in a queue generally about 3 yards. One and a half is enough for a twist or club.' The hair style shown in Plate 70-O is taken from Stewart's *Plocacosmos*.

Since the head was normally shaved underneath the wig, it took time for it to grow out long enough to be properly dressed. As a result, a partial wig was often used for the long back hair. This is clearly shown in the John Adams portrait mentioned earlier (Plate 77-P). Stewart reports that 'The false hair, made up in various shapes, which the gentlemen wear, are not less numerous than the ladies, as the peruke, the false tail, false locks, false natural crown, false top, &c. &c.'

When the natural hair was long enough, the false hair could be discarded. But however it was managed, wigs began to disappear; and by 1790 there was a good deal of natural hair in evidence. Then during the nineties short hair became the fashion, first in France, then elsewhere; and only older men and the very conservative, including some professions, such as the law, hung on to their wigs and wore them well into the nineteenth century.

Since the military, as usual, was not very receptive to new fashions, the men continued to wear their clubs or their pigtails, real or false, with their natural hair. In the garrison at Gibraltar officers were required to have their hair cut the first week of every month according to the following rule:

'The top to be cut as close as possible, being left no longer than is necessary to admit of its being turned with Curling Irons of the smallest size; the back line of the top is not to exceed a line formed by passing a packthread from the back of one ear to that of the other vertically over the crown of the head; the hind hair to be parted from that of the top in the shape of a Horseshoe, which will occasion the sides to extend to half an inch behind the Ear, & which, therefore, forms the extreme breadth of the top; the remaining hair so parted off behind the string is to be combed back, to grow down in one even length, from the crown & the back of the ear, so that the whole of it may tie into the Queue; No part of the hind hair, so parted off from the front, or brush top, is to be thinned off, & none of the short hair in the neck to be cut away.' In addition to all of this, the hair was to be 'moderately filled and mixed with Powder and Pomatum'. There were further instructions on styles of hair to go with various hats.

As for the back hair, it was 'to be covered with soap lather, well beat up with flour in a box, until it becomes a stiff paste, which is to be laid on with a small brush (commonly called by House Painters, a sash Tool) & then, regularly & neatly marked with a comb the teeth of which should be about ten to the Inch, each mark coming directly down from the crown, where the hind hair is parted off from the top, to the tie, after which the whole hair is to be lightly powdered with a thread or cotton Puff, until it is perfectly white; but not so as to fill up the marks of the comb. When this is done, all loose powder that has not attached itself to the paste, where it is directed to be laid on the hind hair, is to be blown off, so that none may by chance fall on the Clothes. The Queue, which is to be made to receive the whole of the Man's hair, & to cover the string with which it is tied, is to be fixed on, so that when the Man has his Coat on, the Queue may be even with the lower row of lace on the Collar, & lastly the Flash is to be fixed on so as to cover the top of the Queue.'

In the American Revolutionary army, on the other hand, there were no regulations beyond that of reasonable neatness until in 1780 Washington ordered that the soldiers 'appear upon the Grand and other Parades shaved, combed and powdered and their Cloaths as clean as Circumstances will admit'. Two years later Washington felt that though near perfection had been achieved, there was still room for improvement; and to that end he suggested that 'to wear the hair cut or tied in the same manner throughout a whole corps would still be a very considerable ornament. Where it cannot be done in a regiment, similarity in a company would add extremely to the beauty of it'.

In the British army it was customary for the adjutant to keep on file, for reference by the barbers, the correct curl patterns to be worn. Sometimes there were actual models to go by. It is reported that on the occasion of a field day in the garrison at Gibraltar, since there was an insufficient number of barbers to attend to all the officers, the junior officers had to have their hair dressed (curled, clubbed, and plastered with pomatum and powder) the day before. And in order not to disturb the hair, they had to sleep face downward all night.

But this was a special problem of the military (and, as we shall see in the next chapter, sometimes of women). It was hardly a deterrent to the passing of wigs and was, perhaps, an added incentive to the return to short hair—the Brutus and the Titus cut, the hedgehog, etc. (see Plate 77-N).

In 1799 a newspaper item mentioned that Dr Randolph, Bishop of Oxford, was the first English prelate to wear his own hair in the eighteenth century. This was considered a scandalous innovation without precedent for more than a century. Even the Church, in the person of one English bishop, was beginning to notice the passing of an era. One must report, unhappily, that Dr Randolph eventually yielded to public pressure and donned a wig for the services.

There were also those in the legal profession who wished to lay aside the wig. Although George III didn't seem to care very much one way or the other what the clergy wore on their heads, he apparently had firm prejudices about the bench. When Eldon was made Chief Justice of the Common Pleas, he did not much want to wear the conventional powdered bush wig. And since Lady Eldon felt even more strongly on the subject, he asked the king to give him a special dispensation on account of headaches caused by the wig. 'No, no,' the king is said to have answered firmly, 'I will have no innovations in my time!' When reminded that the wig itself was an innovation, the king admitted this to be true. But he pointed out to Eldon that the older judges who wore no wigs did wear beards, and he thereupon gave Eldon permission to do as the older judges had done. Eldon continued to wear the wig.

HAIR IN THE THEATRE

Stewart in his book on hairdressing makes some enlightening comments on the theatrical usages of the time:

'In the tragedy of Cato, Mr. Booth is dressed a-la-mode, with the huge peruke; while Mrs. Olfield, in Marcia, is exhibited to view . . . with her hair parted in the middle, hanging carelessly on her shoulders, without the least ornament on her head or in her hair. We even find, and many now living have seen it, that Mr. Quin acted almost all of his young characters, as Hamlet, Horatio, Pierre, &c. in a full-dress suit, and large peruke. But Mr. Garrick's active genius, soon determining on improvement in every department of the theatre, in order to realize the representations, first attacked the mode of dress, and no part more than that of the head and hair. The consequence of this was that a capital player's wardrobe might be compared to a sale shop for all manner of dresses and for nothing more than the various quantities of what they call natural heads of hair; there is the comedy head of hair, and the tragedy ditto; the silver locks, and the common gray; the carotty poll, and yellow caxon; the savage black, and the Italian brown, and Shylock's and Falstaff's very different heads of hair, and very different beards; with the Spanish fly, the foxes tail, &c, &c, &c. But the manners of the stage altering, like the world, these seem to be wearing out, and the hair without powder, simply curled, seems to supply the place of a great many of these artificial hairs.'

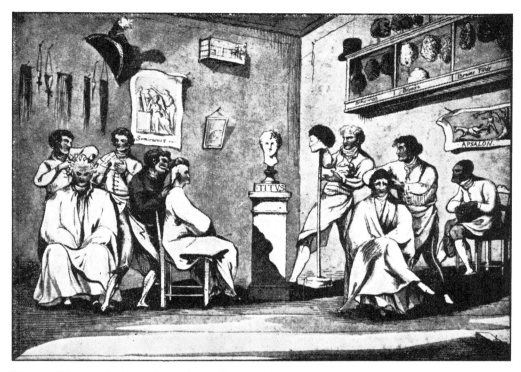

Fig. 81 : Viennese hairdressing and wig shop, 1780

In 1762 a verse by Lloyd indicated one of the contemporary stage conventions:

> To suit the dress demands the actor's art;
> Yet there are those who overdress the part;
> To some prescriptive right gives settled things,—
> Black wigs to murderers, feathered hats to kings.

Garrick made fashionable a wig smaller than Quin's 'with five crisp curls on either side'. This was known as the 'Garrick cut', though it was not the only style he wore. He was aware of the anachronism of wearing eighteenth-century wigs for all periods but was reluctant to attempt any drastic change, admitting quite frankly that he feared the audience would throw things at him if he did. Besides, he was doing quite well by following the convention. As Hotspur he wore 'a laced frock and a Ramillies wig'. There was some objection to this—not, however, because of any anachronism, but because it was considered 'too insignificant for the character'.

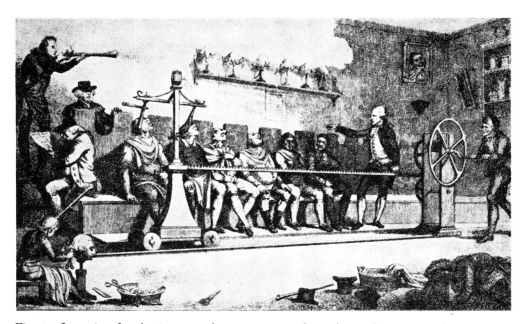

Fig. 82 : Invention for shaving several men at once and powdering their wigs at the same time. English caricature, late eighteenth century

FACIAL HAIR

The few tiny moustaches which remained at the end of the seventeenth century soon disappeared; and in the eighteenth century neither beards nor moustaches, except in military circles, were ever sanctioned by fashion. It was one of the few times in history that almost total beardlessness was ever practised. Still, there were a few here and there who were on the side of the beard, mostly soldiers and eccentrics and occasionally labourers. Military regulations varied from country to country and regiment to regiment. In France, for example, officers shaved, and their men wore curled moustaches. Otherwise, only French coachmen wore hair on the face.

A glance through the plates will show a beard here and there, the most startling probably being the Italian one in 67-I. Plate 68-J shows a Swiss guard with moustache and side whiskers, and 71-B is an eccentric English street musician.

In Plate 69-B we find the Swiss artist, Jean-Étienne Liotard, who grew a beard while in Constantinople and in 1752 appeared in Paris with it full grown, astonishing the populace. Since he was a talented and successful portrait painter, much in demand, his beard was accepted as a curious and fascinating eccentricity, which assuredly did no harm to his career and, in fact, undoubtedly enhanced his reputation. On the other hand, Joshua Evans, an American Quaker, was considered alarmingly eccentric for wearing a beard, was avoided by both friends and enemies and for many years was refused a certificate to travel in the ministry.

Most of the shaving was done in the public barbers' shops. In 1742 it was ordered by the guild of barber-surgeons of Newcastle-on-Tyne that there should be no shaving on Sunday and that 'no brother should shave John Robinson till he pays what he owes to Robert Shafto'.

All this shaving of the beard, though generally accepted, was looked upon with dismay and contempt by a few, among them a Frenchman by the name of Jacques Antoine Dulaure, who in 1786 could restrain his wrath no longer and wrote a book about beards entitled *Pogonologia or a Philosophical and Historical Essay on Beards*, in which he discussed the glorious history of the beard, the folly of shaving, beards and the clergy, and even bearded women. It is not quite clear whether he approved or disapproved of the latter, though it would appear from the general tenor of the work that his feeling was that anyone, regardless of sex, was the better for having a beard. He began his work by saying that 'It must be a strange paradox, perfectly shocking for crazy old beaus, for priests whose beards are always shaved close, in short, for all those that compose the effeminate part of the human species, to hear anyone maintain that a long beard becomes a man's dignity, and that it is beneficial to health and good morals; his ideas must be very different from those of the present age. This, however, is what I have presumed to do. But whether the design of this work be serious or ironical, it has at least the appearance of novelty; and that's a great deal in this age.'

Throughout the long tract M. Dulaure used every means at his disposal to gain his readers' support for his side of the beard question—including quoting Tertullian's opinion on the canons issued by the Fourth Council of Carthage, which, if it actually took place at all, did so nearly two centuries after Tertullian's death.

Having exhausted his invention, he closed his essay on a note of self-satisfaction:

'Well, it's now a whole century since we wore beards. Have we gained by the change? This well merits an investigation. . . . if, as a modern philosopher said, stupor reigns, it is because we no longer wear our beards. But let us console ourselves; the source of these evils is nearly dried up. The fashion of long beards is on the point of being renewed, an epoch which I pronounce to be nearer than people think. . . . You pretty fellows of the present day, Jemmy-Jessamy parsons, jolly bucks, and all you with smock-faces and weak nerves, be dumb with astonishment, I fortel it, you will soon resemble men.'

But it was not to happen quite so soon as M. Dulaure expected.

PLATE 67 : EIGHTEENTH-CENTURY MEN 1700–1735

A   Baron Gottfried Wilhelm von Leibnitz, 1646–1716. German philosopher and mathematician. *Full-bottom* (or *full-bottomed*) *wig.*

B   *c.* 1718. *Full-bottom wig* (see also Plate 73-A).

C   Frederick Augustus I, 1670–1733. Elector of Saxony, 1694–1733. *Full-bottom wig.*

D   Prince Eugene of Savoy, 1663–1736. *Full-bottom wig.*

E   Crown Prince Friedrich Wilhelm of Prussia, 1688–1740. *Full-bottom wig.*

F   *c.* 1705, French.

G   *c.* 1715.

H   *c.* 1720, French. (After Watteau.)

I   1710, Italian government official. The wearing of the full beard with the voluminous wig is most unusual.

J   1735, English.

K   English. *Knotted wig* or *campaign wig* (see also Plates 69-C-K-Q-X-Y-Z-AA, 70-A and 73-I).

L   Child. Natural hair.

M   *Campaign wig* or *knotted wig* (*à nœuds*)—this bushy version is also known as a *physical tie* (see K above).

N, O   *Square wig*, front and back views (see also Plate 69-E-P).

P   Georg Friedrich Handel, 1685–1759. *Full-bottom wig.*

Q   King George II—reigned 1727–60. *Full-bottom wig*—this was no longer a fashionable style, and the enormous full-bottoms had disappeared completely.

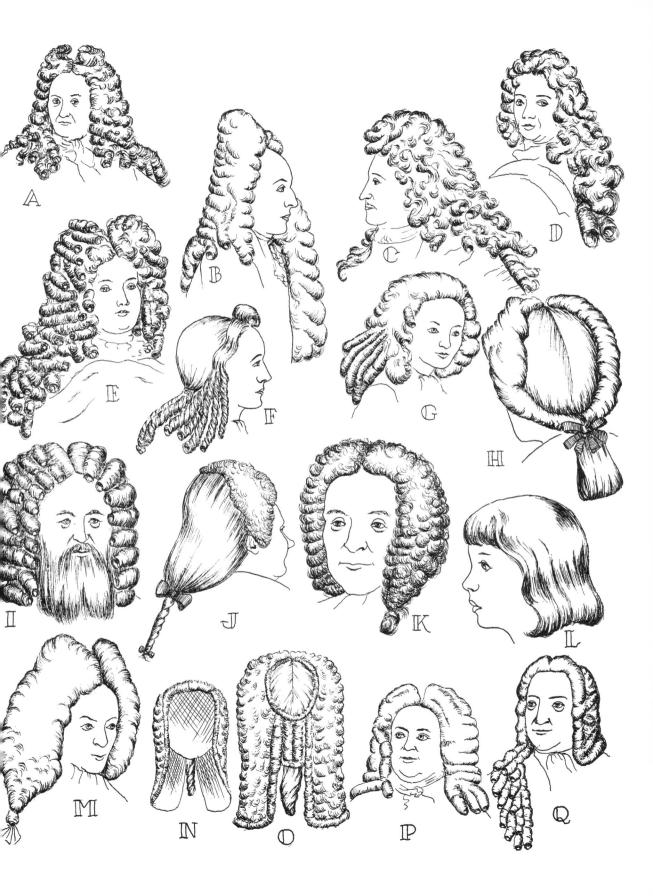

A   B   C   D

E   F   G   H

I   J   K   L

M   N   O   P   Q

PLATE 68 : EIGHTEENTH-CENTURY MEN 1700–1760

(A-E represent Hogarth's satiric five orders of periwigs, Figure 76.)

A   'Episcopal' or 'Parsonic' wig. A *physical bob*—worn by bishops. The foretop was not always so high (see Plate 70-G).

B   'Aldermanic' wig. A *full-bottom wig*—worn by aldermen of the City of London.

C   'Lexonic' wig. A *full-bottom* or *square wig*—worn mostly by 'gentlemen of the Law'.

D   'Foxtail' wig. A *tie wig* (see also 69-J).

E   'Half-natural' wig—worn by some of the nobility.

F   1742, English. (For other braided queues see Plates 71-M, 73-Y, 75-R, 77-J.)

G   Insignium of the Corporation of Wig-makers of Caen, formed in the seventeenth century.

H   1728. Early *bag wig* with *pigeon-wings*. Bag wigs in various styles and sizes continued to be popular throughout most of the century (for other examples see Plates 69-D-I, 70-B-D, 71-T, 72-D-G-L-P, 73-L-M-Q-R-W, 76-E-K, 77-A-D-E).

I   *c.* 1735, English clergyman. *Long bob*—sometimes called a *minister's* or *clergyman's bob* (for other frizzed bobs, see Plates 68-A, 71-J, 72-C, and 73-N; for curled bobs see 69-S-T and accompanying cross references).

J   Swiss guard. Facial hair was frequently worn by the military, rarely by civilians. The queue is probably looped up and secured below the crown with a comb.

K   1740. French workman.

L   1759, English. *Long bob* (see also Plate 69-S-T).

M   *c.* 1745, English. Gentlemen with natural hair in curl papers. (After Hogarth.)

N   *c.* 1744, German. Anton Mengs's portrait of his father. Natural hair.

O   1744, German. Anton Mengs at sixteen. (From a self-portrait.) Natural Hair.

P   Mid-century, English. Probably natural hair. (After Hogarth.)

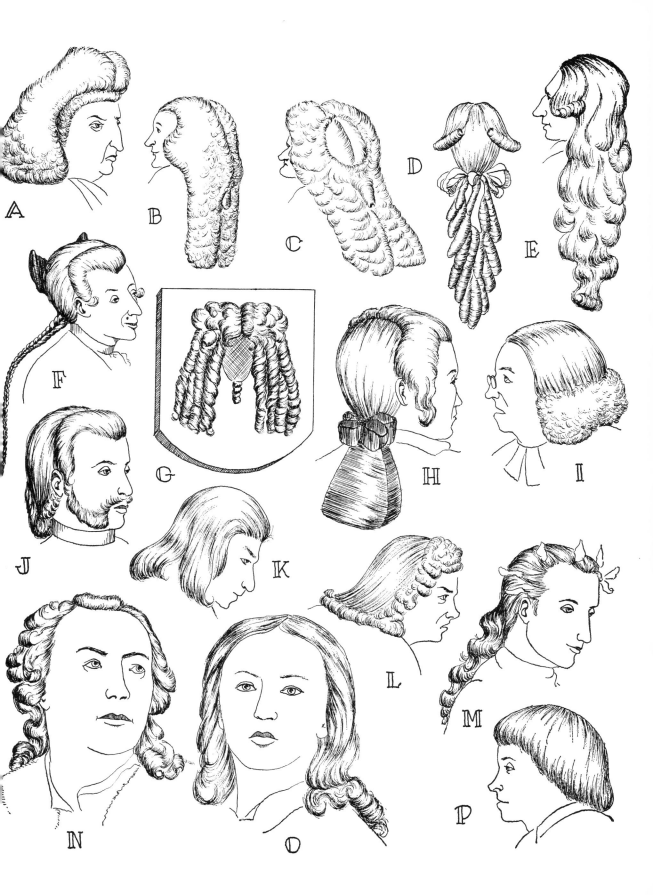

A

B

C

D

E

F

G

H

I

J

K

L

M

N

O

P

PLATE 69 : EIGHTEENTH-CENTURY MEN 1730–1770

A   c. 1730. *Tie wig* with *solitaire* (for other tie wigs see J below, and for other solitaire wigs see W below and Plate 72-L-M).

B   Jean Étienne Liotard, 1702–89. Swiss artist. Natural hair. The beard was decidedly an eccentricity.

C   French. *Knotted wig*, or *perruque à nœuds*, also *à marteaux* (see also Plates 67-K-M, 70-A, and K, Q, X, Y, Z, and AA below).

D   *Bag wig* with *pigeon wings* (see also Plates 68-H, 69-I, 70-B-D, 71-T, 72-D-G-L-P, 73-L-M-Q-R-W, 76-E-K, 77-A-D-E).

E   *Square wig* (see also Plate 67-N-O).

F   1742. Probably a *bag wig* with frizzle.

G   *Scratch bob* or natural hair (see also O and V below and Plate 73-AA).

H   *Bob wig* or natural hair (see S and T below).

I   Jean d'Alembert, 1717–83. French mathematician and philosopher. *Bag wig* (see D above).

J   *Tie wig*—an undress wig (see also 68-D, 71-U, 75-G-H-Q, 76-U-V-X).

K   1735, English. Composer. Powdered *knotted wig* (see C above and Q, X, Y, Z, and AA below).

L   Bellows for applying hair powder (see also Figure 72).

M, N   *Abbot's wig*, front and back—a *bob wig* with tonsure.

O   *Scratch wig* or natural hair (see G above and Plate 73-AA).

P   Johann Sebastian Bach, 1685–1750. *Square wig*.

Q   1745, English marriage broker. *Knotted wig* or *physical tie* (see Plate 73-I as well as C and K above and X, Y, Z, and AA below).

R   Face masks for use when hair was being powdered (see also Figure 73).

S, T   *Bob wig* or *bob major*, back and front—a very popular wig worn by all classes until nearly the end of the century. (Variations, both frizzed and curled, are shown in Plates 68-A-I-L, 70-G-H, 71-A-E-H-I-J-O-S, 72-A-C-Q, 73-C-D-H-I-N, and 76-L-N.)

U   *Bob wig* (see above).

V   *Scratch wig*. Front hair natural (see also Plate 73-AA).

W   1745, English. *Bag wig* with *solitaire*.

X, Y, Z, AA   *Campaign wig* or *knotted wig* (see also C, K, and Q above and Plates 70-A and 73-I).

BB   Dr Samuel Johnson, 1709–84. His wigs were usually rather shabby and singed in front from candle flames.

CC   *Cut wig* or *cauliflower wig*. Popular with coachmen, artisans, etc. (see also Plate 71-F-K).

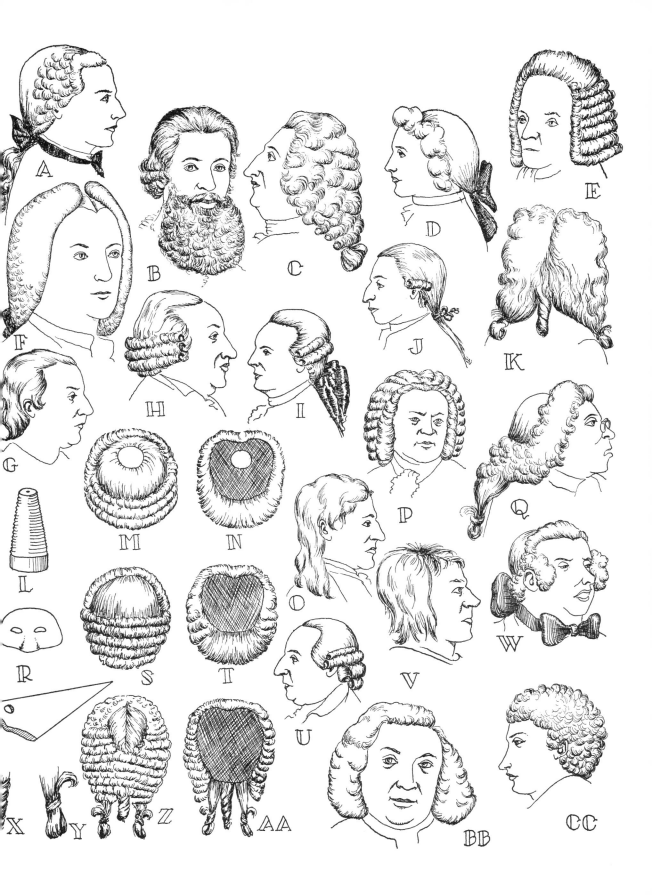

A

B

C

D

E

F

G

H

I

J

K

L

M

N

O

P

Q

R

S

T

U

V

W

X

Y

Z

AA

BB

CC

PLATE 70 : EIGHTEENTH-CENTURY MEN 1730–1800

A   *c.* 1730, Dutch. *Knotted wig*, powdered (see also Plates 67-K-M, 69-C-K-Q, and 73-I).

B   1735, English. *Bag wig* with *pigeon-wings* and *solitaire* (see also Plates 68-H, 69-I, 71-T, 72-D-G-L-P, 73-L-M-Q-R-W, 76-E-K, 77-A-D-E).

C   1736, English. (After Hogarth.)

D   1735, English. *Bag wig* with *solitaire* (for other wigs with solitaire see Plates 69-A-W, 72-L-M, and B above).

E   1751, English. *Scratch bob* (see also Plate 73-AA).

F   1751, English. *Natural bob*.

G   *Physical bob*—the 'parsonic' wig from Hogarth's five orders of periwigs (see Plate 68-A and Figure 76).

H   Benjamin Franklin, 1706–90. Powdered wig. Franklin is more frequently shown without a wig (see Plate 74-P).

I   1762, English. Natural hair. (After Hogarth.)

J   1753, Italian. Manelli, opera singer—'leading buffoon'. Wig is exaggerated for comic effect, but a few years later the raised toupee would have been considered quite fashionable.

K   English. *Scratch wig* or natural hair.

L   1786, Italian. *Pigtail wig* (see also Q below and Plates 72-K, 73-J-Z, 75-J-L-M-U, and 77-L-P).

M   *c.* 1780-90, Dutch.

N   1765, English boy. Natural hair.

O   1782, English. From James Stewart's *Plocacosmos* (see text for Stewart's instructions on dressing men's hair).

P   1786, Italian. *Club wig* (see also Plates 71-M-P-Q, 72-J-M-O, 73-E-F-S, 76-G-H-I-S, and 77-B-C-G-I-M).

Q   1786, Italian. *Pigtail wig* worn carelessly (see L above and cross references).

R   1786, Italian. Tail of wig pinned up (see also Plates 72-F and 77-J).

S   John Adams, 1735–1826. Became president of the United States in 1796. Natural hair with pigtail.

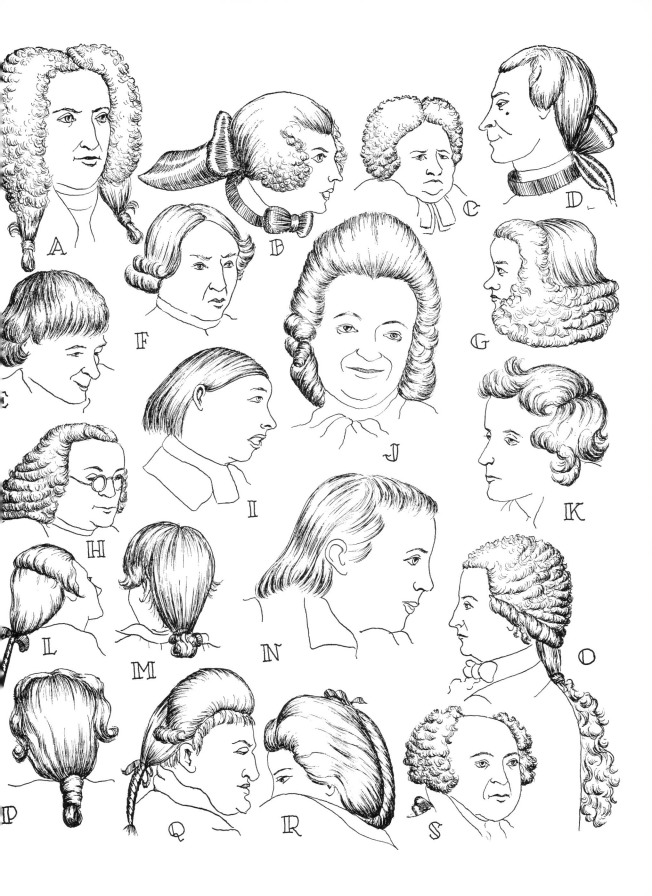

PLATE 71 : EIGHTEENTH-CENTURY MEN 1735–1790

A   1735, English. *Scratch bob* (see also Plate 73-AA).

B   1741, English. Itinerant street musician wearing *scratch wig* over natural hair (for other scratch wigs see Plate 73-AA).

C   1735, English. *Scratch wig* (see also Plate 73-AA).

D   *c.* 1740. Natural hair.

E   1747, English. Alderman's clerk. *Bob wig* (see also Plate 69-S-T).

F   1747, English. Weaver's apprentice. *Cut wig* (see also Plate 69-CC and 71-K).

G   1776, English. Possibly a one-tailed *major wig* (see text, also L below).

H   1758, English. *Short bob.* (A short frizzed bob is shown in J below, see also Plate 69-S-T.)

I   1773, English. *Scratch bob* (see also Plate 73-AA).

J   *c.* 1760, English. *Short* or *minor bob* (see H above; for other frizzed bobs, see Plates 68-A, 72-A-C, 73-N; for bobs in general see Plate 69-S-T).

K   *c.* 1763, English. Gentleman wearing *cauliflower* or *cut wig* (see also F above and Plate 69-CC).

L   1773, English. *Major wig*, sometimes a *brigadier* (see text, also G above and Plate 76-P; for Diderot's French *brigadière*, see Plate 73-U-V-BB-CC).

M   1772, English. Variation of *cadogan* or *club wig* (for the usual cadogan style see Plate 72-J and cross references).

N   1770, French. Gentleman in dressing-gown. The back hair would be dressed this way only at home. With the comb removed, it could easily become either a tie-wig or, more likely, a *perruke naissante* (see also R below and Plate 77-K).

O   *c.* 1762, English. *Bob wig* askew, showing natural hair (for other bobs see Plate 69-S-T).

P   1773, English. *Cadogan* or *club wig* (see also Plate 72-J and cross references).

Q   1788, French. A variation of the *club wig.*

R   1776, French. Gentleman at home (see N above).

S   1776, French. Physician. *Physical bob* (for earlier versions see Plates 68-A and 72-A-C).

T   1780, French. *Bag wig* with *grecque* (for other bag wigs see Plate 68-H and references).

U   1789, French. *Tie wig* (see also Plates 68-D, 69-A-J, 75-G-H-Q, 76-U-V-X).

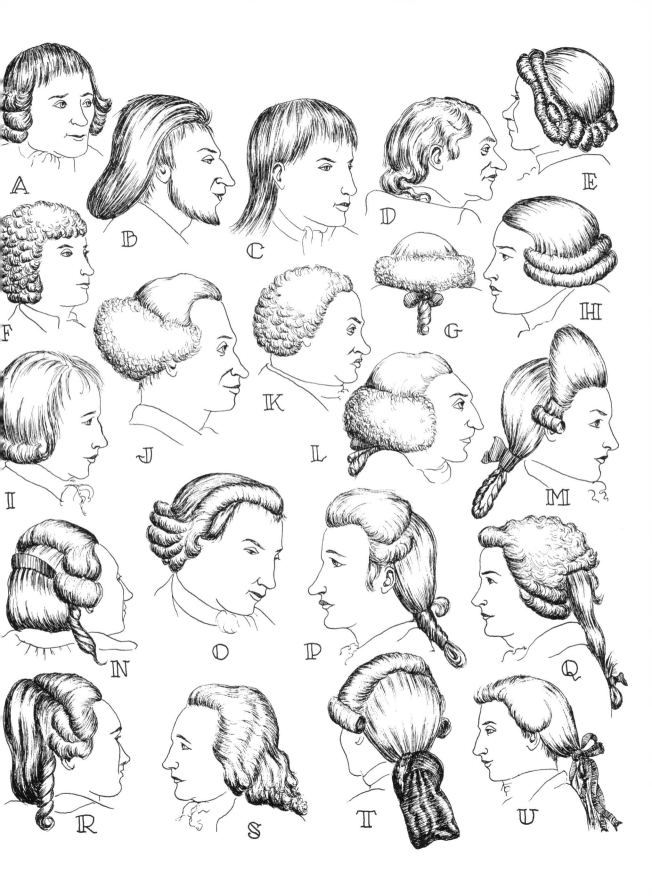

PLATE 72 : EIGHTEENTH-CENTURY MEN 1740–1780

A   Henry Fielding, 1707–54. *Physical bob* (see also C below and Plates 68-A and 71-S).

B   *c.* 1750, English. *Scratch wig* (see also Plate 73-AA and cross references).

C   *c.* 1750, English. *Physical bob*, very popular with the medical profession (see A above).

D   Dr Thomas Augustine Arne, 1710–78. Composer. *Bag wig* (see also G, L, and P below and Plates 68-H, 69-D-I, 70-B-D, 71-T, 73-L-M-Q-R-W, 76-E-K, and 77-A-D-E).

E   Child, French. Natural hair.

F   1770s. French soldier. Wig with horseshoe toupee (*grecque*) and twisted queue, raised and secured with comb (see also Plates 71-N-R and 77-J).

G   1745. Domenico Annibali. *Bag wig* with *pigeon wings* (see D above).

H   *c.* 1755, English. *Spencer wig* (see text).

I   1766. Joseph Wright. English artist. Natural hair in *bob*.

J   *c.* 1772. *Cadogan wig*. Macaroni style with high toupee and very large club (for other cadogans see M and O below and Plates 70-P, 71-M-P-Q, 73-E-F-S, 75-B-C-O, 76-G-H-I-S, 77-B-C-G-I-M).

K   *c.* 1775. Double *pigtail wig* with *grecque*. The double queue was largely French (see also Plates 70-L, 73-J-Z, 75-J-L-M-U, 77-L-P).

L   1770s, French. *Bag wig* with *solitaire* (see D above; for other wigs with solitaire see M below and Plates 69-A-W, 70-B-D and 72-L).

M   1770. Hiacinthe de Rigaud, comte de Vaudreuil. *Cadogan* with tie (see J above).

N   1770s, French. Wig *à l'enfant* or *à la naissance* or *naissante*—popular primarily in France in the latter part of the century (see also Plates 73-O-P, 75-D, and 76-R).

O   1774, English. *Club wig* or *cadogan* (see J above).

P   1772, English. *Bag wig* (see D above).

Q   *c.* 1775, German. *Bob wig* or, more likely, natural hair. The beard is uncommon (see Plate 69-S-T).

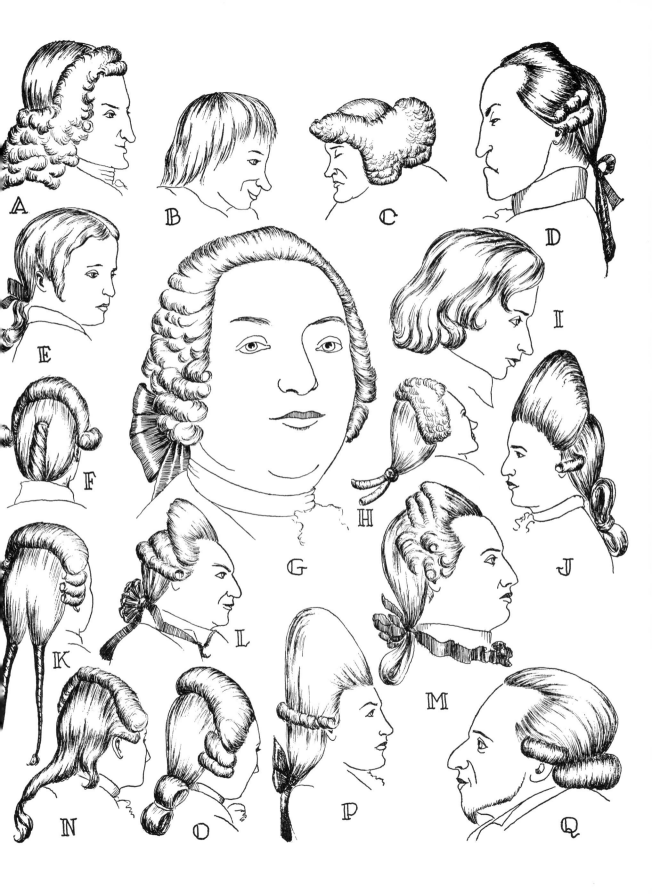

A

B

C

D

E

F

G

H

I

J

K

L

M

N

O

P

Q

PLATE 73 : EIGHTEENTH-CENTURY MEN 1760–1780

A   English. *Full-bottom* powdered judicial wig (see also Plates 67-A-B-C-D-E and 68-B-C).

B   Charles Thomson, 1729–1824. Secretary of the Continental Congress. Probably natural hair.

C   Joseph Priestly, 1733–1804. English theologian and scientist. *Bob wig* (see also Plate 69-S-T).

D   *c.* 1780. *Bob wig* (see also Plate 69-S-T).

E   John Howard, 1726?–90. Powdered *cadogan* or *club wig*—popular after the late 1760s (see also Plate 72-J).

F   *c.* 1775. *Club wig* (see Plate 72-J).

G   Immanuel Kant, 1724–1804. German philosopher.

H   1769, English politician. *Short bob*, powdered (see also Plate 69-S-T).

I   *c.* 1775. *Physical tie* or *knotted wig* (for physical bobs see Plate 68-A, 70-G, and 72-A-C; for knotted wigs see Plates 67-K-M, 69-C-K-Q-X-Y-Z-AA and 70-A).

J   *c.* 1780. Powdered wig or natural hair with short pigtail (see also Z below and Plates 70-L-Q, 72-K, 75-J-L-M-U, and 77-L-P).

K   *c.* 1775. Probably natural hair.

L   1773. *Bag wig* (see Q and R below).

M   1771, German. Child wearing powdered *bag wig* with high toupee. Children of the upper classes often wore fashionable wigs.

N   *c.* 1780, English. *Bob wig* (see also Plates 69-S-T and especially 68-I).

O, P   *c.* 1770, French. *Peruke naissante*, back and front views (see also Plates 72-N, 75-D, and 76-R).

Q, R   *c.* 1770. *Bag wig*, back and front views—a dress wig, always powdered (see also Plates 68-H, 69-D, 70-B-D, 71-T, 72-D-G-L-P, 76-E-K, and 77-A-D-E).

S   1771, German. Powdered *club wig* with *grecque* toupee (see also Plate 72-J).

T   Voltaire, 1694–1778. *Long bob* (see also 69-S-T).

U, V   French. *Brigadier wig*. A military style, and also called a *major* in England (see BB and CC below and Plate 71-L).

W   Wig bag with draw strings and rosette (see Q and R above). Bags and bows were always black.

X   Carolus Linnaeus (Carl van Linné), 1707–78. Swedish botanist.

Y   *Ramillies wig* (for other braided queues see Plates 68-F, 71-M, 75-R and 77-J).

Z   1770s. *Pigtail wig* (see also J above).

AA   Denis Diderot, 1713–84. French philosopher. His *Encyclopédie*, published in 1772, is a classic source of eighteenth-century wig styles, all of which appear in these plates. *Scratch wig*.

BB, CC   Rosette and spiral curls for *brigadier wig* above.

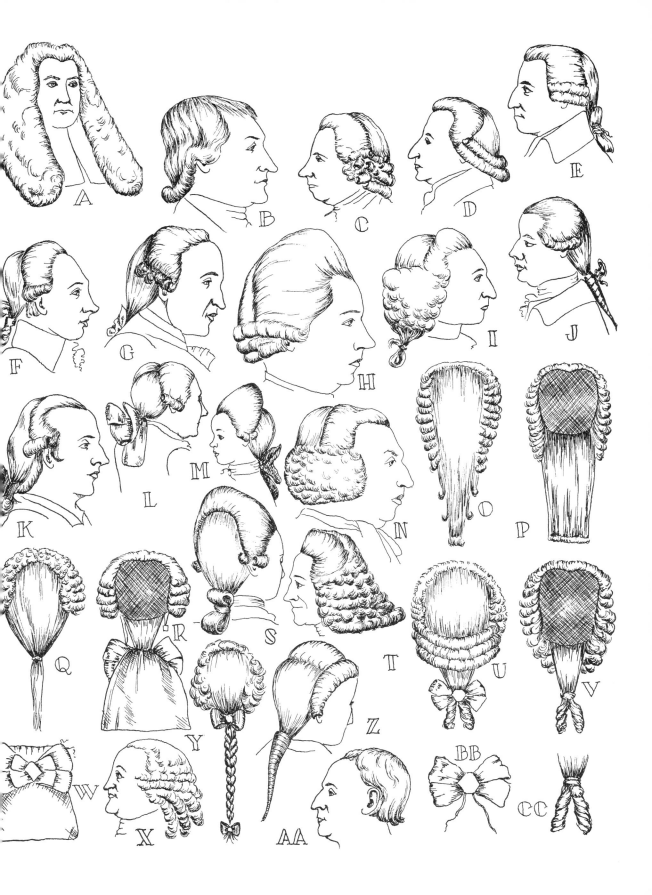

PLATE 74 : EIGHTEENTH-CENTURY MEN 1760–1800

A-G   French wigs fashionable in 1761.

H   1773. *Bob wig* (see Plate 69-S-T).

I   Giovanni Jacopo Casanova de Seingalt, 1725–98. *Tie wig.*

J   Shaving basin.

K   1775, American. James Duane. Congressman.

L, M   1793. Bishop Thomas. Front and back.

N   Adam Phillippe, 1740–93. French soldier.

O   1787, French.

P   Benjamin Franklin, 1706–90. Natural hair (see also Plate 70-H).

Q   1794. George Washington. *Tie wig.*

R, S   c. 1800. James Stuart McKenzie. Side and back.

T   1787. French peasant.

U   Casimir Pulaski, 1748?–79. Polish soldier and general in the American army.

V   James Madison, 1751–1836. American president, 1809–17. *Tie wig.*

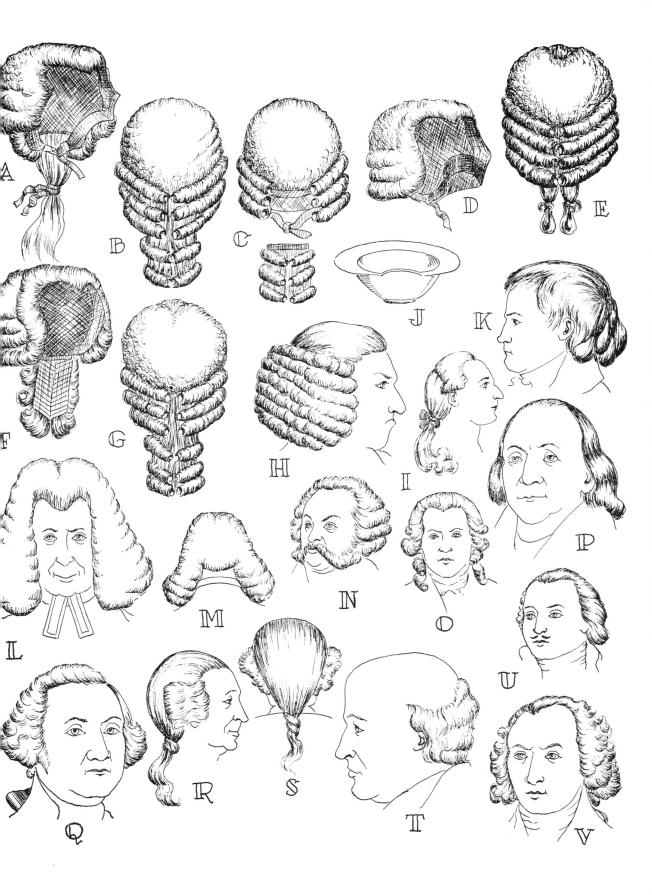

A B C D E

F G H I J K

L M N O P

Q R S T U V

PLATE 75 : EIGHTEENTH-CENTURY MEN 1760–1800

A   1779, French (see also Plates 69-I, 72-D-L, 73-G-K-L, 76-E-K, 77-A-E).

B   1776, French. *Tie wig.*

C   1770s. *Club wig* (see also Plate 72-J and cross references).

D   1778, French. *Peruke naissante* or *à l'enfant* (see also Plates 72-N, 73-O-P, and 76-R).

E   1777, French. Perruke *en médaillon*—a *bag wig* (see description in text).

F   1770s. Natural hair or *scratch wig* (see also 73-AA).

G   1780. *Tie wig* (see also Plates 68-D, 69-A-J, 71-U, 76-U-V-X).

H   Italian. *Tie wig.*

I   1780, French working class. Natural hair or *scratch wig.*

J   *c.* 1760. *Pigtail*—military style (see also L, M, and U below and Plates 70-L-Q, 72-K, 73-J-Z, and 77-L-P).

K   Twisted queue with bedraggled *pigeon wings.*

L   French. Double *pigtail wig*, front and back (see also J above).

M   Late 1780s. *Pigtail.* Probably natural hair (see J above).

N   Franz Joseph Haydn, 1732–1809.

O   1760s. *Cadogan.* Probably natural hair.

P   Partial wig, intended to be worn with natural front hair.

Q   Wolfgang Amadeus Mozart, 1756–91. Powdered *tie wig* (see G above).

R   1794, William Bligh. British admiral, captain of *The Bounty.* Natural hair.

S   1797, American. Natural hair.

T   1796, French. Natural hair in the Napoleonic style (see also 77-N).

U   1795, English. Partial wig with pigtail.

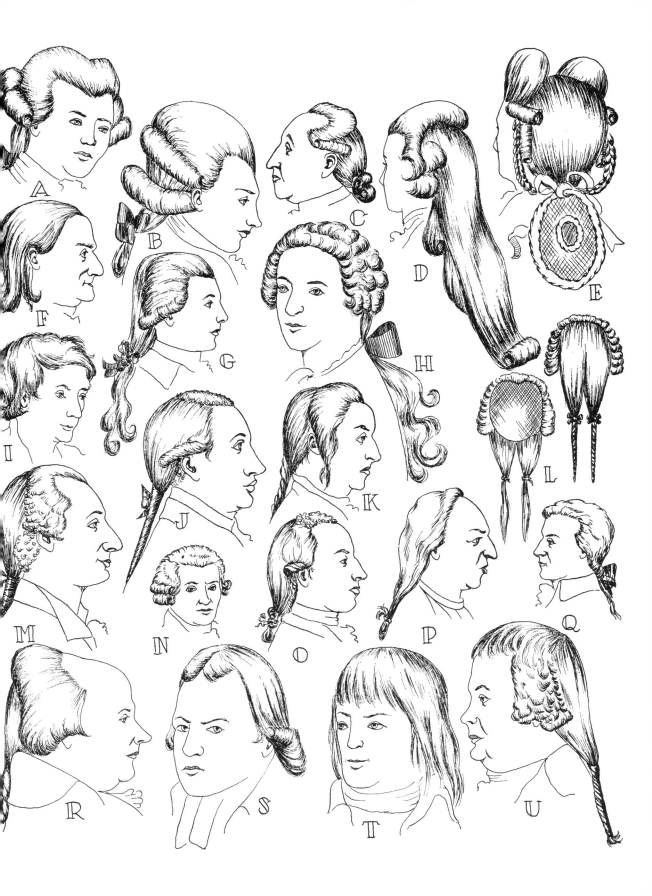

A

B

C

D

E

F

G

H

I

J

K

L

M

N

O

P

Q

R

S

T

U

PLATE 76 : EIGHTEENTH-CENTURY MEN 1770–1800

A   1790s. Natural hair with tie or possibly partial wig.

B   Comte de Provence, 1755–1824, later Louis XVIII.

C   Henry Fuseli (or Heinrich Fuessli or Füssli), 1741–1825. Anglo-Swiss artist. Natural hair.

D   John Wesley, 1703–91. Founder of Methodism. Wig.

E   Jacques Necker, 1732–1804. French banker and financial expert, minister of state under Louis XVI. *Bag wig* (see also Plates 68-H, 69-D-I, 70-B-D, 71-T, 73-L-M-Q-R-W, 77-A-D-E).

F   *Cut wig* or possibly natural hair.

G   Adam Smith, 1723–90. Scottish economist. *Club wig* with frizzed toupee (for other club wigs see Plate 72-J).

H   Benedict Arnold, 1741–1801. American general and traitor. *Cadogan.*

I   Honoré Gabriel Riquetti, comte de Mirabeau, 1749–91. French statesman and revolutionist. *Club wig* with frizzed toupee (or frizzle). (Compare with G above and S below; see also Plate 72-J.)

J   *Scratch wig* or natural hair (see also 73-AA).

K   1771, German. *Bag wig* (see E above).

L   1779, Josiah Wedgwood. Celebrated English potter. *Long bob* (see also 69-S-T).

M   Wolfgang Amadeus Mozart, 1756–91. Powdered wig (see also Plate 75-Q).

N   Johann Kaspar Lavater, 1741–1801. Swiss preacher, theological writer, and pioneer in the study of physiognomy. Natural hair in *bob*.

O   1790s. Partial wig or natural hair in *tie*.

P   *c.* 1778, German. One-tailed *major wig* (see Plate 71-L).

Q   1792, French.

R   1792, Louis XVI. *Peruke naissante* (see also 72-N, 73-O-P, 75-D).

S   Maximilien Robespierre, 1758–94. French revolutionist. *Frizz-wig* or *frizzle* with *club*. (see G and I above and Plate 72-J).

T   *c.* 1790. Natural hair (see also W below, 75-T, and 77-N-O).

U   Emperor Paul I of Russia, 1754–1801—reigned 1796–1801. *Tie wig* (see X below).

V   1789, Mirabeau. *Tie wig.*

W   Robert Burns, 1759–96. Natural hair (see also 75-T and 77-N-O).

X   1789, Louis XVI. *Tie wig* (see also R above; for other tie wigs see Plates 68-D, 69-A-J, 71-U, 75-G-H-Q).

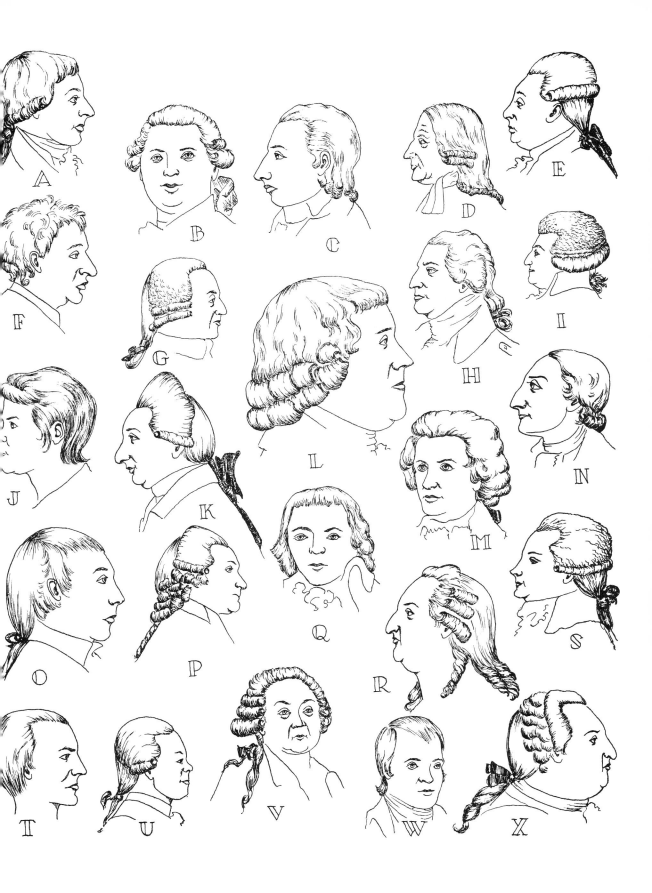

Plate 77 : Eighteenth-Century Men 1770–1800

A   1772, German. *Bag wig*. The bag tended to be quite large in the 1770s (see also Plates 68-H, 69-D, 70-B-D, 71-T, 72-D-G-L-P, 73-Q-R-W, and 76-E-K).

B, C   c. 1770. Powdered *club wig*. Back and front views (see also Plates 72-J).

D   1770s, German. *Bag wig* (see note under A above).

E   c. 1780, French. *Bag wig*. Note unusual bow.

F   Marquis de Lafayette, 1747–1834.

G   c. 1790, French. *Cadogan* (see also Plate 72-J).

H   1780s, French.

I   c. 1790, French. *Cadogan* (see also Plate 72-J).

J   1790s, French.

K   c. 1789, French. Gentleman's valet.

L   1790s. Variation of *pigtail wig* (see also Plates 72-K, 73-J-Z, 75-J-L-M-U).

M   1791, English. *Cadogan* (see also Plate 72-J).

N   1799. Natural hair (see also 75-T and 76-T-W).

O   Late 1790s. *Hedgehog* style, wig or natural hair.

P   John Adams, 1735–1826. American president. Note where natural hair meets false hair with pigtail just below crown.

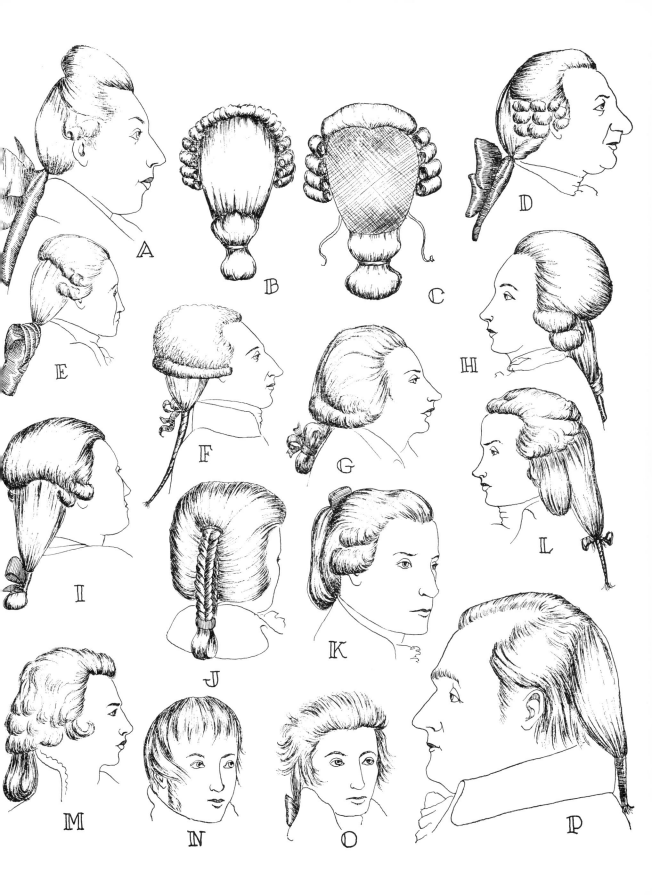

A

B

C

D

E

F

G

H

I

J

K

L

M

N

O

P

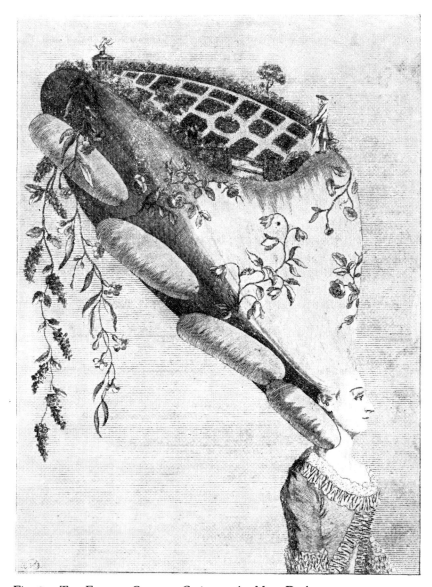

Fig. 83 : THE FLOWER GARDEN. Caricature by Mary Darly, 1777

10 · The Eighteenth Century—Women

Lady S.'s head was the most beyond the
bounds of propriety, she having so
many plates of fruit placed on the top
pillar, and her being without powder,
it was not so delicate a mixture.

The Lady's Magazine

Whereas men's hair styles of the eighteenth century seem to involve a bewildering medley of curious wigs and even more curious names for them, with little apparent logic and only a vague and erratic fashion line to follow, the women's styles move in a clearly defined pattern from a peak of artificiality at the end of the seventeenth century through a disarming trough of simplicity in the first half of the eighteenth, rising at last to a crescendo of excess which could scarcely have been imagined, let alone anticipated, a few years before.

1700–1760 (Plates 78, 79)

At the beginning of the century the constructions of curls had reached their peak. Commodes and tours were still being worn but not so universally as they had been, and the hair was often powdered. The style was hardly one to go unremarked by men, whose opinions broke into print from time to time. The English ladies voiced their defence about 1700 in a rallying ballad entitled *The London Ladies' Vindication of Top-knots*:

> Young Women and Damsels that love to go fine,
> Come listen awhile to this ditty of mine;
> In spite of all Poets, brave Girls we will wear,
> Our Towers and Topknots, with Powdered Hair.
>
> We see the young Misses & Jilts of the Town
> Have six Stories high, as they walk up & down;
> Then pray tell me why should not honest Wives wear
> Rich Towers & Topknots with Powdered Hair.
>
> If we an't as fine and as Gaudy as they
> Who knows but our Husbands might soon run astray;
> Consider this, Women, and still let us wear
> Our Towers & Topknots and Powdered Hair.

> Some young men may flout us, yet mark what I say,
> There's no Woman living now, Prouder than they;
> Observe but the many knick-knacks which they wear
> More costly than Topknots or Powdered Hair.
>
> Their Wigg, Watch, & Rapiers we daily behold,
> And Embroidered Waistcoats of Silver & Gold:
> Likewise, Turn Up Stockings, they constantly wear
> More costly than Topknots or Powdered Hair.
>
> If Pride be a sin & a folly, why then
> Han't we a far better Example from Men?
> If Gaudy Apparel those Gallants do wear,
> We will have our Topknots and Powdered Hair.

But despite the spirited defence, the high constructions were on their way out; and in 1711 we find Addison writing in *The Spectator*:

'The whole sex is now dwarfed and shrunk into a race of beauties that seem almost another species. I remember several ladies who were once nearly seven foot high, that at present want some inches of five. How they came to be thus curtailed, I cannot learn; whether the whole sex be at present under any pennance which we know nothing of, or whether they have cast off their head-dresses in order to surprise us with something in that kind which shall be entirely new; though I find most are of the opinion they are at present like trees lopped and pruned that will certainly sprout up and flourish with greater heads than before.'

In 1712 he was still puzzling over the change and still waiting with considerable curiosity, perhaps with some impatience, for the next act. He wrote:

'The ladies have been for some time in a kind of moulting season with regard to that part of their dress, having cast off great quantities of ribbon, lace, and cambric, and in some measure reduced that part of the human figure to the beautiful globular form which is natural to it. We have for a great while expected what kind of ornament would be substituted in the place of those antiquated commodes. But our female projectors were all the last summer so taken up with the improvement of their petticoats, that they had not time to attend to anything else; but having at length sufficiently adorned their lower parts, they now begin to turn their thoughts upon the other extremity, as well, remembering the old kitchen proverb, that if you light your fire at both ends, the middle will shift for itself.'

But the women were having a rest from extravagance and artificiality; and as a glance at Plate 78 will show, the first half century was a period of relatively simple coiffures dressed more or less close to the head. About 1710 there was a fashion for dressing the front hair horizontally across the forehead or building it up over pads, the hair then being plastered down, powdered, and combined with ribbons and gauze (the Hanover cut); but that was the last of the contrived coiffures.

The following description is of an evening coiffure, probably before 1720:

'She wore her hair not in the extent of fashion, but in a manner far more becoming to her regular and beautiful features. It was raised from her forehead to her temples and brought over a crape cushion, and a small portion was confined and curled at the top of the head, whence a plume of ostrich feathers fell gracefully over the left side, while a single curl waved on her neck beneath, which was exquisitely fair. The remaining quantity was divided into ringlets and brought back over the right shoulder, leaving the back of the neck unshaded.'

Once the hair had been lowered, the emphasis began to move toward the back of the head. This is particularly evident in the thirties, forties, and fifties, when the front hair tended to be pulled back simply and the greater part of the hair arranged in curls, a simple twist, or a braid at the back of the head. For evening wear, curls were allowed to fall over the shoulder.

Stewart, writing in 1782 in England, tells us that 'From the beginning of the century to the year 1745, the hair in private life was worn in the most simple manner. About the above period we find the toupee irons first made use of for the front of the hair, which was curled and then turned back under the cap, which cap was also a new plan: this was the first stage of wire caps, which reached about the middle of the head behind, with small wings on each side, and the hair in a few buckles, hanging carelessly in the neck.'

In mid-century the Greek revival in architecture was reflected in the hair styles. Various ornaments were used in the hair by fashionable ladies—ribbons, pearls, and jewels, as well as flowers and decorative pins. Powder was often used for dress occasions and particularly at court.

In the autumn of 1754 *Connoisseur* reported that 'The long lappets, horse-shoe cap, the Brussels head, and the prudish mob pinned under the chin have all of them had their day. The present mode has rooted out all these superfluous excrescences, and in the room of a slip of cambrick or lace, has planted a whimsical sprig of spangles or artificial flowerets. We may remember when for a while the hair was tortured into ringlets behind: at present it is braided into a *queue* (like those formerly worn by the men, and still retaining the original name of Ramillies) which, if it were not reverted upwards, would make us imagine that our fine ladies were afflicted with the *Plica Polonica*.'

Probably no one person was more influential in determining hair styles during the reign of Louis XV than Madame de Pompadour. 'A hundred entrancing ways did she arrange her hair—now powdered, now in all its own silken glory, now brushed straight back, ears showing, now in curls on her neck . . . till the court nearly went mad attempting to imitate her inimitable coiffures.'

Although her coiffures were for the most part relatively simple and tasteful, other ladies went a bit further; and as early as 1756 there were rumblings of things to come:

'It has for a long time been observable that the ladies heads have run much upon wheels; but of late there has appeared a strange kind of inversion, for the wheels now run upon the ladies heads. As this assertion may probably puzzle many readers, who pay no attention to the rapid and whimsical revolutions of modern taste, it will be necessary to inform them that instead of a cap, the present mode is for every female of fashion to load her head with some kind of carriage; whether they are made with broad wheels or not I cannot determine; however, as they are undoubtedly excluded in the Turnpike Act, it is by no means material. Those heads which are not able to bear a coach and six (for vehicles of this sort are very apt to crack the brain) so far act consistently with prudence as to make use of a post-chariot, or a single-horse chaise with a beau perching in the middle.'

The writer then describes one of the vehicles he has examined at a local milliner's. It was, he said, 'constructed of gold threads and was drawn by six dapple greys of blown glass, with a coachman, postilian, and gentleman within, of the same brittle manufacture. Upon further inquiry, the milliner told me, with a smile, that it was difficult to give a reason for inventions so full of whim, but that the name of this ornament (if it may be called such) was a *Capriole* or *Cabriole*, which we may trace from the same original with our English word *Caprice*, both being derived from the French word *cabrer*, which signifies *to prance like a horse*.'

This appeared in *Connoisseur*. Other contemporary reports confirm the fashion. The following verse, called *A Modern Morning*, appeared in 1757:

> Then Coelia to her toilet goes,
> Attended by some fav'rite beaux,
> Who fribble it around the room,
> And curl her hair and clean the comb,
> And do a Thousand monkey tricks
> That you would think disgraced the sex.
> 'Nelly! why, where's the creature fled?
> Put my *post-chaise* upon my head.'—
> 'Your *chair-and-chairmen*, ma'am, is brought.'—
> 'Stupid! the creature has no thought!'—
> 'And, ma'am, the milliner is come,
> She's brought the *broad-wheel'd-waggon* home,
> And 'tis the prettiest little thing,
> Upon my honour!'—'Bring! bring! bring!
> How can you stand and talk about it?
> You know I die, I die without it!'
>   In *broad-wheel'd waggon* thus array'd
> By beaux, and milliner, and maid,
> Dear Coelia treads the toilet round,
> In her fair faithful glass 'tis found,
> And so employs her every sense
> 'Twould take a team to draw her thence.

1760–1770 (Plates 79, 80)

The 1760s mark the laying of the foundations for the 'greater heads than before', which Addison anticipated in 1711. In his *Caricature History of the Georges*, Thomas Wright took a peek inside women's coiffures:

'With the commencement of the reign of George III, hair dressing became an intricate and difficult science and was made the subject of several elaborate publications. To raise up the lofty pile of hair and fill it out with materials to give it due elasticity, and to arrange the vast curls that flanked it, and to give grace to the feathers and flowers with which it was crowned, was not within the capacity of every vulgar coiffeur. The interior of the mass which rose above the head was filled with wool, tow, hemp, etc., and the quantity of pomatum, and other materials used with it, must have produced an effect calculated to disgust all who were not absolutely mad upon fashion.'

As the head-dresses became more intricate, women often resorted to wigs. Plate 79-N illustrates a very popular style. This could be embellished with additional curls, flowers, pompoms, jewels, etc. When frizzed hair, which had been used extensively for men's wigs, became popular with women, there arose further possibilities for decorating the head.

In 1763 there appeared a book called *L'Encyclopédie Carcassière, ou tableaux des coiffures à la mode gravées sur les desseins des petites-maîtresses de Paris*, illustrating forty-four coiffures with such names as *à la cabriolet, à la Baroque, à l'accouchée, à la Pompadour*, and *à la jamais vu*.

About this time Paris was made very much aware of a former cook-turned-hairdresser by the name of Legros de Rumigny, who was known professionally simply as Legros. And with Legros the art and the profession of hairdressing began to flower. Legros was a promoter as well as an indefatigable worker. In addition to dressing ladies' hair, he also created coiffures for thirty dolls which he exhibited at the St Ovide fair in Paris in 1763. In 1765 he had one hundred dolls and twenty-eight original drawings of his designs. He also taught classes at his own *Académie des Coëffures*. The first class was for prospective coiffeurs and coiffeuses and cost six louis. Thirty-eight of his original designs served as models. The second class was for valets who planned to dress milady's hair. They paid four louis and had only twenty-eight designs. The third class was for chambermaids, who paid only two louis and were not shown how to cut hair.

M. Legros made it clear that all students who were guilty of base actions and had 'dishonourable vices' or who betrayed their masters, would be expelled from the academy; and their fees, which they had presumably paid in advance, would be given to the poor.

Classes were not held on Saturday. On weekdays they ran from 10 A.M. to 5 P.M., except in summer, when they lasted from 9 A.M. until 7 P.M., no doubt to take advantage of the additional hours of daylight.

If a student of the academy became ill and could no longer earn a living, each student-teacher (a student having earned certain certificates, that is) was expected to contribute three pounds a year and each master teacher six pounds a year to his support. Anyone who went back on his promise to do this would be considered 'a coward and unfit to be a member of the human race'. M. Legros looked after his own.

In addition to all this, he wrote what is now an exceedingly rare and valuable book called *L'Art de la coëffure des dames françoises*, which was published in Paris in 1768 with supplements in 1769 and 1770. The original volume contained his thirty-eight coiffures (seven of which will be found on Plate 80), information about his academy, a recipe for pomatum, advice and instruction for hairdressers, with diagrams, some words of praise for himself, and a denunciation of his enemies, whom he seemed to feel were legion.

Here is his own recipe for pomatum: 'To make beef pomatum, take some beef marrow, and remove all the bits of skin and bone, put it in a pot with some hazel nut oil, and stir it well with the end of a rolling pin, adding more of the oil from time to time until it is thoroughly liquefied, and add a little essence of lemon. This pomatum will keep 3 or 4 months, and one uses it like ordinary pomatum.'

He had his own method for touching up grey hair: 'To stain the roots of white or gray hair, put a little ivory black powder with white pomatum, and mix well. Using a brush, stain the roots with this pomatum.' He also informed his readers that in order to preserve the natural hair one must cut the ends at every new moon 'except the red moon', when the hair should not be cut at all.

He advised putting a little pomatum on the ends of the hair before putting it in curl papers, but not on the roots since the oil would become hot and burn the scalp. He says that all kinds of curls can be made with the curling iron (illustrated on Plate 80) but that they won't last as long as when made with curl papers.

M. Legros sent copies of his book to all the courts of Europe and claimed to have received gratifying replies, as no doubt he did. It was his conviction (apparently justified) that he was the foremost coiffeur in Europe and that coiffeurs other than his own students were impostors and beneath contempt.

M. Legros' brilliant and influential career came abruptly to an end during the celebrations in honour of the marriage of Marie Antoinette and Louis XVI, when he was accidentally crushed to death in the Place Louis XV.

In 1766 Lady Sarah Lennox wrote revealingly of the hair styles of the period: 'I think that by degrees the French dress is coming into fashion, tho' 'tis almost impossible to make the ladies understand that heads bigger than one's body are ugly; it is growing the fashion to have the heads *moutoné*; I have cut off my hair, and find it very convenient in the country without powder, because my hair curls naturally, but it's horrid troublesome to have it well curled; if it's big it's frightful. I wear it very often with three rows of curls behind, and the rest smooth with a fruzed *toupé* and a cap, that is, *en paresseuse*. There is nobody but Lady Tavistock who does not dress French, who is at all genteel, for if they are not French they are so very ill dressed, it's terrible. Almost everybody powders now and wears a little hoop; hats are vastly left off; the hair down on the forehead belongs to the short waist, and is equally vulgar with poppons, trimmings, beads, garnets, flying caps, and false hair. To be perfectly genteel you must be dress'd thus. Your hair need not be cut off, for 'tis much too pretty, but it must be powdered, curled in very small curls, and altogether be in the style of Lady Tavistock's, *neat*, but it must be high before and give your head the look of a sugar loaf a little. The roots of the hair must be drawn up straight, and not fruzed at all for half an inch above the root; you must wear no cap, and only *little*, *little* flowers dab'd in on the left side; the only feather permitted is a black or white sultane perched up on the left side, and your diamond feather against it.'

Giving us a closer look at the construction of the coiffure, Redfern, writing of the styles of 1768, reports that 'the substratum was composed of wool, tow, pads, and wire, over which was drawn the natural or false hair; and on this again were arranged gauze trimmings, ribbons, feathers of enormous size, and of all the colours of the rainbow, artificial flowers, etc., adding 24 to 36 inches to the actual height of the fair wearer. Ropes of pearls, small models of sows, coaches and horses made of blown glass, also added to the grotesque appearance of the pile.'

All of this, not surprisingly, brought forth a flurry of comment in the press, all of it unfavourable. The women were no doubt too busy having their hair done to reply. Or perhaps it would not have been seemly for them to have done so. At any rate, 1768 seems to have been a banner year for this sort of thing. It began fairly quietly in February with a short and dignified letter of mild protest to the *London Magazine*, signed by 'Lothario, A****N':

'As the principal aim of ladies in their dress is to attract the regard of the men . . . I would acquaint them, through the trumpet of fame, that men . . . are not fond of the present enormous and preposterous headdress (especially in those whose station it is quite inconsistent with) which seems to be the centre of all their pride, with the addition of pearl-powder and carmine, to destroy that natural beauty and sweetness which I and everyone else must own to be most engaging.'

A somewhat less restrained comment appeared during the year in verse form:

> When he views your tresses thin,
>   Tortur'd by some French friseur,
> Horse-hair, hemp, and wool within,
>   Garnish'd with a diamond skewer.
>
> When he scents the mingled steam
>   Which your plaster'd heads are rich in,
> Lard and meal, and clouted cream,
>   Can he love a walking kitchen?

Since neither the sincerity of the prose nor the satire of the poetry had any effect, something a bit more drastic seemed to be called for. The following letter appeared in the *London Magazine* in July 1768, and is quoted here in its entirety:

To the PRINTER, &c.

SIR,

Having seen some pretty lively remarks on the present fashionable way of dressing ladies heads, I take the liberty to send you some advertisements which appeared in the Dublin Universal Advertiser about twelve years ago. Signior Florentini and Mr. St. Laurent were the two rival frizeurs and had practiced some years with pretty equal success and reputation. The Frenchman, however, by his talent at agreeable satire, with which he entertained every lady under his hands, at the expense of her absent aquaintance, during the time of his operation, had manifestly gained a great ascendant over the Italian. This induced Florentini to make a bold effort to raise his own reputation and ruin his rival, whose great character he envied, and whom he wished to be undone.

"Advertisement I

Signior Florentini, having taken into consideration the many inconveniences which attend the method of hair-dressing formerly used by himself and still practiced by Mr. St. Laurent, humbly proposes to the ladies of quality in the metropolis his new method of stuccowing the head in the most fashionable taste, to last with very little repair, during the whole session of parliament. Price only five guineas.

FLORENTINI

N.B. He takes but one hour to build up the head and two for baking it."

Answer by St. Laurent

"Whereas dere have appear vone scandaleuse advertisement of Signior Florentini, moch reflection on Mr. St. Laurent's capacite for hair-dressing, he defy said Signior Florentini to tell any inconvenience dat do attend his methode; odervise he shall consider said Florentini *boute-feu* and caluniateur.

ST. LAURENT"

Florentini, who was not so good at English as the other, replied by his interpreter:

"Whereas Mr. St. Laurent has challenged Signior Florentini to produce an instance where his (St. Laurent's) method of hair-dressing is inconvenient to the ladies, he begs to observe that three rows of iron pins thrust into the skull will not fail to cause a constant itching, a sensation that much distorts the features of the face and disables it, so that a lady, by degrees, may lose the use of her face; besides, the immense quantity of pomatum and powder, laid on for a genteel dressing will, after a week or so, breed *mites*, a circumstance very disagreeable to gentlemen who do not love cheese, and also does afford a foetid smell not to be endured; from which, and other objections too tedious to mention, Signior Florentini apprehends his new method is intirely free and will admit of no reasonable exception whatever.

FLORENTINI"

St. Laurent replies:

"Hah! Hah! Hah! Dere is no objection den to Signior Florentini's vay of frizing de hair of fine ladie? I shall tell him von, two, three; In de forst place, he no consider dat his stuccow will be crack and be break by de frequent jolts to vich all ladies are so subject, and dat two hour baking vil spoil de complekshon and hort de eyes. And as to his scandaleuse aspershun, dat my method breed a de *mite*, so odious to gentleman who do not love de cheese, I say 'tis false and malitieuse; and to make good vat I say, I do envite all gentlemen of qualitie to examine de head of de countess of ——, (vich I had de honour to dress four weeks ago) next Monday at twelve o'clock, through monsieur Closent's great mikroscope, and see if dere be any *mite* dere, or oder thing like de *mite* vateeer. N.B. Any gentleman may smell her ladyship's hede fen he please."

The controversy ended in a duel; but no hurt, as the combatants behaved like Flush and Fribble; but whatever was the cause, it is certain the monstrous fashion soon ceased; and in a few months the ladies heads recovered their natural proportion and became a piece of themselves.

I am, Sir, your's, &c

Although this exchange of advertisements has since been reported as fact, the writing in dialect, if nothing else, leads one to suspect that here is another case of satire being confused with factual information. In any event, the ladies' heads did not recover their natural proportion, nor did they give any evidence of being about to.

At about this time a London hairdresser named Peter Gilchrist published *A Treatise on the Hair or Every Lady her own Hair-Dresser*, in which he quite naturally defended the art of hairdressing:

'Upon the whole, it is evident that dressing is of great benefit to the hair; for the pomatum and powder nourish it; frizzing expands and gives it a larger body; and while it remains in dress it hath rest at the roots, which saves large quantities that would fall off by frequent combing; yet it is very detrimental to let it remain long without being refreshed; for the lacquer of the pins and the powder, gathering in lumps, are apt to make it tear off in the combing out. Likewise, perspiration, the moisture of the hair, and its being long confined from the air, may occasion effluvia rather disagreeable.'

Later on he describes various methods of dressing the hair:

'By a Full Dress is generally understood the hair is dressed in one or two rows of curls, either regular or promiscuous, according to fancy, or as it is most becoming: the hind part may be done either smooth, in a broad plait, or in irregular curls; but for the latter the hair ought to be about seven or eight inches long; though some dress it at full length, by wrapping it up and confining the curls with pins; which is both hurtful to the hair and painful in combing it out.

'If the hair is of a tolerable thickness in the front, two or three curlings will be sufficient for the winter, as frequent pinching is not only painful, but very pernicious to the hair; and it is in a great measure owing to this disagreeable operation that hair-dressing, which is so requisite, makes such slow progress. . . .

'To keep the hair in dress, it ought to be pressed back from the face and carefully filleted at night, but not so tight as to crowd the curls upon one another; in the morning touch the curls gently with the powder-puff, press the friz in front with the left hand, and with the right raise gently, with the piqued end of the comb, those curls which may be lower than the rest; and then, by pressing gently the tail of the comb between each curl, they will appear clean and detached from one another.'

Mr Gilchrist then informs his readers that a crepe toupee, 'though not so dressy, is to most faces very becoming, keeps long in dress, and is never out of fashion, but, without powder, has a rusty look.

'All that is necessary to keep it in dress is to fillet it tight at night, and in the morning rub a little pomatum between the palms of the hands, and when it is of the consistence of oil, stroke it gently over the hair, then put a little powder on it with a swanskin puff; pick it out with the piqued end of the comb, till it is regular in height and free of lumps; give it the last powder, and clip the loose hairs.'

The smooth toupee he finds 'most becoming to ladies of a dark complexion, whose hair is of an agreeable colour, as it looks better without powder than in any other fashion; but it is attended with several inconveniences.

'First, If the hair is not very long in the front, with a fine skin and gloss, it will never dress smooth. Secondly, If the hair is not remarkably thick, it will not dress full, unless supported by wool, which, after the first day, will be distinguished through the hair, and appear very ill.

'This last inconvenience, together with that of not having hair-dressers in the country, hath brought artificial toupees into repute, which are made to appear as the natural hair, and to suit it under all the different accidents to which it is subject.'

He then gives instructions for a smooth dressing of the back hair:

'Comb the long hair clear, first with a wide, then with a smaller toothed comb; then hold it down with a piece of glazed pack thread or silk bobbin, and, taking a little lock of hair under each ear, tie them in a close knot: this makes it feel tight and prevents it from puckering, which it is very apt to do at each side.

'Then take all the hair in the left hand and turn it up; but hold it in the mean time rather slack; every hair will thereby slide gradually and be in a straight line from its root: then you may pull it tighter, but not so much as to strain or distort the skin in the neck; and then smooth it with the smallest teeth of the comb. . . .

'When the hair is quite smooth and spread close to the front part, pin it at the top with a bit of love-ribband and some blanket-pins; then let loose the string;

and, in order that the head may have its proper shape behind, take the two ends of the string and tie them tight in a loop-knot, till you fix each side close behind the ear with a hair-pin; then pull the string out.'

In August of 1768 there appeared in the *London Magazine* a letter destined for posterity. It is frequently referred to but has rarely, if ever, been quoted in full, perhaps for fear of distressing the squeamish. It gives a picture of the seamier side of the eighteenth-century coiffure which has never been equalled:

'In all this mutability of modes, my fair countrywomen have always outshone all others in splendid cleanliness as well as beauty, till very lately, that invention being perhaps exhausted, the reverse of the characteristical neatness has at last had its turn.

'You easily guess, Sir, that I allude to the present prodigious, unnatural, monstrous, and dirty mode of dressing the hair, which, adorned with many jewels, makes them at once shine and stink upwards. Attracted by my eyes to approach as near as I could to these beautiful creatures, I have soon been repelled by my nose and been obliged to retire to a respectful distance. For (I will speak it out) I had the honour of smelling in the most unsavory manner very many heads of the first rank and condition, thus verifying the Newtonian doctrine of attraction and repulsion.

'I went the other morning to make a visit to an elderly aunt of mine, when I found her tendering her head to the ingenious Mr. Gilchrist, who has lately obliged the public with a most excellent essay upon hair. He asked her how long it was since her head had been opened or repaired. She answered, not above nine weeks. To which he replied, that was as long as a head could well go in the summer, and that therefore it was proper to deliver it now; for he confessed that it begun to be a little *hazarde*. He then asked my aunt how she chose to be *coiffée*, whether *à la Cybele*, *à la Gorgonne*, or *à la Venus* [Plate 82-A]. Here I could not help interrupting the conversation by desiring Mr. Gilchrist to expound to me those terms of art which he had mentioned; which he did in the following most obliging manner. *À la Cybele*, Sir, said he, is to raise the hair true or false together, about a foot high, and towerwise, as you see Cybele represented in ancient Bustos. That *à la Gorgonne* required the curls to be looser, more moveable, and to serpent with all the motions of the head. But that *à la Venus* admitted but of few curls, because Venus was supposed to be risen out of the sea and consequently not to have her hair very crisp. My aunt interrupted our conversation by telling Mr. Gilchrist that she desired not to be *coiffée* in the highest extreme of the fashion, for that when a woman was turned of fifty (by the way, she is seventy-three), the dress should be modest to a certain degree.

'When Mr. Gilchrist opened my aunt's head, as he called it, I must confess its effluvias affected my sense of smelling disagreeably, which stench, however, did not surprize me when I observed the great variety of materials employed in raising the dirty fabrick. False locks to supply the great deficiency of native hair, pomatum with profusion, greasy wool to bolster up the adopted locks, and gray powder to conceal at once age and dirt, and all these caulked together by pins of an indecent length and corresponding color. When the comb was applied to the natural hair, I observed swarms of animalculas running about in the utmost consternation and in different directions, upon which I put my chair a little further from the table and asked the operator whether that numerous swarm did not from time to time send out colonies to other parts of the body? He assured me that they could not; for that the quantity of powder and pomatum formed a glutinous matter, which like lime twiggs to birds, caught and clogged the little natives and prevented their migration. Here I observed my aunt to be in a good deal of confusion, and she told me that she would not detain me any longer from better company; for that the operations of the toilette were not a very agreeable spectacle to bystanders, but that they were an unavoidable evil; for, after all, if one did not dress a little like other people, one should be pointed at as one went along.

'If this plain narrative of a matter of fact may contribute to restore my dear countrywomen to their primitive cleanliness, I shall think my time well spent, and I believe you will think your press well employed; but if not, we must e'en leave them to the care of the scavengers, now that the city of Westminster begins to have *some police.*'

So far as is known, the letter had no more effect than the others; and correspondence on the subject seems to have fallen off.

What the various gentlemen apparently failed to realize was that no amount of logic or pleading or scorn or revilement would have the slightest effect in England so long as the French continued to create new and more preposterous head-dresses. Hairdressers were multiplying so rapidly in Paris (1200 of them in 1769) that legal action was taken against them by the guild of Master Barbers, Wig-makers, Bathers, and Washers; but the coiffeurs, contending that they dealt with *living* hair, won.

Even before the unfortunate death of Legros, a rival named Frédéric had appeared and to some extent eclipsed Legros in popularity. But Legros or Frédéric, the hair continued its upward climb.

1770–1780 (Plates 81–85)

At the beginning of the decade the coiffures were still egg-shaped, sometimes with the admirable simplicity of Madame du Barry, more frequently with extensive additions of false curls and various kinds of decoration. Even as early as 1771 Grimm, the celebrated English caricaturist, was taking note of the height of the coiffures (Figure 85). And with an abundance of hairdressers vying with each other in creating new styles, variations on the theme seemed endless. In 1772 there was on file in Paris a monumental work called *L'Éloge des coiffures adressé aux dames*, in thirty-nine volumes and containing illustrations of 3,744 styles of dressing the hair.

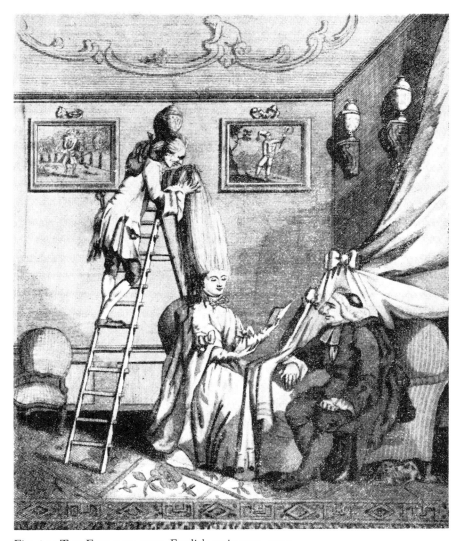

Fig. 84 : THE FOLLY OF 1771. English caricature, 1771

According to *Godey's Lady's Book*, 'In 1772 the *coiffures d'apparat* or *loges d'opéra* appeared and in 1773 those called *à la comté*. The year 1774 is celebrated for two famous modes—the coiffure *à la qu'es aco* [Plate 84-A] and the "sentiment puff". The first was composed of three plumes worn at the back of the head and was a great favorite with the princesses. The other was composed of an infinite variety of matters. Some faint idea of it may be formed from the following description: "In the room was a woman with an infant, the Duke of Valois. On one side of the room was a pet parrot the lady (the Duchess of Chartres) was very fond of. A table was covered with locks of hair from the head of the Duke of Chartres, her husband, of the Duke of Penthievre, her father, of the Duke of Orléans, her father-in-law. These were used in making a sentiment puff for the Duchess of Chartres. It is useless to say all the ladies wore puffs, either *à la reine* or *à la Junon* [Plate 82-D]; and it was a matter of great pride to have been one of the first to wear hair *en parterre galant* [Plate 82-B], *en moulin à vent*, or *en chien couchant* [Plate 84-F]."'

A small pocket book of useful hints for ladies, published in the 1770s, makes the following suggestion:

'Every lady who wishes to dress her hair with taste and elegance should first purchase an elastic cushion, exactly fitted to her head. Then having combed out her hair thoroughly, and properly thickened it with powder and pomatum, let her turn it over her cushion in the reigning model. Let her next divide the sides into divisions for curls, and adjust their number and size from the same models. If the hair be not of a sufficient length and thickness, it will be necessary to procure an addition to it; which is always to be had, ready made, and matched to every colour.'

James Stewart, writing in 1782, says that 'it is not above twelve or thirteen years since cushions were first wore; then they appeared like an exceeding small woman's pin-cushion; but, from this cushion, the plan of the hair has ever since depended on. The hair has been wore higher since, wider, narrower, lower, heavier, lighter, more transparent, more craped, smoother, &c. &c. With one curl, 2 curls, 3 curls, 4 curls, 5 curls, and no curls at all, but all from the same foundation.'

Stewart mentions the French curls, which were popular in the sixties and seventies and describes them as looking 'like eggs strung in order, on a wire, and tied round the head. At the same time, also, appeared the French crape toupee, and also the strait, smooth, or English dress. All these the English had made in false hair, from a notion of cleanliness, which they improved in being at first averse to powder; but soon after they had their own hair drest in all the different fashions. Some time after came up the scollop-shell, or Italian curls, as also the German. The scollop, or shell, were curls in three rows, done back from the face in their several shapes. The German were a mixture of the scollop-shell and French in the front, curled all over behind or *tête de mouton*. After that came long curls; that is, French, but considerably higher, with the points rising as they went back: also the toupee, with two curls done over wool, were worn at this time.'

In 1775 the head-dresses continued to increase in height and to become more eccentric in design. Plate 81-P illustrates an English example. The development was greeted by rather tepid verse. Perhaps the satirists were still too busy with the Macaronis to give their undivided attention to the women's styles.

But about this time a poem called *The Female Macaroni* appeared:

> No ringlets now adorn the face,
> Dear nature yields to art;
> A lofty head-dress must take place,
> Absurd in ev'ry part.
> Patch, paint, perfume, immodest stare,
> You find is all the fashion;
> Alas, I'm sorry for the fair
> Who thus disgrace the nation.

This is followed by more verses in much the same vein. The subject also came up in Garrick's *May-Day or The Little Gypsy*:

> The ladies, I vow,
> I cannot tell how,
> Were now white as curd, and now red.
> Law, how you would stare
> At the huge crop of hair;
> 'Tis a hay-cock at top of their head.

A contributor to the *Irish Quarterly Review* seemed to take a somewhat romantic view of the whole thing:

> Be her shining locks confined
> In a three-fold braid behind;
> Like an artificial flower,
> Set the frissure off before;
> Here and there weave ribbon pat in,
> Ribbon of the finest sattin.

But this was only one small voice (a woman's, perhaps, or that of a young man in love?) against the multitude of protesting males.

It is clear from the various comments that powder was the fashion. But when the hair did appear in its natural colour, it was much preferred that the colour be dark. In June 1775 there appeared in *The Lady's Magazine* a helpful article by Dr John Cook entitled 'Receipt for Changing Yellow Hair', in which the good doctor seems not to distinguish between red and yellow:

'Time was when golden locks were looked upon as very beautiful, and even the lass of golden hair was, for that very reason, the more eligible, and preferred before those of the sex who bore any different color;—but now the case is changed, and red hair is not so agreeable; though this I can say, such women have the finest skins, with azure veins, and generally become the best breeders of the nation.

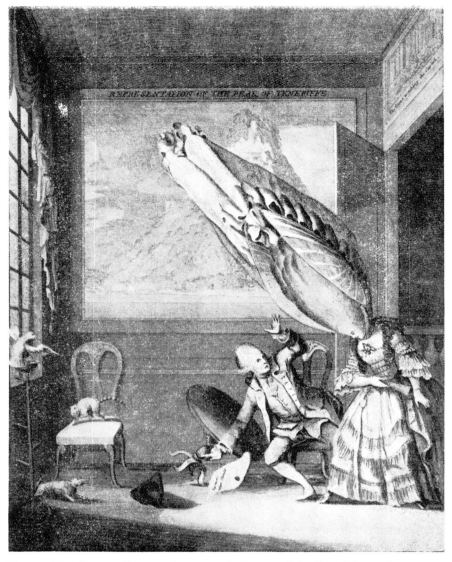

Fig. 85 : THE FRENCH LADY IN LONDON. Caricature of the French hairstyles in 1771. Engraving after J. H. Grimm

'However, for the sake of those of the fair sex not so well satisfied with the present unfashionable color of their hair, I freely proffer them the following short prescription, easily to be had, and as easily prepared, whereby they may privately alter, whenever they please, the disagreeable yellow hue of their hair into an agreeable black, and that without either sin, danger, or shame.

'Squeeze any quantity you choose of the juice of ripe elderberries, or those from the dwarf-elder, as being the stronger; let it stand all night to settle; next day pour off the clear liquor, put into it a cup full (more or less) of red wine, let them simmer together gently, 2 or 3 minutes, over a slow fire, then bottle it for use.

'With some of this liquor warmed, wash the hair now and then, in time it will safely dye it of an agreeable black colour.

'This is the very prescription I sent to a young lady, who wrote to me from London for advice, for which she complimented me with thanks, and genteelly sent me a guinea for my fee.

'I should be ever proud to serve the ladies with the uttermost of my medical capacity, whenever they shall think fit to honour me with any of their commands.'

Still the head-dresses continued to rise; and according to *Godey's*, 'On February 17, 1776, the queen [*Marie-Antoinette*] being about to go to a ball given by the Duchess of Orléans, had a head-dress so high that she could not get into her carriage, and it was therefore taken off and replaced when she arrived. All head-dresses, however, could not be thus taken to pieces, and the ladies, victims of vanity, were forced to keep their heads out of the window of their carriages, and sometimes even to kneel.'

Feathers were all the rage; and Heath reports that the Duchess of Devonshire, who was exceedingly influential in the world of fashion, wore an ostrich feather more than four feet long. Leloir remarks that advancing ladies at the court gave the impression of Birnam Wood coming to Dunsinane.

In *The Lady's Magazine* a correspondent reported:

'At Ranelagh . . . I saw the Duchess of D.'s fine face ornamented more naturally and with but three feathers instead of seven. Lady S.'s head was the most beyond the bounds of propriety, she having so many plates of fruit placed on the top pillar, and her being without powder it was not so delicate a mixture.'

In August 1776 there appeared a description in verse of the lady of fashion:

> Muse being the comic lay,
> Since the female of today,
> Yet to person be confined,
> Nor dare to meddle with her mind,
> Lest the strange investigation
> Cause thee trouble and vexation,
> 'Twere to seek, alas a-day,
> Needles in a stack of hay.

Void of talents, sense, and art,
Dress is now her better part;
Sing her daubed with white and red,
Sing her large terrific head;
Nor the many things disguise
That produce its weighty size;
And let nothing be forgot,
Carrots, turnips, and what not:
Curls and cushions for imprimus,
Wool and powder for the finis;
Lace and lappets many a flag—
Many a party-coloured rag—
Pendant from the head behind,
Floats and wantons in the wind,
Many a gem, and many a feather,
Choice fanago all together,
By whose wood and wire assistance,
(Formidable at a distance,
As the elephants of yore
A famed Queen to battle bore,)
They with honour and surprise
Strike the poor beholders eyes,
What a quantity of brain
Must he think such heads contain,
Though it prove a false alarm,
Feather brains can do no harm,
Hats that only show the chin,
And the mouth's bewitching grin,
As intended for a shield
To the caput thus concealed;
Surely 'tis an useful art
Well to guard the weakest part.
Shoes that buckle at the toe,
Gowns that o'er the pavement flow,
Or festooned on either side,
With two yellow ribbons tied,
While a peak, like pigeon's rump,
Shows behind she's not too plump.
Heels that bear the precious charge,
More diminutive than large;
Slight and brittle, apt to break,
Of the true Italian make,

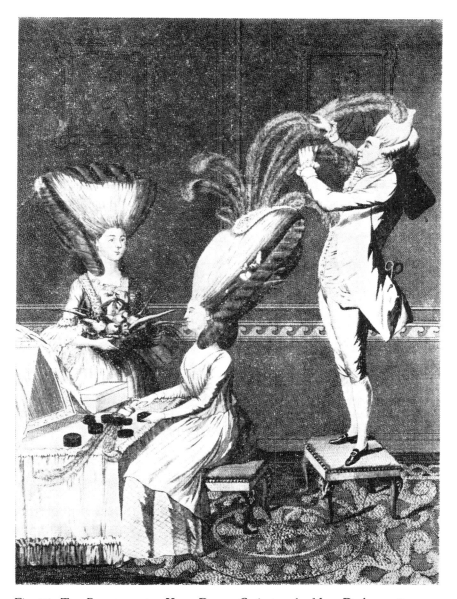

Fig. 86 : THE PREPOSTEROUS HEAD DRESS. Caricature by Mary Darly, 1778

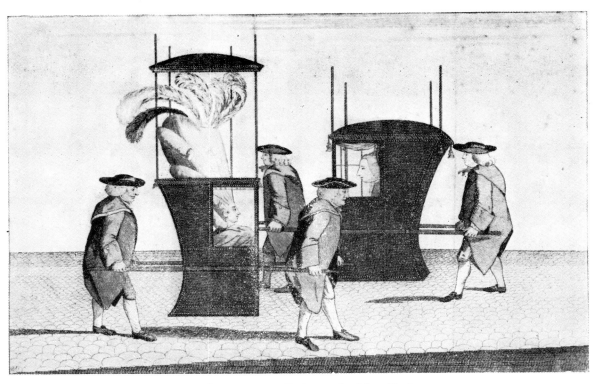

Fig. 87 : THE LADIES CONTRIVANCE. Caricature by Mary Darly, 1777

> For women of bon ton, observe ye,
> Like sugar loaves turned topsy-turvy,
> As their heaviest part's a top
> Rest upon a feeble prop,
> And, that all mankind may know it,
> Toss about their heads and show it!

As to the 'Sing her daubed with white and red', it was not unusual for women of fashion to paint their faces with a sort of white enamel, which was designed to conceal wrinkles along with discolorations and blemishes. The rouge was usually applied in intensely bright spots as unnatural as the white complexion. Although the white paints were notoriously harmful, the women continued to wear them and take their chances. According to *The Art of Beauty*, the chances were exceedingly slim:

The white paints 'affect the eyes, which swell and inflame, and are rendered painful and watery. They change the texture of the skin, on which they produce pimples and cause rheums; attack the teeth, make them ache, destroy the enamel, and loosen them. They heat the mouth and throat, infecting and corrupting the saliva, and they penetrate through the pores of the skin, acting by degrees, on the spongy substance of the lungs, and inducing diseases. Or, in other cases, if the paint be composed of aluminous or calcareous substances, it stops the pores of the skin, which it tarnishes, and prevents the perspiration, which is, of course, carried to some other part, to the peril of the individual. . . . To the inconveniences we have just enumerated, we add this, of turning the skin black when it is exposed to the contact of sulphureous or phosphoric exhalations. Accordingly, those females who make use of them ought carefully to avoid going too near substances in a state of putrefaction, the vapours of sulphur, and liver of sulphur, and the exhalation of bruised garlic.'

Darly, never one to miss an opportunity, managed to combine the enormous height, the feathers, and the fruit all in one caricature (Figure 86). And one of the most famous of all caricatures of the period is the fashionable English lady with most of her head-dress sticking out through the top of her sedan chair (Figure 87).

In the same year there appeared in *The New Bath Guide* a verse by Christopher Anstey:

> A cap like a bat,
>   (Which was once a cravat)
> Part gracefully platted and pinn'd is:
>   Part stuck upon gauze,
>   Resembles mackaws,
> And all the fine birds of the Indies.
>
> But above all the rest
>   A bold amazon's crest
> Waves nodding from shoulder to shoulder;
>   At once to surprise,
>   And to ravish all eyes,
> To frighten and charm the beholder.
>
> In short, head and feather,
>   And wig altogether,
> With wonder and joy would delight ye:
>   Like the picture I've seen
>   Of th'adorable queen,
> Of the beautiful, blest Otaheite.
>
> Yet Miss at the rooms
>   Must beware of her plumes:
> For if Vulcan her feather embraces,
>   Like poor Lady Laycock,
>   She'll burn like a haycock,
> And roast all the Loves and the Graces.

Although Mr Anstey refers to a wig, the term did not necessarily mean what is now considered a wig but was used to refer to any head of hair, false or not. Wigs, however, were being worn by women although not to the extent that they were by men. The problem of living with and maintaining the extremely large and intricate constructions, nearly all of which required a certain amount of false hair, would seem almost to require the use of wigs. But since Marie-Antoinette preferred whenever possible to wear her own hair, wigs were not worn proudly and forthrightly as they were by men but were accepted when necessary as a practical solution to an otherwise almost insoluble problem. Those who could manage to, usually followed the Queen's example.

The Queen's mother, Maria Theresa, was unimpressed with her daughter's position as a leader of fashion; and on receiving from her a portrait in a particularly preposterous head-dress, she returned it, suggesting there must have been some mistake—that she had received a portrait of an actress, not a queen of France.

In referring to English fashions of 1777, Hannah More wrote: 'The other night we had a great deal of company—eleven damsels to say nothing of men. I protest I hardly do them justice when I pronounce that they had, amongst them, on their heads, an acre and a half of shrubbery, besides slopes, grass plots, tulip beds, clumps of peonies, kitchen gardens, and greenhouses.'

Coiffures were often allegorical and represented rustic poems, settings for an opera, or perhaps just a flower garden, a field with sheep and shepherds, miniature models of Paris, or the garden of the Palais Royal, including all details. According to Goncourt, widows sometimes requested tasteful representations of tombs with cupids playing with torches. Others wanted the entire solar system—in movement. Romantically inclined young ladies might ask for the Bois de Boulogne replete with animals.

Topical head-dresses were always popular—*à l'inoculation*, for example, representing the triumph of vaccine, and the *ballon* style, which came about, according to an article in the *Gentleman's Magazine* a century later, as a result of the Montgolfier balloon experiments. Although it is not in the least surprising that such a relationship should exist, it ought to be pointed out that the engraving and description of the style (Plate 83-J) were published in England in 1777, and the first successful public demonstration of the Montgolfier brothers' balloon did not take place until 1783. It is entirely possible, however, that preliminary experiments were sufficiently well known to affect the hair styles.

Every coiffure had a name—*à la candeur, à la frivolité, le chapeau tigré, la Baigneuse, des migraines, à la Mappemonde* (showing the five parts of the world), *à la Zodiaque* (Plate 83-J), *l'aigrette* (a built-in parasol of ostrich feathers, possibly the same coiffure as that shown in Plate 83-F under another name), *à la Minerve, à la Flore, aux insurgents* (with a snake so realistic that the government prohibited it out of deference to ladies' nerves), *au berceau d'amour, les ailes de papillon, la voluptueuse, au mirliton, à l'oiseau royal*—the list is endless.

Although the names sound glamorous enough, we have already had a look inside. A contributor to the *London Magazine* in 1777 (clearly an unromantic type) failed to see the glamour and took a more realistic view:

Give Chloe a bushel of horse-hair and wool,
Of paste and pomatum a pound,
Ten yards of gay ribbon to deck her sweet skull,
And gauze to encompass it round.

Of all the bright colours the rainbow displays
Be those ribbons which hang on her head,
Be her flounces adapted to make the folks gaze,
And about the whole work be they spread.

Let her flaps fly behind, for a yard at the least:
Let her curls meet just under her chin:
Let these curls be supported, to keep up the jest,
With a hundred, instead of *one* pin.

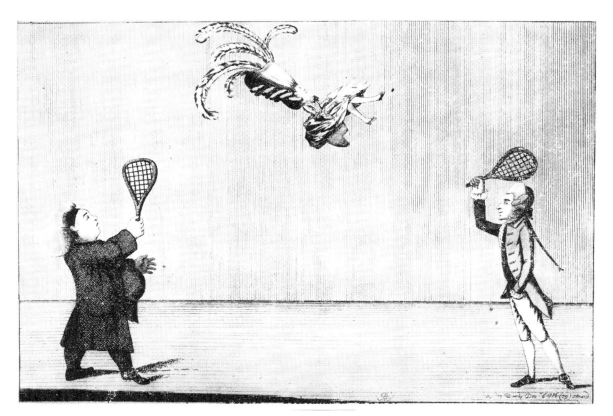

Fig. 88 : Miss Shuttle-Cock. Caricature by Mary Darly, 1776

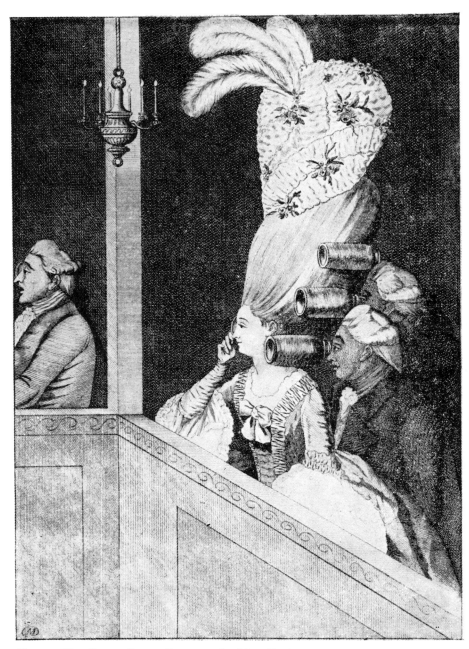

Fig. 89 : THE OPTIC CURLS. Caricature by Mary Darly, 1777

Let her gown be tuck'd up to the hip on each side;
Shoes too high for to walk, or to jump;
And, to deck the sweet creature complete for a bride,
Let the cork-cutter make her a rump.

Thus finish'd in taste, while on Chloe you gaze,
You may take the dear charmer for life;
But never undress her—for, out of her stays
You'll find you have lost half your wife.

But the ladies were hypnotized and seemed to see only the beauty of their decorations. In her memoirs Mme d'Oberkirch included this page from her diary:

'This blessed 6th of June she awakened me at the earliest dawn. I was to get my hair dressed, and make a grand toilette, in order to go to Versailles, whither the Queen had invited the Comtesse du Nord, for whose amusement a comedy was to be performed. These Court toilettes are never-ending, and this road from Paris to Versailles very fatiguing, especially where one is in continual fear of rumpling her petticoats and flounces. I tried that day, for the first time a new fashion—one, too, which was not a little *génante*. I wore in my hair little flat bottles shaped to the curvature of the head; into these a little water was poured, for the purpose of preserving the freshness of the natural flowers worn in the hair, and of which the stems were immersed in the liquid. This did not always succeed, but when it did, the effect was charming. Nothing could be more lovely than the floral wreath crowning the snowy pyramid of powdered hair!'

When the coiffures became so high that doorways had to be enlarged and ladies had to bend double in carriages, a man named Beaulard invented a mechanical coiffure which could, when circumstances required it, be lowered a foot or two by touching a spring. Duvisme, director of the Paris opera, refused entry of all high coiffures into the amphitheatre. But they were still welcome in the boxes. (See the English caricature in Figure 89.)

By this time the chignon had dropped quite low and was sometimes pulled together in the middle, giving what was known as a *banging chignon*, shown in Plate 84-A.

1778 was the year of the victory of the French ship *La Belle Poule* over the English *Arethusa*. The event, naturally, was commemorated in a head-dress (shown in Plate 83-K), which has become considerably more famous than either the ship or the battle. It was not worn by the English.

Other contemporary head-dresses were named *Spaniel's Ears, Drowned Chicken, Indian Chestnut Tree, the Round Table, the Chest of Drawers, the Cabriolet, the Mad Dog, the Sportsman-in-the-Coppice*, and so on. In addition to the gardens and the landscapes and the waterfalls, there was also what is sometimes called the 'kitchen-garden' style, in which vegetables were attached to the side curls. The opportunity for satire did not go unnoticed. (See the caricature in Figure 86.)

A contemporary journalist described the *cabriolet* style as follows:

'Conceive two great wings on either side of the face, sticking out seven or eight inches beyond it, and three or four beyond the biggest noses in the kingdom, the said wings fastened at the back to a full linen bag containing the voluminous collection of hair which ladies at this moment regard as their most precious ornament. Above all this is piled a sort of framework of ribbon puffings, which looks as if it were tied together with a rosette of the same ribbon near the back of the skull.'

And in this same year there appeared in France what Heath describes as 'a certain headdress of prodigious height which represented precipitous hills, enameled fields, silver streams, foaming torrents, symmetrical gardens, and an English park'. Perhaps the caricature in Figure 83 is not really a caricature at all.

Speight tells of a late eighteenth-century Siberian hairdresser named Ivan Peter Alexis Knoutschoffschlerwitz, who, in offering his service to the ladies of London, 'engages to execute it in a manner peculiar to himself, rejecting the use of black pins, hair cushions, and the like cumbersome materials, so dangerous in their effects. He avoids the use of a great many abominations, which he enumerates, but which we abstain from mentioning. Instead of these, he fills the hollows of the hair with soft aromatic herbs, which "prevent the disagreeable effect of perspirations now so generally complained of". He dresses hair in every mode, and engages to make any lady's head appear like the head of a lion, a wolf, a tiger, a bear, a fox, or any exotic beast which she would choose to resemble. He does not, however, confine himself to beasts, for to anybody who happened to prefer the form of a peacock, a swan, a goose, a Friesland hen, or any other bird, he engaged to give a perfect likeness. He also offered to give any colour to the hair that a lady might judge most suitable to her complexion, for as every single hair is an hollow tube, though imperceptible to the naked eye, he, by injecting a certain liquid, communicated the finest shades, and rendered the use of powder unnecessary, thereby effecting, as a wag of the day observes, a great saving in bread corn. Ladies whose hair indicates the time of life which they wished to conceal could be secretly and safely accomodated by this interesting Siberian. He could change their locks into a fine chestnut, blue, crimson, or green, according to the mode which might generally prevail.'

Speight reports the whole matter in complete seriousness, and possibly there was such a Siberian. On the other hand, Speight may have been misled, as other writers have been, by a contemporary tongue-in-cheek magazine piece. Several details, including the Siberian's name, rather incline one to that suspicion. Without the original material it is difficult to be sure. However, it is perhaps characteristic of the period that it is no longer always easy to distinguish between the real thing and the satire of it.

Schools for hairdressers were naturally flourishing, and a letter from Paris to the editor of *Gentlemen's Magazine* gives one Englishman's reaction:

'Mr. Urban, among the oddities which present themselves every minute to the eyes of a stranger in the fluttering city, I have been highly entertained with one in particular, i.e., the academy for teaching the art of female hair-dressing according to the present high *gout*. In my walks I have seen several of these, where a large room with its contents is laid open to public view, and wherein you see a great number of the dirtiest female drabs the streets afford, hired to sit (as we phrase it) not for their pictures, but their patience, and to have their heads and their hair twisted and turned about in various forms, according to the taste of the operator. Some of these ladies in high dress have been so wonderfully picturesque that I have been more than once in danger of breaking a blood vessel; nor is it less entertaining to observe with what astonishment and delight some of them look into the glass under their elegant coiffeure. Yet I must confess that I have seen others who have exhibited well-bred faces, looked full as like women of fashion as their betters, a look which no dress can give to a low educated woman of our nation. When a head is finished, the whole chamber of artists examine the workmanship, and after each has given his opinion, the pyramid is thrown down and re-erected by some other student. Before I have well recovered from the soarness and a fit of coughing, which laughing is apt to produce on me, my eyes are struck with two golden angels sounding trumpets, and which in the joint actions of flying and walking, support their trumpets with one hand, each holding a well-combed perruque with the other. By this you will perceive, Mr. Urban, that the head and hair are the two main objects of a French-woman's attention.'

The *hérisson* or *hedgehog* style (Plate 85-I) appeared about this time and became extremely popular in both France and England and lasted for some years. It seemed for a while as if it might threaten the tall structures, which had reached a clearly unmanageable height; and though there was evidence of some decrease in height, there was a corresponding increase in width. This was the direction the hair was to take in the following decade.

1780–1790 (Plates 84-86)

According to Heath, 'In 1780 there was a vast difference between head-dressing in London and Paris. The English ladies were wearing enormous plumes of feathers of all colors, with chains of pearls or beads hanging round the mass of hair, which formed the outside covering of the "bushel of horsehair and wool" within. Bunches of flowers were stuck about the head surmounted by large butterflies, caterpillars, &c. in blown glass, as well as models of coaches and horses. This last fashion was the subject of caricature. In one of the year 1777 the hair is drawn up and extends backwards perhaps a yard. In the summit a hearse, drawn by six horses and loaded with plumes, is seen slowly crawling down the mountain of hair. At the base of the print is the legend: "A safe and effectual preparation for the next world".'

In the eighties the toupee, which was fuller than it had been, was often frizzed, along with the side hair, to stand out away from the head; and it usually covered the ears, which had previously been at least partially exposed. Drawings C and K on Plate 82 are typical.

In France there was an unexpected change in the fashions when Marie-Antoinette, following her confinement, lost her hair. Obviously, the enormous head-dresses had to go. Léonard designed a simple coiffure for the Queen called *à l'enfant*; and that, with endless variations, became the style for a while. Plate 85 shows some of the low coiffures of the period. But as the Queen's hair grew again, so did the head-dresses.

Although Larseneur was the official hairdresser of the Queen, she much preferred Léonard Autié, who was commissioned in 1779. But rather than dismiss Larseneur or even hurt his feelings, she let him do her hair as he wished; and then for special occasions she had it dressed by Léonard. It was customary for the great ladies to have at least two coiffeurs. For every day Du Barry had Berline, whereas for balls and other special events she relied on the artistry of Nokelle.

From 1780 to 1783 the Queen had the services of Legay, who was also a wig-maker. Léonard's brother, Jean-François, was commissioned in 1783. Then in 1784 Jean-François took over the duties of Legay; and after 1788 only Léonard remained.

With all the frizzing and masses of small curls, hairdressing became more of a problem than ever before. About 1835 the following description of some of the problems appeared in Watson's *Annals of Philadelphia*:

'Ancient ladies are still alive who have told me that they often had their hair tortured for four hours at a sitting in getting the proper crisped curls of a hair curler. Some who designed to be inimitably captivating, not knowing they could be sure of professional services where so many hours were occupied upon one gay head, have actually had the operation performed the day before it was required, then have slept all night in a sitting posture to prevent the derangement of their frizzle and curls. . . . This formidable head work was succeeded by rollers over which the hair was combed above the forehead. These again were superseded by cushions and artificial curled work, which could be sent out to the barber's block, like a wig, to be dressed, leaving the lady at home to pursue other objects—thus producing a grand reformation in the economy of time, and an exemption too from former durance vile.'

The use of large amounts of false hair and the increasing problems of dressing the hair led inevitably to a more widespread use of wigs. Mme Tallien is said to have had more than fifty of assorted colours.

Heath, writing in the *Magazine of Art* exactly a century later, expressed the opinion that in 1786 'the Paris head-dress was really awful, absolutely a lion's mane, frizzed with regular curls, and a great garland at the top, with an enormous plume of three feathers arising out of some drapery at the back'. He might have been referring to the style shown in Plate 85-O.

Certainly the feathers were more in evidence than ever; and bushy, frizzed hair with loose, sleek curls was beginning to turn into a somewhat disorganized mass of small tight curls topped with tiffany and ribbon and feathers and flowers and jewels. Although the hair itself did not rise so high as in the seventies, the things that were

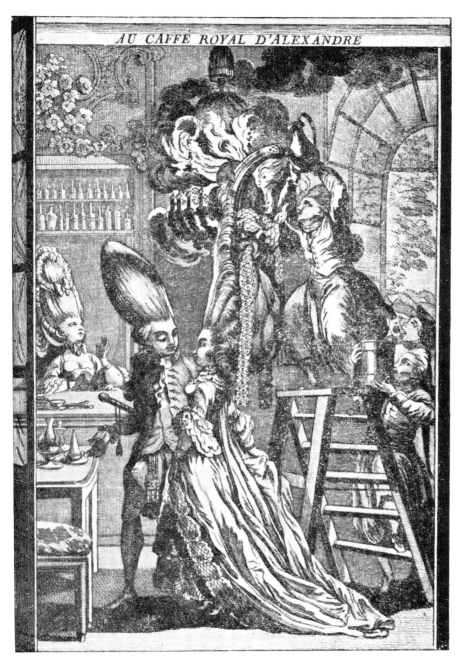

Fig. 90 : Au Caffé Royal d'Alexandre (sic). French caricature, 1787. There are in England records of at least two fatalities resulting from head-dresses being set on fire by chandeliers stuck into it more than made up the difference. After 1786 the hair was lowered somewhat and began to hang farther down the back (Plate 88-D). The 1789 style shown in Plate 86-N gives a preview of the decade to come.

Not all of the hairdressers were as irresponsible as the styles seem to indicate. One of them, William Barker, of No. 6 King Street, Holborn, wrote a short *Treatise on the Principles of Hair-Dressing; in which the Deformities of Modern Hairdressing are pointed out, and an elegant and natural Plan recommended, upon Hogarth's immortal System of Beauty*. Although no date of publication is given, one is led to the conclusion that it must have been written about 1786. Mr Barker was understandably distressed by the current styles and said so repeatedly:

'Many females, whose fronts and shoulders are adorned with tresses, waving or curling naturally, which must rank them in the number of Nature's most beautiful works, by their own false taste, by pursuing fashion to the very extreme, or injudiciously adopting some favourite mode of the dresser, render themselves highly ridiculous. If the hair is forced up in the front, and glued up, as it were, by the dresser, the curls, however managed by the most skilful hand, will only serve as appendages to a bold head; and the lady's head-dress will provoke witticisms by no means favorable to female delicacy. . . .

'The present mode of forming the toupee is the most unaccountable and strange that ridiculous custom ever introduced. In the formation of even the smallest curl, the greatest attention should be paid to ease, grace, and a close imitation of Nature; the contrary mode of extending the hair to the utmost at the side of the head and dragging it from the face backward in a straight line, is not only stiff and unnatural, but there is scarce one face in a thousand that will bear such a mode of dressing. . . . When the head is dressed in the present taste and the toupee made in the Parisian style, it forms a flat as even as the foundation stone for the erection of an edifice, while it presents a disagreeable angle to the eye.

'In the present fashion, that part of the front which forms this awkward toupee, rises more than an inch and a half plain, whilst the hair on the sides serves to form the toupee in a kind of mathematical proportion. Now this adherence to a square form is wandering from Nature; for instead of tending to embellish, it serves only to disfigure her most perfect works; and for the truth of this, I appeal to the opinions and productions of the most eminent artists.'

Mr Barker was also distressed by the stiff side curls which were fashionable at the time and complained that they obscured 'the beautiful neck of our lovely country-women. I am at a loss to represent these curls by any natural allusion; if they resemble any thing, it is the appearance of the head of the private soldier, who when called upon guard, by the management of a piece of leather, obtruded from the side of his head, exhibits something extremely whimsical; with only this difference, that his expedient is not half so indelicate and offensive; the female curls being much flatter and broader. . . . The *things*, or curls . . . (as they are falsely called) are only imprisoned hair, clogged by the grease of pomatum and smothered with a profusion of powder.

'Pomatum and powder, when employed in the hands of a man of taste, who has a genius for style, will considerably augment the beauty of the hair; but these two powerful ingredients in the hands of an ignorant or negligent dresser, are like the pallet and pencil in the hands of an unskilful painter. . . .

'A lady's hair dressed in the present enormous style . . . is rendered more unnatural and ridiculous by the hair being dressed very low and in a strait line of exclusion, so formed as totally to hide the ears, as if our modern ladies intended to rival the ancient Mandarins of China, who cut off their ears as a mark of dignity.

'Mr. Garrick, so universally admired for his very extraordinary theatrical talents, caricatured this ludicrous and disguising mode of dress, about eight years ago, so effectually in wearing a tête, which I made by his orders, so preposterously fashionable, for the assumed lady of Sir John Brute, that many of the fair creation, who had been deaf to the voice of reason, and of Nature, were laughed out of the absurdity, and reduced the size of their head-dresses within the compass of moderation.'

One of Mr Barker's many objections was to the practice of frizzing or craping the hair, which, he suggested, might 'be used in some trifling instances, but is surely a great deformity in general. When it is considered that the craping of the hair is the greatest destruction to that fine ornament of the head, it is to be hoped that ladies will abstain from a practice which eventually must deprive them of this fine embellishment. . . . Indeed, the practice of craping is now on the decline; and it is hoped it will be intirely abolished.'

Mr Barker did not miss the opportunity for a few jibes at the French, whose styles were so influential in England:

'If it is the ambition of my fair country-women to imitate the French ladies, I sincerely wish they would desist from the pursuit of what is impossible to attain. The French ladies being in general of a dark complexion, are very similar to each other when dressed for public appearance; for the fashion of wearing their rouge is systematical; and that fashion, when it does alter, alters always with a very remarkable variety. From a little below the eye there is sometimes drawn a red streak to the lower temple and another streak in a semicircular form to the other line. If the eyebrows are not naturally dark, they make them so; and unless ladies have very striking personal singularities, it is difficult to distinguish them asunder: their manners too so widely differing from the reserve of the English, renders imitation in that particular as burlesque and ridiculous as in the article of dress. Sometimes the French ladies, like the pallid Italian women of the Opera, put on rouge of the highest colour in the form of a perfect circle, without shading it off at all; this is done to give a fire to the eye, which they think adds a spirit to conversation and a force to the art of ogling.

'But the English ladies set a value upon the characters of chastity, modesty, and virtue, to which the *married* ladies of France claim no pretensions; nay, the very supposition would be an insult to them; I infer therefore upon the whole, that the females of our island can never affect a similarity to the French ladies, with

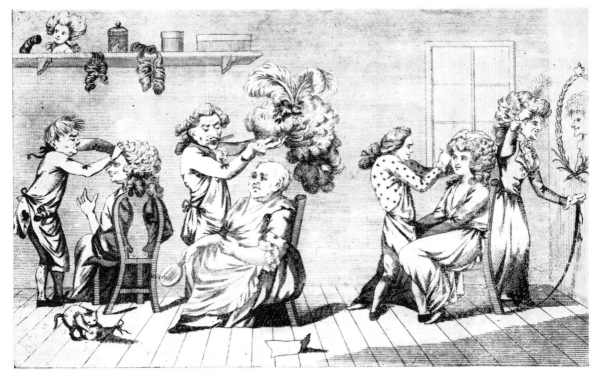

Fig. 91 : THE FEMALE WIG SHOP. English caricature, 1786

propriety, either in dress or manners, till our morals and our notions are totally changed.'

But Mr Barker, in giving the devil his (or her) due, admitted indebtedness 'to the French ladies, in a great measure, for one of the finest ornaments, as a powder to the hair, that this century ever produced. It is matter of little importance whether a Doctor of the Sorbonne or an Abbé first disclosed this brown powder to a Princess, or her waiting woman; and we are much more indebted to the Queen, for introducing the fashion of wearing a kind of orange coloured powder, which, by an artificial light, looks like what is vulgarly called red hair, but which has a very good effect in an assembly, if the lady's complexion should be bad. On the heads of some fine women, it has quite a contrary effect, as powder of such an hue, even with the assistance of rouge on her cheeks, must give her face a livid cast, and her neck must appear as if painted a dead white.

'The Queen of France has also discovered the utmost taste by discountenancing the stiff, starch, and unnatural mode of craping the hair and torturing it into an infinity of side curls, as also by adopting the graceful ease which *once distinguished* the head-dresses of the ladies of this country. Strange, however, as it may appear, it is an uncontrovertible fact that no sooner had the French queen discarded the "absurd" *mode* of *hair-dressing* than the English ladies renounced for once their usual predilection for French fashion and now adhere to the ridiculous mode which the Queen is endeavouring to abolish. With respect to the use of rouge also, the above personage is introducing a more natural mode of laying it on the face, instead of the broad semicular streaks which the French ladies have so long practiced.'

Various colours of powder were used throughout the decade, and Mr Barker had obviously given considerable thought to the choice of the right one for a particular lady under particular circumstances. Reluctant to generalize, however, he suggested that the choice be left to the dresser—provided he was a man of taste. But he did offer a few helpful suggestions:

'White powder is regaining its general use and promises to be the universally adopted taste, but the use of white powder in the extreme is an error that a nice distinguishing taste for elegance can never altogether adopt, because the colour of the powder must ever be governed by the prevailing tints of the person's complexion. A brown beauty and a fair beauty should not use the same coloured powder;—the reason must be self-evident. Ladies who take exercise and have the lovely glow of health in their cheeks, however fair and beautiful the complexion may be, should not use white powder alone, as the effect ever must be that the light acting on white without absorbing one ray, the reflected rays cast a shade on the face that discolours the real complexion and gives it the semblance of a dusky brown. On the contrary, a lady who leads a sedentary life and is little exposed to the air will have a rather languid aspect; a very little brown mixed with white powder will therefore give great assistance to such a complexion, enliven the appearance of the eyes and face, and animate the whole form. There is a coloured hair (I mean the yellow, vulgarly called red, of a more than common bright tinge) to which a deep brown or chocolate powder gives the happiest cast, infinitely surpassing the grey powder, and saving the trouble and expense of staining the hair by advertised nostrums of a mineral, poisonous, destructive effect, which are generally applied by persons wholly ignorant of the nature and quality of hair. This powder, judiciously applied, has the same happy effect on flaxen and grey hair, with this difference as to the latter, that it must be used in its pure state, not lowered by the least mixture of white. . . .

'There are very few heads of hair which do not require the aid of colouring, as well as enriching. Pomade and powder are the best materials for that purpose I know of and have hitherto been so approved, none better having been yet discovered; but the profusion with which these articles, valuable in themselves, is too frequently used, is productive of as injurious effects as the inordinate application of rouge. When ladies, desirous of a florid complexion and out of humour with Nature for having been rather unkind in that particular, first begin the use of that imaginary ornament, they apply it with a sparing hand; but daily habit and the love of admiration tempting them by degrees to enlarge the portion, those articles, which applied with discretion would tend to embellish, are laid on in such profusion, and particularly the rouge, that the beholder turns aside, the eye declining to encounter so glaring an object.'

Mr Barker then explained that his method of dressing the hair for Mrs Siddons and other theatrical clients 'tends principally to the setting off the features of the face and the hue of the complexion, and that my curling also, as well as powdering hair, are governed not by fashion, but by the formation of the face and neck, the colour of the skin, and the lights, whether natural or artificial, by which the face and neck are to be viewed. The hair, in an artificial light, is only to be considered as a mean to give a fine colour to the complexion by such shade and light as the stage affords, which will, in every possible instance, alter the face and natural colour of the complexion. This may be demonstrated by the absolute necessity which stage performers are under of using colour on their faces; and it is evident that young men who perform old characters, by a judicious application of white and red and a few black lines drawn with Indian ink, often wear the appearance on the stage of eighty or ninety and are altogether so much altered that their most intimate friends do not know them.'

1790–1800 (Plates 87, 88)

The high, constructed head-dresses were gone by 1790, and great masses of curls had taken their place. Sometimes the curls hung to the shoulders or below, sometimes not. But in either case they were likely to be combined with a broad cadogan of smooth hair. The head was nearly always bound with some sort of ribbon or tulle and was frequently decorated with beads, feathers, and flowers—especially feathers. They were particularly popular in England and were worn in all varieties and all colours—black, blue, yellow, green, lilac, white, gold, silver. Engravings of court affairs or balls of the period look as if the ladies had all stepped off the same assembly line, in which the last operator had stuck a tall, curling feather or two in the top of each one (see Plate 87).

Although the English imported most of the hair styles from France, it required clever (and busy) hairdressers to copy them and turn out a few of their own on the side. It is reported that at the coronation of George II there were only two hairdressers in London; in 1795 it was estimated that there were fifty thousand in Great Britain.

When hair powdering was taxed in 1795, its use in England rapidly declined for women as well as for men. About this same time there was a dramatic change in the styles when the Titus cut (Plate 87-C) ushered in the fashion of short hair. According to La Mésangère in *Le Bon Genre*, the Titus mode consisted 'in having the hair cut close to the roots so as to restore its natural stiffness and make it grow in a perpendicular direction'.

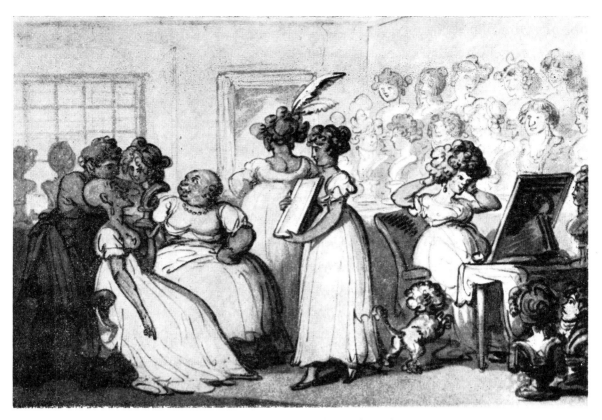

Fig. 92 : A Wig Shop. Caricature by Thomas Rowlandson, late eighteenth century

Thus the women entered upon a whole new era of hair styles, managing to find an astonishing number of things to do with short hair, including naming each new style just as they had in the past. Many of the names, such as *à la victime* or *à la sacrifié*, were associated with the Revolution. The hair for these was combed up from the back in disorder, leaving the neck bare as if for the guillotine. And then around the white neck they wore a blood red ribbon. There was in Paris even a *Bal de Victimes*, to which people came appropriately coiffed and to which no-one was admitted who had not lost a close relative to the guillotine.

But as with all fads for very short hair among women, this one, though extremely popular while it lasted, soon lost its novelty and was discarded by the fashionable. Restless for a change and unwilling to wait for their short haircuts to grow out, women once again began wearing wigs, which they called, appropriately enough, *cache-folies*. The fashionable and influential Madame Tallien, who liked to change the colour of her hair several times a day and was able to do so through the use of her large collection of wigs, in 1796 made black the popular colour. Frequently the natural short hair was worn in the morning; and a wig, often of a different colour, was donned for the evening.

As the century ended, the women, still exulting in their new freedom in hair styles with the endless possibilities for frequent changes, were experimenting in a variety of directions (see Plate 88). But the hair in general followed the natural shape of the head and tended toward a revival of classic styles.

PLOCACOSMOS

In 1782 James Stewart, a London hairdresser who has already been quoted at some length in Chapter 9, published a book called *Plocacosmos: or the Whole Art of Hair-dressing; wherein is contained Ample Rules for the Young Artizan, more particularly for Ladies, Women, Valets, &c. &c. as well as Directions for Persons to dress their own Hair, also Ample and Wholesome Rules to preserve the Hair.* Nor is that all, for we are further informed on the title-page that the hair is 'completely analyzed as to its Growth, Nature, Colour, &c. and all and every Article used in the Hair, on the Head, Face, &c. as, False Hair, Perfumery, Cosmetics, &c. clearly analyzed and examined with a History of the Hair and Head Dress, from the earliest Ages to the present Time, particularly as they have appeared upon the English Stage for these last Two Hundred Years; with Strictures on the present Performers belonging to each Theatre'.

This is followed by an intriguing paragraph outlining further contents:

'The Plan of this Work requiring it, there are also complete Rules for the Management of Children and Education of Youth; and excellent Rules for the Preservation of the Health and Happiness of Age; being a Guide through the Seven Ages of Man: the whole interspersed with Moral Thoughts, being necessary for all families.'

Whatever his qualifications for the management of children and the education of youth may have been, Stewart was a successful hairdresser; and fortunately he set down in great detail the exact procedure he used in cutting and dressing a lady's hair. Although the instructions are much too long to be included in their entirety, they provide such an accurate and precise picture of hairdressing at the time that they deserve to be quoted at some length. But since the technical details presented by Mr Stewart will not be of interest to all readers, this special section has been placed here at the end of the chapter.

He begins with an entreaty against engaging in conversation during the operation and then continues:

'With a large silk puff, beat into the hair a moderate quantity of powder; then take your large wide comb, which should be made of tortoise-shell or good horn properly seasoned, white or green; this comb should be from 7 to 8 inches long, from 2 to 3 deep in the teeth; at most there should not be above 4 teeth in the inch lengthwise. . . . Comb the hair all clear down, beginning at the roots. Supposing now you have combed it all round from the crown, part hangs over the lady's face, ears, neck, and each side. You must now change your comb for your dressing one; this comb should be from 8 to 9 inches long and of the same stuff as the greater wide one. It is cut into the wider or buckling end, and the narrow or frizzing end decreasing gradually in the width, from the beginning of the great teeth to the extremity of the narrow end, or little teeth; the depth of the wider part should be full an inch and a half, the narrow about seven-eighths. With this comb you are to part the hair. . . . The depth of the parting depends a good deal on the quantity of hair. If very thick, the parting must be narrower, in order that the hair may dress light and transparent; if thin, the shade must be wider, in order to give a proper substance to the forepart. The usual breadth of the shade, just in the front, is from 2 to 3 inches, or more, and must gradually increase, so as to be from 5 to 6 at the temples; from thence the line must run almost directly down, about an inch and a half behind the ear. . . . You must now place the narrower or close end of the comb in the palm of your hand, directly at the root of your thumb. . . . With the end and teeth of the comb you must draw a line along the head, about the before-mentioned distance from the forehead. When this line is drawn about 3 inches long, without taking your comb from the hair, turn your wrist inwards to your body, the teeth of the comb all the while touching the head; with this turn of the hand there will appear a small opening, through which you put the forefinger of the left hand, all the length of the line you have drawn; then, by taking the comb out, you separate the hair, and you find a line as smooth as if pencilled or squared, not a hair being out of its place. . . . In this manner you are to proceed, in parting from the very middle of the forehead, winding down each side of the head, till you come to that part of the neck where the extremities of the hair grows, not forgetting to take the distance before-mentioned for your guide.'

He suggests pinning up the front half and then continues:

'Comb well the shade you left down into your left hand; then, with a roll of good hard pomatum, bolt it pretty strongly from each ear to the centre of the neck. Undo the hair from the top, and proceed in the same manner with the comb and pomatum; this do to all the shades. . . . When you have combed it all well and got it smooth and tight in the neck, tie it very hard to keep it out of your way. . . . This done, take your large scissars and cut off the points and straggling ends of the long hair.'

This is followed by detailed instructions for barbering, after which Stewart says that the hair, when properly done, 'should rise from an inch and a half in the front to 4 inches, more or less, on the back part, and so regular that there should not be 2 hairs of one length. . . . When this is done, you must fix it with a pin or comb, so as not to interfere with that uncut. You are then to proceed as you did with the middle parting, but with singular attention that, as you move from the centre to the ears, you cut it more freely in front and leave it gradually longer behind. Thus the short hairs will not be perceptible above half an inch back, just on the middle of the forehead, while they gradually increase as you reach the temples, and from the temples to the ears to be full 2 inches of perceptible short hairs. That is, this short hair may be from half an inch to an inch and a half or 2 inches long; so from the centre of the under part of the front it is from 4 to 5, 6, 7, 8, or 9 inches as it comes down the side

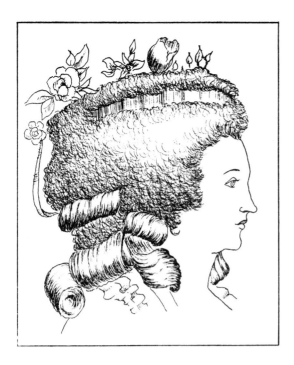

Fig. 93 : Coiffure illustrated in James Stewart's
Plocacosmos, published 1782

of the head. At the same time, the curls, being part of the front, are left about the same length with that just described; they are cut in the same shaded manner, but not to such a degree, the end of their cutting being not for beauty, but to make them frize and fasten together better.'

Stewart then proceeds to give instructions for making various types of curls, recommending that the hair be put in papers. 'You are therefore, it is to be supposed, furnished with a proper quantity of French curling paper. . . . Now take the paper and, with your large scissars, cut it into pieces 4 inches square; cut them transverse, like a half handkerchief, which are the most convenient, and answer all sizes best. After you have cut the papers, . . . begin in the middle—that is, directly in front. Make a small parting, not wider than three quarters of an inch; you must have 2 combs to carry the rest of the hair clearly from you, by drawing it to each side and checking these combs in the hair behind. I think the hair cannot dress well unless there is a good curl in the points. I would recommend the back row to be curled instead of craped; this there is various ways of doing, some with their fingers, others with pointed instruments, &c. &c. . . . The parting you have in your hand I would have 4 rows deep—that is, 4 papers in a regular row under each other.'

The curious appearance of the head in curl papers, as illustrated by Hogarth (Plate 68-M), is explained by Stewart:

'After you have parted your back paper, you must draw the fine teeth of your comb through it while you hold it in your hand, directly upright, or your arm rather leaning back to the crown of the head. In that manner hold the hair between the finger and thumb of your left hand, drawn tight up from the head like a piece of silk ribbon. While you thus hold the hair with your hand, leaning back, let the end of the tail-comb, from your right hand, press between the finger and thumb of your left hand over the points of the hair, and when you have drawn it to the extreme points, turn it quick over till it has catched; then roll the tail-comb up to the roots of the hair, as close as can be to the head; then applying again the finger and thumb of your left hand to guide and keep the curl firm while you draw the tail-comb out, which you will easily do, if well done. You have now got the curl fast between your finger and thumb; lay the tail comb down, take a paper and press the edge of it close to the head and to your left finger and thumb, which has hold of the curl. The paper and curl being in this position, turn over the end of the paper upon the curl; by that means you take hold of the curls with your right finger and thumb, the paper being between both; that is, under and over the curl in the right hand. Therefore, turn the other end of the paper with your left thumb tight over the neck of the curl; then, bringing both ends beyond the curl, twist them very firmly, and so let it go. If it stands right up, or rather leans back, and the paper firm around the neck, you are sure it is well done and will not be in your way. If it lays down upon the head, and is in the way of your future paper, and the paper shabbily put on, it is very badly done and ought not to go. . . . The first curl being done, it ought to be the largest, as being the longest; for the nearer you come to the face, you must have the less hair in the paper, because shorter.

'The next curl is to be twisted or craped; you have now separated it, as before directed, and are to dip the finger and thumb of each hand in brick-dust or pipe-ashes or anything gritty; then you must roll or twist the hair in a regular direction, as if twisting a pack thread or fringed silk. This you must do between the finger and thumb of both hands till it rolls itself up to a finall twisted ball, quite up to the roots of the hair; you must then draw it with some strength, in order to make it firmer, and then with the points of your finger and thumb of your right hand, compress it, and roll it up in as small a compass as possible, down to the head; then take it between the finger and thumb of your left-hand, and apply the paper with your right, as before directed. The other two are to be done in the same manner, but very close to the head, standing upright, with their heads bending backwards. . . . You are to remember that when the hair is short, it cannot take less than 15 or 18 papers for the front row to be well done, and the same proportion all the way backwards.

'The hair that is allotted for the curls must not be put up so strong, but done with the fingers, or else over a well-turned pair of toupee-irons . . . in order to give them the proper buckle without cramping. To do it with the fingers, you must hold it at the points and keep constantly turning it over with the points of your right finger and thumb, and keep them so close as to prevent the hairs from touching each other, though curled, your left fingers guiding your right all the way down to the roots of the hair, when, as usual, you take the curl between your left finger and thumb, and apply the paper.

'When all is done, they look like regular rows of trees, truly set, with their heads bending to the crown, as if blown thence by a gust of wind from the face. . . .'

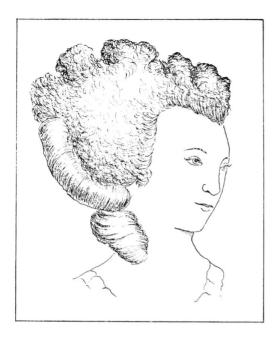

Fig. 94 : Coiffure illustrated in James Stewart's *Placa-cosmos*, published 1782

In explaining the use of the irons, Stewart instructs one to 'take the whole paper in the irons, but take care the irons do not go beyond the paper. . . . The length of time ought to be till the paper smoaks.'

He also gives instruction for using toupee irons directly on the hair, though he prefaces his instructions by deploring the method, which he considers extremely harmful to the hair. In this direct method, each lock of hair was simply rolled on the iron and held till it smoked. Then the curl was released and pinned till it cooled. He concludes his reluctant instructions by commenting that 'if the hair is all curled properly, it looks very pretty, being like so many rows of tubes, pipe above pipe, like the small flutes of an organ, only placed horizontally'.

Stewart then proceeds to the chignon, instructing the operator first to have available soft pomatum and powder, with a swans-down puff and a large silk puff. This is accompanied by a strict caution on choosing a good quality of pomatum made from the fat of 'a young and healthy animal'. He recommends the fat of calves, hogs, and bears. This seems to lead quite naturally into a digression packed with useful information:

'Deer's grease is good to fortify the nerves against the rheumatism, sciatica, gout, and fractures. Hare's grease applied externally promotes digestion, and a suppuration of abscesses; that of rabbits is nervous and resolutive; that of cocks and hens dissolves and softens induration; that of geese has the same qualities and likewise abateth haemorrhoids, assuages pains in the ear, being applied within the same, and opens the belly, being taken inwardly. Eel's fat is esteemed good against roemeroids and deafness, to take away the pits of the small-pox, and to make the hair grow. . . .'

The comments on powder are equally instructive and somewhat more to the point:
'The powder should be perfectly free from adulteration, which the fresh duties

have so much encouraged, particularly from lime, or plaister of Paris, as, by a long continuance, it will not only bring the hair off, so as to make them as bald as coots, but breed a terrible disease, not unlike the scald-head. In order to guard against this, you may judge of powder from the following. The colour of pure powder is like that of the clearest cream, without a speck, and so light and feathery as to look like snow falling, or ice imbossed; the least adulteration of any kind will change it to a darkish hue, and look like soiled writing-paper, appear solid and heavy, as if it were egg-shells ground down very small; even that tinged with pink is exceeding unhealthy, if coloured with rose pink; to prove this, if the forehead is rubbed at the roots of the hair but 5 or 6 mornings, it will come out all in a rash, or heat, and appear very red to the look, as well as painful; therefore, though the direct or immediate effects of the pink powder now used is not felt from the small quantities required to tinge it, yet it must prey upon the pores, though slowly, and bring the hair off.'

Stewart is equally specific about the puffs to be used:

'The silk puff you use, the filament of which should be 6 or 7 inches long, the knotted kind is best, powdering much finer, as it rejects the coarsest particles, while taking up the powder.

'The swan-down to be good should be at least 3 inches long, and the purest white, without the least cavity, hole, or unevenness, but appeare, when you blow on it, like a tall field of corn, bending before the wind. It will retain the powder, and powder more regular than those of a worse quality, which look gray and ragged, as if moth-eaten.'

At last he comes to the chignon:

'Now open the hair behind, and it will easily part into the same breaks you used the hard pomatum in; begin with the bottom one as you did before, while you check the last with your large comb at the top of the head. Take now about the bigness of a walnut of soft pomatum, put it in the palm of your left hand, as directed heretofore, and, with the points of your left fingers, rub it into the head and roots of the hair. . . . There must be a cloth pinned to the lady's shoulders at two corners, and the other two round the back of the chair she sits in; this will form a bag into which you may put part of your powder, as you want. Now take the wide end of your comb, and shelve it into the powder, bringing up as much as will lie on the comb; this you lay upon the stripe of hair just pomatumed, with your left hand under it, and shove part up to the roots, and part fall lower, in order to mix properly with the pomatum; this you must repeat till it is intirely free from the greasy look from root to point, and let the wide end of the comb pass gently through it, that all the loose powder may fall from it, and no more. This being done, proceed to the next parting, and do it in the same manner quite to the last, taking care that the long hair, as it were, incorporates and grows together.

'If there is a false chinong wore, you must frize the root of the last stripe but one, next the top, pretty strong; after that put a quantum extraordinary of powder and pomatum, then check firmly the small comb of the false chinong into this constituency, and let the last stripe of hair, or top one, effectually cover it; if it is well made, it cannot be told there is false hair placed on. This done, take all the hair firm in your left hand, and comb it a good deal with the widest comb, and strain it hard down with both your hands in the neck; then take a smallish quantum of soft pomatum, well separated and rubbed in your hands, and draw both your hands from the top of the head to the bottom of the hair; grasping it after very firm, tie it up afresh.'

With the chignon (or 'chinong') finished, the next step is to comb out and powder the toupee, which is still pinned or in curl papers. The instructions quoted here are for hair curled directly with the iron. A similar procedure is followed for hair curled in papers once the papers have been removed.

The instructions are that 'between each turning you must rub into the head a little pomatum, as before told, and to each of them powder sufficient; and then, before you take any of the pins out, rub a little soft pomatum, well broke in your hands, all over them; after that beat the swan down puff full of powder over them. The first row you turned you must first frize; therefore, take the pin out of it, and draw it through the wide part of your comb, and while you hold it between your two first fingers . . . about 5 inches from the head, you must put the comb into the hair close to your left hand, and beat it in a regular succession down to the roots of the hair, till you, as it were, weave it into a mat. Remembering to do it effectually, the left hand is to exert itself exceedingly against the efforts of the right. Thus the hairs that the comb force from the left fingers must be so sparing that the more power the comb gains, the more the left hand must pull against it as if it forced the hair from your fingers by mere violence. . . . There is a double reason for this firmness, as without it the hair would not have a proper consistency to stand erect and keep together, and at the same time appear to have the same length it originally had. If it is well done, it appears like the stripe of hair-cloth well wove, transparent, yet strong, and stand as high as the length of hair.

'Before you proceed further, it may be necessary to part the curls, as the full dress is now in 3 curls. We will part them as such, having it in our power at all times to take 1 or 2 into the toupee, either as half-dress or undress.

'With the wide end of the comb draw a line 3 inches back from the front hair at the ear, slanting from the crown of the head, inclining to the top of the ear. The line should advance from the ear near 4 inches, more or less, towards the back, parting so as the top of this division is about 6 inches, more or less from the centre of the forehead. The hair thus severed from the front, you are to part it in 3 regular divisions, rather inclining most to the bottom curl; begin with the top one, and hold it in the direction given for frizzing, which you are to perform on this, in the same manner, inclining the curl to lay to the face.

'As the curls must be frizzed still firmer than the front, you must take your hard pomatum and run it along the small teeth of the comb and friz it from the roots to the points, after that a little powder, and friz it over afresh. When this is done, take a little soft pomatum, and bathe the curl in your hands from the ends to the roots; then use a proper quantity of powder, but putting it in with the wide end of the comb till the black or greasy look entirely vanishes; after that friz it again firmly all along, with your comb stuffed with hard pomatum, then a little powder; then stripe firmly your hard pomatum along the curls from the roots to the points, on both sides, taking care to collect every straggling hair. Stripe it like a piece of silk half a dozen times through your fingers, and roll it up close to the head and pin it. All this mixture is very necessary to make the curls pliable and fit well at first, which set they always keep. If well done, it appears like a slip of buck or doe's skin. . . . The curls of each side being thus far done, the front is to be finished, frizzing in every row quite to the face, as before directed. When thus frizzed, if clearly and well done, it looks like a quickset hedge in June; but instead of growing perpendicularly, slanting regularly from the face.

'The hair having got thus far, you are to take a small quantity of soft pomatum, well rubbed in your hands, and with one hand on one side of the hair, and the other on the other, pomatum it quite from the growing of the hair round the forehead to the points; then beat a sufficient quantity of powder with the swan-skin puff till there is not the least darkness or greasiness to be seen, and till there is enough to thicken and make the hair feel of a proper body. Now use the powder knife and take off all the loose and dirty stuff from the forehead and the root of the hair. If the hair grows bad, use the roll or hard pomatum; if not, there is no necessity. . . . You must now use a fourth comb, the same as your dressing one, but a full size finer in the small teeth, unless you can make you tail-comb do. . . . With this comb you must friz the back part of the hair, particularly the points, in order to keep them in a body at the ends. . . . Take the front of the hair in your left hand, within half an inch of the forehead, the back of your hand being to your face; both your hands being thus placed, you must begin and heat or friz the hair down towards the face, in a regular friz, your left hand giving way imperceptibly as your right hand gains upon the hair. . . . After you have reached the ends of the hair, begin to the next on either side you please till it is all gone over in this manner; if well done, it looks now like the hedge before mentioned, but considerably polished. . . . Again take some soft pomatum, but in a small quantity, and gently touch the front all over with it; after that, take your machine and blow a considerable quantity of powder in the hair from the front and from behind, in order to give it a light, clear, clean look. When this is done, to render it as complete as possible, the same frizzing as the last should be gone through regularly all over, as it polishes the hair and makes it look finer and more graceful. . . .

'The hair now being ready for the cushion thus far, you may proceed almost invariably. What follows depending altogether on the mere whim and fancy of the day, of which I shall mention further hereafter. The cushion to be used cannot be too small, its shape nearly that of a heart, or rather between that and the head of a small dart or spear; it should be made clean and delicately neat, or else, being placed on the warmest part of the head, it may breed and become troublesome. Be careful to place your cushion entirely in the centre. . . . Place your left thumb upon the front of the cushion when it is on . . . then take your cushion pins and use one directly in front and one at each side, which will be sufficient. . . . The cushion being fixed, begin in the front, and with a thin, slender, well made hair pin, hang the hair to the cushion; this is done by pushing the pin in the friz and catching the back friz by lifting it, as it were, then pushing the pin in the cushion. . . . Go on doing this down the side of the toupee, which may take 7 pins for the whole front, one the middle, and 3 for each side. . . . The hair being hung well round the cushion, place your left hand open behind the points of the toupee, and with the comb in your right hand, raise your left hand as you smooth the points with the comb, that they may fall back in a buckle; this do all around, and, if possible, without a break; this not only makes it appear elegantly finished but keeps it much more compact and makes the curls last three times as long as it otherwise would.'

The author then leaves the top hair for the moment and goes back to the chignon:

'First, it is to be untied, then rub a little soft pomatum in your hands, that it may be mellowed as you proceed; you are to comb it very well once more, and get it with all your power as clean and tight as possible into the hollow of the neck, while one of your hands keeps it firmly down; you are to cross it above your hand with the string that tied it, and give one end of each into the lady's hands, which she is to pull with all her strength. . . . While it is thus held, take your large comb, and in the underside push the teeth quite up to you, and endeavour to bring it down to the points; so by combing it a good many times on the under and upper side, first with this comb, and then with your dressing comb, you will make it incorporate and, as it were, grow together, that it will hang well any way you chuse to wear it. When this is done, place the back comb in the centre of the back part of the cushion and pin it to it with one short pin of each side. This is a small comb, with a slender back to it, stitched somewhat like stays and worn at present by the ladies to keep the hind hair from falling too near the head, as well as in some measure to support the cap and hat. . . .

'You now proceed to do the hair up behind, in which there is many ways, as the hair is now held, and such pains taken with it; particularly if there is no short hairs in the neck, there is no occasion for tying, therefore, to do it in one plait, it must be parted in 3 even divisions, and each division pretty well smoothed and combed then, with a little soft pomatum on the hands to lull the straggling hairs; you proceed to plait it by first dividing pretty well each slip from the other, then cross from the left first, and so on, in one plait. If the hair is good, there never should be above 3 or 4 crossings. When done, place one hand at the bottom, where you would have it turned from—that is, how low you would have it, and with the other turn it quick and strong over the hand, and tie it with, or fix it to the string of the thin cushion above mentioned; and, to make sure, draw a pretty strong double black pin through the knot into both cushions. Let the lady draw the string out after you have adjusted the plait a little, by pulling it broader if required. . . . If writhed or lappet curls are

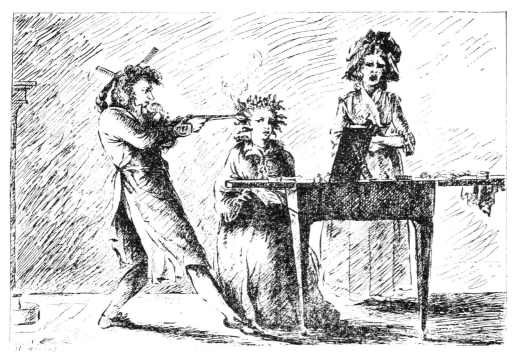

Fig. 95 : Curling the hair with irons. English caricature, 1787

wore, they are generally made from false hair, into a single bit, wove about 3 inches long, placed at the back point of the cushion, from which 4, 5, or 6 small corkscrew curls, hanging loose and dangling at the distance of 7 or 8 inches from the head.'

Other methods of dressing the chignon are then given, after which Stewart returns to the front hair, which he had left hung on the cushion.

'The hair is left as it is, but with a very slight curl in the points. . . . As to the various shaping of the hair, some like the head to look oval, in the shape of a pearl, others in that of an urn, and others again in that of a heart, &c. &c. But I will direct as I think it looks best, either for the undress cap, half-dress, or full-dress.

'And first, if undress, begin in the centre of the front, and with the end of your tail-comb, draw it forward from root to point. This swell regularly decreasing, as you reach each temple; if the forehead is very high, the swell in a greater degree; if very low, hardly any swell. You will now unpin the curls which have been so long close to the head. The two uppermost you must join to the back part of the toupee, by well frizzing and incorporating both curls and toupee together and to make the swell backwards handsome. Check the 2 hairs together with one or two long single pins, at least long enough easily to reach the cushion; they are to be put in much in the manner you hung the front to the cushion, and they are meant to keep the back hair falling from the front. This being completed, the toupee appears without the least break or defect quite down behind the ear. You next take your tail-comb, and with the end of it by degrees wear the short hairs above the ear, over three parts of it, as it is at present wore, going regularly back, drawing it down at the same time, without appearing at all severed, from the front quite to the extremity of the bottom of the toupee, which may be 6 inches depth from the temples, more or less; this hair you can very easily wear down over the ear, without the least danger of breaking the toupee or making it look ragged, as the hair has been so well cut and so thoroughly curled, frizzed, and prepared. Again, begin at the front, and with your fingers gently turn it down as far as you intend; then take firmer hold and drag it up a little from the roots with the left hand, and with the right take a small pin about 4 inches in length; push the pin through the front, and assisting the back hair with it, drive the pin into the cushion, at the same time lifting the hair up, as it were, with the pin. . . . Thus you are to proceed along the side of the toupee. The height you may finish it at may be about 4 inches in the front; from that gradually rising to the corner till it is 7 inches. . . . After you pass the corner, you are to take care the hair is turned remarkably smooth round, and every hair in its place, in one regular large curl, as it were turned back from the face. To keep it in this position, put your thumb from the root to the point in the curl, and the rest of your fingers bending round it; then take in your right hand a very long slender double pin, the points of which you must nearly close together; then, just before your thumb, put the points in the hair, and shove it so as to be able to check the under part of the hair which your fingers are round; that done, put it up to the cushion so as to have a good hold. Three of these pins in regular succession, well put in, from the top of your thumb to the bottom, will fully answer; when you may drag it as low as you please, without breaking the toupee or pulling out of shape; and the bottom curl, which has been taken so much pains with before in preparing, now only wants smoothing with the comb. And with a little soft pomatum on your fingers, you stripe it through your hand 5 or 6 times, but held so close to the neck, as your hands to touch the shoulders; you are then to turn it round your fingers like a piece of silk ribbon, the common size they are wore, and place it about 2 inches back from the bottom of the ear, and quite low and easy, else they look awkward. They are at present wore short and small, and not pinned so as to look stiff, or too near the head. When you have rolled it up, put your thumb in the curl, and take an exceeding short slender pin, not above an inch in length, and warp it 7 or 8 times in the under part of the curl; this one will do as well as an hundred, and hardly look as if pinned at all if properly done.

'The hair now completed on both sides in this fashion, it is to be powdered either with the machine, or silk, or swan-down puff. After it is quite finished, and you have cut any straggling hairs with the large scissars, that may hang about, use a small quantum of soft pomatum, well rubbed in both your hands, and touch your hair with it in the gentlest manner all over, behind and before; that done, take the machine and fill it about half full of powder; after that, see that both ends are well screwed on; then let the smallest end of it lay in your left hand, and the mouth just projecting to your fore finger, which encircles the mouth on the under side, while your thumb rests upon the extremity of the mouth on the other side; whilst it thus lays in your hand, with your right hand grasp the bottom round, but so as not to touch the leather, while your right arm is raised considerably higher than the left; the machine looks half bent, or falling, in the middle; in this position you point the mouth of your machine to the root of the hair or forehead, seldom advancing much higher, as it will rise sufficiently of itself to powder the upper parts of the hair; in this manner you will keep moving directly backwards and forwards with your right hand, your left being quite still, and only guiding the machine; the powder, if properly blown, will come out in a regular smoke, which should be a considerable quantity, whether white, pink, brown, or yellow. The lady having wore a mask all the while, you use the powder knife in the gentlest manner round the roots of the hair, without at all touching it. To powder with the silk puff is to fill it very full of powder and let it be nearly shook out, again filled and again shook out, 2 or 3 times, till the finer parts of the puff is filled with the finest powder. Grasp then the root of the puff in your hand, and with your arm raised pretty high and the back of your hand toward your face, direct the body of the puff to the head and hair, and then shake and jerk it quickly with your hand and arm as before. . . . Continue till this is done, then finish as before directed. When powdered with the swan-down puff, you must also bury it very much in the powder, and shake it well out 2 or 3 times, the same as the silk puff. . . .

'For the half-dress cap only, the top curl is placed in the toupee and the second curl so formed as to make the toupee look in the same shape it was in with one. If they are meant to be hanging curls, that is, the two like one long one broke, you must stand very back, your left hand stretched very high, when you must roll the curl up as before directed, pointing directly to the face, and with the small double pin warp it or darn it as before told. After that, use a very long double pin at the root that will well reach the cushion, or sometimes not so, in order to bear it up to be seen from the face; the other is in a regular direction under it, and the whole head is the same shape it was before.

'For full-dress, the 3 curls are left out of the toupee, as at first parted, and sometimes four is worn, but the top one usually false. If it is to be worn in the present fashion, with a number of small curls round the face, the hair must have been turned with the irons, as before told, instead of craped or twisted. . . . If well done, they look like a small plot of ground, thickly planted with small tulips or daisies, bending their heads to the ground, but more commonly compared to a bull's forehead, hence it may well be called *en tauro*. . . . The head is now powdered complete for full-dress.'

This exhausting description is followed by directions for putting on caps or hats or, when none is worn, on adding fake curls and feathers. The special instructions for care of the coiffure at night are interesting:

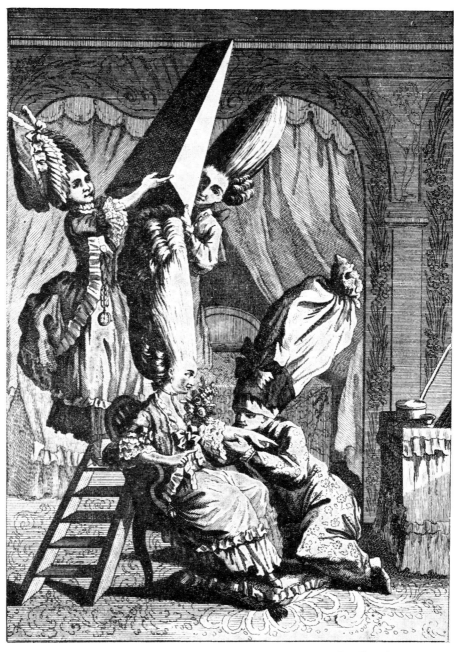

Fig. 96 : Contraption for preserving ladies' head-dresses at night. French caricature, late eighteenth century

'Nothing need be touched but the curls; you may take the pins out of them and, with a little soft pomatum in your hands, stroke the hairs that may have started; do them with nice long rollers, wind them up to the root, and turn the end of each roller firmly in to keep them tight, remembering at the same time, the hair should never be combed at night, having almost always so bad an effect as to give a violent head-ach next day. After the curls are rolled up, touch them with your pomatumy hands, and stroke the hair behind; after that take a very large net fillet, which must be big enough to cover the head and hair, and put it on, and drawing the strings to a proper tightness behind, till it closes all round the face and neck like a purse, bring the strings round the front and back again to the neck, where they must be tied; this, with the finest lawn handkerchief, is night covering sufficient for the head.'

Directions are then included for combing out the curls and the back hair and resetting them with more pomatum and powder. Stewart then adds, 'In this manner you may proceed every day for 2 or 3 months, or as long as the lady chuses, or till the hair gets strait and clotted and matted with dirty powder; then it is absolutely necessary to comb it out, when you must be provided with 2 very wide combs.

'In order to hurt the lady the least, you must endeavour to separate it in as many slips as you can; this you must do with the end teeth of your large comb, drawing a line along the head, and trying to sever it at the roots, partly by humoring it, and partly by strength.'

It is suggested that 'to dress hair without powder in the present day, you must proceed exactly in the same manner, as with only omitting craping or twisting, and omitting the various applications of powder and pomatum'.

Stewart says finally that he 'would inform those ladies who wish to dress their own hair, that they will find it very troublesome and tedious, as well as exceeding tiresome for the arms, and straining for the eyes, sometimes not only making them tender but even blood-shot'.

PLATE 78 : EIGHTEENTH-CENTURY WOMEN 1700–1750

A   *c.* 1700. Hair dressed over a frame, decorated with pearl hairpins and a large, pendant pearl.

B   *c.* 1700, French. Mlle de Varenne. *Fontange* style with pearls, jewelled pins, and *favorites* (curls at temple).

C   *c.* 1702, English. Queen Anne.

D   *c.* 1700, English. *Fontange* style.

E   1710, French.

F   *c.* 1701.

G   1712, French.

H   1732, English.

I   *c.* 1730, French. Known as the 'Dutch coiffure', and usually powdered. Popular into the 1750s.

J   *c.* 1735, French.

K   1730s, French.

L   *c.* 1720.

M   French.

N   1743. *À la grecque.*

O   1745, French.

P   *c.* 1750.

Q   *c.* 1750, French.

R   *c.* 1750.

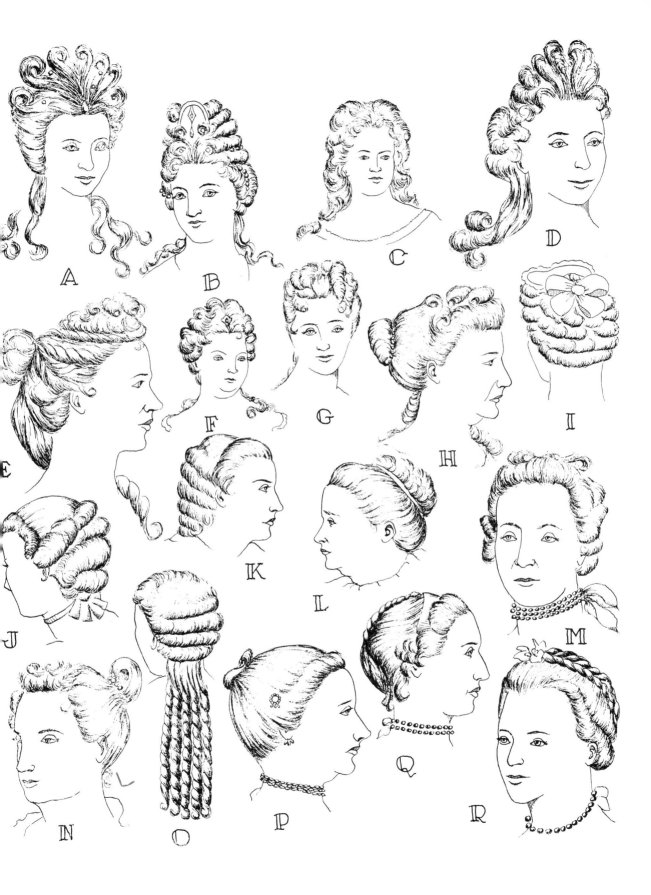

A

B

C

D

E

F

G

H

I

J

K

L

M

N

O

P

Q

R

PLATE 79 : EIGHTEENTH-CENTURY WOMEN 1750–1778

A   1750s. Style worn by Marie Joseph of Austria.

B   1750s. Child.

C   1760, French. Susanne Jarente de la Reynière.

D   1764.

E   1764. Style of Mme de Pompadour.

F   1760s, French.

G   1767, German.

H   1760s, French.

I   *c.* 1765, French.

J   *c.* 1765, French.

K   *c.* 1760, French.

L   1778. Child (see also Plate 84-C).

M   1774, French.

N   1760s, French. Wig. Natural front hair was dressed over the wig and extra curls and decoration added. It was also worn earlier.

O   1760s, French. Curls are false (see Plate 81-G).

P   1770, French. Style of Marie Antoinette at 15.

Q   *c.* 1770, French. Madame du Barry.

R   1771, Russian. Catherine the Great.

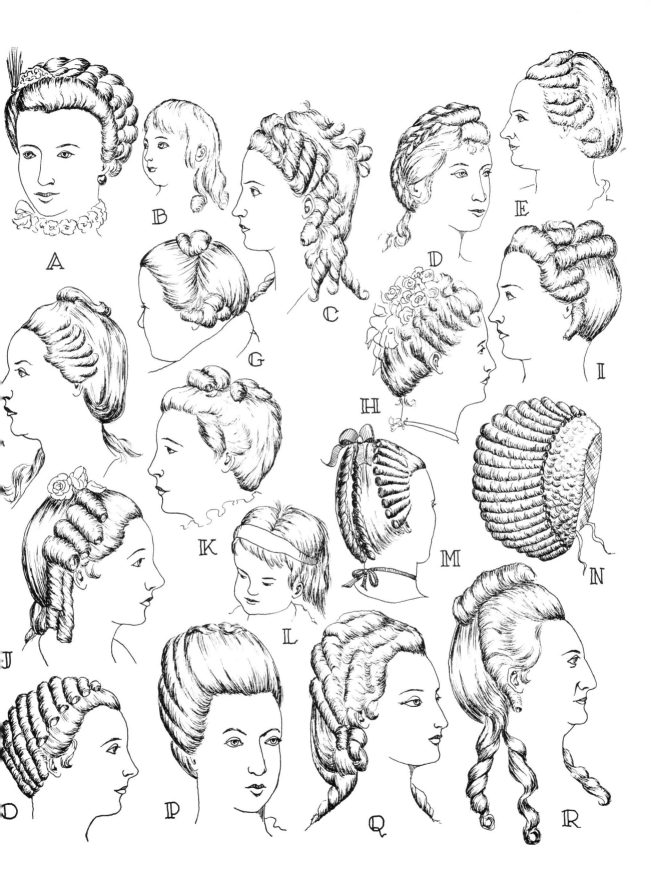

A

B

C

D

E

G

H

I

J

K

L

M

N

D

P

Q

R

Plate 80 : Eighteenth-Century Women's Styles depicted by Legros, 1768

All hair styles and equipment shown on this plate are from Legros' *L'Art de la coëffure des dames françoises*, published in 1768 and containing drawings of 38 hair styles. For further details about Legros and his book, see text.

A   *Hair style No. 7.* '2 rows of 7 curls, 2 shells and a sword-knot, made with 2 locks of hair drawn from the top of the head, and reversed curl made with the end of the chignon. The sword-knots are used only for balls or the theatre.'

B   *Hair style No. 26.* 'Broken curls and rosettes . . . and 2 half-plaited puffs, made with 2 locks of smooth hair drawn from the top of the head or the end of the chignon.'

C   *Hair style No. 38.* 'The 38th coiffure is the bouquet of the art of the French hairdressers.'

D   *Hair style No. 6.* 'A row of diagonal curls and a *coque* and a 3-fold knot of smooth hair, made with the end of the chignon, to serve as a crest.'

E   *Hair style No. 19.* 'A row of semi-diagonal curls . . . a *coque*, and the chignon braided in a parquet pattern, and a long reversed curl made with the end of the braid.'

F   *Hair style No. 35.* '5 *coques* and an enclosure of hair in 3 parts, with a *Sultane* drawn from the top of the head, and 3 puffs made with the end of the chignon the same as the 3 rosettes.'

G   *Hair style No. 15.* 'A frizzled chignon with broken curls making the Hungarian stitch.'

H   First and second patterns 'for the width of the roots which one must follow in order to dress a lady's hair with 3 side curls made of false hair.'

I   'Type of compass essential to hairdressers in order to regulate hair cutting, following the system of *L'Art de la coëffure des dames françoises*.'

J   Four of the combs used by M. Legros.

K   Curling iron used by M. Legros.

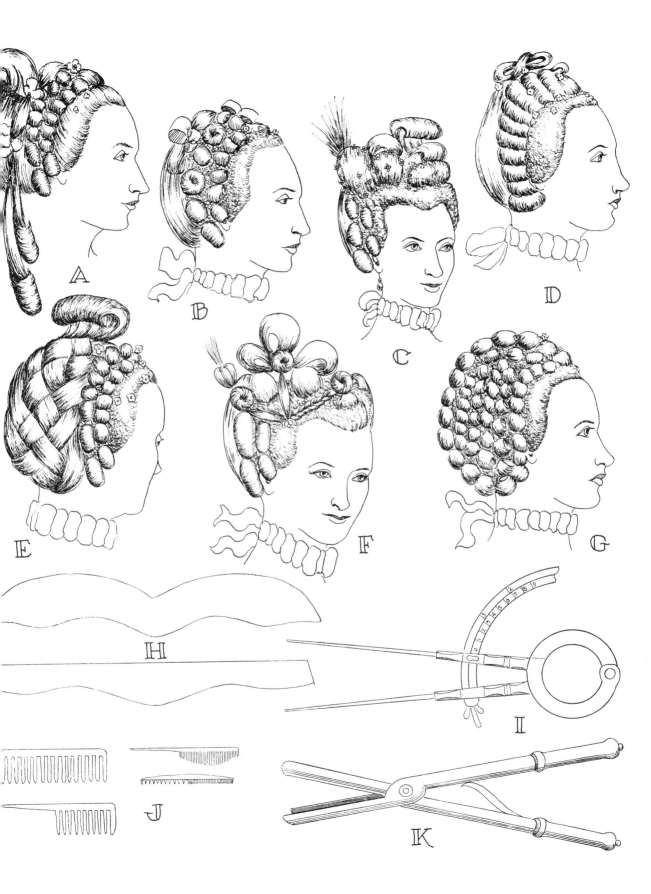

A

B

C

D

E

F

G

H

I

J

K

PLATE 81 : EIGHTEENTH-CENTURY WOMEN 1770–1775

A   *c*. 1770, French. Mme du Barry, 1743–93. Last mistress of Louis XVI and eventually guillotined. Toupee built up over pads. Hair powdered.

B   *c*. 1770, French.

C   *c*. 1770, French. The top curls and the long hanging ones are detachable (see G below).

D   1770s. Marie Adelaide, Queen of Sardinia.

E   *c*. 1770, French.

F   *c*. 1770, French.

G   French. Detachable curls to add to coiffures of natural hair. Also worn in previous decade (see C, D, E, and F above and Plate 79-O).

H, I, J   1773, German. These seem to tally well with a description in *Lady's Magazine* of the fashion of 1774: 'The hair is dressed very backward and low, with large flat puffs on the top, toupee not so low . . . three long curls or about six small puffs down the sides. Powder almost universal.'

K   1773, French. Style of Madame du Barry.

L   1774 (see Plate 82-I for a French style of the same year).

M   *c*. 1772, English.

N   1774, Marie Antoinette.

O   Marie Christine of Austria.

P   1775, English. The hair is 'dressed in a great club, surmounted by rows of overhanging curls of large dimensions, above which an ornamental bandeau is placed, from which hang two lace lappets' (see Plate 83-D for another English style of the same year).

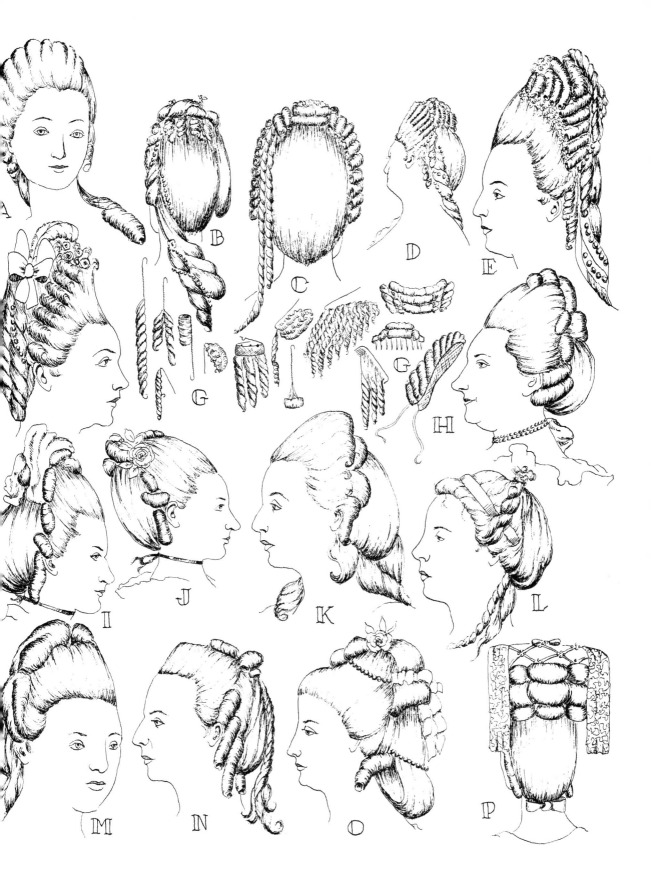

A

B

C

D

E

F

G

G

H

I

J

K

L

M

N

O

P

PLATE 82 : EIGHTEENTH-CENTURY WOMEN 1770–1780

A   *c.* 1777, French. *À la Venus* (see similar styles on Plates 83 and 84).

B   1774, French. *Le parterre galant.*

C   1780, French. *Le bandeau d'amour.* Frizzed toupee and sides. This style is sometimes shown with smooth hair; but with the amount of fullness required, the frizzle is more likely. However, even with frizzed front hair, the chignon and the hanging curls were always smooth, as shown here. The stiff, partially unrolled curls are typical. Later in the eighties these side curls were not always worn.

D   1774, French. *À la Junon.*

E   1780, French. Marie Antoinette.

F   *c.* 1778, French. *À la Driade* (see also Plates 83 and 84 for additional styles of the same period).

G   *c.* 1780, French. Probably the Princesse de Lamballe (see also Plate 86-I).

H   *c.* 1780.

I   1774, French (see also Plate 81-H-I-K-L-M-O).

J   1776, Italian. Lady's maid. Note similarity to men's styles.

K   1780, French. Frizzed toupee and side hair.

L   Silk-covered wool cushion over which hair was arranged. These could be of various shapes and sizes and were also made of other materials. Wire frames were also used, especially for the very high coiffures.

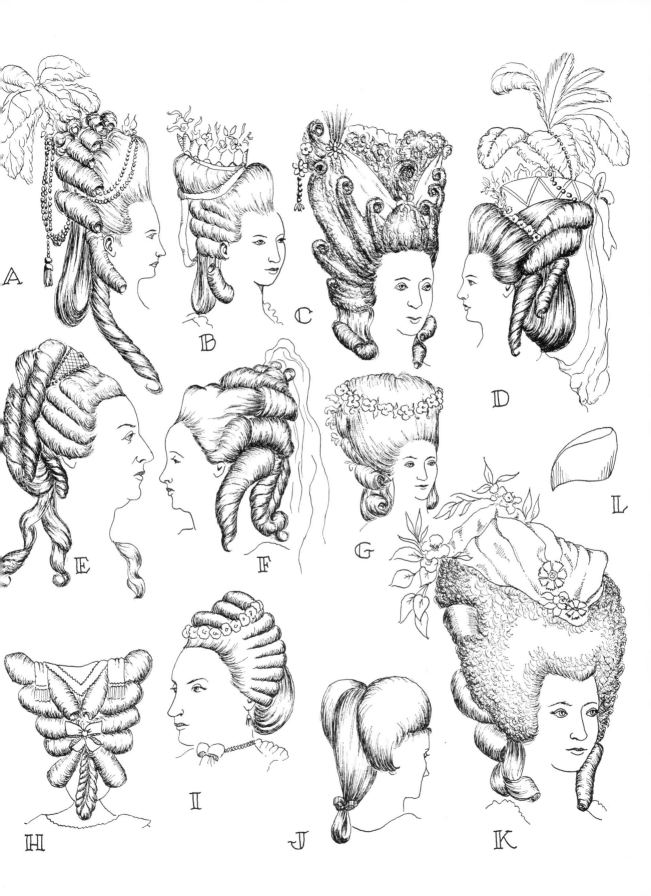

A

B

C

D

E

F

G

L

H

I

J

K

PLATE 83 : EIGHTEENTH-CENTURY WOMEN 1775–1779

A   Marie Antoinette.

B   1778. Coiffures were beginning to show greater width.

C   *c.* 1777, French.

D   1775, English. 'The head dress was ushered in at the beginning of the spring with a small tuft of feathers, which was soon changed to 2 or 3 distinct ones of the largest size, some pink or blue, but most generally white, and placed remarkably flat, with a rose of ribbons on the fore part. . . . The hair low before, yet rising on the forehead nearly perpendicular in a small round toupee. The sides down to the ears combed smooth, very far back and broad behind. The corners raised but a little above the front, with 2, 3, or 4 large curls down the sides, the bottom curl nearly upright. The bag not so low as the chin, small, and smooth at bottom, in general. . . . 2 or 3 rows of large curls.'—*Lady's Magazine.*

E   *c.* 1776.

F   1777, French. *À la persane.* Chignon in club. Sunshade of ostrich plumes.

G   1778, German.

H   1778, French. *En rouleaux.*

I   1778, German.

J   1777, French. *À la zodiaque.* 'The toupee is about 6 inches high. Just over the eyes a small curl of about 4 inches long and 1½ inches in diameter. The next curl over the ear is 6 inches long and 2½ inches in diameter. The third curl falls just behind the ear and is 5 inches long. The fourth descends toward the chignon and measures 6 inches in length and 2½ or 3 inches in diameter. The fifth falls toward the bosom just as low as the shoulder and is the same dimension as the last. The chignon is pretty full and descends rather lower than it used to do. The upper part or crown of the head is all hair, dressed in a globular form, representing the hemisphere, interspersed, as well as the toupee, with jewels representing stars, and over the ear a half moon. Just over the toupee a broad white or sky-blue ribbon is drawn from one side to the other, upon which the twelve signs of the zodiac are either painted or embroidered with silver or gold, or woven in (all which sorts of ribbons may be had ready made in Paris) and tied behind in a large knot, the bows of which ascend, and the streamers are left flying.'—*Lady's Magazine.*

K   1778, French. *À la Belle Poule.* One of the most famous of the eighteenth-century styles, commemorating a victorious French ship.

L   1778, German.

M   1779, French. Probably Madame St Aubin, wife of the artist. *À la capricieuse.*

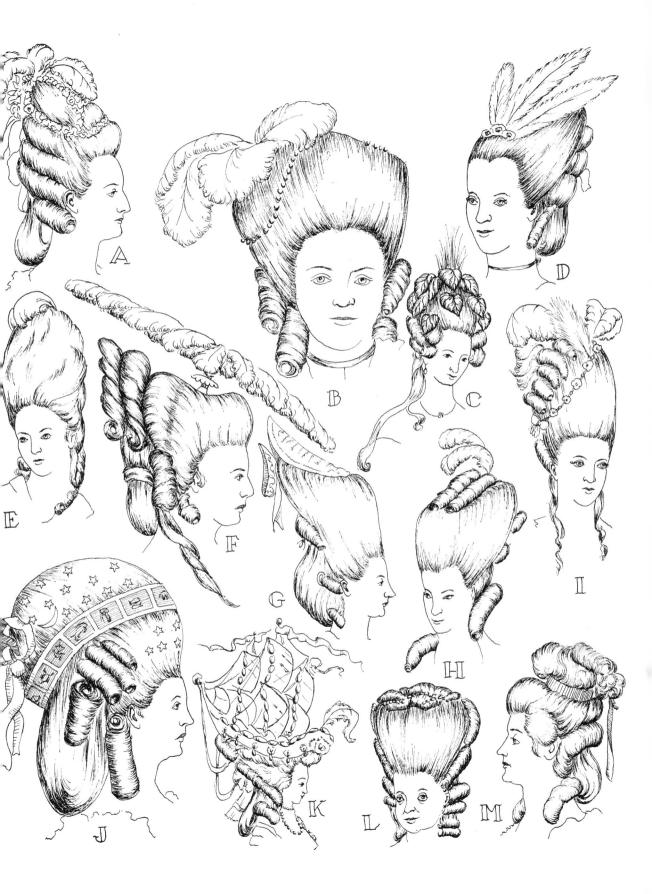

PLATE 84 : EIGHTEENTH-CENTURY WOMEN 1774–1785

A   1774, French. *En qu'es aco.* Note banging chignon. This is one of two particularly famous coiffures which appeared in Paris in 1774, the other being the 'sentiment puff'. (See text.)

B   1778, French.

C   1780, French. Young girl (see also Plate 79-L).

D   1778, French.

E   1778, French.

F   1778, French. *Chien couchant.* 'Asiatic coiffure composed of a sleeping dog with his tail hanging down behind; a double rope of pearls, ending in tassels, and held in place with a bow of ribbon similar to that of the trimmings and holding up a heron plume. On top of the head is placed a kerchief puff, held in place by a second rope of pearls. The unattached end of the chignon falls under the point of the kerchief and flies about like streamers.'–*Galerie des Modes.*

G   1780, French.

H   1778, French. *À la Dauphine.* 'Two side curls and two shoulder curls match the queue of the Dauphin; this coiffure is held together by a stiff ribbon with a rose of diamonds and crossed by a row of pearls. The chignon is in the form of a *croix de chevalier* from which escapes a curl *à la Sultane,* which falls to the neck, where it ends.'—*Galerie des Modes.*

I   1778, French.

J   *c.* 1776, French.

K   *c.* 1785, French. Wig. This is a reflection of the men's styles and was worn for riding.

L   1780. Probably a wig. However, it is slightly out of fashion—coiffures were wider in 1780 (see Plate 82-K, for example).

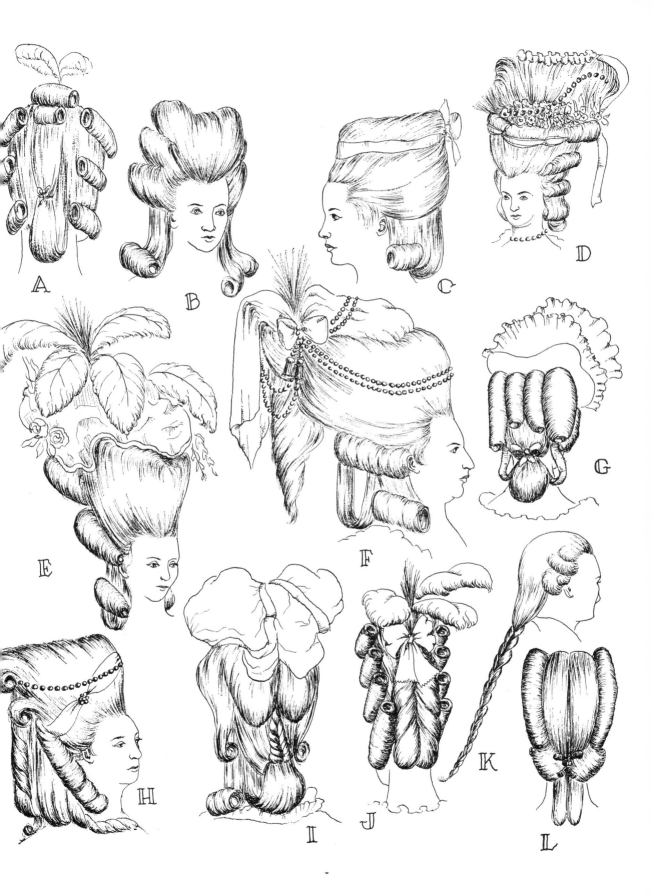

A

B

C

D

E

F

G

H

I

J

K

L

PLATE 85 : EIGHTEENTH-CENTURY WOMEN 1776–1789

A, B   1789, French and English. *Oreilles de chien*. These are two different versions of the same style. It can be surmised that A is probably the French original and B an English copy. However, both may have well been worn in England. The style seems to have been popular enough in England to elicit several derisive comments in print.

C   1782, German.

D   1781, English.

E   French. *À la reine*.

F   1776, French. Coiffure *à la Syrienne*. The coiffure originated in 1775. 'It is a familiar *hérisson*, encircled by a ribbon, which joins with a rope of pearls; from the centre of this join rises a black feather tuft, held in place by a diamond clasp. The two ends of the ribbon, having formed a love-knot in the back, fall free on either side in the form of little bands and cross the second curl and come to rest on a breast whiter than alabaster, which a neckerchief of gauze hides from too curious eyes.'—*Galerie des Modes*.

G   1783, English.

H   French. *À la Janot*.

I   1781, English. *Hérisson* or *hedgehog*. Originated in Paris. It was an extremely popular style and lasted for some years in both France and England. There were many versions of it. The essential was the bouffant frizzle, which gives the style its name (see also M below and Plate 88-D).

J   French. *À la sylphide*.

K   *c.* 1780, French. Style of Marie Antoinette.

L   *c.* 1781, French. Style of Marie Antoinette (see text for explanation of low hair styles about 1780).

M   *c.* 1781, English. Variation of the *hedgehog* (see **I** above).

N   *c.* 1782, French (see also Plates 86-B and 88-A).

O   1785. Coiffure *aux charmes de la liberté*.

P   1783.

Q   French. *À la distinction*.

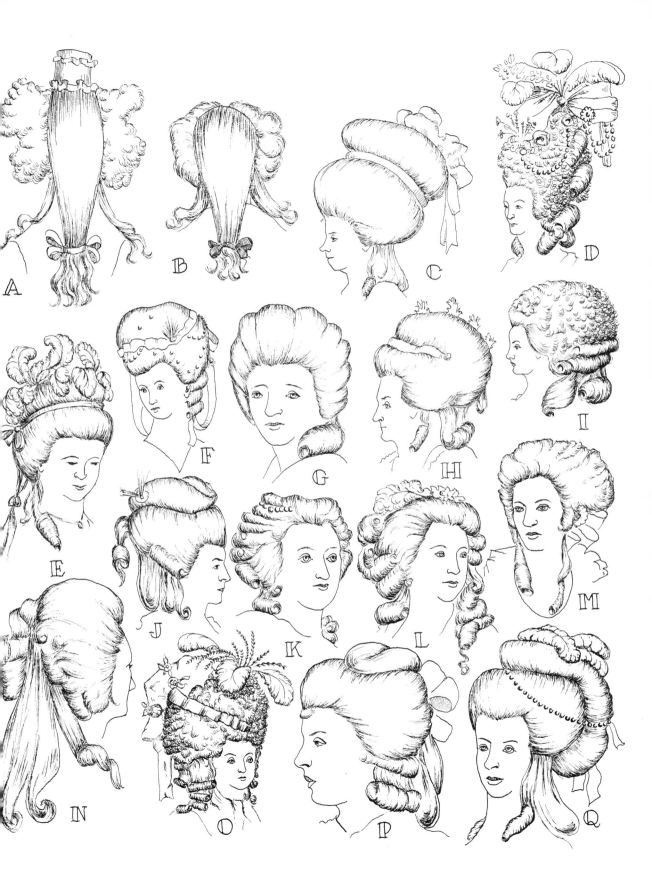

A

B

C

D

E

F

G

H

I

J

K

L

M

N

O

P

Q

PLATE 86 : EIGHTEENTH-CENTURY WOMEN 1780–1794

A   French.

B   French. Princesse de Talleyrand (see also Plate 85-N).

C   French. Powdered wig.

D   French.

E   *c.* 1790, English.

F   1793, French. Charlotte Corday.

G   English.

H   1790, English. Variation of the *hedgehog* (see Plate 85-I).

I   1792, French. Princesse de Lamballe, 1749–92. From a sketch made a few hours before her death. Having refused on September 3 to take the oath against the monarchy, she was torn to pieces by the mob. Her hair was then dressed and her head mounted on a pike for the Queen to see.

J   *c.* 1794.

K   1794.

L   1794, English. 'A turban made of light blue satin fringed with gold. The hair dressed in light curls; the chignon turned up plain, the ends turned back over the turban, falling down in ringlets; and the side curls falling easy on the neck. Three white feathers, the edges cherry-colored from the top down to the middle, and a black heron feather placed in the turban to incline forwards.' (Although this description from *Gallery of Fashion* refers to 3 white feathers, only 2 appeared in the accompanying drawing, as shown here. Probably the third is assumed to be hidden by the other two.)

M   Marie Antoinette.

N   1789, French.

Note: An indication that a style is English means only that it was worn in England or appeared in an English publication. Most of the styles originated in Paris.

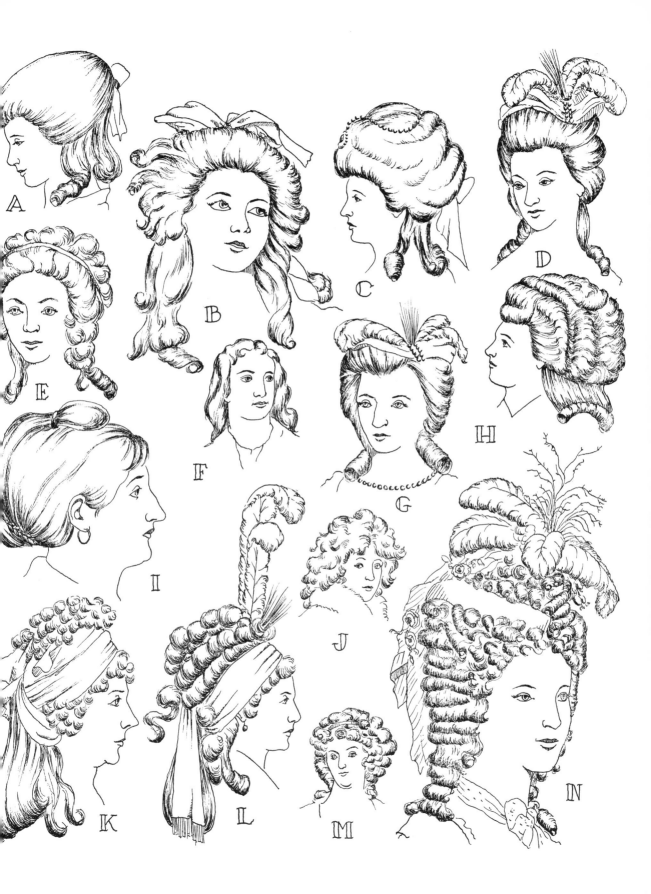

A

B

C

D

E

F

G

H

I

J

K

L

M

N

PLATE 87 : EIGHTEENTH-CENTURY WOMEN 1794–1799

A   1794, English. Court dress. 'A chiffonet of Italian gauze, the bandeau composed of 3 rows of white pearls, 2 rows of the same pearls twisted round the chiffonet. 3 plain white feathers and 2 edged with lilac placed in the head-dress. Bell lapets of gauze, tied in different parts with pearls. The hair very lightly frizzed, thrown into a variety of curls and ringlets and intermixed with the chiffonet. Plain chignon.'

B   1794, English. For afternoon wear. 'Toupee and side hair frizzed and thrown into large curls; bandeau of black and white ribband, cut out and formed into a wreath of flowers. 1 black and 2 white ostrich feathers placed in the front. Plain chignon, falling very low upon the back.'

C   1796, French. *Titus cut.* This style signalled the end of long hair (see also 88-F).

D   *c.* 1794, English.

E   1796, English.

F   *c.* 1798.

G   *c.* 1797.

H   1797, English. 'The toupee dressed very high in small curls, the skirts cut short and combed forward in easy curls around the face; the hind hair turned up plain, and the ends turned into loops upon the back of the toupee. Bandeau of white silver spangled crêpe, formed into a large bow on top of the head and confined at the side with a diamond pin.'

I   *c.* 1796.

J   1794, French.

K   1797, English. 'The toupee dressed very full upon the forehead and on the sides, straight lock upon the cheek, so that the ear remains uncovered; the hind hair turned up in chignons, fixed with small combs, the middle one set with diamonds; bandeau of the hair drawn through the toupee, and part of the sides and the hind hair drawn up in a variety of loops. Bouquet of lilies of the valley placed on top of the headdress.'

L   1798, English.

M   1799, English. 'The front and hind hair cropped and combed into bushy curls, ornamented with hair bandeaux, and a tassle of black bugle on the crown of the head; 1 black curled ostrich and 2 black *esprit* feathers placed in the front.'

Note: The descriptions are taken from the *Gallery of Fashion.*

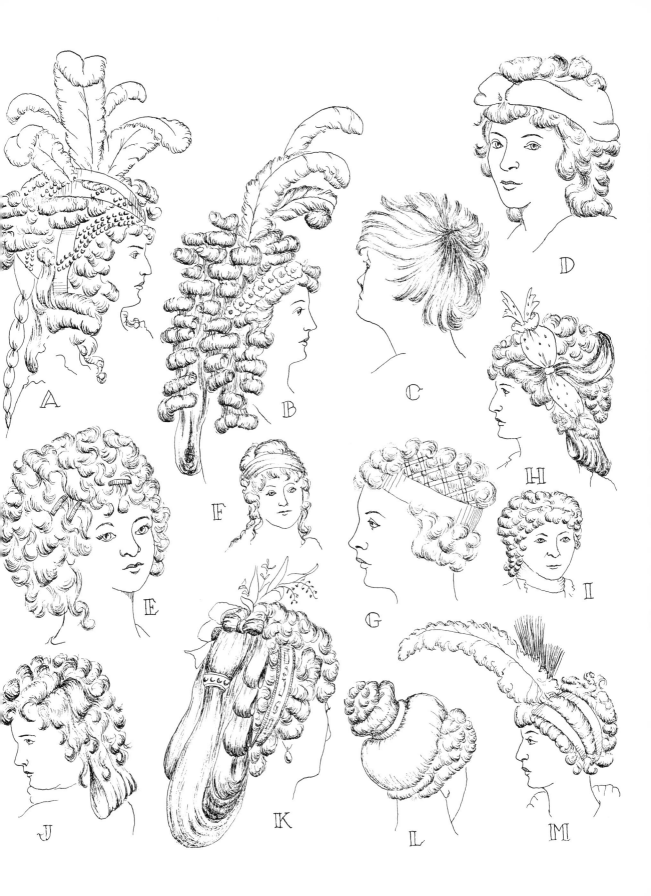

A

B

C

D

E

F

G

H

I

J

K

L

M

PLATE 88 : EIGHTEENTH-CENTURY WOMEN 1781–1799

A   *c.* 1785, English (see also Plate 85).

B   1781, French. Femme de chambre (see Plate 85 for fashionable styles).

C   Late 1780s, French. Marie Antoinette.

D   1788, French. *Hérisson* (see also Plate 85-I).

E   1798, German.

F   1798, French. *Titus cut* (see also 87-C).

G   1799, French.

H   Late 1790s, French.

I   *c.* 1788, French.

J   1797, French. Wig *à la grecque*.

K   1798, French. 'Raised chignon with net.'

L   1798, French. 'Garland of flowers and moss.'

M   1798, French. *À la caracalla*.

N   1798, French. *Chevelure en porc-épic* or *porcupine* head-dress.

O   1799, French. *À l'antique*.

P   1799, French. Note similarity to men's military style, in which queue was held up with comb.

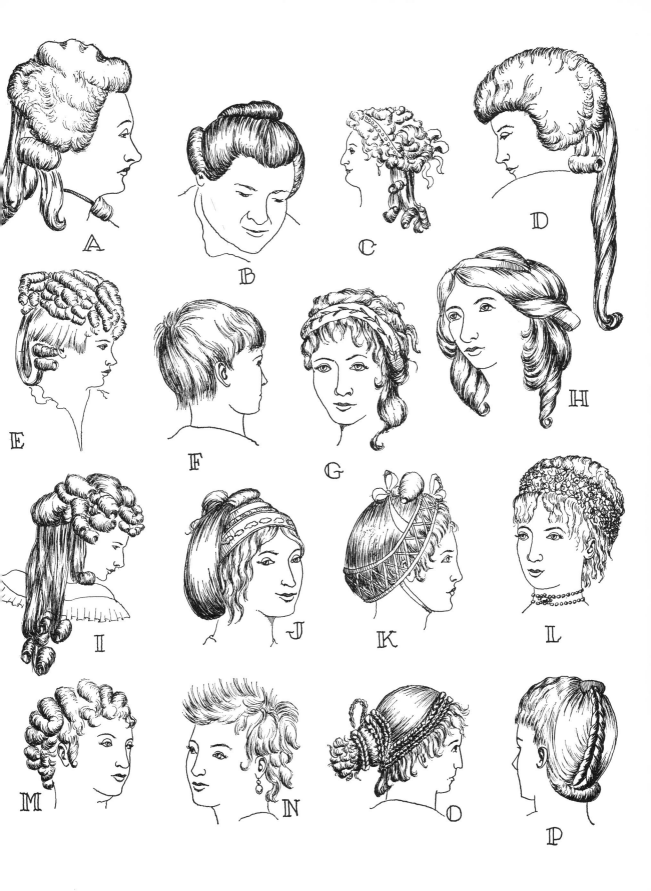

A

B

C

D

E

F

G

H

I

J

K

L

M

N

O

P

11 · The Nineteenth Century—Men

> I call upon the Military Prefects to take
> prompt and efficacious measure to the
> end that the detestable usage of wear-
> ing beards may be repressed and that
> the inhabitants abandon this indecent
> and subversive innovation.
>
> *Proclamation by His Majesty*
> *the Emperor of all the Russias*

Men's fashions in this century contrasted sharply with those of the preceding century in several ways. The hair was natural, it was unpowdered, it was considerably shorter, and, eventually, facial hair was almost universally worn.

The Early Years (1800–1840)

At the beginning of the century wigs were sometimes worn by older men, lawyers, clergymen, and others; but they were not fashionable. Military traditions in hair styles were more difficult to change than civilian ones and were usually fairly rigid.

Baron de Marbot tells of joining the Hussars, who prided themselves on looking as much alike as possible; and 'as the hussar regiments at that time wore not only a pigtail but also long "love locks", locks on the temples, and had their moustaches turned up, everyone belonging to the corps was expected to have moustaches, pigtails, and locks. As I had none of them, my mentor took me to the regimental barber, where I purchased a sham pigtail and locks. These were attached to my hair, which was already fairly long. . . . I was embarrassed at first by this make-up, but in a few days I got used to it and enjoyed it because I thought it gave me the air of an old hussar. With regard to moustaches the case was different. Of them I had no more than a girl, and as a beardless face would have spoilt the uniformity of the squadron, Pertelay, in conformity with the practice of the regiment, took a pot of blacking and with his thumb made two enormous hooks covering my upper lip and reaching almost to my eyes.' Marbot was expected to wear the painted moustaches until he could grow his own.

In 1804 the British army reduced the length of its pigtails and in 1808 cut them off entirely. According to Repton, 'when the order was given to the army, each regiment was drawn out, and the soldiers, who are always quick in obeying the orders of the commanding officer, when the word was given, *faced*, and each man cut off his comrade's Pig-tail, and all the Pig-tails were cut off in ten minutes'.

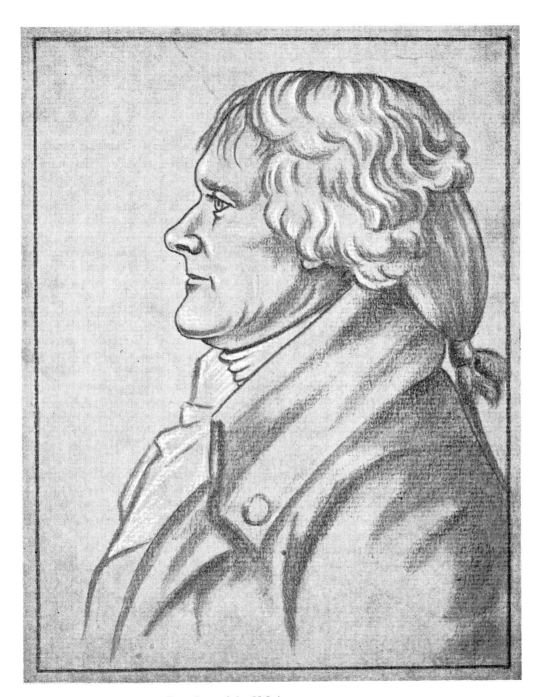

Fig. 97 : Thomas Jefferson, President of the U.S.A. 1801–9

Not all soldiers, however, were so eager for the freedom of short hair. Capt. Frederick P. Todd, writing in the *Infantry Journal*, relates the story of Thomas Butler, an American lieutenant-colonel of the Fourth Infantry, who clung with fierce determination to his long hair, defying the order of General Wilkinson on 1st April, 1801, that all military hair 'be cropped, without exception of persons'. Although many officers were dismayed, only Butler refused to obey the order, continuing to appear uncropped. Finally, on 2nd August, Wilkinson ordered that Butler 'at his particular request, and in consideration of his infirm health, has permission to wear his hair'.

The outraged Butler, bursting with health and vitality, became even more openly defiant and in 1803 was court-martialled and found guilty. In April of the following year he was released, still wearing his long hair. Once again he refused to crop it, defying even President Jefferson. Again he was arrested, tried, and found guilty. Two weeks before the findings of the court were made public Butler died of yellow fever, his long hair still intact.

Among civilians, older men, even though they had in many cases discarded their wigs, often still wore their hair in eighteenth-century styles—as for example, Thomas Jefferson, shown in Figure 97. Young men wore their own hair, sometimes clipped very short, sometimes longer and brushed forward, falling in natural or artificial curls over the forehead, sometimes both at once, and occasionally arranged in a curious style involving short hair, long hair, and a sort of topknot. (See Plate 89.) Fops of the period were known as *les incroyables*. Whatever the details of style, the fashionable hairdos, following the classic revival, were based on the Greek and the Roman. Normally, the hair was brushed away from the crown in all directions and allowed to fall naturally over the forehead. Straight-haired men often achieved fashionably curly locks with a crimping iron.

Gradually the side parting was adopted, and by the thirties hair was becoming longer and curling irons were used less. With the longer, straighter hair it was customary to use some kind of oil or grease to keep it in place and make it shine. In a curious little volume called *The Whole Art of Dress! or, The Road to Elegance and Fashion at the Enormous Saving of Thirty Per Cent!!!*, published in London in 1830 by 'a Cavalry Officer', there is included a recipe for hair oil:

'The following recipe for making an economical beautifier of the hair, I am indebted to a friend for, and as I have had so long a tried proof of its virtue, I can with pleasure impart it to others.

RECIPE FOR THE HAIR

Of fine Beef Marrow take $\frac{1}{4}$ lb.
Of Burnt Brandy two table spoonfuls
With the same quantity of the best Flask Oil.

'These should be mixed and allowed to simmer over the fire, when it should constantly be skimmed until it boil; when, after boiling a little time, the perfume bergamot, musk, lavender, or rose, as preferred, should be added, when it should be potted and tied up. This, if properly managed, will keep any time, and will be found to impart a beautiful freshness to the hair.'

For those who wanted a preparation ready-made there was always Macassar Oil, for which antimacassars were provided by neat housewives. The author of *The Art of Beauty*, published in 1825, had, however, some strong reservations about the popular Macassar Oil:

'We are assured that this is advertised at the rate of some hundreds, if not thousands, annually. The public, of course, pay smartly for this as well as for the cheap materials of which it is composed. The following we believe to be the genuine recipe for its preparation:

> Take three quarts of common oil, half a pint of spirits of wine, three ounces of cinnamon powder, two ounces of bergamot. Put it in a large pipkin, and give it a good heat. When it is off the fire, add three to four pieces of alkonet root, and keep it closely covered for several hours. Filter it through a funnel lined with blotting paper.

'The commonest oil is used; and, when rancid, it is remedied by putting in two or three slices of an onion. Not an ounce of Macassar oil is imported from Macassar, or it would be entered at the Customs, which it is not.'

As for the popular 'bear's grease', the author, who obviously considered it a sort of *pomatum non gratum*, nevertheless supplied a cryptic description: 'There are two sorts of it; one of the consistence of thick olive oil, which is procured by boiling from the fat about the caul and the intestines of the animal; the other, much harder and, in appearance, like frozen honey, obtained from about the kidneys. Both sorts have a rank, rancid, and intolerable smell.'

The apprentice system in the barbering trade seemed to have changed little over the years. Richard Wright Procter, in *The Barber's Shop*, quotes the document given to him in 1826 upon his indenture as a barber's apprentice at the age of nine:

'BARBER's HALL—It is proper and necessary for me to explain to you (my lad, who have this day been bound) the nature and obligation of the agreement you have entered into with your master. You are henceforth to look upon your master as your parent, and as such to love, honour, and obey him. You are, during the seven years of your servitude, to consider your time no longer as your own, but the property of your master, and accordingly to employ it all in his service, except only that part of it which the laws of your country have set apart and dedicated to public worship. You are, in everything else, to consult your master's credit and advantage; to be sober, careful, and diligent in his business, and neither to wrong him yourself, or suffer him to be wronged by others; always remembering that you hope in time to become a master yourself, and that you must in reason expect to be treated by your apprentices and servants as you shall behave to your master during the course of your apprenticeship. Lastly, to enable you to continue in the performance of your duty, let me advise you to avoid the company of the idle, the vicious, and profane,

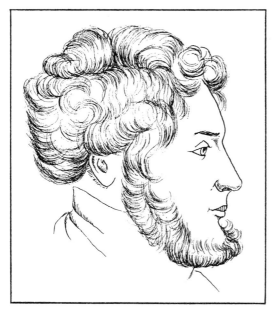

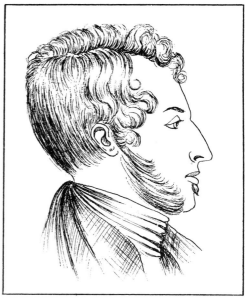

Fig. 98 : Count d'Orsay in 1833. His sketches of contemporaries are the source of several illustrations of hair styles.

Fig. 99 : Edward Lytton Bulwer in 1837. After a sketch by Count d'Orsay

whose conversation and example cannot fail, sooner or later, to debauch your principles and drive you into unjustifiable and destructive practices, such as must end in your inevitable ruin. By pursuing the advice now given to you, you will, among other advantages, secure to yourself the favour of your master, the good opinion of the world, and what is above all—the blessing of Almighty God.'

It was customary for apprentices to place Christmas boxes in view of the customers with gentle reminders, usually in verse. This was Procter's own:

> My Christmas-Box, kind gentlemen,
> I hope you will remember;
> And I will shave and lather well
> Until the next December.

Side-whiskers appeared early in the century. Usually they were wispy at first, occasionally fuller; and by 1810 they were commonplace. Then, for a while, instead of being allowed to follow the beard line straight down along the jaw, they were shaved diagonally across the cheek. Gradually they became fuller and longer, and by the thirties some men were even letting the hair creep around under the chin. A few Englishmen were beginning to wear moustaches, but they were rather ahead of their time. In some cases these were undoubtedly military men. Even in the beardless eighteenth century, the military had often hung on to their moustaches. The French and the Belgians, however, were wearing moustaches in the thirties. Apparently they were beginning to do so in Bavaria too, for in 1838 the king forbade them. In France the young Romantics had gone even further by growing beards; and the younger ones, who couldn't manage to grow them fast enough, occasionally resorted to false ones for special occasions. On the other side of the Atlantic, at about the same time, a completely unrelated event took place, causing quite a commotion in New England.

In 1830, at the age of forty-two, a quiet, unobtrusive, God-fearing man named Joseph Palmer moved to Fitchburg, Massachusetts. Normally, such an event would have caused no great stir in the community, the newcomer would have settled down and been accepted, and life would have gone on as before. Only one thing prevented matters working out that way—Joseph Palmer wore a beard. And in 1830 beards were not worn in Fitchburg. Had he been merely passing through or stopping off for a few days, he would undoubtedly have been merely an object of curiosity and perhaps some thoughtless finger-pointing. But he had come to stay, to settle among these people, to become one of them; and this was intolerable. The unthinkable had happened—Fitchburg was harbouring a non-conformist. Derision changed to outrage and outrage to anger. Palmer's windows were repeatedly broken, and somehow the culprits were never found. Women crossed the street to avoid him, and their sons threw stones at him. Even the Reverend George Trask admonished him; and eventually, all else failing, the Church refused him communion.

Shortly afterwards, Palmer was set upon in the street by four men, who threw him down, injuring his back, and attempted to shave him. Palmer managed to drive off the assailants with his pocket knife and was thereupon arrested, beard and all, for unprovoked assault. When he refused to pay the fine, he was imprisoned for a year in Worcester.

But this was not the end of his story. In prison he nourished his beard and wrote letters, which he managed, with the help of his son, to smuggle out. The letters protested that he had really been imprisoned not for assault, but for wearing a beard. They were published in various newspapers, the case was widely discussed, public opinion shifted to his side, and Joseph Palmer and his beard became a *cause célèbre*. After a time, he became such an embarrassment to the local constabulary that they suggested he forget the whole thing and go home. He refused as a matter of principle, saying that if they wanted him out, they'd have to carry him out. And that is what they finally had to do.

Before he died in 1875, Joseph Palmer had the satisfaction of seeing practically the entire male population bearded, including the local clegy. Palmer's tombstone, on which there is a likeness of his beard (Figure 100), reads: 'Persecuted for wearing the beard'.

THE MIDDLE YEARS (1840–1860)

By the 1840s the neo-classic influence could be seen only on older men who had worn their hair combed forward in their youth and had simply continued to do so, often

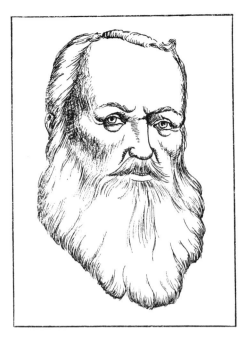 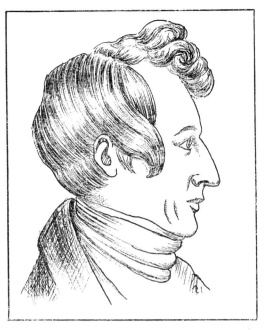

Fig. 100 : Joseph Palmer (1788–1875). 'Persecuted for wearing the beard'

Fig. 101 : William Henry Lytton Bulwer in 1845. After a sketch by Count d'Orsay

deliberately, in order to conceal a receding hairline. The hair was usually parted on the side with the side hair brushed straight down, then slightly forward. It tended to be fairly full to the neck in back. Centre partings were occasionally seen but were not fashionable until much later. Hair during this period was longer than at any other time in the century (see Plates 94 and 95).

The centre partings, fashionable or not, were defended in 1859 in *The Habits of Good Society*:

'Of course the arrangement of the hair will be a matter of individual taste, but as the middle of the hair is the natural place for a parting, it is rather a silly prejudice to think a man vain who parts his hair in the centre. He is less blamable than one who is too lazy to part it at all, and has always the appearance of having just got up.'

Wigs had virtually disappeared, but the few remaining ones were a sufficient aggravation to call forth occasional but firm criticism. In 1852 in a lecture on sculpture, a Mr Westmacott had a few words to say on the subject:

'When King Charles was the pensioner of Louis XIV, the French court rejoiced in the peruke; our king and his court servilely adopted this strange piece of costume, with the other follies, and worse than follies of that court; and the fashion was transplanted into England. All—princes, peers, and commoners, adopted it; the church, medicine, law, gentry, all imbedded their heads in this most absurd dressing. By slow degrees, good sense, and it may be hoped better taste, have led to the discontinuance of this unsightly piece of French costume, amongst many who, so late as our own times, indulged in it. Among the most eminent of those who have discarded it are our bishops, who now exhibit without disguise the natural development of their heads. Even parish beadles and workmen (except state coachmen!) have repudiated the wig—be it buzz, full-bottomed, bag, or scratch. And who now wears it as a dress appendage? dandies or dancing masters? Alas, no! The judges of the land, and counsel "learned in the law",—and, still more strangely, the "first commoner" (as his official badge)—are now the only supporters of this most ridiculous disguise. What a reflection it is on the *taste* of a nation, which alone, I believe, tolerates such a monstrous absurdity!' The criticism had, of course, no effect.

At about this same time a patent was taken out 'for a Forensic Wig, the curls whereof are constructed on a principle to supersede the necessity of frizzing, curling, or using hard pomatum; and for forming curls in a way not to be mauled; and also for the tails of the wig not to require tying in dressing; and further, the possibility of any person untying them'. This last in the list of virtues gives rise to interesting speculation on pastimes of the advocates. At any rate, there seems to be no record of the success of this admirable wig.

The most striking development was the gradual acceptance of beards and moustaches. The revival, as always, met with considerable resistance at first, and there were strong opinions on both sides. In 1844 in a contemptuous article in the *New Monthly Magazine*, it was suggested that the French were turning razors into swords:

'They seem more disposed to slaughter others than to shave themselves. . . . When a party of young Frenchmen approach one, it is like the advance of a herd of goats. . . . We never remember our neighbors so irritable as they are at present. The reason is obvious; they were never so exposed to be plucked by the beard. Fortunately, it is easier just now for England to pluck France by the beard than for France to return the affront. We are still respectable and razored.'

And yet in this same year Charles Dickens wrote in a letter to a friend: 'The moustaches are glorious, glorious. I have cut them shorter and trimmed them a little at the ends to improve their shape. They are charming, charming. Without them Life would be a blank.'

In 1847 there was published a book bearing the title: *Beard Shaving and the Common Use of the Razor; an Unnatural, Irrational, Unmanly, Ungodly, and Fatal Fashion Among Christians.* And in 1860 there was another called *Shaving a Break of the Sabbath and a Hindrance to the Spread of the Gospel.*

In 1850 a certain John Waters, who could barely contain his loathing for beards, wrote three articles for *Knickerbocker* on the subject. In the first he wrote:

'I would not object to the soft, silky, well-trained moustache of one of our leisurely lads who has nothing else in the world to do but attend to his toilette and spend gracefully the money that his father acquired and perhaps went to the devil for . . . and I might well admire a pair of moustaches like those of the late renowned Ali Pasha of Egypt that were taught to grow upward, diminishing in volume, until the fine master-hairs of the ends mingled with the long lashes of his brilliant eyes . . . but to see our yard-wide men, who in their youth have never imagined a beard at full-length except upon a maniac or a religious enthusiast . . . coming forth in this community of sober merchants with their strait, stiff, red or pepper-and-salt bristles, occupying the thoughts of peaceful men and disgusting ad nauseam those of a more refined class, is an enormity no longer to be endured in silence. . . . There is a fellow that it is my mischance to be acquainted with, with a form of body carved out of a cheeseparing after dinner who wears a red stiff brush at the extremity of his chin, of the very hue and wirey consistency of the beard of Judas Iscariot. . . . It is impossible to look at him and at his eyes, which are also red, without thinking at once of "treasons, stratagems, and spoils!" Do you know that this animal, who ought never, under any circumstances, to have lived elsewhere for a moment than in the solitude of a crowd, where he might hope by the uniformity of his equipment to escape observation, or else in some darker place of concealment—could you believe that he wears it (this badge) because without it he is "hardly satisfied", he says, with the profile of his chin?'

Having thought the matter over for a month before his second article, Mr Waters decided he had not changed his mind. He confessed:

'The longer the time may be that I spend in reflection the more fixed and perfect is the conviction that . . . I *only* am altogether in the right. Taste! say I, Taste!— Suppose a wretch should decide upon going home and shooting his father and mother—shall it be considered a matter of *Taste* whether of the two he shall first plump over? . . . Then neither are these brushes of Beards . . . in any degree defensible upon the pretext of the *Taste* of the owners of them. There exists no right whatever to exhibit to the community on any such plea a disgusting object of this sort, upon every principle of comity and social order they ought to be abolished. . . . Trim your Imperials. Subdue your Moustaches. Banish your Beards. And look after the half-concealed Saucers that you cherish under your chins.'

The saucer beard (Plate 94-Y) he reserves for special vilification in his third article:

'The Saucer or Trencher Beard then is affected and cultivated mainly by those to whom nature hath denied a growth of hair upon the cheek, the lip, and upper part of the chin; and often in these instances it renders the appearance of the wearer eminently vulgar and grotesque.

'I have before me in my mind's eye while I write, a short stout thickset clumsily-built man with hardly any neck, who cherishes a broad layer of black hair from the deep throat to the chin as a cushion for his jaws to repose upon. He has neither moustache nor whisker. The hair of his head is of a sandy brown and is made to hang in long loose disheveled morsels down his head and one side of his face, and is endeavored to be controlled behind the ear, where its ends mingle with the back outskirts of this trencher beard. . . . The *effect*, when seen in the distance of the strong contrast between the complexion and the black isolated undergrowth of hair seen like a streak beneath it, is to sever the head from the body; and the spectator beholds in front a head of John the Baptist brought before Herod in a black charger. . . . This is a trencher, or a saucer beard! It is that of a publick speaker, whose appearance beyond that of other men ought to be marked in every respect by the nicest possible rules of propriety, neatness, decorum, elegance, and grace.'

Mr Waters closes his article with a salute to the Emperor of Russia, arch-enemy of beards. 'May the gracious shadow of His Imperial Majesty never be less!'

It seems that His Majesty the Emperor of all the Russias had recently issued a proclamation (Reynolds questions this), according to which he, 'having graciously turned his attention to an unfortunate habit' which had begun to prevail among the nobility of his empire, namely, the habit of allowing the beard to grow, had deigned to order all his noble subjects to abstain from that 'impropriety'.

'The Council of Administration of the Kingdom of Poland, his Highness the Prime Lieutenant presiding, after having maturely deliberated on this affair, have declared that the same disposition ought to be applied to the nobility of the Kingdom of Poland.

'His Majesty having permitted the Russian nobility to wear uniform, a privilege which he has graciously extended to the Polish nobility, it is evident that the beard, being incompatible with the uniform in Russia, cannot be tolerated in Poland.

'In consequence of this decision . . . I call upon the Military Prefects to take prompt and efficacious measures to the end that the detestable usage of wearing beards may be repressed and that the inhabitants abandon this indecent and subversive innovation.'

Beards, no matter what their distinguished history, were somehow, in the nineteenth century, considered a corrupting influence. Yet only two years later *Tait's Edinburgh Magazine* declared:

'We have had visions of things looming in the future . . . and we are enabled to prophesy that beards are coming back again. Civilized chins shall again repose in the shadow of perennial pilosity; and the barber, no longer condemned to reap the barren crop of a stubble-field, shall be restored to his pristine dignity as the artistic cultivator of man's distinguishing appendage. Already the martial mustache, the haughty imperial, and the daily expanding whiskers, like accredited heralds, proclaim the approaching advent of the monarch Beard; the centuries of his banishment are drawing to their destined close, and the hour and the man are at hand to re-establish his ancient reign.'

In the following year, Alexander Rowland, in his book called *The Human Hair*, rose feelingly to the defence of beards:

'Deprive the lion of his mane, the cock of his comb, the peacock of the emerald plumage of its tail, the ram and deer of their horns, and they not only become displeasing to the eye, but lose much of their power and vigor. . . . The caprice of fashion alone forces the Englishman to shave off those appendages which give to the male countenance that true masculine character indicative of energy, bold daring, and decision.'

An article had already appeared in the *London Methodist Quarterly Review* strongly supporting the beard faction:

'It may surprise not a few when we say that the bronchitic affections under which ministers of the gospel so frequently labour, are often due to the violation of a hygienic law. The fact that the creator planted a beard upon the face of the human male, thus making it a law of his physical being, indicates, in a mode not to be mis-understood, that the distinctive appendage was bestowed for the purpose of being worn. Moreover, physiologically considered, those views are corroborated by experience; for diseases of the throat have, in many instances, been traced directly to the shaving of the beard. . . . Let, then, all our ministers of religion wear beards, for the Bible and nature are in favour of it; nor is the great head of the Church, Christ himself, ever seen in a painting without a beard; and it was said by the early Christian father, Tertullian, that to shave the beard is "blasphemy against the face".'

Those who wished to maintain the *status quo* were saying very little, at least in print. After all, they had the inertia of nearly two centuries of beardlessness on their side. But the tide was turning nonetheless; and the non-conformists, who evidently did not really have the courage of their convictions, rushed into print to try to persuade the rest of the male population to join them so that they would no longer be non-conformists. In many cases they campaigned for the beard long before they had the courage to wear one.

A British correspondent wrote feelingly to the *Irish Quarterly* on the subject, asking 'Why should men cut off what nature has given them for use, comfort, and ornament, and as a distinguishing characteristic of their sex! Is shaving a pleasing operation?' He clearly felt that it was not, and he stated flatly that 'if the fashion of wearing beards was to come in, we should have no more sore throats'. He then expounded on the ornamental value of the beard and declared that it gives to the face 'dignity and conveys the idea of strength, decision, manliness, depth of intellect, solidity—in short everything may be said in its favour—nothing against it. "What!" I hear a fair friend exclaim, "would the wretch have our husbands, our brothers, our sons, and our nephews wear nasty beards and look like Frenchmen?"' This was obviously a sore point in those days, but our correspondent's answer was unequivocal and bursting with patriotism: 'Certainly not, Madam; and one reason why we should *not* look like Frenchmen is that our beards would *not* be nasty. If we ceased to shave, we should not cease to use soap and water, and I venture to say that the English beard would be the cleanest, glossiest, handsomest thing in the world.' Nor would he be content with anything less than a full beard. 'You very seldom see a foreigner,' he wrote, 'with the beard, the whole beard, and nothing but the beard. He shaves off his whiskers or moustache, or in some way or other manages to disfigure himself. Now what I want is, the whole or none. Once admit that the use of the razor may be advantageous to some extent, and I am as far off my end as ever. Dear Madam, you know not the pain of shaving and the beauties of the beard.'

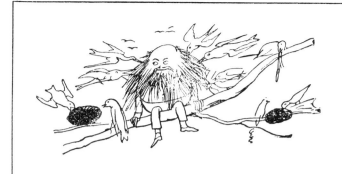

There was an Old Man in a tree,
Whose Whiskers were lovely to see;
But the Birds of the Air
Pluck'd them perfectly bare,
To make themselves nests in that tree.

Fig. 102 : Limerick and drawing by
Edward Lear (1812–88)

Southey, presenting a general discussion of beards in *The Doctor*, expresses his own reaction:

'I myself, if I wore a beard, should cherish it, as the Cid Campeador did, for my pleasure. I should regale it on a summer's day with rose water, and without making it an idol, I should sometimes offer incense to it, with a pastille, or with lavender and sugar. My children, when they were young enough for such blandishments, would have delighted to stroke and comb and curl it, and my grandchildren in their turn would have succeeded to the same course of mutual endearment.'

In Naples there was considerable hullabaloo over the wearing of moustaches. The government objected to them; and the police, when it was necessary, shaved them off, whereupon the wearing of the moustache became a *cause célèbre*. The following quotation from Lorenzo Benoni gives some idea of the persecution:

'I am now twenty one, and a thick circlet of hairs has grown under my chin. I should also have a pair of beautiful moustaches—the object of my ambition as a child—if moustaches were not unmercifully proscribed. I have made several attempts towards wearing them, but they were all frustrated. One day, a long, long time ago, M. Merlini, meeting me in the peristyle of the University, with a show of down upon my lip, protested, with sundry indescribable nods, jerks, and grimaces, that he had taken me for a pioneer. I understood the hint, and my budding moustaches fell under the razor. Twelve months later, the moustaches having reappeared thicker than ever, the Director of Police had the kindness to send me word through my father, that if I did not shave them off of my own accord, he would have them cut off for me; a very simple ceremony not at all unprecedented. Two carabineers would take you by each arm, force you into a barber's shop, and stand present during the operation.'

The American army resisted the early spread of facial hair and ordered that side whiskers were not to extend below the bottom of the ear. The order, widely ignored, was repeated in 1835. On March 16, 1840, a new order specified that 'officers and men of the dragoons are permitted to wear mustachios of a fashion to be regulated by the Colonels of their respective regiments'. In 1853 the War Department virtually gave up the losing battle and permitted the beard to be 'worn at the pleasure of the individual' so long as it was 'kept short and neatly trimmed'. The permission arrived after the fact, and the reservation was, of course, ignored in the glorious splurge of facial hair which adorned the middle of the century. In the British navy orders were issued against 'unseemly tufts of hair under the chin'. The moustache was strictly prohibited.

In 1854 the *Westminster Review* summed up the situation dispassionately:

'The beard is at present in what we must venture to call an unnatural position in Europe. Once the symbol of patriarch and king, it is now, it would seem, that of revolution, democracy, and dissatisfaction with existing institutions. Conservatism and respectability shave close. The mustachio enjoys military honor, indeed. But the beard itself is from sea to sea in disfavor with power and order. It is hated at once by the King of Naples and by Mrs. Grundy. In England, too, public opinion . . . is perhaps harder on the beard than it is anywhere else. All kinds of offices discourage or prohibit it; only a few travellers, artists, men of letters, and philosophers wear it, and to adopt it places you under the imputation of Arianism or dissipation or something as terrible with the respectable classes. Yet this opposition proves unable to stem the rising agitation. Pamphlets accumulate on the question; and the curiosity about it has reached that degree of livliness which authorizes us to pronounce it a movement.'

In this same year, according to *The Spectator*, a Preston firm politely requested the young men in its employ not to wear their moustaches during business hours. And the parishioners of an English county parish refused to attend church because the clergyman had taken to wearing a beard.

In mid-year the *Westminster Review* felt called upon once again to publish an article on beards:

'So far from the beard's requiring an apology . . . it would not be difficult to show that in every age it has had a philosophical relation to institutions. Thus, once it was a symbol of patriarchal majesty; next, of general manliness; then, of devotion to speculative pursuits. It has risen and fallen as empires have risen and fallen. And its being an object of so much contest and dispute just now is profoundly natural.

'We approach the subject with the impartiality of Cicero's friends at the New Academy. All that we claim is freedom from tyranny on the one side and on the other, that he who wears a beard and he who rejects it may equally be permitted liberty of conscience. So that we neither advocate nor do we oppose its adoption.'

The author states, in concluding, that 'it will be observed that the very reason which would induce us to sanction the wearing of the beard would also, in a vast number of cases, forbid its assumption. As certain dresses do not become diminutive women and must, in order to display their wonted effect be worn by those of noble

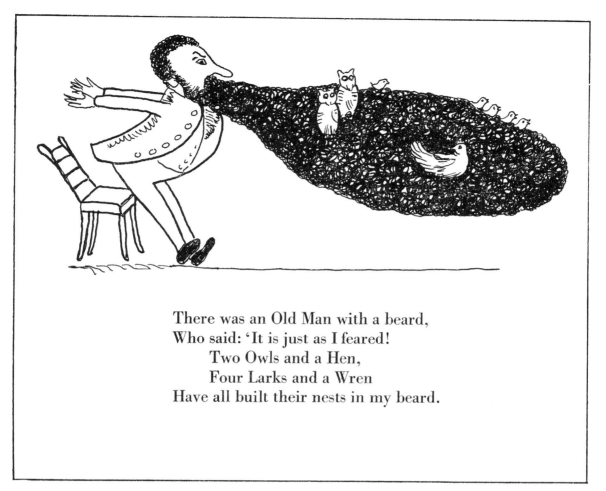

There was an Old Man with a beard,
Who said: 'It is just as I feared!
Two Owls and a Hen,
Four Larks and a Wren
Have all built their nests in my beard.

Fig. 103 : Limerick by and drawing after Edward Lear. From *A Book of Nonsense*, first edition 1846

stature, so the beard—identified as it is with sternness, dignity, and strength—is only the becoming complement of true manliness. If we are not mistaken, therefore, the cultivation of the beard is a perilous experiment for all degenerate sons of Adam and may produce in the wearers the most ludicrous incongruity. We trust that the noble association with the beard will never be degraded, and we would advise all beard-loving aspirants to be well assured of their worthiness—physically and mentally—to wear it before they show themselves in a decoration so significant of honor. . . . Let him who assumes it plant himself on what he conceives the sense and right of the matter; his moral courage will then sustain him until his friends, who may now amuse themselves at his expense, shall esteem him for his brave fidelity to his convictions.'

Still in the same year, the magazine published an article by Erasmus Wilson, in which he quoted Edwin Chadwick on the subject of beards: 'There can be no doubt that the moustachio is a natural respirator, defending the lungs from the inhalation of dust and cold . . . and it is equally, in warm climates, a protection of those parts against excessive heat'. He also points out that it is a protection against burning desert sands should they prove to be a problem. He further suggests it is helpful in preventing toothache, colds, bronchitis, and mumps. He reminds his readers that the arguments against the beard are based largely on the question of cleanliness; and although he feels that these arguments could hardly apply to the army and navy, they might be valid where the lower classes are concerned. And he admits that in excessively warm climates there is the special problem of keeping vermin out of one's beard. He makes no suggestion as to how women are to avoid the numerous ills which are likely to result from not wearing a beard.

The movement was clearly well under way; for not only was the reading populace bombarded with articles on the subject, but theatre-goers were subjected to a slightly different form of propaganda in an English play by Robert Barnabas Brough called *The Moustache Movement*. The scintillating dialogue includes the following exchange:

> LOUISA (*looking at his moustaches rapturously*): Yours are such loves! (*Caressing them.*)
> SOSKINS (*putting up his hand nervously*): D-don't pull them about.
> LOUISA (*passionately*): I wouldn't injure a hair of them for worlds! They are the lodestar of my existence!
> SOSKINS (*aside*): Ahem! (*Seriously, taking her hand*) Louisa, I fear it is the moustaches and not the man you love.
> LOUISA: Oh, don't say that, Anthony—though I own it was they that won me two months ago, when we met at the Eagle.

And so it goes. The moustaches, unfortunately, are false; but Louisa bears up, and all ends happily. At the final curtain Louisa says: 'If it be true that a good face needs no whiskers, 'tis true that a good farce needs no tag—yet to good faces they do use good bushes, and good farces prove the better by the help of good tags'.

Apparently the anti-beard faction had been complacent too long. The handwriting was on the wall. But the pro-bearders were anything but complacent and kept pressing their advantage to the limit.

One Martin van Butchell, who was vehemently opposed to shaving, tended to take out advertisements, not always entirely intelligible, but always having something to do with hair. One of these read, 'Girls are fond of hair; (and love *comforters*), see their *bosom friends*:—large waists, *muffs*, tippets. Let your beards grow long, that ye may be strong in mind and body; Jesus did not shave, for he knew better. Had it been proper our chins should be bare, would hair be put there by wise Jehovah, who made all things good?'

Even more confusing, if possible, is the following: 'Am I not the first healer (at this day) of bad fistula? With a handsome beard, like Hippocrates'. The combine I sell one guinea each hair. (Of use to the fair that want fine children:—I can tell them how; it is a secret.) Some are quite auburn; others silver-white;—full half-a-quarter long, growing (day and night) only fifteen months.'

This clearly was written early in his sixteen years of eschewing the razor. Two years later he described himself as 'a British Christian man, with a comely beard full eight inches long'.

By 1858 the wearing of facial hair of some sort was well established. According to the *Irish Quarterly Review*:

'British whiskers . . . have grown up like all the great institutions of the country, noiselessly and persistently. . . . Let us take the next half-dozen men passing by the window as we write. The first has his whiskers tucked into the corners of his mouth as though he were holding them up with his teeth. The second whisker that we descry has wandered into the middle of the cheek, and there stopped, as though it did not know where to go to, like a youth who has ventured out into the middle of a ball-room with all eyes upon him. Yonder bunch of bristles twists the contrary way, under the owner's ears; he could not, for the life of him, tell why it retrograded so. The fourth citizen, with the vast Pacific of a face, has little whiskers, which seemed to have stopped short after two inches of voyage, as though aghast at the prospect of having to double such a Cape Horn of a chin. We perceive coming a tremendous pair, running over the shirt collar in luxuriant profusion.'

The Habits of Good Society; A Handbook of Etiquette for Ladies and Gentlemen, published in London in 1859, was firmly on the side of the beards:

'Whatever *Punch* may say, the moustache and beard movement is one in the right direction, proving that men are beginning to appreciate beauty and to acknowledge that Nature is the best valet. . . . Above all, the whiskers should never be curled nor pulled out to an absurd length. Still worse it is to cut them close with the scissors. The moustache should be neat and not too large, and such fopperies as cutting the points thereof or twisting them up to the fineness of needles—though patronized by the Emperor of the French—are decidedly a proof of vanity.'

The author's enthusiasm for beards, and especially beards in their natural state, led him eventually to turn on the entire barbering profession:

'As for barbers, they have always been gossips and mischief-makers, and Arkwright, who invented spinning by rollers, scarcely redeemed his trade from universal dishonor. They have been the evil spirits of great men too, whom they shaved and bearded in their private closets. . . . Who, in fact, can respect a man whose sole office is to deprive his sex of their distinctive feature?'

THE LATER YEARS (1860–1900)

According to Lewis Gannett, the Harvard classes in the 1870s were thoroughly bewhiskered. Gradually the beards disappeared, leaving only the moustaches. In the class of 1900 there were no beards.

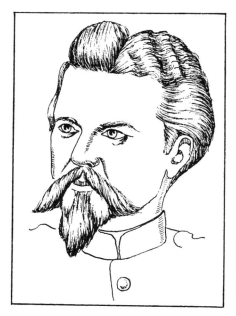

Fig. 104 : Ludwig II (1845–86), King of Bavaria

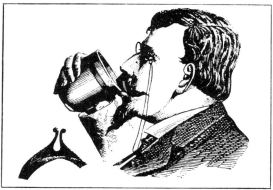

Fig. 105 : A device, patented by Eli J. Randolph in 1872, for keeping food and drink out of the moustache

A look at American presidents tells a somewhat similar story. They were clean shaven until Lincoln, who campaigned without a beard but grew one after his election. According to Carl Sandburg, he did so at the suggestion of a little girl named Grace Bedell in Westfield, New York; or, at least, he gave her the credit. Five other presidents followed suit. Grant's is described by Edith Effron in a retrospective article in the *New York Times Magazine* as 'short and utilitarian'. This was followed by 'the long, flowing Rutherford Hayes beard, the proletarian bush of James Garfield, and Chester A. Arthur's sprightly whiskers. The last was Benjamin Harrison's beard. It ended the series with charm and dignity.'

Two of the presidents in that bewhiskered period were clean shaven—Andrew Johnson and William McKinley. Cleveland, Roosevelt, and Taft wore moustaches.

Clearly, whiskers were well established; for in 1861, in an article entitled *Proposed Alterations in Our Military Dress, Arms, and Equipment*, Lt.-Col. E. Napier recommended, among other things, that soldiers be permitted beards and moustaches and then added:

'This will no doubt by many be pronounced very "un-English" and unbecoming; it is, however, only likely to be considered such because we are not accustomed to the sight of the beard and mustache, which . . . are doubtless most efficient protections to the face in extremes of either heat or cold; besides enabling the soldier to lighten his kit of scissors, razors, razor-case, razor-strop, soap-box, and shaving brush—to say nothing of the loss of time entailed, particularly whilst on service, of a poor fellow being obliged daily to rasp his countenance—to effect which may likewise be supposed to carry a looking-glass. Should a most competent authority be required as to the feasibility of wearing what Providence has no doubt, for wise purposes of His own, planted on the face of man—if such authority for sanctioning this patriarchal usage be required, we would beg leave to refer to the opinion and example of Gen. Sir Charles Napier [Plate 96-L], who whilst in India, not only sported himself a beard of which a Persian need not have been ashamed, but, I understand, likewise allowed all those under his command to do the same.'

Resistance to facial hair, especially the moustache, was still strong; and in 1862 a will made by one Henry Budd specified that 'in case my son Edward shall wear moustaches, the devise hereinbefore contained in favour of him, his appointees, heirs, and assigns of my said estate, called Pepper Park, shall be void; and I devise the same estate to my son William, his appointees, heirs and assigns. And in case my said son William shall wear moustaches, then the devise hereinbefore contained in favour of him, his appointees, heirs, and assigns of my said estate, called Twickenham Park, shall be void; and I devise the said estate to my said son Edward, his appointees, heirs, and assigns.' An upholsterer in Pimlico, who also had convictions in the matter, left ten pounds each to his employees who did not wear moustaches and only five pounds to those who did.

Dr Belcher, an Irishman who felt, not unreasonably, that the beard still required defending, did so on the ground that it 'makes a countenance, which would without it appear weak, appear full of reflection, force, and decision'—surely a persuasive argument for the recalcitrant.

By 1871 it would probably not have occurred to anyone that beards required defending. In that year there appeared a serene editorial in *Every Saturday*:

'Since Nature is above Art, and the work of God of more certain worth than any device of man, it is something remarkable that beards have been under the control of Fashion, as absolutely as boots and bonnets. Sometimes, indeed, conscience has claimed jurisdiction of beards, as, at other times, of apparel; and men have been deemed pious or profane according to the cut of their hair. But religious scruples have proved, in the long run, no match for the caprice of *La Mode*.

'Time was when the clergy were unshaven, save on the one spot devoted to the sacerdotal tonsure,—when a Romish priest with a full beard would have lacked one of the most prominent outward credentials of his holy function. Yet the present Pope rejects the beard of the primitive Peter. . . . Puritan beards have been subject to changes no less extreme. Cromwell and his psalm-singing soldiers wore mustaches of fierce aspect; and John Knox thundered his denunciations against Pope, Cardinal, and Bishop, through a beard as voluminous as that of a Turkish sultan. . . . The clergy, advancing by discreet graduation,—a hair's breadth at a time, so to speak— have at last come into the full freedom of their lay brethren and now wear their beards, if they like, and *as* they like, without peril of the parochial Inquisition. Nevertheless, mustaches, we believe, are still deemed unbecoming a parson; and in all cases, except when worn as an army regulation, are generally thought to savor of dandyism.'

The question was no longer whether or not to wear whiskers but simply what kind. Side-whiskers, beards, and moustaches were all being worn in any combination

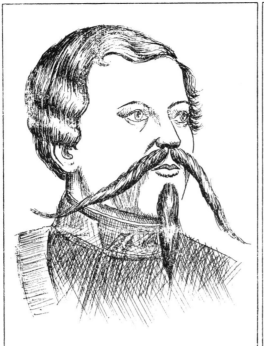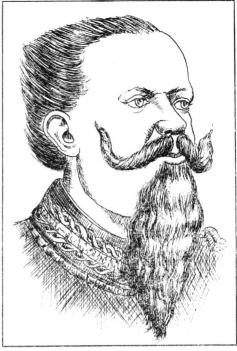

Fig. 106 : Victor Emmanuel II (1820–78), first king of Italy

and in whatever shape happened to suit the individual fancy. But it was the side-whiskers which distinguished the nineteenth century from previous periods in history. The timid sproutings of the early years had flourished and often developed into flowing, luxuriant growths, frequently unaccompanied by any beard or moustache.

Mutton chops were very full at the bottom, curving around to the mouth, giving the general shape of a mutton chop. The chin was bare (Plate 103-I). *Piccadilly weepers* (or simply *weepers*) were long, flowing side-whiskers (100-E). *Dundrearies*, named after Lord Dundreary in *Our American Cousin*, were a particular form of the Piccadilly weeper worn by the actor playing Lord Dundreary (Figure 107). It seems, however, that the two terms became interchangeable, though perhaps semanticists aimed at a distinction. In any event, *weepers* appears to be the more general term. A writer in *Harpers Weekly* refers to 'Piccadilly weepers of the Lord Dundreary kind'. It also appears that *weepers* was used more in England and *Dundrearies* in America.

Burnsides, a heavy growth of side-whiskers curving across the cheek and joining the moustache, took their name from the style of whiskers worn by General Ambrose Burnside in the American Civil War (see Figure 108). Most authorities, including Webster's *New International*, as well as other dictionaries and encyclopedias, state that the term *sideburns* evolved from *burnsides*. Reynolds attributes this explanation to a guess by F. J. Hudleston and refuses to take it seriously. Although the two terms have been used interchangeably to some extent, the tendency appears to be to reserve the term *burnsides* for the particular style worn by the general and to use *sideburns* for less luxuriant growths covering a smaller area of the cheeks.

The 1909 supplement of the *Century Encyclopedia* defined *Burnsides* as 'a style of beard such as that affected by General Burnside, consisting of a mustache, whiskers, and a clean-shaven chin'. In other words, *all* of the hair on the face was included, not just that on the side. Even earlier, in 1875, the *Cincinnati Enquirer* referred to a gentleman whose 'whisker was of the Burnside type, consisting of mustache and "mutton-chop", the chin being perfectly clean'. In 1917 Walter Pritchard Eaton, in *Green Trails and Upland Pastures*, described a man who had 'ample Burnside whiskers which gave him a most benevolent expression'. With the passing of the beard, however, the word fell into disuse.

Precisely when the term *sideburns* came into being is not known, but on August 1, 1887, it was used by the *Chicago Journal*: 'McGarigle has his mustache and small sideburns on'. *Sidebar whiskers* apparently meant the same thing. In 1882 George Peck in *Sunshine* described 'a red-faced man, with these sidebar whiskers'. *Sideboards* was another and probably synonymous term which was in use at least as early as 1890.

As for beards, the *imperial*, worn by Napoleon III (Plate 93-H), became extremely popular and lasted for many years. The traditional *Vandyke* was also worn; and as Reynolds points out, it was especially popular with physicians around the turn of the century. Both the *swallow-tail* and the *forked beard* were to be found. Then there was the *Horace Greeley* (Plate 103-K), an American beard which merely framed the bare face with a fringe of whiskers, and the full *Nokomis* beard (see Plate 99-Z).

Fig. 107 : E. A. Sothern as Lord Dundreary in
Our American Cousin.
After a photograph of 1881

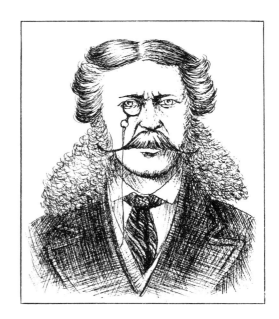

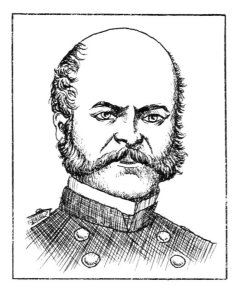

Fig. 108 : Brigadier-General A. E. Burnside
(1824–81)

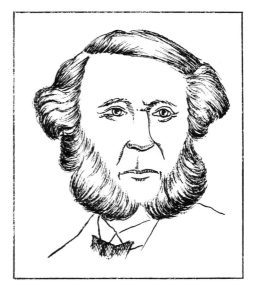

Fig. 109 : John Tyndall, British physicist
(1820–93)

The general term *goatee* was used for any small beard confined to the chin. In the United States a long, goat-like chin beard was sometimes called an *Uncle Sam*, whereas a very tiny one (Plate 99-W) was a *breakwater*. The full but relatively short chin whiskers were known as *billy whiskers* or *billies* (Plate 98-T).

Moustaches were also given special names. The popular full moustaches which drooped down over the mouth were called *soup strainers* (Plate 96-X), whereas a moustache which curved around the mouth was known as a *horseshoe* (Plate 96-U). The curled moustaches shown in Plate 105-F were sometimes called *bullet heads*.

Despite the early support of the *Methodist Quarterly Review*, the clergy had not rushed to adopt the beard. It is said that the first prelate of the Church of England to appear in a full beard was John Ryle, first Anglican Bishop of Liverpool.

A Milwaukee barber, looking back fondly on the bearded days of the late nineteenth century, spoke rapturously of 'glorious grizzled ornaments of lovely hues of red' and continued: 'Some clung to the Dundrearys or sideburns—small tufts of orange which protected the ears and lent dignity to the face. Came the spikey imperials which decorated the chin, falling away in a pie-shaped drop from under the lip, giving an austere and somewhat severe expression to the face. Red whiskers were always about three shades lighter than the shock of hair, perhaps because of exposure to the sun. The red beard never attained its beauty unless allowed to grow wild. The wild dense growth of a full beard gave color and lent distinction to the owner.'

Sometimes, when moustaches and beards became distressingly grey, often before the hair on the head, a little touching up was resorted to. In 1867 it was reported that 'nitrate of silver—lunar caustic—has . . . acquired a certain celebrity as a hair dye, and if the colour be not objected to, the nitrate is effectual . . . but nitrate of silver used as a hair dye ultimately bestows, in addition to black, a certain play of irridescent colours, which makes one look ridiculous. I happen to have seen a physician, a very celebrated physician too, whose whiskers are resplendent in sunshine with all the rainbow tints one sees on the neck of a pigeon or the tail feathers of a barn-door cock. He had been dyeing his whiskers with nitrate of silver: the fact stood revealed. . . .

'To dye hair a natural-looking brown is almost beyond the competence of art. For the most part, the so-called dyes are only mitigated black dyes; but a true brown result can no more be expected from this treatment than a black dress, when worn till shabby, shall change to brown. If only a small hair mass has to be treated, as a moustache or imperial, for example, chloride of gold may be used to impart a colour between ruddy and brown, not unnatural to begin with. Ultimately, however, gold solutions give rise to the same irridescent tints that were adverted to when silver was in question.'

Usually one's barber was entrusted with the dyeing. In fact, it was often he who suggested it in the first place. When there were no beards to trim or to dye, the barbers were kept busy shaving. In the 1880s the usual price of a shave in the United States was ten cents. After the turn of the century the *Barber's Journal* looked back at the good old days:

'A barber of twenty years ago, being blessed with low rent, cheap labor, and ordinary appliances, needed but to invest small capital in his enterprise. People were not so particular in those days, and the barber used a single towel on as many customers as he chose, or as long as the absorbent qualities of the linen held out. The face-wash consisted of a few drops of bay rum in a pint of water; the shampoo mixture was composed of a little borax or salsoda mixed liberally with water, with a small piece of shaving soap at it. At that time also hair dye-ing was quite a feature of the trade. A barber could earn more in one hour dyeing hair than a man could take in in one day at the present time.'

By the nineties, beards, though still worn by older men, were no longer fashionable. And even the men who did wear them were sometimes beginning to feel a certain dissatisfaction. An 1891 article on beards in *All the Year Round* probably summed up the feeling of a good many men:

'Like all other excellent things—except mushrooms—the beard does not spring up in a single night. In its transitional stage, it is not altogether a thing of beauty. The man then feels that he is hardly fit for the society of his fellow creatures. . . . He has many humiliating moments to endure ere the time of his dignity has come. And it is just conceivable that when he is duly bearded like the pard, he still retains such a recollection of the slights he has suffered in quest of his ambition that pique makes him dissatisfied with the reality. For it is often with beards as with the other goals towards which we aspire: the pleasure lies mainly in expectation. Happily, the

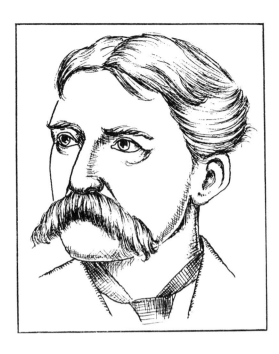

Fig. 110 : E. A. Sothern (1826–81),
who created the role of
Lord Dundreary

barber will, in a trice, be able to set his petitioner yet again at the foot of the ladder which he has been so long in scaling.'

Although beards were on their way out, men of all ages wore an astonishing variety of moustaches (see particularly Plates 105, 107, and 108). Edith Effron, writing of the moustache in America, points out that 'it was a subsidiary part of the early beard for many decades and slowly, almost surreptitiously, it began to appear as a solo with the waning popularity of the beard. It reached erratic and unpredictable heights in the Gilded Age. Young city dandies of the Nineties grew mustaches rapturously. Prosperous and impoverished business men caught the virus. Even the farmer's son cultivated a small stubble beneath his nose.' But, as Miss Effron puts it, 'something about those brassy, black handles of the mustache did not symbolize the worrying, marrying American. Almost without warning, after the turn of the century, this splendor vanished. It had no cultural roots.'

Whiskers had crept in slyly on the sides of the face very early in the century, had slowly blossomed into a display equalling that of any period in history, and by the end of the century were quietly fading away.

As for the hair on the head, it waxed and waned along with the beards. The fairly short Roman clip of the early years developed very nearly into a fifteenth-century bob, then subsided into the medium short cut which was to last with minor varia-tions for years to come. Perhaps the most notable characteristic of the hair at the end of the century, apart from the length, was the centre parting. This was by no means universally worn (see Plates 104-108), but it was fashionable for a while and seemed to go with the handlebar moustache. Antimacassars were still in use and still needed.

The anonymous, though presumably English, author of *The Habits of Good Society* could 'see nothing unmanly in wearing long hair, though undoubtedly it is inconvenient and a temptation to vanity, while its arrangement would demand an amount of time and attention which is unworthy of a man. But every action and every age has had a different custom in this respect, and to this day even in Europe the hair is sometimes worn long. The German student is particularly partial to hyacinthine locks curling over a black velvet coat; and the peasant of Brittany looks very handsome, if not always clean, with his love-locks hanging straight down under a broad cavalier hat.' Ten years later an unidentified English countess, author of *Good Society*, stated unequivocally that long hair was never indulged in 'except by painters and fiddlers'.

'When once the head has been properly arranged', wrote Robert Tomes in 1877, 'it is well to avoid all farther interference with it. The practice, so common with men, of passing the hands through the locks . . . is filthy and not becoming before company. The use of a comb, or even its habitual carriage in the pocket, is irreconcilable with all nicety of manners.'

Mr Tomes regarded dyeing the hair as 'the most preposterous of all attempts at human deceit; for it deceives no one but the deceiver himself, whose vanity leads him to believe that his artifice is successful. There is no one who has once commenced this practice of giving an artificial color to his hair but must regret it. . . . The wig and dyepot are, we are pleased to announce, going out of fashion.'

The legal profession stuck to its wigs in spite of sporadic attempts to discard them. In the London *Times* of July 24, 1868, the following item appeared:

'During the last two days the learned judge and the bar have been sitting without their wigs; and in opening a case, Sir Robert Collier called attention to the innovation and apologized for not appearing in full forensic costume. His lordship said he had set the example of leaving off the wig in consequence of the unprecedented heat of the weather, as he thought there were limits to human endurance. Sir Robert Collier expressed a wish that this precedent might be generally followed, and hoped that the obsolete institution of the wig was coming to an end,—a hope in which many members of the bar heartily concur.' However, this new phase was short lived.

In 1872 one writer took a critical look at stage wigs in the contemporary theatre:

'The light comedian still indulges sometimes in curls of an unnatural flaxen, and the comic countryman is too often allowed to wear locks of a quite impossible crimson color. . . . But in what are known as "character wigs" there has been marked amendment. The fictitious forehead is now very artfully joined on to the real brow of the performer without those distressing discrepancies of hue and texture which at one time were so very apparent, disturbing credibility and destroying illusion. And the decline of hair in color and quantity has often been imitated with very happy ingenuity. Heads in an iron gray or partially bald state—varying from the first slight thinning of the locks to the time when they come to be combed over with a kind of "cat's-cradle" or trellis-work look, to veil absolute calvity—are now represented by the actors with a completeness of a most artistic kind.'

PLATE 89 : NINETEENTH-CENTURY MEN 1800–1810

A   English.

B   Alexandre Sabès Pétion, 1770–1818. Haitian general and president of Haiti, 1807–18.

C   1802, French. Fashionable young man—an *incroyable*.

D   1801, French. Fashionable young man.

E   *c.* 1800. Fops of the period, with their extreme hair styles, were known as *incroyables*.

F   1803, English.

G   *c.* 1800. Napoleon Bonaparte (for later portrait see O below).

H   Sir Walter Scott, 1771–1832.

I   1802, French. Fashionable young man—an *incroyable*.

J   1803, French.

K   Joseph McKeen, 1757–1807. First president of Bowdoin College, 1802–7. Long hair was still worn by conservative men but was not fashionable.

L   1807, English.

M   English.

N   Samuel White, 1770–1809. U.S. Senator. Back hair is false.

O   Napoleon Bonaparte, 1769–1821 (see G above).

P   Henry Dearborn, 1751–1829. American soldier. Back hair is false.

Q   1801, English.

R   Jonathan Dayton, 1760–1824. Speaker of the House and U.S. Senator. Back hair is false.

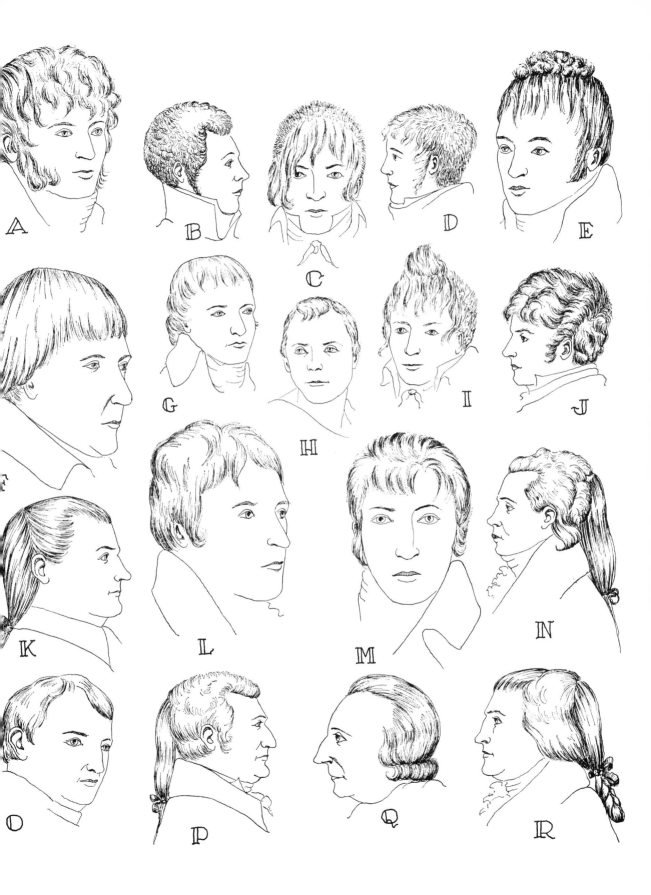

PLATE 90 : NINETEENTH-CENTURY MEN 1810–1820

A   1813, French. Fashionable young man.

B   1815, English. *Physical wig*. This is an eighteenth-century style, but it was worn by some older men in the early nineteenth century.

C   French. George Cuvier, 1769–1832. Zoologist and geologist.

D   *c.* 1820, German.

E   *c.* 1810. Army officer.

F   1812, French. Fashionable young man.

G   *c.* 1817, German.

H   1810, German. Philipp Otto Runge. (From a self-portrait.)

I   American. Andrew Jackson, 1767–1845. President of the U.S., 1829–37.

J   1810, French. Fashionable young man.

K   1811, French. Fashionable young man.

L   1812, French. Fashionable young man.

M   1810, French. Fashionable young man.

N   1815, French. Fashionable young man.

O   1818, French. Fashionable young man.

P   George IV, 1762–1830—reigned 1820–30.

Q   1812, French. Fashionable young man.

R   1814, English.

S   1814, French. Fashionable young man.

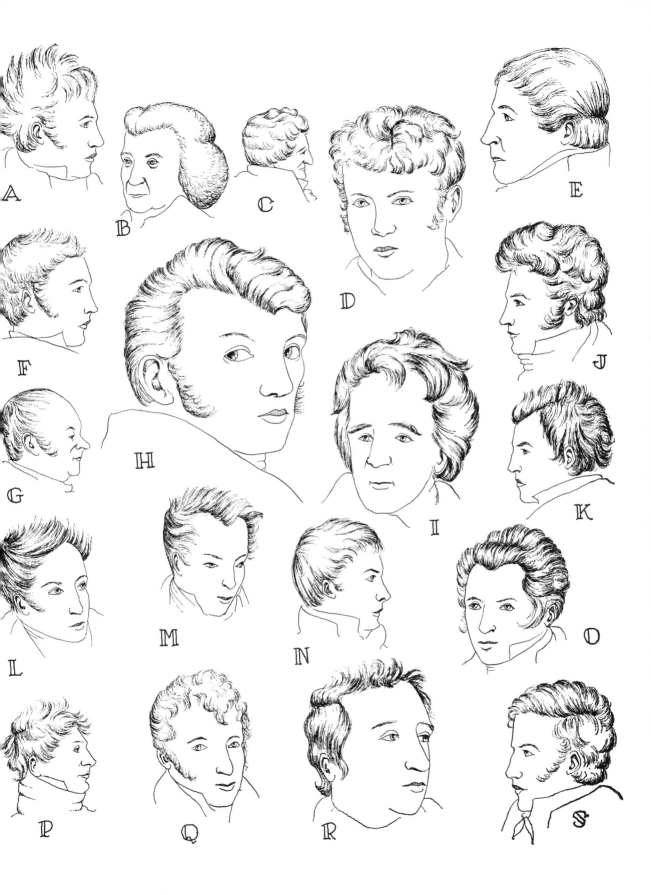

A

B

C

D

E

F

G

H

I

J

K

L

M

N

O

P

Q

R

S

PLATE 91 : NINETEENTH-CENTURY MEN 1820–1830

A   French. Jean Louis André Théodore Géricault, 1791–1824.

B   English. Percy Bysshe Shelley, 1792–1822.

C   1820, English.

D   English. Lord Byron, 1788–1824.

E   1820, English.

F   1820, English.

G   Simón Bolívar, 1783–1830.

H   German. Alexander von Humboldt, 1769–1859. Explorer, scientist, natural philosopher.

I   *c.* 1825.

J   1820, English.

K   *c.* 1827, German.

L   *c.* 1828, German.

M   Austrian. Franz Schubert, 1797–1828.

N   1820, English. Judge's wig. The style is not restricted to this period but happened to be taken from a painting of 1820 (see T below).

O   German.

P   1822, English.

Q   *c.* 1827, German.

R   English. John Keats, 1795–1821.

S   American. John Quincy Adams, 1767–1848. 6th president, 1825–29, and son of John Adams.

T   1820, English. Barrister's wig (see N above).

U   1828, English. Fashionable young man.

V   1828, English. Fashionable young man.

W   1822, French.

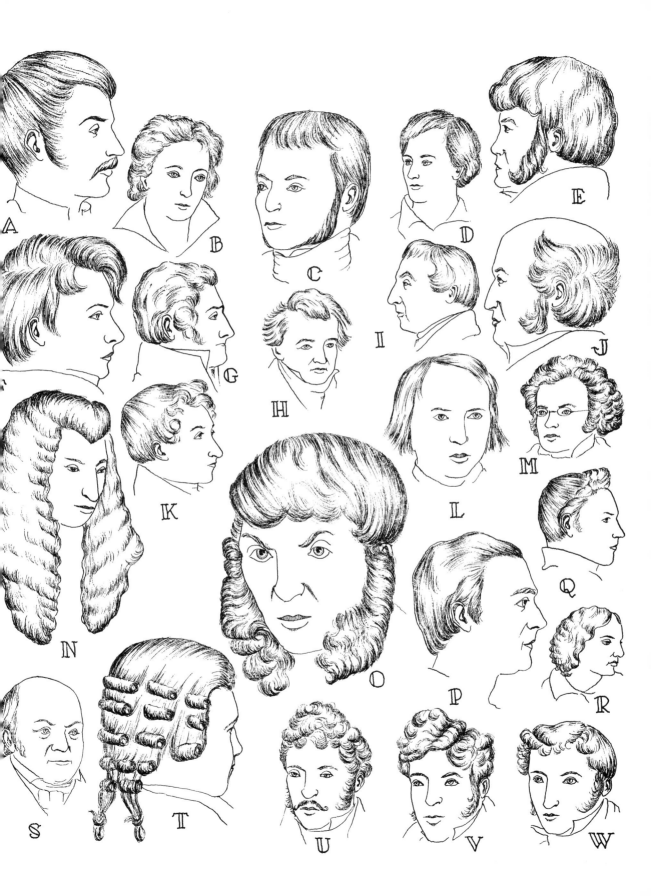

PLATE 92 : NINETEENTH-CENTURY MEN 1830–1840

A   1833, English.

B   American. Washington Irving, 1783–1859.

C   Scottish. Christopher North (John Wilson), 1785–1854. Writer.

D   1830, French. Victor Hugo, 1802–85.

E   1833, English. Moustaches were not common in England this early.

F   Professor George Bush.

G   American. Lorenzo Dow, 1777–1834. Evangelist.

H   *c.* 1830.

I   English. Benjamin Disraeli, 1st earl of Beaconsfield, 1804–81, who became prime minister in 1867 (for later portrait see Plate 99-W).

J   *c.* 1835.

K   English. William Wordsworth, 1770–1850.

L   French. Louis Jacques Mandé Daguerre, 1789–1851. Painter and physicist, inventor of the daguerrotype.

M   English.

N   Irish. Thomas Moore, 1779–1852. Poet.

O   *c.* 1835. Nathan Covington Brooks. Writer, teacher.

P   *c.* 1838, German.

Q   *c.* 1830. James Sheridan Knowles.

R   English. Lord Brougham.

S   1833, English.

T   1838, German.

U   1839, English.

V   German. Justus, Baron von Liebig, 1803–73. Chemist.

W   1833, English.

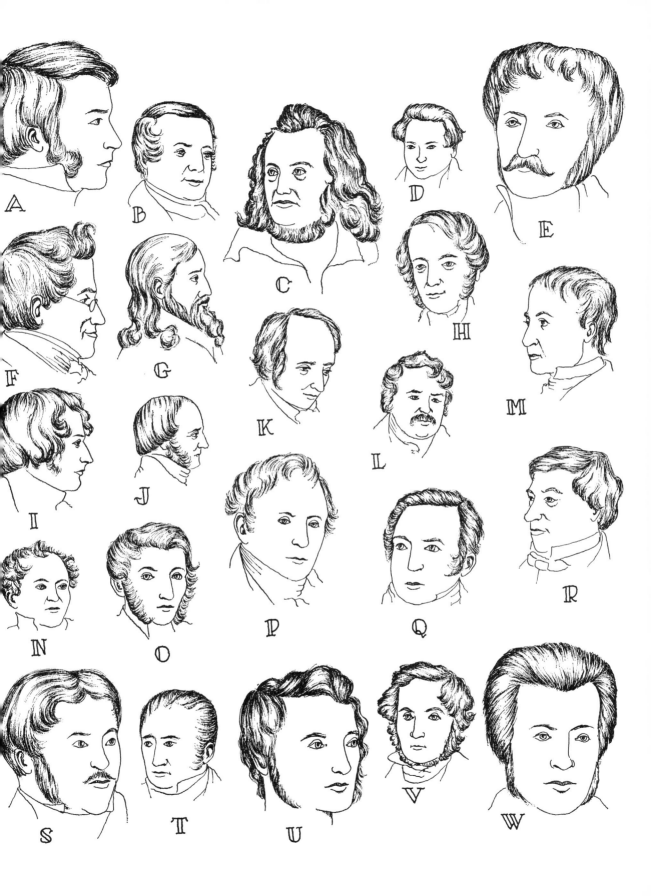

A   B   C   D   E

F   G   H

K   J   I

L   M

N   O   P   Q   R

S   T   U   V   W

PLATE 93 : NINETEENTH-CENTURY MEN 1840–1865

A   Frédéric Chopin, 1810–49 (see also 94-T).

B   Karl Ferdinand Gutzkow, 1811–78. German writer.

C   James K. Polk, 1795–1849. 11th U.S. president, 1845–49.

D   Millard Fillmore, 1800–74. 13th U.S. president, 1850–53 (see also I below).

E   Nathaniel Hawthorne, 1804–64.

F   Rufus Choat, 1799–1859. American lawyer.

G   John Brown, 1800–59. American abolitionist.

H   Napoleon III, 1808–73. Emperor of France, 1852–70. *Imperial.*

I   Millard Fillmore, 1800–74 (see also D above).

J   Mikhail Ivanovich Glinka, 1803–57.

K   1845, Danish. Niels Wilhelm Gade, 1817–90 (for later portrait see Plate 98-U).

L   *c.* 1860. E. A. Sothern, 1826–81, as Lord Dundreary in *Our American Cousin* (see Figure 107).

M   Johann Peter Eckermann, 1792–1854. German writer.

N   *c.* 1860.

O   1860. *Dundrearies.*

P   Charles F. A. Hindrichs, born 1814. American merchant. *Imperial.*

Q   John McLoughlin, 1784–1856. Canadian physician.

R   Benjamin Franklin Kelley, 1807–91. *Uncle Sam* beard.

S   Robert Toombs, 1810–85. Confederate general.

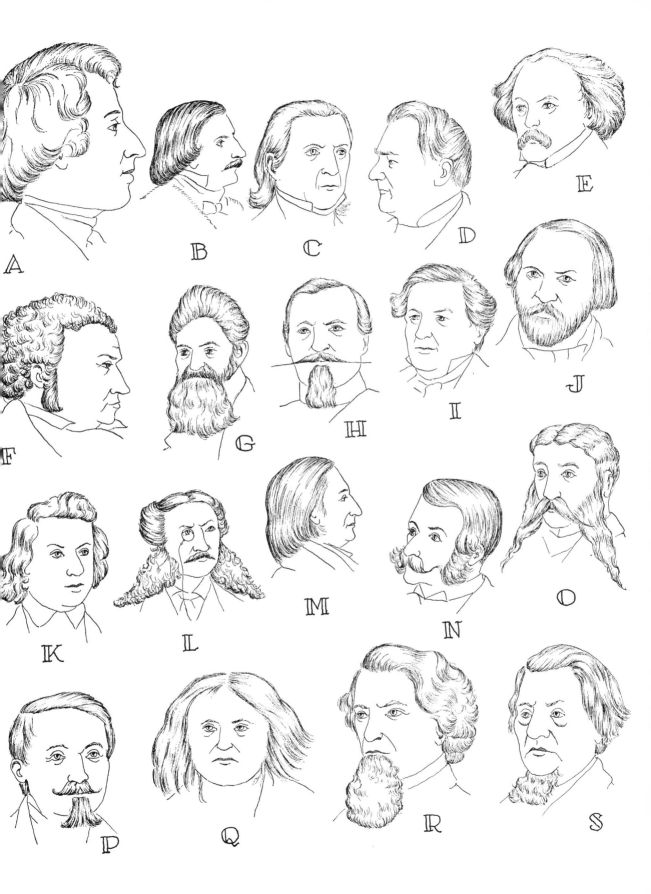

A

B

C

D

E

F

G

H

I

J

K

L

M

N

O

P

Q

R

S

PLATE 94 : NINETEENTH-CENTURY MEN 1840–1850

A   1842. Fashionable young man.

B   *c.* 1840, English.

C   American. Daniel Webster, 1782–1852.

D   American. Matthew Brady, 1823–96. Pioneer photographer (for later portrait see 99-F).

E   Victor Emil Jannings. (From a self-portrait.)

F   Clergyman.

G   1843, American. William C. Borah, 1865–1940. Senator from Idaho, 1907–40.

H   American. Zachary Taylor, 1784–1850. 12th U.S. president, 1849–50.

I   American. Andrew Jackson, 1767–1845. 7th U.S. president, 1829–37.

J   1843.

K   American. William H. Prescott, 1796–1859. Historian.

L   American. John C. Calhoun, 1782–1850.

M   American. Edgar Allan Poe, 1809–49.

N   Scottish.

O   1844.

P   1840, English.

Q   American. James Fenimore Cooper, 1789–1851.

R   1843. Boy.

S   German.

T   Frédéric Chopin, 1810–49 (see also Plate 93-A).

U   American. William Henry Harrison, 1773–1841. 9th U.S. president, 1841.

V   1840, English.

W   Italian. Gioachino Rossini, 1792–1868.

X   German. Felix Mendelssohn, 1809–47.

Y   1846, German. *Saucer* or *trencher* beard.

Z   1846, English.

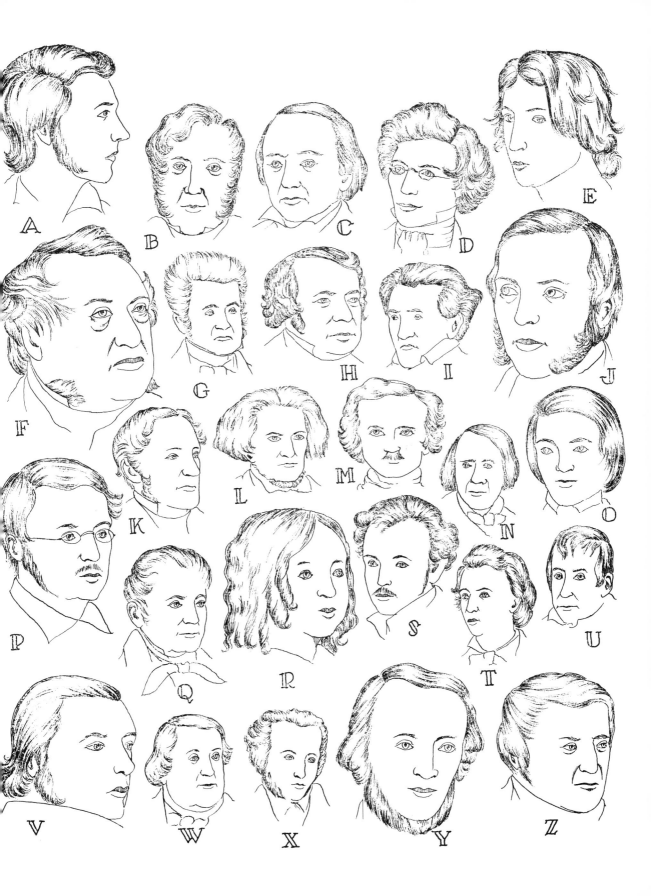

PLATE 95 : NINETEENTH-CENTURY MEN 1850–1860

A   American. Cyrus W. Field, 1819–92. Promoter of the first Atlantic cable. *Saucer* or *trencher* beard.

B   1858, French.

C   English. Earl of Derby, 1799–1869. Statesman.

D   American. Samuel F. B. Morse, 1791–1872. Inventor and artist (for later portrait see Plate 97-B).

E   Hon. William H. English.

F   Frederick William Louis, Prince Regent of Russia.

G   American. N. P. Willis, 1806–67. Journalist.

H   French. Jean Auguste Dominique Ingres, 1780–1867.

I   American. Senator Brown, Mississippi.

J   British. Thomas Carlyle, 1795–1851.

K   Hungarian. Franz Liszt, 1811–86 (for later portrait see Plate 99-U).

L   French. François Delsarte, 1811–71. Elocution teacher and originator of the Delsarte system.

M   1854, French.

N   William Winston Seaton.

O   American. General John A. Quitman, 1798–1858.

P   1859, Fashionable young man.

Q   1854, French.

R   German. Robert Schumann, 1810–56.

S   American. Cornelius Vanderbilt, 1794–1877.

T   William Lyon Mackenzie, 1795–1861. Canadian journalist and insurgent leader.

U   1851, American.

V   1854. Artist.

W   1852. Boy.

X   1858, British. *Saucer* or *trencher* beard.

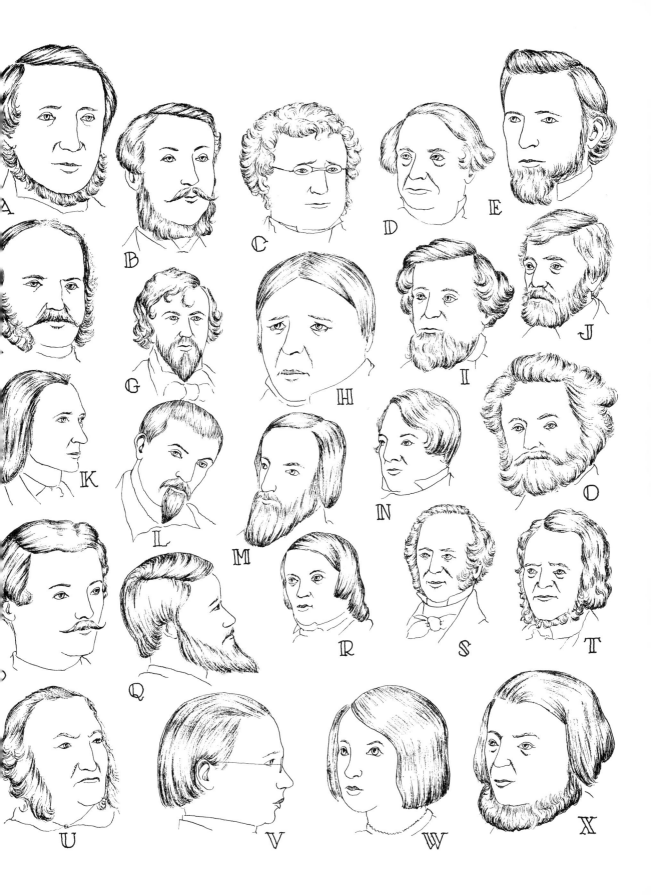

PLATE 96 : NINETEENTH-CENTURY MEN 1860–1870

A   American. William H. Seward, 1801–72. Secretary of State under Lincoln.

B   American. *Piccadilly weepers* or *Dundrearies*.

C   American. Rev. Lyman Beecher, 1775–1863. Protestant minister. Father of Henry Ward Beecher (see E below).

D   American.

E   American. Henry Ward Beecher, 1813–87. Congregational minister.

F   American. General A. S. Johnson.

G   American.

H   Child.

I   Child.

J   Fashionable young man.

K   American. General George Custer, 1839–76.

L   British. General Napier.

M   American.

N   Russian. Alexander II, 1818–81—reigned 1855–81.

O   American. General Philip Henry Sheridan, 1831–88.

P   John Pierpont.

Q   American. Major General David Hunter.

R   British. John Stuart Mill, 1806–73.

S   Scottish. David Livingstone, 1813–73. Missionary and explorer.

T   American. Benson John Lossing, 1813–91. Historian and journalist.

U   American. *Horseshoe* moustache.

V   American. General Alvin P. Hovey. Modified *imperial*.

W   American. Raphael Semmes, 1809–77. Confederate naval officer.

X   American. Major General Daniel Butterfield. *Soup strainers* or *walrus* moustache.

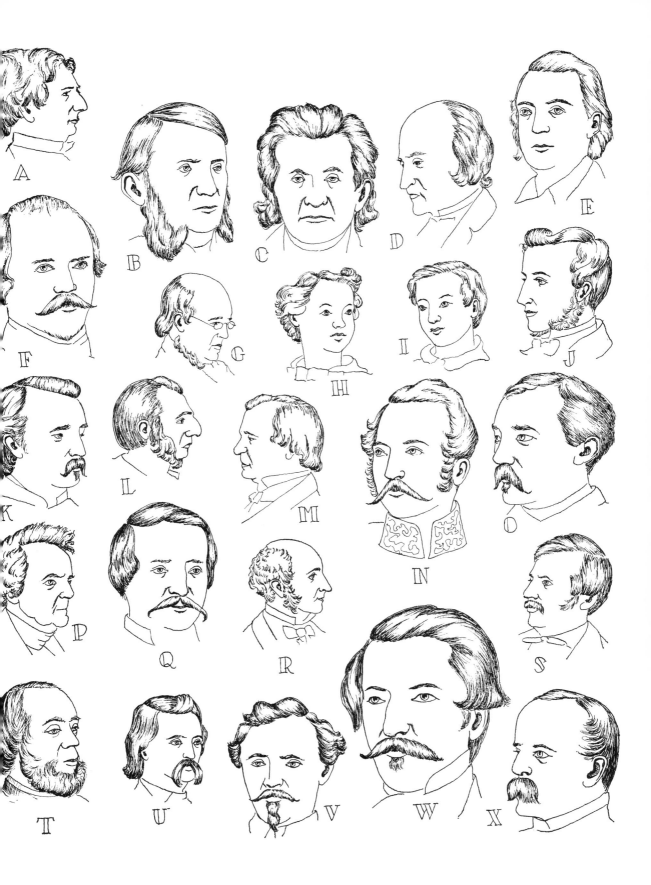

PLATE 97 : NINETEENTH-CENTURY MEN 1860–1870

A   *c.* 1860.

B   American. Samuel F. B. Morse, 1791–1872 (for earlier portrait see Plate 95-D).

C   1863, American. General Alfred Pleasonton.

D   Hungarian.

E   American. Ulysses S. Grant, 1822–85.

F   *c.* American. Samuel R. Wells. Physiognomist, 1860.

G   *c.* 1870.

H   Italian. Giuseppe Garibaldi, 1807–82. Patriot and soldier.

I   American. Samuel F. DuPont, 1803–65. Naval officer.

J   American. General Winfield Scott Hancock, 1824–86.

K   American. Civil War general.

L   American. Major General George Stoneman.

M   American. William Cullen Bryant, 1794–1878. Romantic poet.

N   American. George Edward Pickett, 1825–75. Confederate general.

O   1863. *Piccadilly weepers.*

P   American. George Bancroft, 1800–91. Historian and statesman.

Q   American. Ambrose E. Burnside, 1824–81. Union general.

R   *c.* 1869.

S   Abraham Lincoln, 1809–65 (see also Plate 98-C-D).

T   American. Civil War general.

U   General Law.

V   English. Anthony Ashley Cooper, 7th earl of Shaftesbury, 1801–85.

W   American. John Hunt Morgan, 1825–64. Confederate general. *Vandyke.*

X   American. Jefferson Davis, 1808–89. President of the Confederacy. *Goatee.*

Y   American. Edwin M. Stanton, 1814–69. Secretary of War under Lincoln.

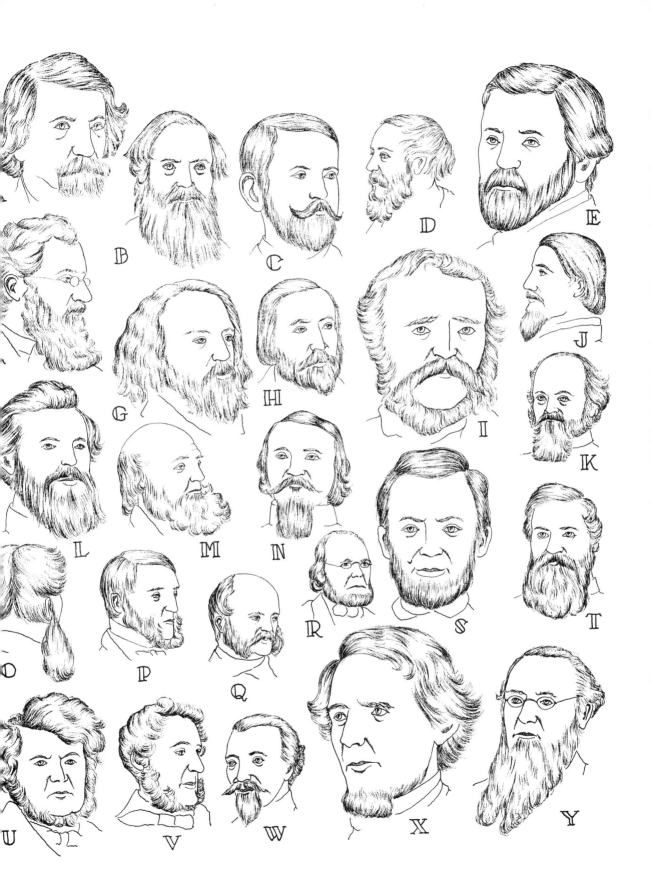

Plate 98 : Nineteenth-Century Men 1860–1880

A   Algernon Charles Swinburne, 1837–1909.

B   John Slidell, 1793–1871. American politician.

C   1860. Abraham Lincoln (see also Plate 97-S).

D   1864. Abraham Lincoln.

E   Stephen A. Douglas, 1813–61.

F   Sir Francis Grant, 1803–78. Scottish portrait painter.

G   Johann Strauss the Younger, 1825–99. Austrian composer.

H   Elisha Graves Otis, 1811–61. American inventor.

I   John Wilkes Booth, 1838–65.

J   John A. Sutter, 1803–80. Swiss-American pioneer and trader.

K   Maximilian, archduke of Austria, 1832–67.

L   Franz Sigel, 1824–1902. German-American general.

M   James Buchanan, 1791–1868. U.S. President, 1857–61.

N   1877, German. Richard Wagner.

O   William Wilson Corcoran, 1798–1888.

P   Peter Cornelius, 1824–74. German.

Q   Alexander II, 1818–81. Emperor of Russia, 1855–81.

R   Georg Johann Meyer, 1813–86. German painter.

S   John A. Logan, 1826–86. American general and statesman.

T   Andrew Adgate Lipscomb, 1816–90. Author and educator. *Billies.*

U   Niels Wilhelm Gade, 1817–90. Danish (see also Plate 93-K).

V   Cornelius K. Garrison, 1809–85. American capitalist.

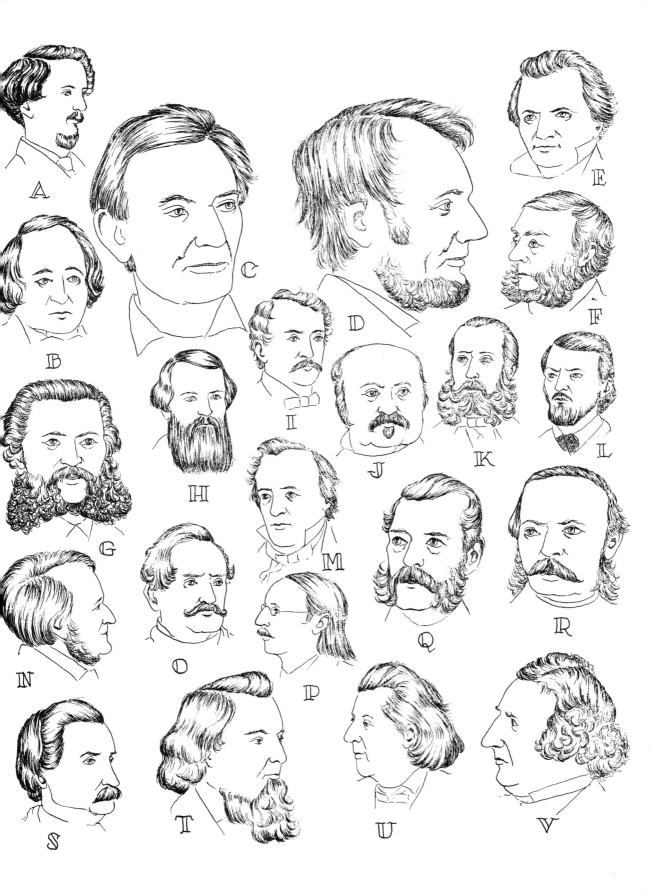

A

B

C

D

E

F

G

H

I

J

K

L

M

N

O

P

Q

R

S

T

U

V

PLATE 99 : NINETEENTH-CENTURY MEN 1870–1880

A   American. Bayard Taylor, 1825–78. Writer and world traveller.

B   *c.* 1880, American. Public official. *Soup strainers* or *walrus* moustache.

C   American. Wendell Phillips, 1811–84. Reformer and orator.

D   *c.* 1880. *Mutton chops.*

E   American. Philip Henry Sheridan, 1831–88. Union general in the Civil War.

F   American. Matthew Brady, 1823–96. Pioneer photographer (for earlier portrait see Plate 94-D).

G   *c.* 1880, American. C. E. Cady. Teacher of penmanship and business education.

H   *c.* 1880, American. John Davis. Associate Justice of the U.S. Court of Claims.

I   Edwin Booth, 1833–93. American tragedian.

J   *c.* 1880, American. Politician.

K   American. Ralph Waldo Emerson, 1803–82.

L   1872, English. *Piccadilly weepers.*

M   American. Oliver Wendell Holmes, 1809–94. Writer and physician.

N   French. Louis Pasteur, 1822–95.

O   *c.* 1880, American. Public official.

P   1872, English.

Q   1873, American. Senator J. B. Gordon.

R   John Tyndal.

S   Cardinal Manning.

T   English. Charles Darwin, 1809–82.

U   Hungarian. Franz Liszt, 1811–86 (for earlier portrait see Plate 95-K).

V   *c.* 1880.

W   English. Benjamin Disraeli, 1804–81 (for earlier portrait see Plate 92-I). In America this small beard was called a *breakwater.*

X   American. Martin Milmore, 1844–83. Sculptor.

Y   1877, American. Wade Hampton, 1818–1902. Confederate general.

Z   *c.* 1880. C. M. Hovey. *Nokomis* beard.

AA   Thomas S. Hunt. Scientific writer.

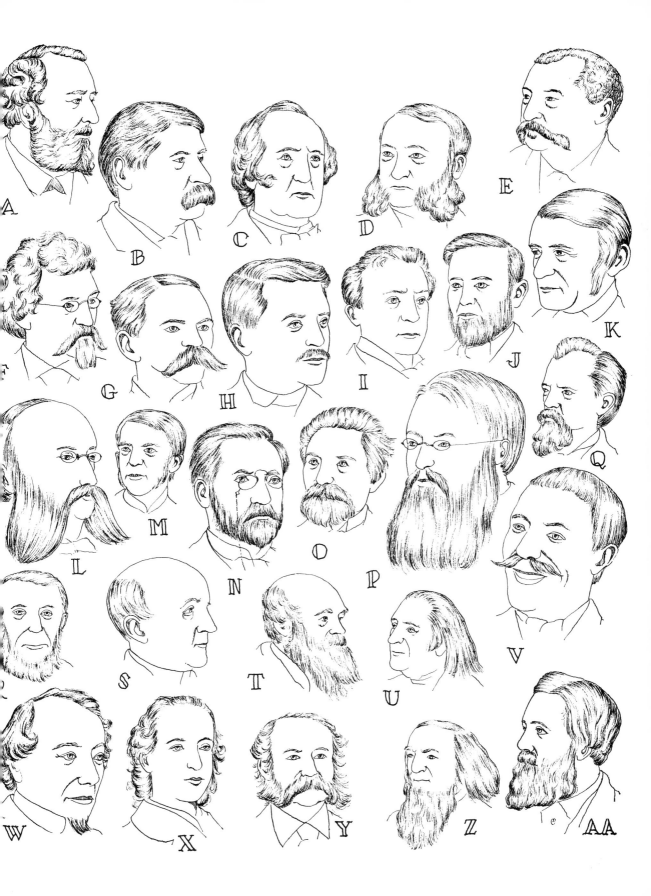

A
B
C
D
E
F
G
H
I
J
K
L
M
N
O
P
Q
S
T
U
V
W
X
Y
Z
AA

PLATE 100 : NINETEENTH-CENTURY MEN 1880–1890

A   Amos Henry Worthen, 1813–88. American geologist.

B   Edvard Grieg, 1834–1907.

C   Simon L. Brewster, 1811–86. American banker.

D   James G. Blaine, 1830–93. American statesman.

E   Hiram Ricker, born 1809. American hotel proprietor. *Weepers.*

F   Aleksandr Borodin, 1834–87. Russian composer.

G   Watson Robertson Sperry, born 1842. American journalist.

H   Pierce Manning Butler Young, born 1839. American congressman.

I   Irving Ramsay Wiles, born 1861. American artist.

J   Martin B. Leisser, born 1845. American artist.

K   Horace Gray, born 1838. Associate Justice of the U.S. Supreme Court.

L   Benjamin Harrison, 1833–1901. 23rd U.S. president, 1889–93.

M   Chester A. Arthur, 1830–86. 21st U.S. president, 1881–85. *Weepers* or *Dundrearies.*

N   Franklin Carter, born 1837. President of Williams College. *Weepers.*

O   John Meredith Read, 1837–96. U.S. Minister to Greece. *Imperial.*

P   George Soule, born 1834. Educator and author.

Q   James A. Garfield, 1831–81. 20th U.S. president, 1881 (see also Plate 101-O).

R   American clergyman. *Goatee.*

S   Washington C. DePauw, 1822–87. Founder of DePauw University.

T   Charles Butler, born 1802. American philanthropist.

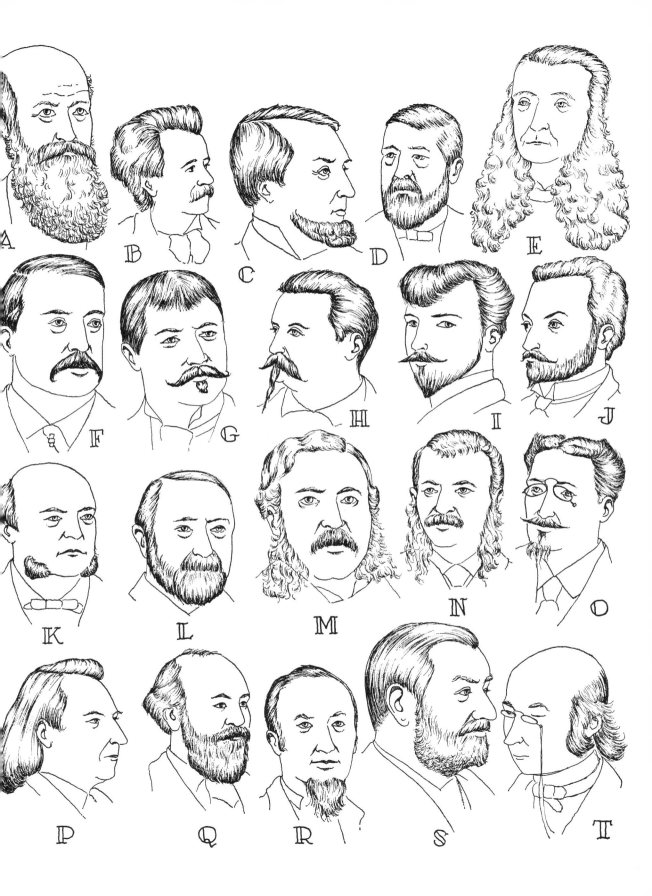

PLATE 101 : NINETEENTH-CENTURY MEN 1880–1890

A   American. Isaac Bell, Jr. U.S. Minister to the Netherlands. *Mutton chops.*

B   English. Sir Edward Frankland, 1825–99. Chemist, discoverer of helium.

C   Spanish. Alfonso XII, 1857–85—reigned 1870–85.

D   John W. Garrett.

E   American. David B. Hill. Politician. *Soup strainers* or *walrus* moustache.

F   British. William Thomson, 1st Baron Kelvin, 1824–1907.

G   English. T. H. Huxley, 1825–95. Biologist.

H   English. Alfred, Lord Tennyson, 1809–92.

I   American. Henry Wadsworth Longfellow, 1807–82.

J   American. General George Crook, 1828–90.

K   English. Lord Rayleigh. President of the British Association for the Advancement of Science.

L   American. John Greenleaf Whittier, 1807–92.

M   American. John C. Cook. Congressman. *Dundrearies* or *weepers.*

N   American.

O   American. James A. Garfield, 1831–81. 20th U.S. president.

P   American. Montgomery Blair, 1813–83. Postmaster-General, 1861–64.

Q   American. Pvt Henry Biederbeck. Member of the Greely Expedition.

R   American. Pvt Maurice Connell. Member of the Greely Expedition.

S   American.

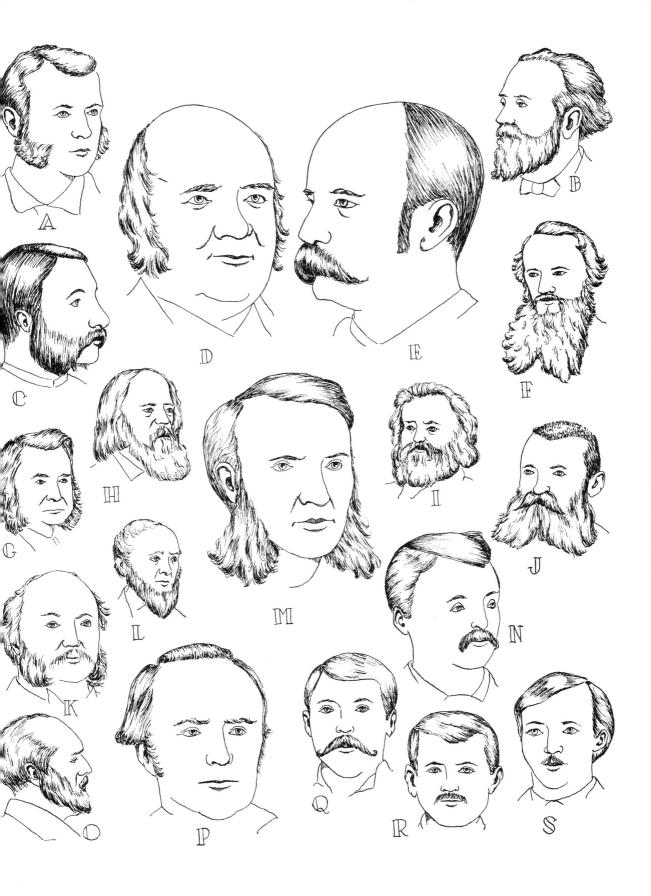

PLATE 102 : NINETEENTH-CENTURY MEN 1880–1890

A   American. Henry J. Pearson. Postmaster of New York.

B   American. Lyman W. Redington.

C   American. Robert E. Odlum—jumped from the Brooklyn Bridge.

D   French. Alphonse Marie de Neuville. Painter.

E   American. General E. C. Walthall. Senator from Missouri.

F   American. Robert M. McLane. Governor of Maryland.

G   Thomas M. Waller. Consul-General.

H   American. Frederick T. Frelinghuysen, 1817–85. Secretary of State, 1881–85. Notice especially the very curious form of beard (see also Christopher North, Plate 92-C).

I   American. Alfred C. Chapin. Politician.

J   American. Captain Webb.

K   American. Joseph' Jefferson, 1829–1905. Actor, remembered particularly for his Rip Van Winkle.

L   Dominick J. Ryder. Life guard.

M   American. R. D. Sears. Lawn tennis champion.

N   American. Seabury Brewster.

O   English. Sir Henry Irving, 1838–1905. First English actor to be knighted (for later portrait see Plate 140-D).

P   American. Honorable John P. St John.

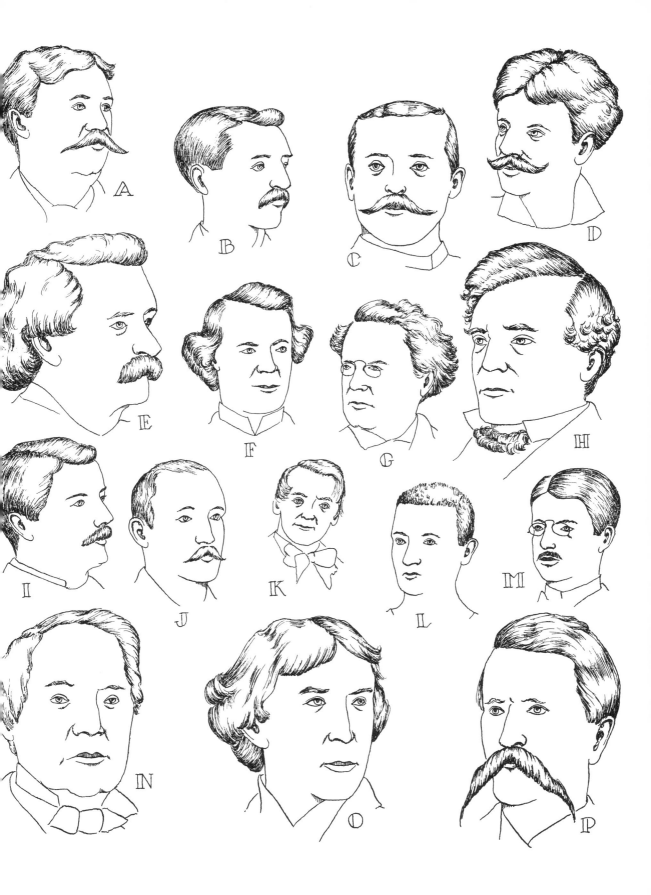

PLATE 103 : NINETEENTH-CENTURY MEN 1880–1890

A   American. Buren R. Sherman. Governor of Iowa.

B   American. Lt Adolphus Washington Greely, 1844–1935. Army officer and explorer, who directed relief operations after the San Francisco earthquake. *Swallow-tail* beard.

C   American. Richard Grant White. *Dundrearies*.

D   American. Army officer.

E   English. Sir Joseph Dalton Hooker.

F   American. Jesse R. Grant, son of U. S. Grant.

G   Frederick Kaulbach.

H   English. Earl of Carnarvon.

I   American. William Dorsheimer. U.S. District Attorney. *Burnsides*.

J   Russian. Ivan Sergeyevich Turgenev, 1818–83.

K   American. Walter C. Palmer, M.D. *Horace Greeley* beard.

L   American. Peter C. Olney. District Attorney. *Dundrearies*.

M   American. Silas W. Burt of the U.S. Navy.

N   American. Dr Octave Pavy of the Greely expedition. *Forked* beard.

O   Canadian. Sir Francis Hincks, 1807–85. Journalist and statesman.

P   Honorable W. Q. Gresham.

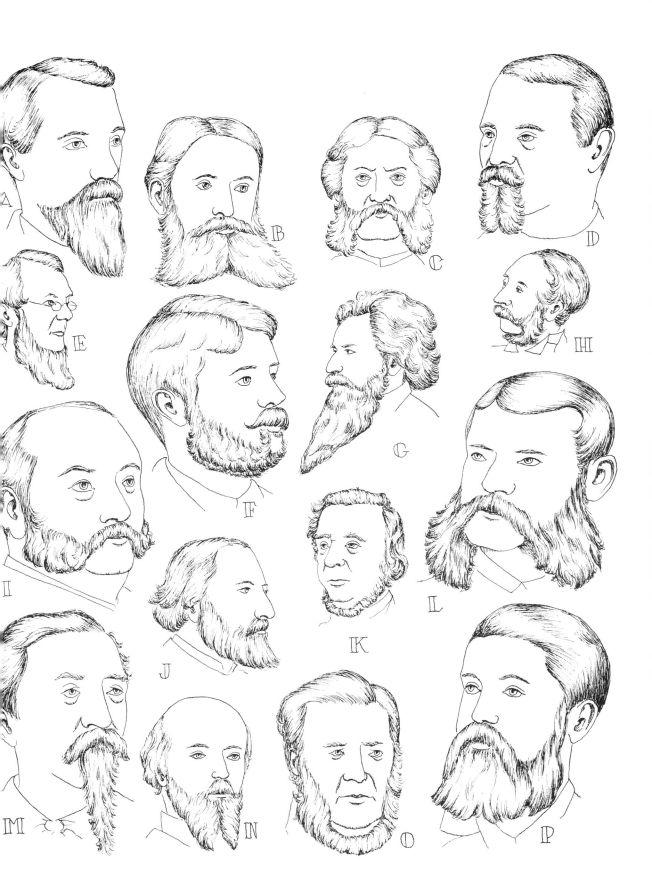

PLATE 104 : NINETEENTH-CENTURY MEN 1890–1900

(All of the following were New Yorkers who were to some degree prominent during the nineties, though most of the names are no longer remembered. An attempt has been made to include not only a variety of beards, but also a variety of occupations. All of the sketches are taken from photographs.)

A Drygoods manufacturer.

B Reverend Henry Van Dyke.

C William Allen Butler. Lawyer.

D S. E. Lane. New York City Commissioner. *Swallow-tail* beard.

E David McAdam. Judge.

F John F. Shera. Stockbroker.

G Banker.

H Paul L. Thebaud. Shipping merchant. *Swallow-tail* beard.

I Hugh J. Grant. Lawyer, mayor of New York.

J Joseph Hirsch. Drygoods manufacturer.

K Reverend William M. Geer.

L Reverend J. N. Hallock. Editor, writer.

M Bank president.

N William H. Arnous. Judge.

O Editor.

P Nelson Sizer. Phrenologist.

Q Edmund C. Stedman. Stockbroker, writer, editor.

R Daniel Frohman, 1851–1940. Theatrical producer.

S John Philip Sousa, 1854–1932. Composer, conductor.

T Architect.

U Lawyer.

V Editor.

W Arthur Burdett Frost, 1851–1928. Illustrator and cartoonist.

X James B. Pond. Publisher, lecture manager for Mark Twain and many others.

Y Hiram Hitchcock. Hotel proprietor.

Z Abraham O. Hall. Mayor of New York.

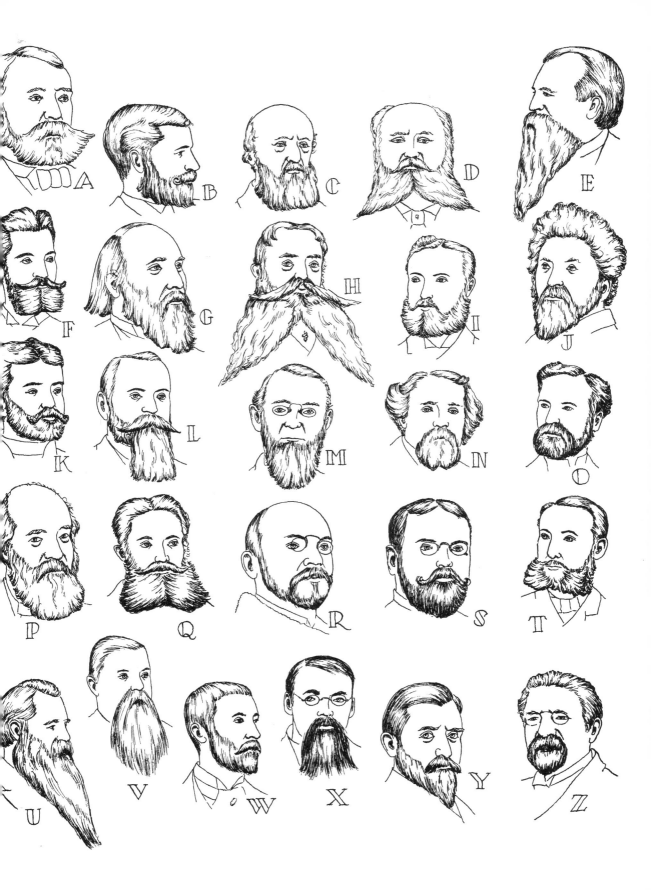

PLATE 105 : NINETEENTH-CENTURY MEN 1890–1900

(All of the following were Americans, and all except Admiral Dewey were New Yorkers. Mark Twain lived in New York for a time.)

A   Alfred de Cordova. Broker.

B   Lawyer.

C   Bruce Crane. Landscape painter.

D   Grosvenor Atterbury. Architect.

E   Admiral George Dewey, 1837–1917.

F   Gilbert Smith Coddington. Capitalist. *Bullet heads.*

G   Importer.

H   President of an electrical company.

I   Clarence A. Seward. Lawyer, judge.

J   Walter S. Logan. Lawyer, lecturer.

K   F. S. Flower. Broker.

L   John R. Dos Passos. Lawyer.

M   Edward Mitchell. Lawyer.

N   Mark Twain (Samuel Clemens), 1835–1910 (see also Plate 108-S).

O   A. W. Peters. New York borough president.

P   Name and occupation unknown.

Q   Howard Gibb. Drygoods merchant.

R   John Howard Van Amringe. Professor of Mathematics and dean of Columbia University.

S   Clayton Platt. Underwriter.

T   Attorney.

U   Henry Miller, 1860–1926. Actor-manager (for later portrait see Plate 140-Q).

V   Executive.

W   Hillary Bell. Artist, journalist.

X   Reverend George P. Mains. *Soup strainers* or *walrus* moustache.

Y   William N. Cromwell. Lawyer.

Z   Clergyman.

AA   Joseph I. C. Clarke. Journalist and playwright.

BB   C. Bainbridge Smith. Attorney.

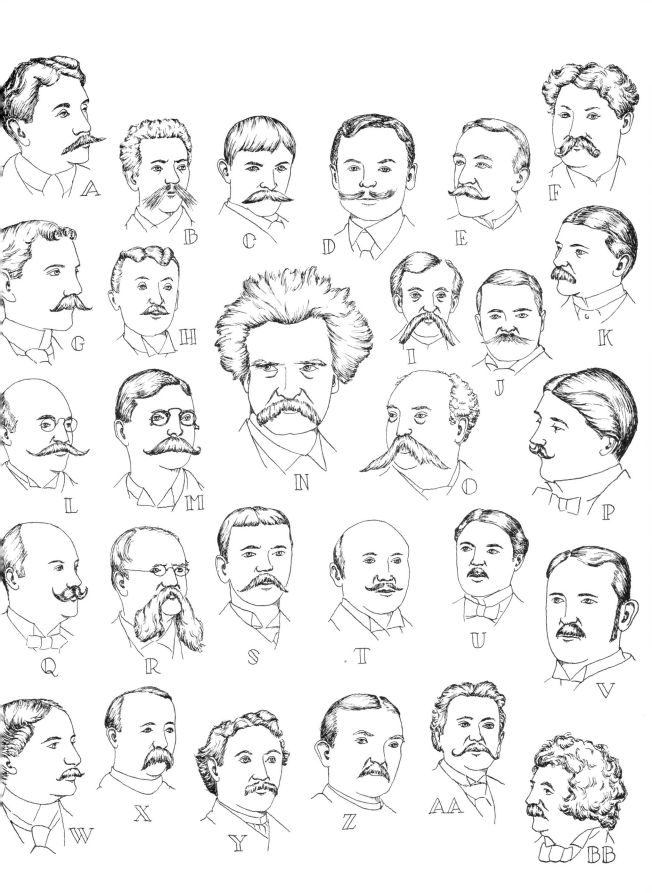

PLATE 106 : NINETEENTH-CENTURY MEN 1890–1900

(Most of the following were New Yorkers.)

A   Singer.

B   Reverend Morgan Dix.

C   Maurice Barrymore (Herbert Blythe), 1847–1905. First of the distinguished acting family. He was English, but in 1875 he joined Augustin Daly's stock company.

D   James K. Hackett. Actor.

E   Anton Seidl. Musician, composer.

F   Walter Damrosch, 1862–1950. Conductor, composer.

G   Thomas S. Hastings. President of the Union Theological Seminary.

H   Le Grand Bouton Cannon. Banker.

I   James Roosevelt. Steamship official.

J   Reverend William T. Sabine.

K   Shoe merchant.

L   Child.

M   S. B. Dutcher. Banker. *Piccadilly weepers* or *Dundrearies*.

N   Reverend A. E. Kittredge. *Piccadilly weepers* or *Dundrearies*.

O   Banker.

P   William Rumney. Judge. *Dundrearies* or *ladykillers*, perhaps *weepers*.

Q   Lawyer. *Weepers*.

R   J. M. Deuel. Attorney, city magistrate. *Burnsides*.

S   Emile Henry Lacombe. Lawyer, judge.

T   Executive of an electric company. *Burnsides*.

U   H. M. Alexander. Attorney.

V   Lawyer.

W   Engineer.

X   Reverend J. T. Beckley.

Y   Banker. *Dundrearies*.

Z   Reverend Thomas Gallandet.

AA   President of a milk company.

BB   Reverend Jacob S. Shipman.

CC   Thomas Denny. Broker. *Dundrearies*.

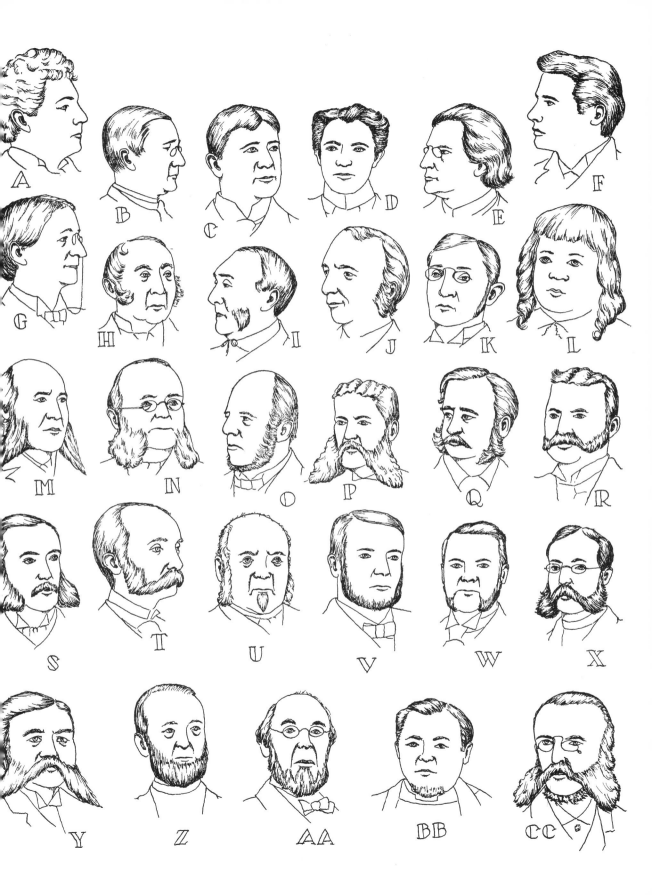

PLATE 107 : NINETEENTH-CENTURY MEN 1890–1900

(All of the following except the first were Americans.)

A   Norwegian. Fridtjof Nansen, 1861–1930. Explorer, scientist, statesman, humanitarian, and first Norwegian minister to Great Britain; awarded Nobel Peace Prize in 1922.

B   William T. Sampson.

C   Painter.

D   Merchant.

E   Broker.

F   Broker. Variation of the *imperial*.

G   Merchant, philanthropist. *Imperial*.

H   Reverend W. T. Smith.

I   Journalist.

J   Bank director.

K   Merchant, soldier.

L   John H. McCarthy. Congressman, judge.

M   George W. Cable, 1844–1925. Writer noted for his stories and novels of Louisiana.

N   Manufacturer.

O   Journalist.

P   Reverend Charles H. Parkhurst.

Q   Wauhope Lynn. Lawyer, judge.

R   Lloyd Stephens Bryce. Writer, congressman.

S   Hubert Vos. Portrait painter.

T   Thomas Whittaker. Publisher.

U   William Holbrook Beard. Painter, writer.

V   Simeon Ford. Hotel proprietor.

W   Wine merchant. *Rimmers*.

X   Broker.

Y   Steamship official.

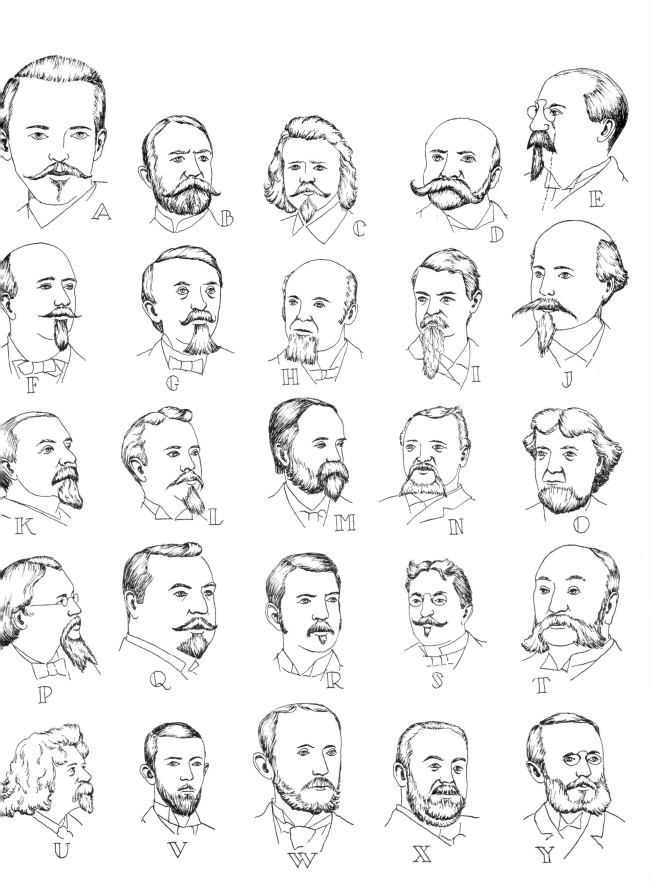

PLATE 108 : NINETEENTH-CENTURY MEN 1890–1900

A Chief Joseph (Shahaptian family)—died 1904.

B Alexander Graham Bell, 1847–1922.

C Chief Sitting Bull.

D Walter L. Bragg. Member, Interstate Commerce Commission.

E 1896. Andrew D. White. Member, Interstate Commerce Commission.

F Nikolay Rimsky-Korsakov, 1844–1908.

G Edward Gay. Irish-American artist.

H Armand Capdervielle. American editor and publisher.

I 1892. William Collins Whitney. Secretary of the Navy, 1885–89.

J Ward McAllister, 1827–95. American lawyer.

K Guy de Maupassant, 1850–93.

L Charles Carroll Walcutt, 1838–98. American soldier.

M Sir Arthur Sullivan, 1842–1900.

N John Mason Loomis, 1825–1900.

O William T. Sampson, 1840–1902. American naval officer.

P Scottish. Robert Louis Stevenson, 1850–94.

Q 1897. Práxedes Mateo Sagasta. Premier of Spain.

R Don M. Dickinson. Member of Cleveland's cabinet. *Dundrearies* or *weepers*.

S Mark Twain, 1835–1910 (see also Plate 105-N).

T Daniel Smith Lamb, 1843–1929. American pathologist and anatomist. A variation of the *imperial*.

U Hermann Sudermann, 1857–1928. German dramatist and novelist.

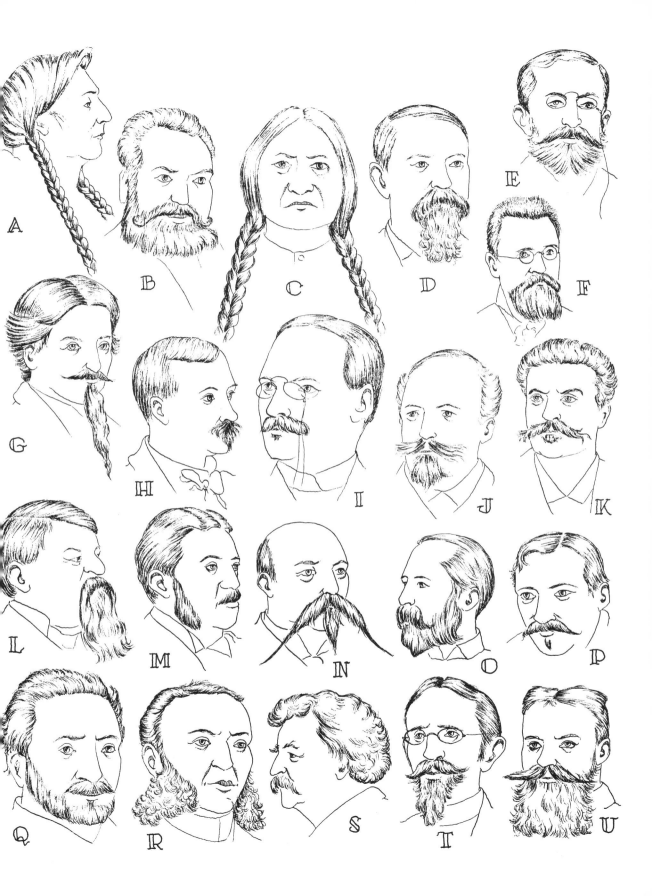

A

B

C

D

E

F

G

H

I

J

K

L

M

N

O

P

Q

R

S

T

U

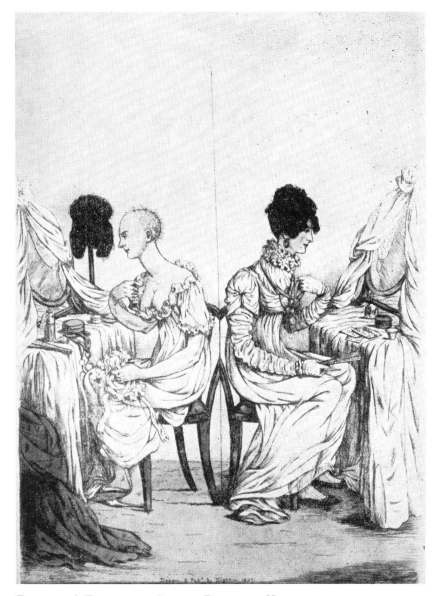

Fig. 111 : A Fashionable Lady in Dress and Undress.
English caricature, 1807

12 · The Nineteenth Century—Women

> It almost goes without saying that a
> well-bred woman does not dye
> her hair.
>
> ISABEL MALLON

The nineteenth century, with its well-established hairdressers, brought forth in rapid succession an astonishing variety of hair styles, never quite matching those of the preceding century in extravagance but coming close in some cases. And the amount of hair required for a fashionable coiffure increased steadily until nearly the end of the century.

1800–1810 (Plates 109-111)

Referring to the dramatic change of hair styles in France at the end of the eighteenth century, Lafoy says, 'Shortly after this, the taste for Greek and Roman fashions gave rise to those Alcibiades, Titus, Agrippina, Aspasia, and Julian headdresses, which are now the admiration of the world and will be handed down to the wonder of posterity.' Plates 109-111 give some idea of the variety of detail—short curls, long curls, braids, chignons, combs, jewels, feathers, diadems, chains, flowers, ropes of pearls. The relative simplicity of the gowns was compensated for rather than matched by the highly ornamented hairdos.

The Titus cut (Plate 109-J-N), which Lafoy expected to be handed down to the wonder of posterity, was so popular that in 1813 a Frenchman named D. Rothe de Nugent published a 135-page book entitled *Anti-Titus ou Remarques critiques sur la coiffure des femmes au XIXe siècle*, in which he pleaded eloquently for a return to more feminine hair styles. Many of the women obviously regretted cutting off their hair long before the book appeared, and wigs of various styles were flourishing—*à la Vénus, à la Sappho, à la Caracalla, à l'anglaise, à l'espagnole*, etc.

In 1802 Maria Josepha, Lady Stanley, wrote to a friend: 'I have a commission or two for you. I enclose a bit of my hair for you to hand over to Marshall as a pattern for a fillet of hair for the front; I have cut off my tail for comfort, and as my front hair is always coming out of curl in the damp summer evenings, and as I find everybody sports a false toupee, I don't see why I should not have the comfort of one too. I wish it to be as fashionable and as deceiving as possible.'

Cosmetics were still being applied over-generously by many women, as noted disapprovingly in *The Habits of Good Society; A Handbook of Etiquette for Ladies and Gentlemen*, published in London in 1859:

'Until the first twenty years of this century had passed away, many ladies of *bon ton* thought it necessary, in order to complete their dress, to put a touch of rouge on either cheek. The celebrated Mrs. Fitzherbert was rouged to the very eyes; those beautiful deep blue eyes of hers. The old Duchess of R— enamelled, and usually fled from a room when the windows were opened, as the compound, whatever formed of, was apt to dissolve and run down the face. Queen Caroline (of Brunswick) was rouged fearfully; her daughter, noble in form, fair but pale in complexion, disdained the art. . . . I once knew a lady who was bled from time to time to keep the marble-like whiteness of her complexion; others, to my knowledge, rub their faces with breadcrumbs as one should a drawing. But, worst of all, the use of pearl powder, or of violet powder, has been for the last half century prevalent.'

1810–1820 (Plates 111-113)

During the second decade, the wild experimentation of the early years gave way to more clearly marked trends. The hair was usually straight and dressed close to the head, and a topknot of some sort was customary. It tended to be fairly large, sometimes high, sometimes low. It might be fashioned of braids, curls, a large bun, or a combination of any or all of them. The topknot continued to grow in importance; and during the last half of the decade, the simpler forms were frequently abandoned by the ultra-fashionable for very ornate constructions (Plate 113-A, for example).

The hair during this period was either brushed straight back and up, the ends forming the topknot or being concealed under it, or else it was parted in the centre and brushed to the back, then up. Even on the rare occasions when it was allowed to hang free in back, a topknot was still required. The hairline was frequently softened with ringlets, covered with a braid, ropes of pearls, a band, or a ribbon, or both. Gradually, the front ringlets, which had started out as mere wisps, took on greater importance; and a larger section of front hair was reserved for them. This led to bandeaux of hair in front with no curls.

Clearly, hairdressers were essential for the more ornate styles; and nobody was more aware of this than the hairdressers themselves. In *The Complete Coiffeur*, published in 1817 and one of the relatively few books ever written (or, at least, published) by practising hairdressers, J. B. M. D. Lafoy refers to hairdressing as the 'noblest and most useful of the arts [and] the most profound'. He then extols its merits in some detail:

'Let it not be attributed to enthusiasm that I have dared to designate this noble profession as an art: it is truly so. . . . To modify, in various forms, the long and graceful filaments, which nature seems to have intended rather for covering than ornament; to impart to these forms a consistency of which, naturally, it appears not to be possessed; to . . . substitute order for confusion; to correct deficiency by factitious elegance, so as to deceive the most penetrating eye; to combine the adventitious with the natural, which it seems to soften and relieve; to sustain the delicacy of figure by light flowing ringlets; to lend to feminine majesty the accompaniments of waving and lengthened tresses; and, withal, to counteract an ungainly aspect, either by contrast or well-timed relief; to bring about these admirable effects by an execution at once graceful and rapid, is what characterizes a master art: and this is but a small proportion of the toils which the artist has to encounter! *His* is no imitation, no servile copy. He is without any exemplar law but that which his own imagination furnishes; without any materials but the slight foundation of the hair; or any other auxiliary but the *Comb*!'

M. Lafoy cannot seem to refrain from bursting into emotional verse from time to time, and the mere thought of a *Comb* sets him off:

> Hail *Mystic Implement*, to whom I owe
> My laurell'd triumphs, at the toilet's side!
> My poems begin with thee! If Pallas' hand
> (Which wrought of you, the spindle's wondrous power,
> And gave the magic needle to the fair,)
> Lent aught beside in aid of beauty's charms,
> 'Twas thee, celestial Comb! thou who doest course
> Amidst the mazy tangles of the hair,
> Educing order, elegance, and grace!
> When to the beauteous Paris was assign'd,
> Amidst contending goddesses, to adjudge
> *The Golden Apple to the fairest she*,
> The Cyprian goddess doubtful of her charms
> Implor'd the aidance of the God of Love,
> 'Twas then, from forth his quiver Cupid chose
> The lightest of his arrows. Hence was form'd,
> Wrought by his plastic hand, the graceful *Comb*;
> And Venus triumphs in the golden prize.

He continues for some thirty-five pages to extol in poetry and prose the coiffeur and his art. His climactic poem, at the end of Chapter 3, ends on an heroic note:

> O! if for honour, fame, yet sigh
> While noble ardour fires the eye,
> Yet let the midnight lamp behold,
> Studious of what these themes unfold;
> 'Til old experience do attain
> 'To something of prophetic strain;'
> Then shall ye *live*, and drink with me
> The draft of immortality;
> And, in the historian's future page
> Shine forth the Coiffeur of the age!

In succeeding chapters he sandwiches in between poems some surprisingly sensible advice. In discussing ornaments for the hair, for example, he cautions his readers: 'Before you place one single ornament, consider the occasion and place where it is to be worn. The same which become the town would be ridiculous in the country; and those which glitter in a side-box would be absurd in the family parlour.'

He then adds some further suggestions for the lady of 1817: 'Do you mean to receive some friends, or pay a neighbourly visit? let a simple ribband negligently infold the irregular plaits of your hair; or let it, like the blindfolding band of love, voluptuously aisle the white forehead, or yet a transparent net may allow some straggling tresses to wave on the snowy neck.'

After this, he seems to drift away from the point. 'But Phoebus impetuous rushes down the expecting billows, and clouds of gold and purple veil his devouring rays, destructive to the pure freshness of beauty.—Zephyrs now wanton in the rustling leaves, and the hour for the walk is come.—Laura, thou playful and innocent, the green fields call thee; lightly thou trippest on the plain, and the eye can scarce follow thy steps—oh, how seducing is thy country attire.' This, naturally, leads to more verse.

In discussing fashion, Lafoy is at his most sensible. After a commendably brief poem on the tyranny of fashion, he says, 'Nevertheless, if the reigning fashion should expose in you some natural defect, if it does not agree with the cast of your physiognomy, you will do wisely not to follow it; for you will infallibly reject it at last. And the ladies, principally, must keep in mind that the best fashion is that which sets them off to best advantage. Their first care must be to modify the fashion of the day from the combined counsels of their looking-glass and hairdresser; and even to give it up, if, in this serious consultation, the majority incline to so painful an effort. . . . Your business is to be as handsome as you can: and you may be certain of pleasing if an artist of sound judgment and classical taste has adapted a proper head-dress to your features, were it even the head-dress of your grandmother.' He is suggesting, in other words, what is called in this book the *Individual* style.

1820–1830 (Plates 113–115)

With the aid and encouragement of hairdressers, the topknot continued to spread upward and outward during the decade. The importance of the front hair also increased until frequently the two became inseparable. As the arrangement of the hair itself became more elaborate, it was complicated still further by the addition of flowers, feathers, pins, ribbons, and pearls. The high flying bows of hair which were to achieve undeserved popularity in the thirties, had to be wired up to hold their shape.

Details of fashion changed from year to year and, for that matter, from month to month. According to the *Pocket Magazine* for July, 1825, 'Flowers in the hair are much worn by young ladies in evening dress parties. They are often in wreaths and consist of ranunculuses, Japanese roses, both white and red, with a few small flowers intermingled. Splendid diadems, in full dress, add to the glitter of a brilliant assembly.'

In September we find that: 'The hair continues to be arranged in large curls around the face. Young persons have the hinder tresses braided or formed into light bows; they have very little other ornament—a richly ornamented diadem comb, a few bows of riband, ears of corn or flowers are the sole embellishments adopted this summer.'

In the November issue it was reported that, 'The hair of young persons is now more ornamented with flowers than it was last month. Ringlets are becoming again in fashion. Bandeaux of pearls, with other valuable ornaments, are expected to ornament the tresses of the young at full dress parties this winter.'

The following February readers were told that 'The hair of young ladies for balls and evening parties is generally adorned with half-wreaths of flowers, the front forming a kind of diadem. Young married ladies in full dress wear plumes of feathers in their hair or rich combs or jewels with an aigrette formed of small feathers on one side.'

In the spring of 1828 a note of relief crept in: 'The very high head-dresses have experienced a very sensible abasement, and our lovely countrywomen now again appear as the fairest of nature's daughters. The large curls round the face are certainly still rather *too* large but not so enormous as formerly. Wreaths of spring flowers often encircle the heads of our most youthful votaries of Terpsichore and are appropriate to their early age. Bandeaux and splendid diadems glitter on the hair of the titled and the wealthy dame at the full evening dress party.'

But the relief was premature, for the lowering of the coiffure was fleeting. The first half of the succeeding decade found it soaring to new heights.

Dark hair, especially black, was much in fashion; and *The Art of Beauty; or, the Best Methods of Improving and Preserving the Shape, Carriage, and Complexion*, published in London in 1825, quotes 'an elegant writer' as exclaiming, 'What spectacle, indeed . . . can be more seducing than that of jet black hair, falling in undulating ringlets upon the bosom of a youthful beauty?' A recipe was included for 'Grecian Water for Darkening the Hair':

'Dissolve two drachms of nitrate of silver in six ounces of distilled water, add two drachms of gum water. Perfume it with any essence you choose, and wet the hair which you wish to dye black. It is dangerous if applied to the skin; and, though it does darken the hair at first, the black colour is apt soon to become purple. It is often sold at a rack price.'

A method for strengthening the hair, reminiscent of the seventeenth century, is suggested. One is instructed to wash the hair daily for at least three days with a lye made from the roots of hemp, the roots of a maiden vine, and the cores of soft cabbage, first having rubbed the head well with honey.

Under 'Methods of Beautifying the Hair', the author recommends first 'a new hair-oil, which has lately been introduced and is coming into great repute'. This is the recipe:

PALMA CHRISTI OIL FOR THICKENING THE HAIR

'Take an ounce of Palma Christi oil, a sufficient quantity of oil of bergamot or
   lavender to scent it;

Apply it morning and evening for three months, or as long as it may be necessary,
   to the parts where you want the hair to grow thick and luxuriant.

The Palma Christi oil is much used, and with great success, for thickening the
   hair, in the West Indies; and, since it has been tried in this country, we have
   heard that it has been equally successful. It has this recommendation besides,
   that it is in the hands of neither monopolist nor patentee, but is open to all
   the world.'

The author's objection to Macassar oil and bear's grease has been mentioned in the preceding chapter. An interesting recipe for a home-made perfumed oil is suggested as preferable to the commercially prepared ones:

'Blanch a quantity of sweet almonds in hot water, and, when dry, reduce them to a powder, sift them through a fine sieve, strew a thin bed of almond powder, and a bed of fresh odoriferous flowers, such as lavender, jasmine, roses, &c., over the bottom of a box lined with tin. Do this alternately till the box is full, and leave them together for twelve hours. Then throw away the flowers, and add fresh ones, in the same manner as before, and repeat the same operation for eight successive days. When the almond-powder is thoroughly impregnated with the scent of the flowers, put it into a new clean linen cloth, and, with an iron press, extract the oil, which will be strongly scented with the fragrance of the flowers.'

A recipe for pomatum calls for two pounds and a half of hog's-lard and ten pounds of flowers.

As for painting the face, the attitude was more permissive than it would be later in Victorian days:

'Ought people to use paint? Why not? When a person is young and fresh and handsome, to paint would be perfectly ridiculous; it would be wantonly spoiling the fairest gifts of nature. But, on the contrary, when an antique and venerable dowager covers her brown and shrivelled skin with a thick layer of white paint, heightened with a tint of vermilion, we are sincerely thankful to her; for then we can look at her at least without disgust. And are we not under obligation to her for being at the pains to render herself in reality more ugly than she is, in order that she may appear less so.'

The author then argues strongly in favour of rouge and asks, 'In an age when women blush so little, ought we not to value this innocent artifice, which is capable of now and then exhibiting to us at least the picture of modesty, and which, in the absence of virtue, contrives, at least, to preserve her portrait . . .

'It is not the present fashion to make so much use of red as was done some years ago; at least, it is applied with more art and taste. With very few exceptions, ladies have absolutely renounced that glaring, fiery red with which our antiquated dames formerly masked their faces.'

It is then suggested that ladies would do well to compound their own rouge and avoid the risk of the dangerous metallic paints by using harmless vegetable dyes from 'red sandal wood, root of orchanet, cochineal, Brazil wood, and especially the bastard saffron, which yields a very beautiful colour when it is mixed with a sufficient quantity of talc. Some perfumers compose vegetable rouge, for which they take vinegar as the excipient. These reds are liable to injure the beauty of the skin; it is more adviseable to mix them with oily or unctuous matter, and to form salves. For this purpose you may employ balm of Mecca, butter of cacao, spermaceti, oil of ben, &c.'

One of the rouges used at the time was called 'Portugese rouge' and was of two types. 'One of these is made in Portugal and is rather scarce; the paint contained in the Portugese dishes being of a fine pale pink hue and very beautiful in its application to the face. The other sort is made in London and is of a dirty, muddy, red colour; it passes very well, however, with those who never saw the genuine Portugese dishes or who wish to be cheaply beautified.'

Spanish wool was frequently mentioned in the eighteenth century as a cosmetic for both men and women and evidently was still in use. Of the several sorts, it is stated in the book that 'that which is made here in London is by far the best; that which comes from Spain being of a very dark red colour, whereas the former gives a bright pale red; and, when it is very good, the cakes, which ought to be of the size and thickness of a crown-piece, shine and glisten, between a green and a gold colour.

'This sort of Spanish wool is always best when made in dry and hot summer weather, for then it strikes the finest blooming colour; whereas, what is made in wet winter weather is of a coarse dirty colour, like the wool from Spain. It is, therefore, best always to buy it in the summer season, when, besides having it at the best time, the retailer can likewise have it cheaper; for then the makers can work as fast as they please, whereas, in winter, they must choose and pick their time.'

The book then describes an interesting variation called 'Spanish papers':

'These papers are of two sorts: they differ in nothing from the above, but the red colour, which in the latter, tinges the wool, is here laid on paper; chiefly for the convenience of carrying in a pocket-book.

'This coloured wool comes from China, in large round loose cakes, of the diameter of three inches. The finest of these give a most lovely and agreeable blush to the cheek; but it is seldom possible to pick more than three or four out of a parcel, which have a truly fine colour; for, as the cakes are loose, like carded wool, the voyage by sea, and the exposure to air, even in opening them to show to a friend, carries off their fine colour.'

There were also Chinese boxes of colours, each containing 'Two dozen of papers, and in each paper are three smaller ones, viz. a small black paper for the eyebrows;

a paper, of the same size, of a fine green colour, but which when just arrived and fresh, makes a very fine red for the face; and, lastly, a paper containing about half an ounce of white powder (prepared from real pearl), for giving an alabaster colour to some parts of the face and neck.

'These are not commonly to be bought, but the perfumer may easily procure them by commissioning some friend who goes to China to purchase them for him.'

As to the application of the colours, the reader is informed that the red powders 'are best put on by a fine camel-hair pencil. The colours in the dishes, wools, and green papers, are commonly laid on by the tip of the little finger, previously wetted. As all these have some gum used in their composition, they are apt to leave a shining appearance on the cheek, which too plainly shews that artificial beauty has been resorted to.'

1830–1840 (Plates 116-118)

The topknot became higher and less wide, consisting of flat loops and bows of hair sometimes intertwined with braids, pearls, leaves and flowers, feathers, etc. The hair was still brushed out flat and sleek and was almost invariably parted in the centre. The decorative curls moved firmly to the sides, usually covered part or all of the ear, and became almost as prominent as the topknot itself.

In 1834 a note from Paris proclaimed that 'Head-dresses of hair are in the *juste milieu*, between high and low; two plaited braids upon the temples are still very fashionable. Instead of a ferronière, a diadem of fancy jewelry or of gold and cameos is placed upon the forehead. Flowers are also in great vogue, particularly those light and beautiful wreathes called *guirlandes à nœuds*.'

This time the hair styles were actually on their way down. The topknot shrank, often to a mere knot, a twist, or a small bow, and moved to the back of the head. The enormous clusters of side curls drooped and became long spiral curls or braids or occasionally disappeared entirely. The parting took on various forms—a centre parting front to crown; a centre parting for the front hair only, forming bandeaux; a parting on either side, the top being brushed straight back; or two short diagonal partings in a V-shape. The body of the hair was still flat and sleek, the softening effect coming from the side curls. By the end of the decade the hair styles had undergone an almost complete transformation and retained very few reminders of those of the early thirties.

That fashionable ladies of the period were not only dependent upon their hairdressers but were grateful to them is indicated by an effusive and presumably unsolicited tribute in *Godey's*:

'There is one art, which I consider of all others the most useful to society, as well as the most arduous in relation to the virtues which it requires: I mean the art of a

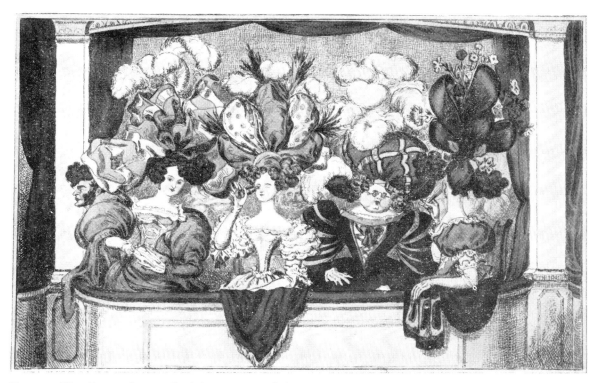

Fig. 112 : THE DRESS CIRCLE. English caricature of the 1830s

Lady's Hairdresser. To modify into pleasing forms those long and slender filaments which nature seems to have intended for the sport of every gale; to lend to them a consistency of which no-one would suppose such materials were susceptible; to give to abundance regular order in the place of confusion, and to supply a want with factitious riches, which would deceive the sharpest inquiry; to soften the coarseness of features; to increase the brilliancy of the eye by contrast of colors, and even sometimes by reflected union: to effect all these miracles, without any other means than a comb and a few essences, these are the characteristics of the art. . . . He [the coiffeur] must have a peculiar genius for invention, a superior taste for combination. . . . The products of his art are more fleeting than those of the spring. Like the bouquet whose brilliancy they possess, they disappear with the day that has seen their growth and find their tomb in the sleep, from whence the beauties they adorned derive new freshness. . . . Every toilette is a fertile field where he scatters his roses, and the prodigality of the evening is only a pledge of the abundance of the next day. . . . The exercise of this art supposes a calm temper, excessive virtue, attention, and inexhaustible patience. As to punctuality, only think a moment what disorder would arise in society upon all such essential occasions as balls and assemblies, spectacles and plays, were a coiffeur to neglect his duty or slip his memory! How many empty boxes, how many distressed families, how many broken engagements, and hence what confusion, what embarrassments both in public and private!'

1840–1850 (Plates 119, 120)

The general style established at the end of the previous decade continued with minor modifications. The hair was still flat and sleek on top with the same variety of partings listed for the previous decade. The bun was sometimes as high as the crown but usually lower. The side hair was still important, consisting ordinarily of one or more spiral curls, especially for evening wear; but frequently the curls became braids, which were dressed in curious long loops, exposing the ears. There is a bust of Queen Victoria in the National Portrait Gallery (London) showing her hair dressed in this style (Plate 119-D). Later, the braids, when used, were more likely to be coiled in front of the ear. Braids were also used extensively at the back of the head or over the top. During the course of the decade side curls or braids became less and less important, though they were still worn in the evening; and the bands of hair were simply brought down over the ears and carried to the back. Sometimes the top of the ear was allowed to show. More and more, the bands were eliminated, and the hair was parted front to back in the centre. Feathers, flowers, lace, cut-out cloth leaves, artificial grapes, etc., were worn in the hair, especially in the evening.

The increase in the length of hair necessary for fashionable coiffures frequently meant supplementing the natural hair, and in 1848 Britain imported 8,766 pounds of hair from France alone. Additional amounts came from other sources. This was only the beginning of a trend which was to continue for some years.

1850–1860 (Plates 121-123)

A Mrs Baillie, in writing from Lisbon, spoke of the long hair of many of the Portuguese and of her particular admiration for the luxurious hair of a young lady named Nina. It seems that during an amateur theatrical performance in her mother's home, Nina 'uncoiled its superb length, and . . . it electrified the audience, being done suddenly and in the most graceful manner'.

Long hair in this era was greatly admired and envied, and hair was beginning to attract attention for its ornamental value off the head as well as on. According to the *Irish Quarterly Review*:

'Among the lighter ornamental works in the Great Exhibition in London of 1851, few were finer or more curious than those executed in human hair; of which there were many exquisite specimens shown by French and English exhibitors.

'In the French department, M. Lemonnière particularly excelled; a portrait of Queen Victoria, worked in hair, being so chaste and delicate, and at the same time so truthful that it was difficult to believe it was not a sepia drawing. There was also shown in an ornamental frame in the south gallery an interesting collection of likenesses, correct and pleasing, worked in hair, of her Majesty, Prince Albert, and all the royal children. Beneath these were emblems of church and state, the army and navy, arts and sciences, commerce and industry, &c., beautifully executed in hair and gold, and exceedingly minute and perfect.'

This decorative hair work, as we shall see, was to flourish as long as the vogue for large quantities of hair on the head continued.

A glance at Plates 121-123 will show the general trend of the hair during this decade. Braids continued in popularity, and in 1853 *Godey's* gave instructions in various ways of plaiting hair. These will be found opposite Plate 121.

In *The Human Hair*, published about this same time, Alexander Rowland reported that 'some distinguished ladies in the Paris fashionable world, who wish to create a sensation, have reintroduced the practice of wearing powder in the hair. Others, carrying the matter still further, have made this fashion more costly by adopting gold and silver hair powder: gold for brunettes, silver for Italian blondes. Several belles have appeared in the first boxes of the theatre with their hair thus glitteringly powdered. There were five or six *merveilleuses* in gold and silver powder. It had a ravishing effect. . . . The fashion of simple perfumed powder, which was worn by the grandmothers of these ladies was resumed some twenty years ago, soon after the revolution of July, and several aristocratic ladies have preserved the fashion and still wear it on great and solemn occasions. . . . But notwithstanding the attempt, it may be presumed that gold and silver powder will hold its place merely among the eccentricities of the day.' The fashion eventually spread to the United States and had a certain vogue, especially after the Civil War.

In this very same year a Mrs Merrifield wrote in the *Art Journal*:

'The improving taste of the present generation is, perhaps, nowhere more conspicuous than in permitting us to preserve the natural colour of the hair and to wear our own whether it be black, brown, or grey. There is also a marked improvement in the more natural way in which the hair has been arranged during the last thirty years. We allude particularly to its being suffered to retain the direction intended by nature, instead of being combed upwards and turned over a cushion a foot or two in length. . . . We do not presume to enter into the question whether short curls are more becoming than long ones, or whether bands are preferable to curls of any kind, because, as the hair of some persons curls naturally, while that of others is quite straight, we consider that this is one of the points which must be decided accordingly as one style or the other is found to be most suitable to the individual.

'The principle in the arrangement of the hair round the forehead should be to preserve or assist the oval form of the face. As this differs in different individuals, the treatment should be adapted accordingly. The arrangement of the long hair at the back of the head is a matter of taste; as it interferes but little with the countenance, it may be referred to the dictates of fashion, although in this, as in everything else, simplicity in the arrangement and grace in the direction of the lines are the chief points to be considered.'

In 1856 *Godey's* gave an enlightening account of the fashions of the period:

'There is no *one* given style—as the once invariable French twist—or the all-pervading plaits. No fashionable woman makes an elaborate hair-dressing for the morning. The different engagements of the day demanding a use of the bonnet would interfere with it. . . . A fashionable woman puts up her hair as simply as possible in the morning—a twist or a knot behind and plain bandeaux in front, unless her hair curls naturally. This is always the most suitable style for home until it is dressed for dinner or the evening. . . . Ribbons are the only suitable decorations (in morning caps, that is). Flowers are used only for dinner or dress caps. . . . In New York the dinner hour is always late—usually five or six P.M. Consequently, it is customary to arrange the hair anew for the evening. In Philadelphia, where earlier hours prevail, this is done for the tea-table.

'For simple home wear there are several favorite styles. The braid passing through the bandeaux or front hair and crossing the top of the head, as the past season, leaves a space behind, which we have lately become accustomed to see filled by a twist or knot. Hence the introduction of the *cache peigne* or "comb concealer". This is much worn, even by young ladies. For everyday wear at home bows of black velvet or plain dark taffeta ribbon are the most serviceable and suitable *cache peigne*. They are usually placed on a foundation of stiff cotton net and ribbon wire and extended across the back of the head from ear to ear. Sometimes a flat bow and ends is placed exactly in the middle so that the streamers fall over the shoulders [Plate 122-R]. Straw gimp or lace mixed with the velvet or ribbon has a good effect. When they surround a small braid or twist, instead of crossing the back of the head, they are held in place by a cap spring, otherwise by hairpins, plain or ornamental.

'For evening or dinner parties, the styles of *cache peigne* are varied and elegant. Some are entirely of flowers—for young married ladies a mixture of flowers and blonde or flowers, blonde, and ribbon. This style of headdress is the most suitable for a young girl whose hair is in that uncomfortable state passing . . . to a woman's graceful length or where the hair is just growing out after sickness or baldness.'

In 1859 the very popular English book on etiquette, entitled *The Habits of Good Society*, declared that 'a lady's hair should, in ordinary life, be dressed twice a day, even if she does not vary the mode. To keep it cool and glossy, it requires being completely taken down in the middle of the day, or in the evening, according to the dinner-hours. The taste in dressing it in the morning should be simple, without pins, bows, or any foreign auxiliary to the best ornament of nature. I do not mean to deprecate the use of pads, as they are called, or supports used under the hair at this time, because they supersede the necessity of frizzing, which is always a process most injurious to the hair; but I own I object much to the ends of black lace, bows of ribbon, &c., used by many young women in their morning coiffure: of course, for those past girlhood, and not old enough to wear caps, the case is different.'

By the end of the decade the supplying of artificial hair had become a major industry. In 1859 there were 950 hairdressers listed in London, along with three hair merchants, seventeen hair manufacturers, and twenty-seven wig-makers. The *Irish Quarterly Review* gave an informative account of the sources of the increasingly large quantities of hair being required:

'Among the many curious occupations of the metropolis is that of the human hair merchant. Of these there are several, and they import between them more than fifty tons of hair annually.

'Both this country and the United States draw a large portion of their supply of human hair and of articles made of hair from France and Prussia. A singular feature on the Continent is this "hair harvest", as it has been termed.

'Young women in England who have beautiful tresses are occasionally, we know, urged by poverty to part with them for money to the hair-workers; but in France and Germany it is a regular system. There are, we are told, hair merchants in Paris who send agents in the spring of each year into the country districts to purchase the tresses of young women, who seek to obtain an annual crop with the same care as a farmer would a field crop. . . . The price paid is about five francs (4s. 2d.) per pound. The agents send the hair to their employers, by whom it is dressed and sorted, and sold to the hair workers in the chief towns of the empire at about ten francs per pound. That which is to be made into perukes is purchased by a particular class of persons by whom it is cleaned, curled, prepared to a certain stage, and sold to the peruke maker at from twenty to eighty francs per pound. The peruke maker gives it the desired form, when, as is well known, it commands a very high price; a peruke is often sold for double its weight in silver. . . . Light hair all comes from Germany. . . . Forty years ago, according to one of the first dealers in the trade, the light German hair alone was called for, and he almost raved about a peculiar golden tint which was supremely prized, and which his father used to keep very close, only producing it to favourite customers. . . . This treasured article he sold at 8s. an ounce—nearly double the price of silver. Now all this has passed away—and the dark shades of brown from France are chiefly called for. . . . The lining of perukes formerly consisted of a coarse net-work, but was afterwards superseded by a fine silk net-work, which for a long time was purchased of the English at fifty francs, and is now so extensively made in France that the English are glad to avail themselves of the manufacture of Lyons, where the same article is sold at ten francs; silk linings and ribbons are made in that city for a million perukes a year; metallic clasps and fastenings are also made and sold to the amount of one hundred thousand francs yearly.

'Black hair comes mainly from Brittany and the South of France, where it is collected principally by an adventurous virtuoso, who travels from fair to fair and buys up and shears the crops of neighboring damsels.'

Francis Trolloppe, in *Summer in Brittany*, describes the process:

'We saw several girls sheared, one after the other, like sheep, and as many more standing ready for the shears, with their caps in their hands and their long hair combed out, and hanging down to their waists. Some of the operators were men, and some women. By the side of the dealer was placed a large basket into which every successive crop of hair, tied up into a wisp by itself, was thrown. . . . The money given for the hair is about twenty sous, or else a gaudy cotton handkerchief.'

During the period of the worst excesses of the eighteenth-century hair fashions, men, as we have seen, kept breaking into print in fruitless protest. Now, in mid-nineteenth century, men were beginning once again to comment in print on ladies' hair fashions; but the tone of the comment, for the most part, was gentle and tolerant. The following is from an article in the *Irish Quarterly Review*:

'In no country in the world is more attention paid to the hair than in Great Britain; and unlike other nations there is no set fashion or uniformity of practice in wearing it, every female exercising her own good taste and taxing her ingenuity in displaying her beautiful hair to the best advantage according to the contour of the face. This variety is pleasing, and one is delighted in a mixed fashionable assemblage to glance from head dress to head dress, witnessing here the hair flowing freely in ringlets, waving unconfined over neck and shoulders;—there crisp set curls, framing the temples and blooming cheeks;—anon braids and plain Madonna bands set off with a simple flower or wreath. Another has elaborately woven and twined masses adorning the back of the head interlaced with ribbon or pearls:—each eye forming its own beauty.

'The natural hair, observes a modern writer, after its long term of imprisonment, seemed for a moment to have run wild. The portraits of the beginning of the century, and even down to the time of Lawrence's supremacy, show the hair falling thick upon the brow and flowing, especially in the young, over the shoulders. . . . At the present moment almost every lady one meets has her hair arranged in "bands"; nothing but bands—the most severe and trying of all coiffures, and one only adapted to the most classic style of beauty. For the face with a downright good-natured pug nose, or with one that is only pleasantly retroussé, to adopt it is quite as absurd as for an architect to surmount an irregular Elizabethan building with a Doric frieze. Every physiognomy requires its peculiar arrangement of hair, and we only wonder that this great truth has ever been lost sight of. There is a kind of hair full of graceful waves, which, in Ireland, is called good-natured hair. There is something quite charming in its rippling line across the forehead. Art has attempted to imitate it, but the eye immediately detects the imposture. . . . This buckled hair is, in short, the same as that denounced by the early churchmen under the name of the *malice of the D - - - l*, a term which it well deserves. . . . But most of all to be admired . . . is that compromise between the severe looking "band" and the flowing ringlet, in which the hair, in twisting coils of flossy silk, is allowed to fall from the forehead in a delicate sweep round that part of the cheek where it melts into the neck, and is then gathered up into a single shell-like convolution behind; the Greeks were particularly fond of this arrangement in their sculpture because it repeated the facial outline and displayed the head to perfection. Some naturally pretty women, following the lead of the strong-minded, high-templed sisterhood, are in the habit of sweeping their hair at a very ugly angle off the brow so as to show a tower of forehead and, as they suppose, produce an overawing impression. This is a sad mistake. . . . The ancients were never guilty of thinking a vast display of forehead beautiful in woman, or that it was, in fact, at all imposing in appearance. They invariably set the hair on low and would have stared with horror at the atrocious practice of shaving it at the parting, adopted by some people to give height to the brow. . . . Least of all is such an abomination as a "fixature" allowable for one moment. He must have been a bold bad man indeed who first circulated the means of solidifying the soft and yielding hair of woman.'

The second comment is by Leigh Hunt:

'Ladies, always delightful, and not the least so in their undress, are apt to deprive themselves of some of their best morning beams by appearing with their hair in papers. All people of taste prefer a cap, if there must be anything; but hair a million times over. To see grapes in paper bags is bad enough; but the rich locks of a lady in papers, the roots of the hair twisted up like a drummer's, and the forehead staring bold instead of being gracefully tendrilled and shadowed!—it is a capital offence— a defiance to the love and admiration of the other sex—a provocation to a paper war; and we here accordingly declare the said war on paper, not having any ladies at hand to carry it at once into their head-quarters. We must allow, at the same time, that they are very shy of being seen in this condition, knowing well enough how much of their strength, like Samson, lies in that gifted ornament. We have known a whole parlor of them who fluttered off like a dove-cote at the sight of a friend coming up the garden.'

A century later the article would have been as timely. Although the papers would be gone, incredibly ugly curlers, growing larger by the year, would have taken their place. There would be no caps, and kerchiefs would never seem quite to cover the front curlers. And, unfortunately, the ladies would never, never flutter off like a dove-cote at the sight of a friend.

1860–1870 (Plates 124-128)

This was the decade of the chignon and, with it, enormous quantities of false hair. At first the emphasis was primarily to the back and very low, usually with no impor- tant detail in front of the ears; but soon the false hair spread like a cancer in all directions until often a lady wore so many different hair pieces that her own hair was completely obscured. Plates 124-128 illustrate the general development and especially the enormous variety of chignons, most of them needing to be professionally made. It is hardly surprising to learn that in 1859–60 between 150,000 and 200,000 pounds of hair, valued at close to a million dollars (about £356,000 in the present day), was imported into the United States. The amount increased steadily during the decade and in 1866 was about triple the amount. Paris was the major hair market of the world and exported as much to Russia as to the United States. It was reported in 1862 that about a hundred tons of hair a year was bought in the Paris market. Hair from France and Italy was considered the most desirable. The price ranged from fifteen to two hundred dollars (about £71 in the present day) a pound, depending on colour, quality, and length. Grey and white have always been the most expensive. Campbell reports a case of a dealer's being offered four hundred dollars for half a pound of seventy-inch hair and refusing the offer. The women who grew the hair were paid, it is said, only about fifteen to seventy cents a pound.

In 1862 *Godey's* reported that 'the *crepé* or waved style of hair is in favor now with our ladies. It is generally very becoming, but as it injures the hair very much, the heavy braids are more worn.'

Apparently Mrs Merrifield's satisfaction, in writing a decade earlier on the willingness of women to live with their natural hair colour, was short-lived; for now we find G. W. Septimus Piesse informing the readers of *The Art of Perfumery* that 'Under the name of "Baffine," a very excellent brown hair-dye has been introduced by Mr. Condy of Battersea. It consists of saturated solution of permanganate of potass. This salt, like nitrate of silver, undergoes decomposition when in contact with organic substances. Hair and skin are stained by it of a good chestnut hue.

'For the purpose of dyeing the hair it is therefore necessary to take the usual precaution nôt to wet the partings of the hair with the manganese fluid. . . . "Fair" persons are seldom, if ever, improved in appearance by the process of hair-dyeing. Such persons who do not exhibit these marked features of Teutonic extraction, in whose veins commingles the blood of a more southern race—whose dark or brown complexion, gazelle-like eyes, and raven hair, tend to form that style of beauty we designate "brunette"—should age trip up youth, or their locks become prematurely grey or silvery white, may call in the aid of art to restore the hair to its original tint, without infringing the principles of the harmony of color. If the hair be too glowing, too bright an auburn to assimilate well with the eyes, or with the blush of the cheek, then its redness can be artificially lowered by the application of an article sold under the name of walnut-water, but which in reality consists of a solution of plumbate of potash. . . .' The colour preference in that era was definitely for dark brown or black hair.

Procter cautioned, however, that in dyeing the hair, one must be exceedingly wary: 'Only the other day a perfumer of Marseilles was sued for damages to the amount of four hundred francs because he unfortunately dyed a lady's hair violet instead of red. And not long ago I observed an elderly, unsuspecting gentleman, whose hair was glittering in the bright sunlight—an unmistakable green.'

As for the unpopularity of red hair, Procter quotes a verse current at the time:

> Oh! Why do you laugh at red hair?
> 'Tis really a great want of charity;
> 'Mongst the Greeks, we are free to declare,
> Two at least of the Graces were χάριτε.

The indispensable *Lady's Book* once again furnishes us with an intriguing picture of contemporary styles, this time for 1863:

'Perfect scaffoldings of hair are now built on the head—roll upon roll—puff upon puff. Some of the styles are extremely odd; not the least odd is that for which are used two rats, two mice, a cat, and a cataract. Lest, however, we should be the means of some pussy being cut off by a premature death from the circle of which she is the ornament, we hasten to explain. The rats are the long frizetts of curled hair for the side rolls; the mice are the smaller ones above them; the cat is for the roll laid over the top of the head; and the cataract is for the chignon at the back of the head—which is sometimes called waterfall, cataract, and *jet d'eau.*

'Little girls are wearing their hair in short frizzed curls, and in some instances we have seen very long hair floating down the back only slightly *crepé.* This, however, is not a pretty style, and we would not advise its adoption.

'For coiffures, the humming bird alone disputes with the butterfly the favor of fashion. These ornaments were introduced by the Empress of the French and bring fabulous prices, many of them being made of precious stones or of enamel worked with gold. They are worn by young ladies as well as matrons. The humming birds, being the natural bird of the rarest plumage, are frequently set with diamond eyes.'

With female hair rampant, as well as false, male comment in the press lost its note of tolerance and became rather more barbed. A satiric piece published in *Punch* in 1867 took the form of a 'Suggested law for the abolition of chignons':

'Whereas it has become necessary and expedient for divers cogent reasons and causes fully developed, brought forth and shewn, that the customs relating to Chignons be forthwith suppressed by special act of Parliament, Be it therefore Enacted, by and with the Approbation of the Lords Spiritual and Temporal and Commons in this present Parliament assembled, and by authority of the same, as follows:

'1. That from and after the passing of this Act, it shall not be lawful for any Female whether single or married, to obtain or become possessed by any means direct or indirect of any Artificial Nobulous, hairy superfluity, or rotunditive protuberance whether the same be for decorative or other purpose.

'2. For what Whereas notwithstanding this is the age of civilization, it has become the custom for the wives and daughters of England, to attire, wear, deck, and bedizen themselves after the manner and in the style, fashion and eccentric mode generally adopted by ferocious and benighted cannibals, therefore from and after the passing of this Act, all Females shall be assumed to know and be acquainted and informed, that the fashionable Chignon by which they consider they adorn themselves, contains foreign and unpleasant elements, fitted only for an Aquarium, where the turbinative movements of the species, would be inoffensive.

'3. That from and after the passing of this Act all Females who shall wear an Artificial Chignon, without a Certificate as hereinafter mentioned, shall upon conviction deposit the same at the Police Station nearest her residence, and the same may and shall be used as artificial Bird Nests, for the intelligent sparrows of large Towns in Great Britain who at present use the gutter spouts on the roofs of Houses, to the stopping up of the same, and each ape and monkey in the Zoological Gardens shall each and every one receive one to be used as a wig for winter wear. Farmers and Naturalists requiring Artificial Nests, to make applications to any Magistrate for a supply.'

Naturally, nobody writing in *Punch* or anywhere else had the slightest dampening effect on current excesses. If they had, certain business men might have been seriously inconvenienced, for in 1867 the advertisement of a New York wig-maker listed the following materials available in his retail department: 'Hair Jewelry, Gold Mountings for Hair Jewelry, Gent's wigs and Toupees, Ladies' Wigs, Switches, Braids, Curls, Waterfalls, Frizettes, Coils, Bows, Fronts, Scratches, Bands, Hair-Nets, Ornamental Hair, Partings, Whiskers, Beards, Mustaches, Puffs, Curling-Irons, Curling-Sticks, Crimping-Irons, Perfumery, Pomades and Creams, Soaps, Hair Brushes, Combs, Hair Oils, Cosmetiques, Crimping-Pins, Face Powders, Rouges, French Enamel, and Hair Powders—Diamond Powder, Gold Powder, Silver Powder', as well as 'Wig Materials and Tools of Every Description'.

Powdering the hair was reported to be all the rage in fashionable circles, with gold and silver powder being considered particularly elegant.

A gentleman writing in *Leisure Hour* had some firm opinions on the matter of hair colour when he wrote:

'Quite recently an insane fashion has run upon golden and other light tints for ladies' hair. Brunettes would seem to have gone out of vogue, and blondes to have come in. Considering the traditional pride of dark ladies, the deference now accorded by them to their fair rivals is the more extraordinary. There is much to offend masculine sensibilities in the over-rigid deference to fashion shown by some ladies in matters of attire; but when it comes to the extreme of setting a fashion for the colour of a head of hair, then we may well exclaim, "What next?". . . .

'There are acted falsehoods as there are spoken falsehoods; and in some respects enacted falsehoods are the worse. Amongst falsehoods unspoken, the dyeing hair of fancy colours seems to me amongst the most contemptible. The poor clerk or shop-man may, perhaps, be excused for trying to beget an impression of greater youth by dyeing his hair, whiskers, or moustaches black. His bread may in some sense depend upon it; but were he to bleach his naturally black or brown hair, only to dye it some fancy colour, one would then call him, among other names, a poor silly fellow. Nothing can palliate the fancy-colour hair-dyeing now prevalent among the ladies. The practice is silly, and worse, morally wrong. Worse still (in the estimation of some, I fear), it is ruinous to the hair, as many ladies will discover to their cost when the fashion changes.'

In the same year there appeared a book by Mark Campbell called *Self-Instructor in the Art of Hair Work*. In the preface Mr Campbell states (writing in the third person), that 'the great consumption and rapidly increasing demand for every description of Hair Goods, will make this work he now presents to the public, one of particular interest to all classes. Heretofore the Art of making these goods has been zealously guarded by a few dealers, who have accumulated fortunes, and would still

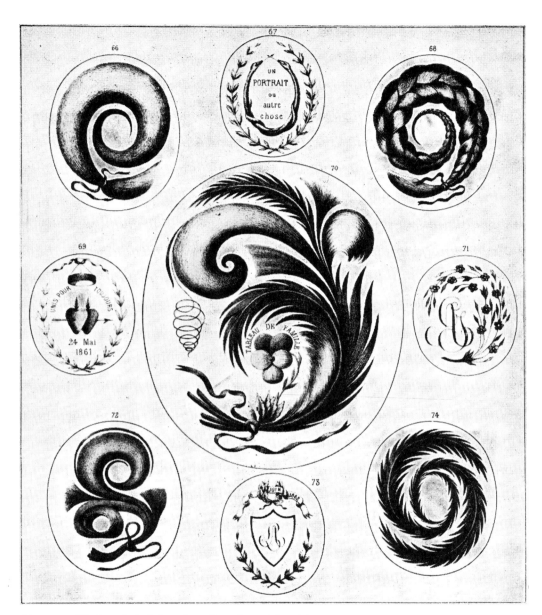

Fig. 113 : Designs in hair based on French models, 1862

retain it as a profound secret but for the publication of this book. This is the only descriptive volume ever published on Hair Work . . . containing over one thousand drawings, devices and diagrams, engraved at great expense by the publisher.' He goes on to say, hopefully, that it 'will prove an indispensable adjunct to every lady's toilet table'. And in one final bid for purchasers he suggests that 'persons wishing to preserve and weave into lasting mementos, the hair of a deceased father, mother, sister, brother, or child, can also enjoy the inexpressible advantage and satisfaction of *knowing* that the material of their own handiwork is the actual hair of the "loved and gone"'.

Not one to miss an opportunity, Mr Campbell closes his book with six full-page advertisements for his own hair establishment. Three of these are for 'Campbell's Chevrolion', which he guarantees for 'Restoring the Color and Growth of the Hair, Purifying, Whitening and Beautifying the complexion'. It is also, he claims, a 'sure cure' for rough skin, freckles, sunburn, and baldness. In one of the advertisements there are two before-and-after drawings, the first showing a dejected lady with straight, straggling hair and an appalling complexion. She is clutching a bottle of Chevrolion. In the second drawing her hair is darker, luxuriant, and beautifully wavy; and all of the horrid skin blemishes have magically disappeared. She has apparently discarded the no-longer-needed bottle of Chevrolion and seems, if not really ecstatic, at least understandably relieved. Mr Campbell virtuously abstains from the prevalent and what he seems to consider vulgar practice of presenting testimonials. Chevrolion, he feels, should be allowed to speak for itself.

With rats, mice, cats, butterflies, humming birds, precious stones, and endless quantities of hair to be piled on the head, it is hardly surprising that one could scarcely keep up with the latest fashion. Each monthly issue of one's favourite ladies' magazine brought something new to try. The following is a series of reports from *The Lady's Friend* for 1869:

February. 'In the matter of hair dressing everybody seems to adopt her own peculiar style, but the hair is certainly not drawn so much away from the nape of the neck as heretofore. Curls are more in favor than ever. One belle wore the hair turned off from the face in front, with a mass of curls falling from the top of the head onto the shoulders. The puff of hair, which seems now the inevitable accompaniment of all kinds of chignons, is brought further forward than it used to be, and bandeaux of velvet or hair are often worn in front of it with gold or pearl, silver or diamond ornaments in the center. Birds, bees, and butterflies are a great deal worn, and sprays of flowers or leaves appear invariably to fall onto the shoulders. The only exception admitted this winter by the elite to the tortoise-shell comb, is the comb enriched with real jewels and precious stones for all coiffures. The high Josephine comb, sparkling with rubies, pearls, and emeralds, is quite the *fureur* this season for full dress toilets.'

March. 'The hair is worn higher than ever. . . . For ball coiffures the ornaments are very few. Ladies wear such a profusion of curls and frizettes that the head would really become overloaded if flowers, feathers, or any other sort of trimming were added to them. A tiny jewelled coronet or a string of pearls, one simple flower or white plume, is all that really looks well in modern coiffures. None but elderly ladies wear head-dresses of any size.'

April. 'Diadems are in great vogue. Who does not like to adorn herself just like an empress, queen, or princess? Diadems of blade-tortoise-shell are carved like diadems of the time of Blanche de Castille, when queens still wore habitually the ensigns of royalty. This diadem comb fastens all the hair brushed upwards from the forehead, leaving the temples free. Other models are in the Grecian style or mere torsades of tortoise-shell.'

May. 'Chignons are to be abolished by the select world of Paris, and ladies who would be thought "good form" are to endeavor to dress their hair themselves or to look as if they dressed it: for "when the work of a professional is manifest on the head, prestige ceases". In the daytime the hair, simply braided, will be confined within the meshes of a net, and far from assuming a pyramidal shape, will rather fall loose, Niobe fashion. For the evening it will be sufficient to place a simple wreath upon the head, a garland of roses, sweet briar, or clematis. All beads and gilding must be discarded. The artificial hair must return to its proper place—a sometimes needful help, but always concealed and not, as it has too long been, the principal, not to say the whole ornament of the head.

'Such are the ideas of our *reactionnaire* ladies, but so far these ideas do not prevail. Chignons are not much smaller than they were, but we must say that the long curls of which they are most frequently composed, especially for evening dress, render them far more graceful than the smooth, round *cushions* of last year.

'A diadem of tortoise-shell fastens the plait or curl upon the top of the head. All faces, however, do not look well under the diadem. A mere bandeau of tortoise-shell is more suited to a laughing, Heke-like countenance. The diadem is always grand. It requires the full-dress toilet, the court train, and a statuesque figure. The tortoise-shell bandeau may be worn with a short toilet. Such details must be noted. The great art of appearing well dressed is to dress in a manner suitable to one's age, style of countenance, and figure.'

This article is followed by a poem, *Going to Milk the Cows*, by Phila H. Case.

Perhaps the decision of Paris came none too soon, for in this same year there appeared a second-hand news item with a familiar ring:

'We learn queer things of American affairs from the journals of London. Here is the *Pall Mall Gazette*, which informs us that Bishop Odenheimer of New Jersey has determined not to lay his hands in confirmation upon any woman, young or old, whose head is adorned with borrowed tresses. The statement may be fact, but if so, we marvel at the indifference with which so remarkable an Episcopal resolve has been received here. To what does it not tend? If chignons are not to be confirmed, may not the marriage rite be withheld from other artificialities? And if false hair be put under the ban, shall stained hair, dyed hair, escape censure and the scissors? If ladies must not wear braids, can gentlemen wear wigs? And must a hairdresser attend at confirmation to decide between false hair and the true? But the matter involves too great an array of questions to be further pursued.'

While the bishop fumed and threatened, others wrote poetry. The two verses following are from *March Winds*:

> See March now in a bluster
>   'Midst chignons and the curls,
> Puts stout mamas a-fluster,
>   And confuses slender girls;
> He showers golden tresses
>   Over faces soft and sweet,
> And raises skirts and dresses,
>   Showing pretty legs and feet!
>
> With chignons so gigantic,
>   Or with falsely-braided tress,
> He'll play some impish antic,
>   I am sorry to confess:
> He'll whirl them where he pleases,
>   And their owners leave appalled,
> When twirled off by the breezes,
>   Winds so love to chill the bald.

And that brings us to the end of another decade.

1870–1880 (Plates 129-132)

Apparently the word from Paris on chignons was premature, for in September, 1870, we find the following report in the *Lady's Friend*:

'With the drooping chignons of curls and the catogans of smooth braided hair, wreaths and garlands of flowers are once more come into fashion for evening coiffures. They are made fuller in front so as to rise into a diadem above the forehead and continued into trailing springs, which fall and mix with the hair at the back.'

A note on children's hair states that 'Blonde hair is most often worn flowing in crimps, prepared by being braided the night before. A blue or brown ribbon confines the fluffy front hair. Dark brown and black hair is braided in two long, thick plaits, tied with ribbons.'

In the October issue we read that 'Rouleaux are taking the place of plaits. In other coiffures the chignon is composed of long, thick curls. The flowers are always placed on the top of the head for evening—coiffures with long, trailing sprays coming very low down in the neck.'

And in November we are told that 'the coiffure is now becoming rather a serious subject with the many who have chosen during the past few years to conform to the extravagant dictates of fashion. Some who commenced with long, luxuriant hair are compelled at last to put on the false in default of the real, while others, fearing a like fate, are endeavoring to "flee from the wrath to come" by discarding all false capillary appendages. Those who really have hair after passing through such a hair-destroying ordeal, are proud to show it now and are beginning to arrange it in very simple and graceful styles. Tight puffs on the top of the head are worn. Braids are also arranged *en diademe*, and with the chatelaine braids at the back, made to appear thick by crimping. This style of coiffure is pretty. Pendant braids are still worn by children and are very becoming for young misses.'

The false capillary appendages were obviously of concern to a good many people. A forthright poem informatively entitled *Chignons* appeared about this time. Here are the last two verses:

> But the fashion that governs the bonnet
>   (Perhaps it is *tout au contraire*—
> I can't make my mind up upon it—)
>   Is the fashion of 'doing' the hair!
> We all of us have our opinions,
>   And mine, I must candidly own,
> Is this: that the things you call chignons
>   Are the ugliest things we have known!
>
>
> They are half of them false as the figure
>   We see in a hairdresser's shop!
> You *must* wear them, because it's *de rigueur*,
>   But you're always in fear lest they drop!
> They are larger than ever this season,
>   And this theory's better than none,
> That two heads—of hair, you may reason,
>   Are certainly better than one!

According to an article in the London *Times*, 'The number of chignons exported from France to England during the past year was 11,954, in addition to which there was exported a sufficient quantity of hair for 7,000 chignons to be made up in England. The total value of the exports of hair and chignons from France during 1856 amounted to 1,206,605 f., or upwards of £45,000 sterling. England took the largest quantity, and the United States figure next on the list.'

Alexanna Speight, writing about this time, adopted a philosophical view to the dyeing of hair, which was still practised:

'The sudden change of hair from all colours into the brightest golden, which astonished and perplexed the male portion of the population some few years since, and required the father to be indeed a wise one who could know his own child . . . was after all but the restoration of a very ancient art, and it really is very questionable whether the glorious golden hues of bright yellow hair have not after all a natural and superior attractiveness, which would account for the constant efforts which one after another are seen repeating themselves, to attain through science what nature has denied.'

The poets and the writers of letters-to-the-editor seemed no more concerned about the colour of the hair than Speight, but they persisted in attacking false hair. A poem of suspicion called *Is It Her Own?* reflects the general attitude:

> Is it her own? through each long afternoon,
>   When airy muslins sweep along the grass,
> Is it her own? when couples sit and spoon,
>   And fairy girls through tents of blossom pass,
> When flower fetes horticultural delight us,
> Or promenades botanical invite us,
>   Then if you list you'll hear
>   Sweet voices whispering near,
>   'Is it her own?'

> Is it her own? when the grand pow'r of song
>   Tears us from dinner and ANINA's side,
> To hear LA MURSKA cadences prolong
>   And watch for tresses which the curtains hide.
> When passionate applause at last is dying,
> And anxious friends acquaintances are eyeing,
>   Then watchful mothers say,
>   'Look, darling, o'er the way,
>   Is it her own?'

> Is it her own? question of shelved maids
>   Viewing with jealous eyes their sisters fair:
> Whisper of damsels whose concocted braids
>   Pass for luxurious wealth by golden hair;
> See in sly corners dowagers conspiring,
> Pleasantly smiling, audibly admiring.
>   Hear how their voices sink,
>   'Quite so; but do you think
>   It is her own?'

Is it her own? smooth tufts and curls distrust,
    And chignons hidden by a silken net,
Beware of ornaments and golden dust,
    Mark well the juncture where the comb is set.
If neat disorder reigns beneath the bonnet,
Friend of my youth! I'll stake my life upon it,
    Then instantly you'll say,
    When wilful tresses stray,
      It is her own!

The *Lady's Friend* for March, 1871, provides us with a more factual report on the situation:

'The few who have abundant hair of their own wear it in thick plaits, turned up and fastened at the top of the head, the arrangement completed with a bow of ribbon. But as scanty hair is the common thing, and fashion still imperatively requires the appearance of plenty, the drooping chignons now à-la-mode, and which are formed of large torsades or loose twists of hair, are thus managed; the pad is a large but soft fluffy thing, composed of a number of long, sausage-like separate pieces, only held together at the top. This is fastened under the back hair, which is divided in as many braids as there are separate pieces. Each of these pieces must be entirely covered with the real hair, after which the torsades or plaits are made, and of an enormous size they are when done up in that way. In front the hair is dressed higher than ever, and towers high above the forehead. No curls are worn, but only frizzles just over the forehead. Few ornaments are worn in the coiffure. One diamond star or one flower is often the only ornament.'

In July the magazine reported that 'The hair is worn straight down the back in waved ripples and confined in a net, the front hair arranged in small bandeaux and brushed back from the temples. Another mode is to wear long braids of hair flat to the head, falling down the back and in a net.'

The year 1872 finds wide ribbons fashionable for head-dresses, with the ends falling almost to the shoulders. 'These ribbons', according to the *Lady's Friend*, 'are made up into bows, which nestle in a fullness or gathering of white lace. The two ends are almost entirely covered with a wide falling loop, which is almost of equal length with them. . . . Gray hair has come to be so much admired that it is displayed rather than concealed. Consequently hair dyes and false fronts are out of fashion. A great many ornamental pins are now worn in the plaits of hair, which are fashionable for evening toilets. These pins have either filigreed gold or silver heads. Some ladies wear antique pins with enamelled heads of butterflies, flowers, etc., studded along the plaits.'

The July styles show more simplicity. 'The bandeaux are now completely raised off the forehead and temples and puffed out, but to soften the curve of these bandeaux the hair is waved in a particular way; just on the top a few curls play over the brow but without covering it. Thus the head is not increased in volume with the absurd exaggeration of most of our modern coiffures; it remains of about its natural size, which is a great condition of elegance. The chignon is composed of the thick drooping loops of hair called marteaux and of one large plait; it is placed much higher than was the case in the winter and fastened with a handsome tortoise-shell comb with elaborate openwork beading.'

The September report, striking a more permissive note, tells the reader that 'the style of hair-dressing is, like everything else, left very much to personal taste, but there is a tendency to a less drooping style of coiffure. The hair is raised off the neck, and the plaits, or large coques, placed much higher and fastened with a tortoise-shell comb, shaped like a coronet or low diadem, while a few stray curls only are allowed to fall in the neck. The ornament, bow, or flower is placed in front, a little on one side, the front hair is either brought low over the forehead in waves or frizzles or drawn quite off the brow. This must depend upon the wearer's style of features. To some faces the hair brushed off from the forehead is exceedingly becoming; to others it is very trying. As a rule, it is suitable only to a youthful face. A lady, however, must judge for herself what will suit her style.'

Although the demise of the chignon had been predicted and awaited (eagerly, in some circles) for a number of years, it was not until 1873 that it was definitely reported that 'the change from the drooping chignon is now a *fait accompli*. And many a fair neck and delicate turn of the neck now appears, the beauties of which were long hidden by massive coils and plaits'.

Readers were also advised that 'when the hair is insufficient in quantity, there is added, here and there, a puff or two, a few floating curls, a bow of ribbon, one or two pins of precious stone, metal, or simply shell, or when the dress permits the ornament, two or three flexible stems with a few flowers'.

As late as 1877 Robert Tomes, in *The Bazar Book of Decorum*, complained about the lingering chignon: 'This tumor-like excrescence disfigures the top of the head with the appearance of a horrid growth of disease which would seem to call for the knife of a surgeon did we not know that it could be placed or displaced at the will of the wearer'. In a footnote Mr Tomes adds that 'the hair of which the *chignon* or *waterfall* is made is mostly brought from Caffreland, where it is cut from the heads of the filthiest and most disgusting population in the world. The former sources of supply, the peasants of Germany and the dead of hospitals and prisons, are incapable of furnishing the excessive demand for hair created by the general prevalence of the present monstrosity of fashion. The Hottentot product is shipped to London, near which there is a place where it was purified. This, however, in consequence of the intolerable stench, has been indicted as a nuisance.'

Although the chignon was officially dead so far as the fashion leaders were concerned, the death throes took longer among the followers. Perhaps the parody of Tennyson called *Lady Chignon Hair of Hair* was intended to speed them up a bit:

LADY CHIGNON HAIR OF HAIR,
  You've won at last a great renown.
You thought to turn a score of heads,
  With fashion when you took the town.
On me you shone, but when you'd gone,
  I knew the dodge that I'd admired,
The head of a prae-Raffaelite!
  Yours is not one to be desired.

LADY CHIGNON HAIR OF HAIR!
  You needs must hide your head in shame,
Your tresses can't compare with mine,
  For now you know from whence they came:
And as I live, I would not give
  A fig for yours, though bald I am,
A simple maiden's pretty locks
  Are worth a thousand lumps of sham!

LADY CHIGNON HAIR OF HAIR,
  I stole the plaits from off your head,
Not many months have come and gone
  Since they adorned a Kalmuck-dead.
Oh! your fine nets, your soft *frisettes*,
  A microscope was brought to me,
And there were those about the ends
  Which you had hardly cared to see.

Trust me, CHIGNON HAIR OF HAIR,
  Though Paris fashions woman apes,
Your great grandfather and his wife
  Smile at the claims of bonnet shapes.
Howe'er this be, it seems to me
  'Tis fair to fascinate the flirt,
Your hair's worth more than coronets,
  And simple braids than Russian dirt.

CHIGNON! CHIGNON HAIR OF HAIR!
  If you have lots of tails and bands,
Are there no pillows in your house,
  Or sofa cushions near your hands?

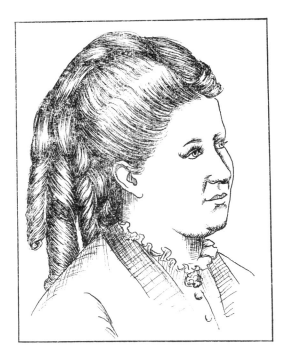

Fig. 114 : Grand-Duchess Pauline of
Sachs-Weimar in 1873

Go! cram an ottoman or stool,
   And stuff your sunny locks with tow,
Ask Paris for another freak,
   But let this nasty fashion go!

But the passing of the chignon did not mean the end of false hair, as a glance at Plates 131 and 132 will show. It merely moved the emphasis upwards. And in 1879 we find Mrs M. R. Haweis complaining impatiently in *The Art of Dress*, 'I have no prejudice, none need have, against false hair used in moderation and *when necessary*, any more than one need have against cosmetics and paint, used in moderation and *when necessary*. But the enormous masses of hair which load fair heads now, like the masses of red and white which smeared fair faces nearly 100 years ago, are purely ugly and ridiculous. When a plait is palpably bigger than one human head can supply, it ceases to be an ornament, and becomes a burden and annoyance.'

We have one final note of complaint to close the decade. G. F. Watts, writing 'On Taste in Dress', remarks that 'the habit of piling up enormous masses of hair, mostly or always false, needs no comment'. He then proceeds to comment:

'Hair is beautiful, and Greek poetry is full of allusions to it and its value as a splendid possession; but it never will be found that the size of the head of a Greek statue is much enlarged by it; it is closely confined to the shape of the head so as not materially to increase the size of it. The relative proportion was felt to be important before all; in the coins hair is more voluminous, but, the head being cut off at the throat, the principle of proportion does not come into play. The Greeks, with their fine taste, reduced art instincts to a science; they never violated by top-heaviness in their sculpture the sense of security which the upright tower of the human form should suggest; and to overweight the upright human figure with an immense quantity of hair massed into a solid lump is to distort that fitness without which there is no harmony or beauty. It will be in better taste, if a large hat or bonnet be worn, to make it of light materials, while one of the denser materials should be small. In a picture any amount of hair may be made to fall or fly about with charming effect, because its lightness may be delightfully suggested; but, excepting in the case of children, the effect of hair flying about is not good, for the suggestion of untidiness and want of cleanliness, with general unfitness. So that, as a rule, it may be said that it is in better taste to braid the hair closely to the head, not, of course, so tightly as to destroy the especial quality of beauty of hair; for notwithstanding the advantage of form and proportion, to plaster the hair down upon the head till it resembles a metal cannot be in good taste.'

1880–1890 (Plates 133-135)

Masses of hair continued to be worn throughout the eighties, occasionally drooping low on the neck but more often concentrated on the top and the back of the head, being held in place with large pins or decorative combs. The hair was softer around the face than it had been. The side hair was usually gently waved, and during the early part of the decade a fringe across the forehead was fashionable. A slightly fluffy effect was the result. Frequently the front hair was false as well as the torsades, puffs, rolls, and curls. Small clusters of fluffy curls could be bought and stuck in wherever there happened to be an empty space. Larger pieces conveniently attached to combs could also be had. Late in the decade the styles were less fluffy and rose higher.

'In the fall of 1888', reported *Hobbies* some sixty years later, 'the jeweled hairpin was in great demand. One of the well known opera singers of that day had a collection of over two hundred, from the black wire pin which she used to button shoes or pick locks to dainty and bejeweled trinkets of great costliness. For morning wear dul and bright jet pins were preferred; during the day amber pins with ornaments of stars and flowers were the favorites; and for teas it was correct to wear shell pins. . . . The Parisian preferred the hairpin with shell foundation which had a spray of leaves or flowers cut in steel to ornament the top. The pin with garnet ornamentation seemed to be the general favorite.' Enamelled pins representing sprays of flowers, silver pins appropriate to a particular sport, and small gold pins decorated with pearls or precious stones were also worn.

With all the crimping and frizzing which was going on, the birth of a new kind of hair treatment called the 'marcel' took place unnoticed in a dingy little hairdresser's shop at Number 87, rue de Dunquerque, in Montmartre. It was actually not so much an invention as an experiment, which, partly through persistence and partly through sheer good fortune, eventually became the rage of Paris, as did its originator, Marcel Grateau, born October 18, 1852, at Chauvigny.

Marcel began his career currying horses, tried his hand at helping out in the hairdressing shop and, presumably owing to his lack of skill, was shortly sent back to the horses. But for want of anything better, he did, at the age of twenty, run his own miserable shop, where he catered to the lowest class of women at a few centimes a head, frizzing the hair with the same sort of curling iron which had been used for centuries. But one day he noticed that a lock of his mother's naturally wavy grey hair was hanging straight and limp. In trying to restore the curl with an iron and make it match the natural wave, he tried turning the iron upside down. *Voilà*—a natural-looking wave. Although Marcel and his mother were pleased with the result, his clients refused to let him experiment on them until he offered to do it free. Even then there were few takers at first; but soon an occasional client would ask for the new style of hair-dressing, which was described as the moiré or watered effect and then as *ondulations*. It wasn't until much later that it took on the name of its creator.

One day when Marcel was busier than usual, a client wanted the new effect; and on being told there was no time that day for free experiments, she offered to pay extra. From then on everyone paid.

All this time Marcel assumed that he could use the technique only on hair with a slight natural wave. But one day when a straight-haired client demanded the new style, Marcel reluctantly obliged, certain that it would not last through the day. A month later the client returned with a soft wave still in her hair.

But it took some time for the wealthy and the famous to become aware of the new style. Madame Gaston Menier, of the chocolate firm, was one of the first. Having seen the style but being unwilling to go into Marcel's exceedingly uninviting shop, she paid him what was then an enormous sum to dress her hair on her private yacht. After a few more such happy circumstances, Marcel was able, in 1882, ten years after his discovery of the new waving technique, to sell his shop in Montmartre and set up a new shop at Number 2, rue de l'Échelle, near the Théâtre français. Although he had gradually accumulated a few clients in the theatrical world, he was virtually ignored by the world of fashion, looked upon with contempt by his fellow hairdressers, and caricatured in the newspapers.

Then one of his clients, Jane Hading, who was at the height of her popularity, opened in *Le Maître des Forges*. Until then he had been dressing her hair in the fashion of the day. Now she wanted a completely new coiffure. Marcel, devoid, as

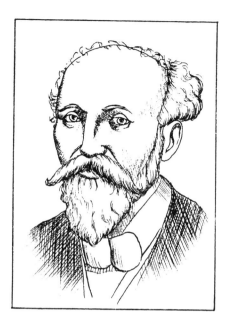

Fig. 115 : The French hairdresser Marcel, originator
of the wave named after him, in 1927

he thought, of ideas but clearly not of inspiration, told Mlle Hading that he was going to dress her hair in the style worn by his mother. The 24-year-old actress was not enchanted with the idea; but reassured by Marcel's own confidence, she reluctantly let him have his way. Without using fancy pins or false curls or piles of hair on the head, he simply waved her hair with his own special technique. The style, which suited Miss Hading admirably, as Marcel must have known it would, was an extraordinary success, and a new era in hairdressing was born.

By the end of 1884 Marcel's clients included such celebrities as Cléo de Mérode, la belle Otéro, Diane de Pougy, Réjane, Melba, and Calvé; and he was in such demand that, as Rambaud puts it, he needed two hundred arms. One day an impatient client offered to pay extra for immediate attention. Other clients offered to pay still more. Marcel's wife, Maria, who evidently had a head for business, saw in this the solution to their problem. From then on Marcel accepted clients on the basis of competitive bidding.

At the age of forty-five, Marcel, satisfied that he and his wife had all the money they needed for the rest of their lives, retired and, it is pleasant to report, lived happily ever after. He died in 1936, beloved and respected by his profession. Figure 115 shows him as he looked in 1927, long after his retirement.

1890–1900 (Plates 136-139)

The nineties showed a marked change in the styles. At first the artificial torsades and curls were used as they had been; but before long most of the false hair was discarded except when really needed, and the natural hair was fluffed up and frizzed and curled and twisted. The topknot, which came back in various guises, was very fashionable late in the decade. Usually it sat squarely on top of the head; occasionally it even moved to the front. In the latter case it was probably a blending of the topknot and the front fringe or puff. It is easy to see, for example, how the style in Plate 139-P could become that of Plate 139-R.

Apart from the topknot, the nineties' hairdo was notable for its volume and width. In the 1820s and thirties, width had been achieved by means of clusters of curls which seemed to be and sometimes were stuck on. But now, for the first time in a century, the body of the hair was voluminous, though it remained relatively flat on top, height being achieved with topknots. Queen Victoria's flat mid-century hair style (Plate 139-G) is in striking contrast to the puffy hairdos of the more fashionable ladies.

In 1892, writing in the *Ladies Home Journal*, Isabel Mallon told her readers that braiding the hair was decidedly in vogue:

'The mistake usually made by the girl in arranging her hair in braids for the first time is that she begins her braids too low. As she wants to loop it or twist it, she must brush it up from the nape of her neck and start to braid it mid-way of the back. Then it is easily turned around and fastened, if she wishes to wear it in that fashion; or if it is to be looped, she lets part of it belong where the plait began making the other curl around the loop and tying the ribbon below that. No other color ribbon is worn but black, and one must beware of having too wide a ribbon or too large a bow.

'A very decided fancy has arisen for parting the hair. It may be just in the center or slightly to one side, as is most becoming, but the part does not need to extend through the bang, so that the soft framing of the face is still retained. . . . The part immediately in the center requires very regular features—so is not attempted by very many women. . . . Women who wear their hair very plainly part it in the back and turn it over like a French twist, drawing it up to the top of the head in such a way that the parting is visible.'

In this same year Mrs Mallon wrote (no doubt straightening her back as she did so), 'It almost goes without saying that a well-bred woman does not dye her hair. If in some moment of, I was going to say temporary insanity, she should be induced to do it, although it would be mortifying and she will have to permit herself to look like a striped zebra for a short time, still it will be wisest to face the situation and allow her hair to grow back to its natural color.'

In 1894 she began one of her columns with an admirably permissive attitude toward fashion: 'There is no reason why every woman should not wear her hair in the manner that is most becoming, for the styles are many and each woman can choose that one which suits her best.

'The woman with very dark hair should never have it very much crinkled or fluffy. If she can wear it quite plain, it will be well to do so. However, if a plain style should be too severe, let it be arranged in close waves and full, not frizzy, locks.

'The blonde or brown-haired woman is at liberty to arrange her hair after a much-fancied fashion which does not depend on her having a very great quantity of it. Nowadays her hair is what used to be called "crimped", but with every change of fashion comes a new name, and so it is spoken of as "undulated". It is done with the iron after the hair has been carefully parted. The hair is parted, waved all over the head, and then is drawn down at each side lightly and allowed to rest just over the top of the ear. At the back it is very softly coiled, the end being turned over like a puff and fastened with a small tortoise-shell pin.'

In referring to a brunette model, Mrs Mallon writes:

'As her forehead is somewhat high, she cannot dispense with the suggestion of a fringe, and therefore the coquettish, simple curl just in the center is pulled a little so that it spreads at the end, although the idea of the one curl is not lost. The hair is then drawn back very softly, and midway of the head it is turned, made to stand out in something not unlike a psyche knot, although about it, making a round outline, the ends of the hair are twisted in what used to be known as a rope coil, which comes out most effectively in black hair. Usually a rope coil, to be an absolute success, must be arranged by a hair dresser, and this is the only objection to it.

'Blondes have found that for daytime wear the low, plaited knot is almost invariably becoming. A blonde whose head is so shaped that a plain arrangement of the hair in front will suggest flatness, has the hair on top of her head cut about halfway back so that it is only sufficiently long to turn over once in soft little curls, best arranged by putting them up in curl papers. At the sides the hair is long enough to be brushed back and then turned over toward the front in a long fluffy curl on each side. At the back the hair is carefully braided and pinned somewhat closely to the head with small gold pins.

'For evening wear there is a decided tendency to arrange the hair quite high so that ribbons, jewels, or whatever hair decorations one may possess or find becoming may be used.

'Where a ribbon or jeweled coronet is to be worn and the hair must necessarily be worn high, it must be very firm so that the tiara may not get out of place. The fluffiness of a puff or a few short curls, no matter how becoming, are not allowable. The cutting of the hair in the back is entirely out of vogue, but the natural short curls are usually made fluffy.'

Mrs Mallon concludes her article with a charming paragraph entitled 'Mistakes that are Made'. One rather suspects that some of her friends may not have been reading her column very carefully, for she asks:

'Who of us is there who has not grieved at seeing a friend, intelligent and pretty, make herself look stupid and ugly by an over-heavy fringe, frizzed like wool, and made to come down so far on the forehead that there is doubt as to her having one? The mode of today permits, where it is necessary, a soft fringe, but this is a short one, allowing the forehead to show and making the looker-on conscious of the intellectual strength of the wearer. Who of us has not seen with horror the friend whose hair a month ago was a pretty brown, appear with it made either a brassy yellow or a fiery red that deceives nobody as to its reality? I cannot say enough against the bleaching or dyeing of the hair. The complexion and the hair are always in harmony, and when you interfere with nature and change the color of your hair, you will suddenly discover that your skin looks dull and faded. Gray hair, which frequently comes to very young women, should not be interfered with, as its tendency is to soften the face and make it look even younger than it is.'

The anonymous author of the *Art of Beauty*, published in London in 1899, was equally disapproving of hair dyes; but for darkening the hair without actually dyeing it, she suggested a mixture of rust of iron, oil of rosemary, and strong old ale (unsweetened), to be shaken daily for a fortnight, each shaking to be followed a few hours later by a decanting of the clear liquid.

She also disapproved of cosmetics but seemed to be on the verge of accepting them, albeit reluctantly, as a fact of life. For those women who refused to use commercially prepared cosmetics on principle, she suggested devious means of achieving the same results—beetroot juice instead of rouge, lampblack for the eyelashes, cologne and cold cream to redden the lips. For ladies whose low-cut gowns revealed skin less white than they might wish, she recommended sponging with perfumed water, thorough drying, then sponging with glycerine and rose water, followed by thickly coating the skin with powder. Then she added, 'The practice of "shading" and accentuating the bosom, though often indulged in, is to my mind neither necessary nor a nice one, and therefore I shall not refer to it.' Outlining the veins, she warned, should be attempted only by experienced hands. As a final caution, she added, 'Remember always to have plenty of light in the room while "making up". To attempt to do without it will prove disastrous and may result in one cheek being perceptibly rosier than the other and the eyebrows of different shades and arches.'

In 1898 Mrs Mallon reported that 'the thick, tightly curled, heavy bang no longer obtains, but there is a decided tendency toward a few loose curls on the forehead. The "blouse roll" remains in favor, but it is usually waved or given what is called the natural ondule, which makes it appear soft and frames the face well. When the hair is arranged high in the back, it is waved from the nape of the neck up, but the waves are not as close as they were. There is a fancy shown for one, two, or even three small curls on the neck. Fillets of ribbon, tortoise shell, or steel are liked, and when the fillet is worn, a comb, a pin, or an aigrette is added.'

As for children's hair styles, she had this to say: 'The little child, whether it be a boy or a girl, is just now wearing its hair in soft ringlets—ringlets that a wise mother has trained in the way they should go.' Mrs Mallon advised the side parting for both boys and girls. 'Older children', she told her readers, 'wear the hair in one or two long braids or loose; crimped hair for children is no longer seen.' In those days it was a wise father who knew his son from his daughter.

PLATE 109 : NINETEENTH-CENTURY WOMEN 1800–1804

(All of the following styles were fashionable in the years indicated.)

A   1800, French.

B   1800, French.

C   1800. French. For afternoon wear.

D   1800. French. For afternoon wear. 'The hair full dressed, light curls around the face, crossed with a silver bandeau, ornamented with diamonds. Esprit feather.'

E   1801, French.

F   1801, English.

G   1801, French. Morning coiffure.

H   1802, French. Wig.

I   1802, French.

J   1802, French. *Titus cut.*

K   1802, French.

L   1803, French.

M   1803, French.

N   1803, French. *Titus cut.*

O   1803, French.

P   1803, French.

Q   1803, French. For evening wear.

R   1803, French. For evening wear.

S   1803, French.

T   1803, French.

U   1804, French.

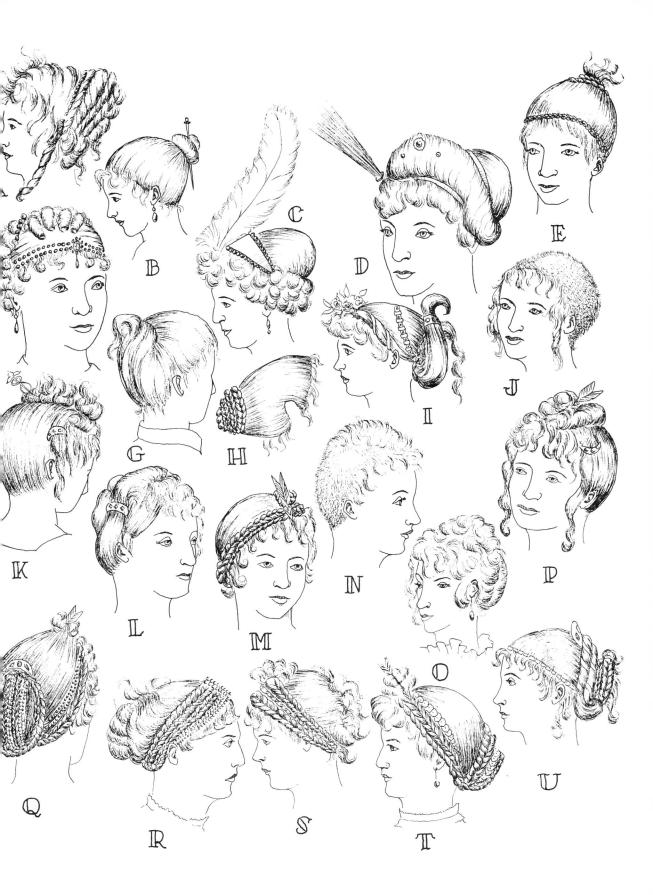

A

B

C

D

E

F

G

H

I

J

K

L

M

N

O

P

Q

R

S

T

U

PLATE 110 : NINETEENTH-CENTURY WOMEN 1804–1807

(All of the following styles were fashionable in the years indicated.)

A 1804, French.

B 1804, French.

C 1804, French.

D 1804, French.

E 1804, French.

F 1804, French.

G 1804, French.

H 1804, French.

I 1804, French. Coiffure of a *demi-élégante*.

J 1804, French.

K 1805, French.

L 1805, French. Combs ornamented with topazes and pearls.

M 1805, French.

N 1805, French.

O 1805, French.

P 1806, French.

Q 1805, French.

R 1806, French.

S 1806.

T 1806, French.

U 1806, French.

V 1806, French.

W 1807.

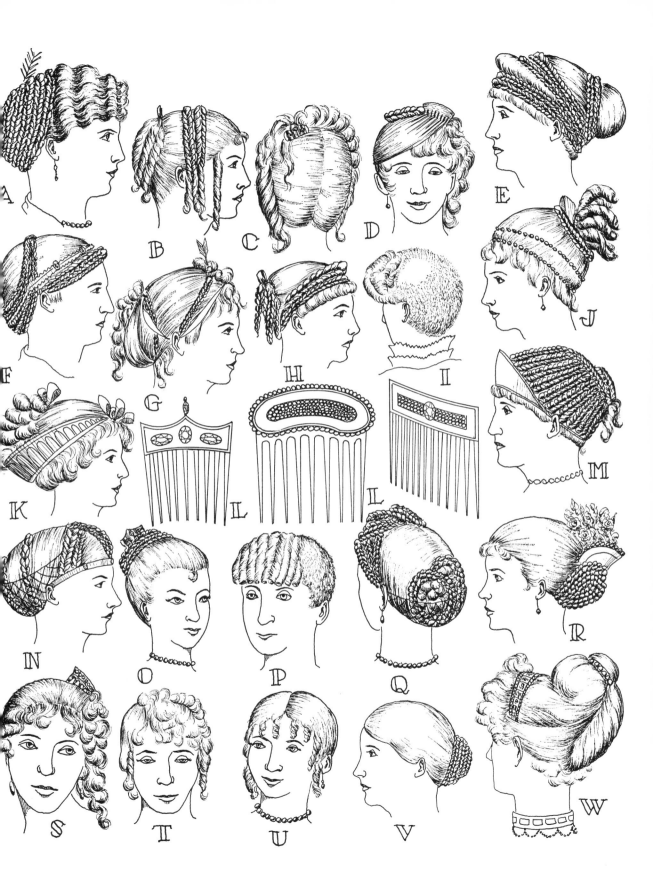

A B C D E
F G H I J
K L L M
N O P Q R
S T U V W

PLATE III : NINETEENTH-CENTURY WOMEN 1807–1811

(Most of the following styles were fashionable in the years indicated.)

A 1807.

B 1807, French.

C 1807, French.

D 1807.

E 1807.

F 1807.

G 1807.

H 1808, French.

I 1808, French.

J 1809, French. *À la Ninon* (after Ninon de Lenclos, who is supposed to have clipped off her curls and sent them to her lover, M. de Villarceaux).

K 1809. *À la Ninon.* Wig.

L 1809, French.

M 1810, French. *À l'enfant.*

N 1810, French. *À l'enfant.*

O 1810, French.

P 1810, French.

Q 1810, French.

R 1810.

S 1811, French. Wig.

T 1811, French.

U 1811, French.

V 1811, French.

W 1811.

X 1811, French.

Y 1811, French.

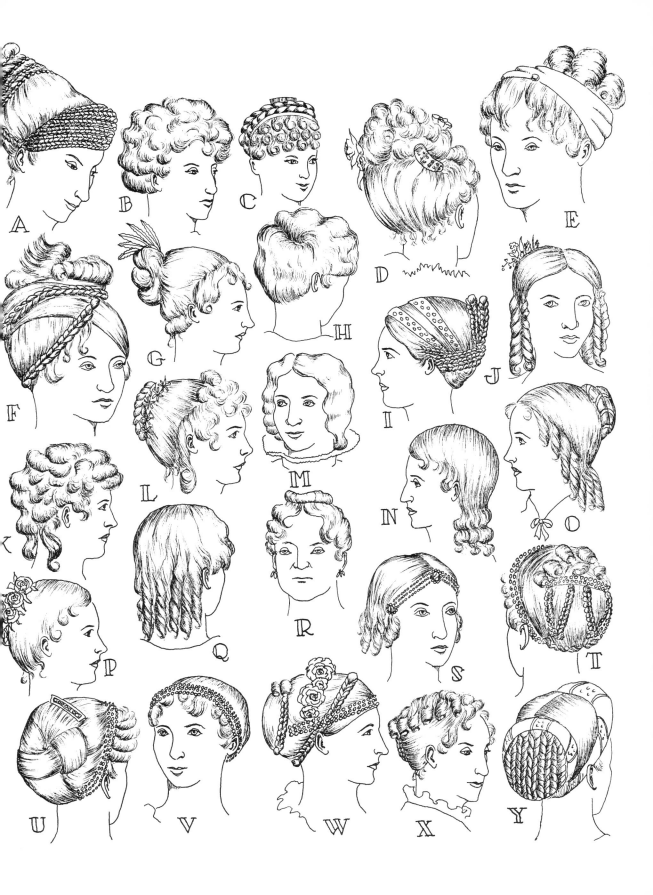

PLATE 112 : NINETEENTH-CENTURY WOMEN 1812–1815

A 1812, French. *À la chinoise.*

B 1812, French.

C *c.* 1812, French.

D 1812, French.

E 1812, French. *À la chinoise.*

F 1813, French. *À la demi-chinoise.*

G 1813, French.

H 1813, French. *À la chinoise.*

I 1813.

J 1813, French. *À la chinoise.*

K 1813, French.

L 1813, French.

M 1813, French. *À la chinoise.*

N 1813.

O 1814, French.

P 1814.

Q *c.* 1814.

R 1814, French.

S 1814, German.

T 1814, French.

U 1814, French.

V 1814, French.

W 1814, French.

X 1815.

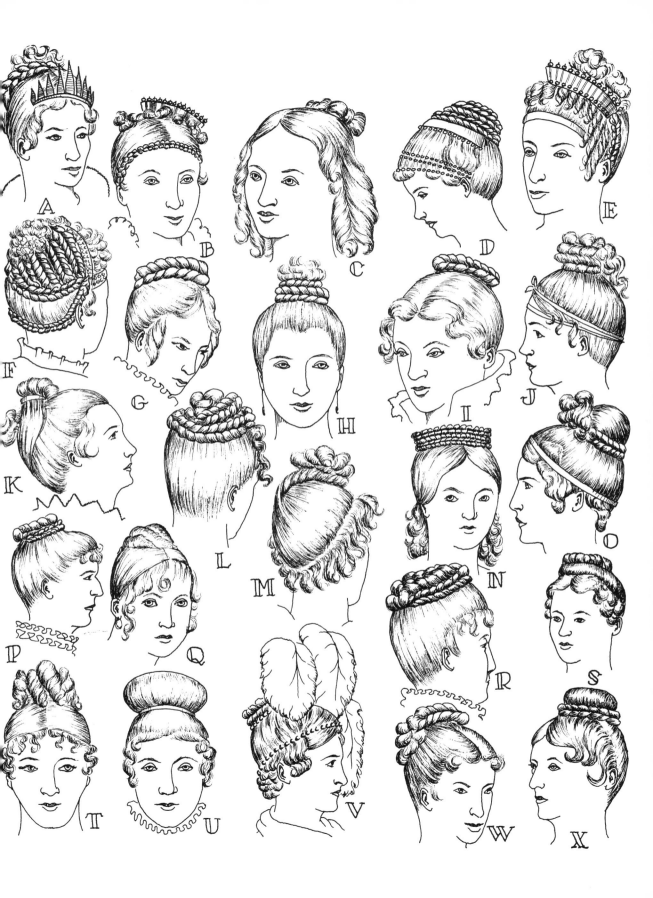

PLATE 113 : NINETEENTH-CENTURY WOMEN 1815–1821

A   1815, French.

B, C   1815, French.

D   1815.

E   1815, French.

F   1815, French.

G   1816, French.

H, I   1816, French.

J   1816, French.

K   1816.

L   1816, French.

M   1816, French.

N   1817, French.

O   1817, French.

P   1817, English.

Q   1817, German.

R   1818, French.

S   1818, French.

T   1819.

U   1819, French.

V   1820, French.

W   c. 1820, American. Maria Monroe Gouverneur, daughter of James Monroe.

X   1820, English.

Y   1821, French.

Z   1821, French.

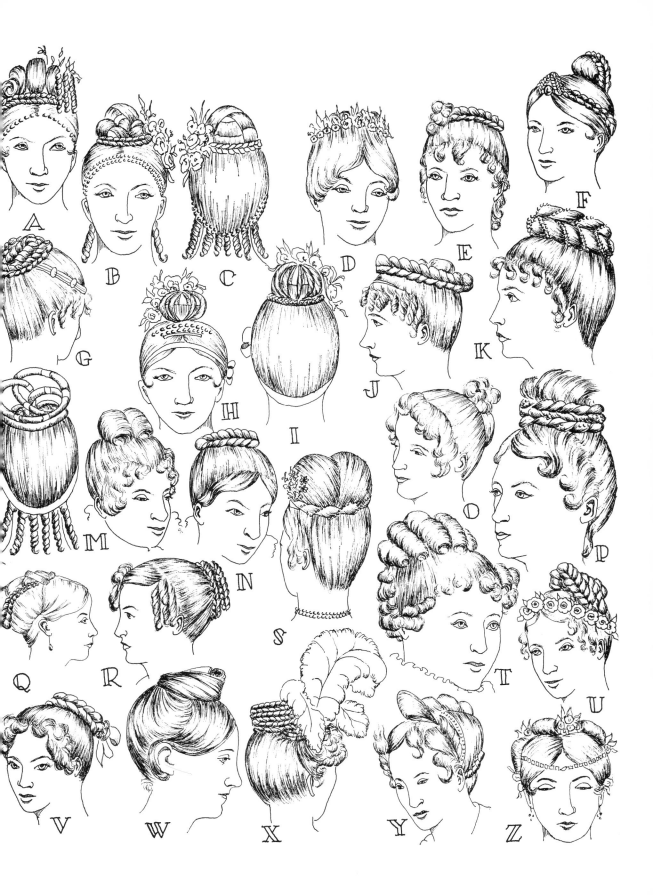

A

B

C

D

E

F

G

H

I

J

K

M

N

O

P

Q

R

S

T

U

V

W

X

Y

Z

PLATE 114 : NINETEENTH-CENTURY WOMEN 1821–1825

A   1821, French.

B   1821, French.

C   1822, French.

D   1822.

E   1822.

F   1823, French.

G   1823.

H   1823.

I   1824. For evening wear.

J   1824. Coiffure with Apollo knot, to be worn to a ball.

K   1824.

L   1824. For evening wear.

M   1825, English.

N   1824.

O   1825, American. Louisa C. Adams.

P   1824, English. Duchess.

Q   1825, French.

R   1825. To be worn to a ball.

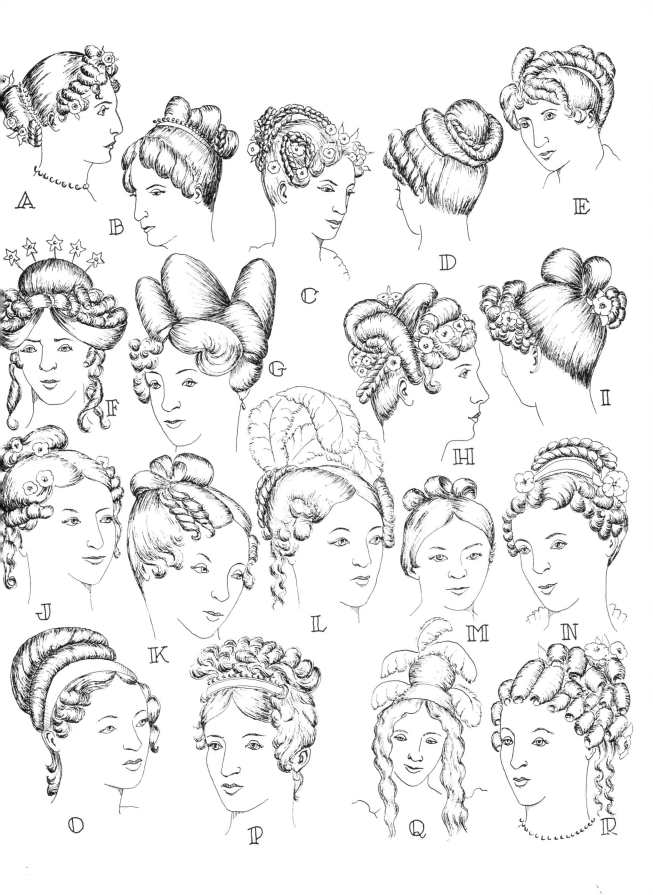

A

B

C

D

E

F

G

H

I

J

K

L

M

N

O

P

Q

R

PLATE 115 : NINETEENTH-CENTURY WOMEN 1825–1829

A   1825. For evening wear. Apollo knot and circular gold band.

B   1825. For evening wear.

C   1825. For the theatre.

D   1825. Coiffure for a ball.

E   1825, French.

F   1825. For a dinner-party.

G   1826. For an evening at home.

H   1825.

I   1826. For an afternoon at home.

J, K   1826.

L   1827. For evening wear.

M   1827. Coiffure for a ball.

N   1828.

O   1828.

P   1828, English.

Q   1828. For evening wear.

R   1829.

S   1829. For evening wear.

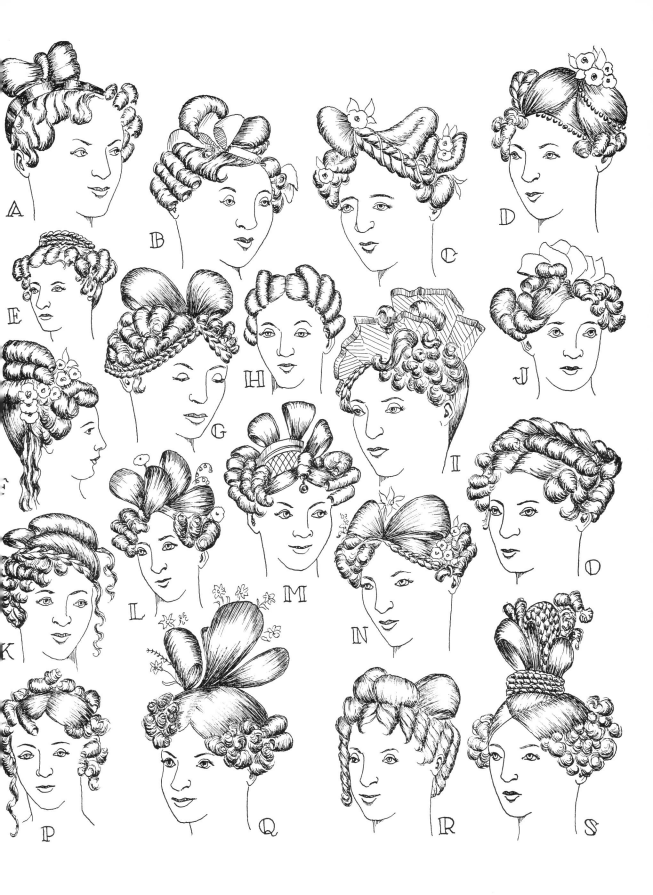

A

B

C

D

E

G

H

I

J

K

L

M

N

O

P

Q

R

S

PLATE 116 : NINETEENTH-CENTURY WOMEN 1830–1834

A   1830.

B-D   1831.

E-H   1832. *Godey's Lady's Book* reported in the spring of 1832 that 'The low Grecian arrangement of the hair in the severe classic taste of the antique is universally adopted by ladies whose outline will admit of this often most unbecoming style. Coronets of pearls, cameos, or flowers are worn very low on the brow. Gold beads or pearls are woven with the braided hair. The high gallery shell combs are now as vulgar as the ferronnière. In place of carved shell combs, combs on which four or five classic cameos are arranged en couronne, are worn in full dress.' A vulgar ferronnière is shown in F above. For an arrangement to be worn with a ball gown, *Godey's* suggested 'hair braided with gold beads in Grecian bands and a low coronet and large knot, ornamented with plumes or silver barley, à la Ceres'. The following arrangement for evening was also described: 'The hair is banded à la Grecque, small knot on the crown, from which depend a number of ringlets à la Sévigné, is ornamented with a high crown of small field flowers; two half garlands of the same nearly meet on the brow'.

I-N   1833.

O   1834. In this year *Godey's* reported that 'Although there is a good deal of variety in headdresses of hair, yet we observe that low ones are in a majority. Several are adorned with a diadem of gold enriched with precious stones, brought low upon the forehead. Others are trimmed with two *gerbes* of flowers. The one is placed on the curls on the right side and rises in the style of a feather. The other is placed on the left side, drooping over it and mingling with the curls. In some instances the hair is disposed in plaited braids, which fall low and doubled at the sides of the face; but this fashion is very partially adopted, curls being much more general.'

P   1834. 'The hair is divided on the forehead, falls in loose curls at the sides of the face and is combed up tight to the summit of the head, where it is arranged in a cluster of light bows, in which a sprig composed of coloured gems is inserted. A bandeau composed also of colored gems is brought from the sprig round the forehead.'

Q, R   1834.

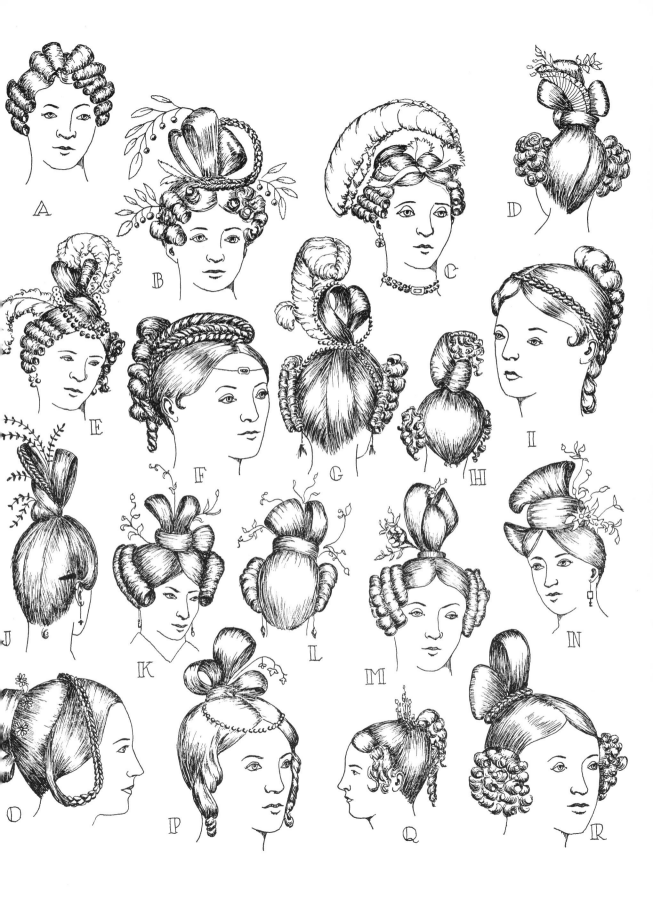

A

B

C

D

E

F

G

H

I

J

K

L

M

N

O

P

Q

R

PLATE 117 : NINETEENTH-CENTURY WOMEN 1835–1837

A   1835. Style of Maria Christina, Queen of Naples.

B   *c.* 1835. Empress Augusta of Germany.

C   1835.

D   1835.

E   1835.

F   *c.* 1835–38, German. Frau von Vernus. *A la Clotilde* (see also Plates 118-A-J and 119-C-D).

G   1835.

H   *c.* 1835.

I   1835. For evening wear.

J   1835. For evening wear.

K   1835.

L   *c.* 1835. Polish.

M   1836, French.

N   1836, French.

O   1836. For evening wear. 'The hair is parted *à la madonna* in the forehead, arranged in a round knot behind, and ornamented with a full-blown rose and foliage, placed two on one side.'

P   1837. Child.

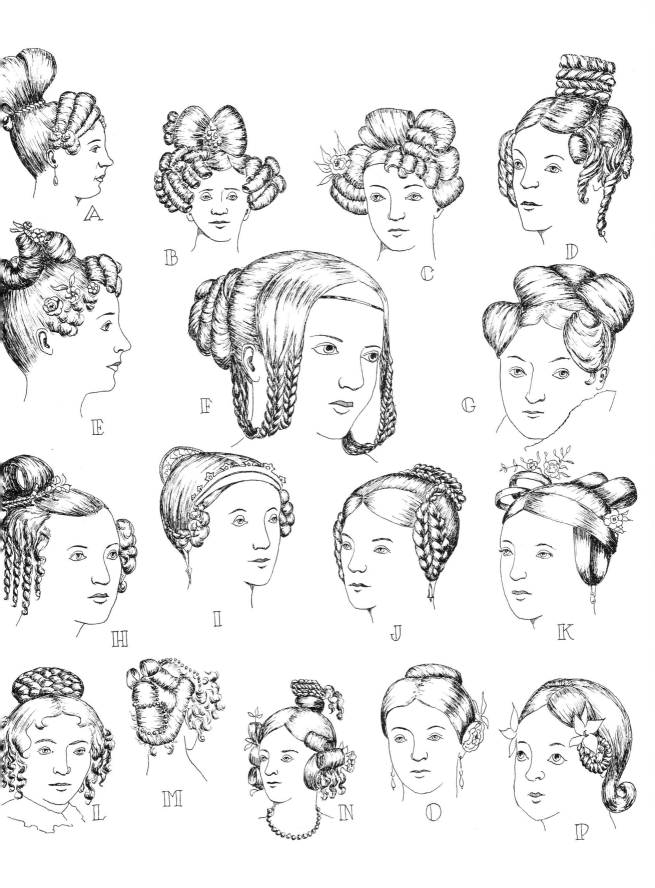

PLATE 118 : NINETEENTH-CENTURY WOMEN 1837–1840

(According to *Townsend's Monthly Selection of Parisian Costumes* for 1837, 'some coiffures are very low, quite in the Grecian style; others are raised up *à la Chinoise*. Some have the hair in bands in front, others again in large tufts, or in ringlets, on each side of the face. Many ladies adopt the two large twists, named *à la Clotilde*, which descend half down the cheeks and then are carried up towards the top of the coiffure.' All of these styles are illustrated on the opposite page. Plates 117 and 119 show additional examples.)

A   1837. *À la Clotilde* combined with elevated bows (see also J below as well as 117-F and 119-C-D).

B   1837. Child.

C   1838. *À la Chinoise*. Front hair in bands with ringlets.

D   1838.

E   1838.

F   1838. Front hair in bands. Note V-shaped parting (see also O below).

G   1838.

H   1838. Front hair in bands.

I   1838. Lydia Huntley Sigourney. Poetess.

J   1839. For a child's coiffure the braid can be let down and allowed to hang free from the crown with a ribbon bow at the end.

K   1839.

L   1840.

M   1840.

N   1840. Little girl.

O   1840.

P   1840. Note double parting, front to back.

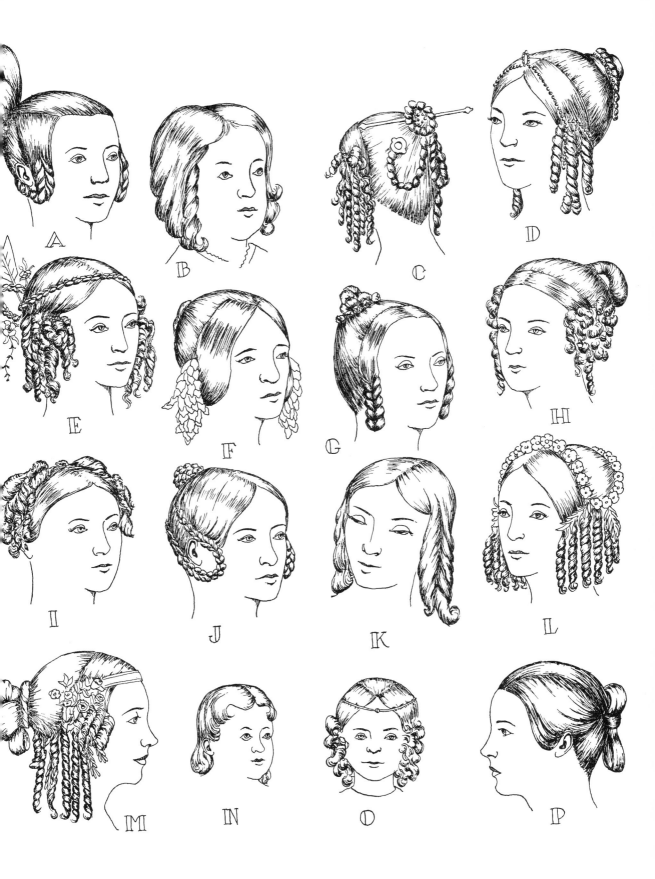

A

B

C

D

E

F

G

H

I

J

K

L

M

N

O

P

PLATE 119 : NINETEENTH-CENTURY WOMEN 1840–1844

A 1840.

B 1841.

C 1841.

D 1841, English. Queen Victoria, 1837–1901 (for later portrait see Plate 139-G).

E, F 1841. Front and back views.

G 1841.

H 1842.

I 1842.

J 1842.

K 1842. Servant or middle-class housewife.

L 1842.

M 1842.

N 1843.

O 1843.

P 1844. Servant. Note how the current style has been followed but has not been carefully executed or maintained. This happens in all periods and is very useful in suggesting personality, social position, etc.

Q 1844.

R 1844.

S 1844, French.

T 1844. Coiffure for a ball.

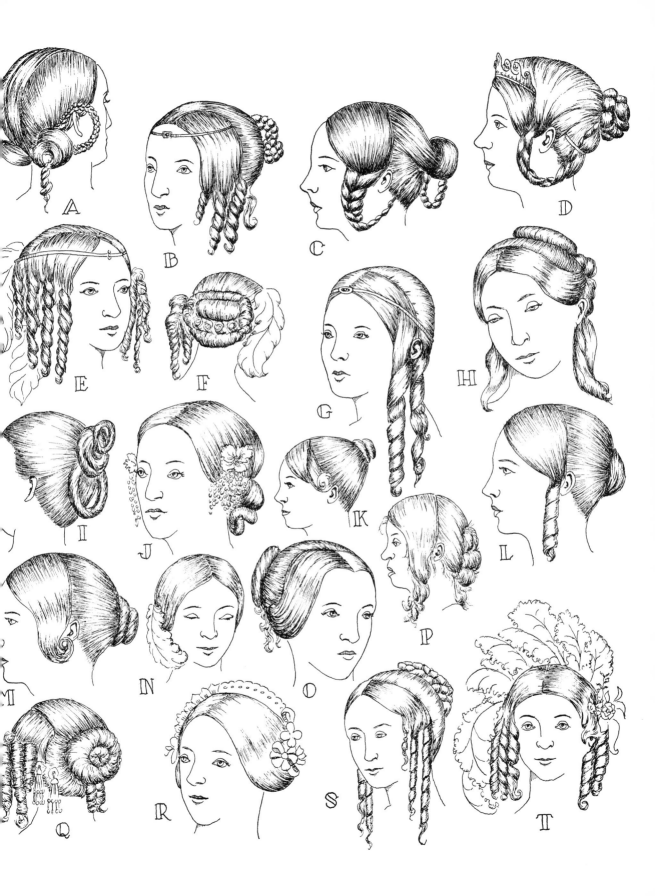

A   B   C   D

E   F   G   H

I   J   K   L

M   N   O   P

Q   R   S   T

A   1844.

B, C   1845.

D   Mrs Charles Dickens.

E, F   1846.

G   Charlotte Brontë.

H, I, J   1847.

K, L   1848.

M, N   1848. Back and side views.

O, P, Q   1848.

R, S   1849. Front and side. 'The first curl is next to the face. Above it is a row of lace, over which is the second curl, surmounted by a second row of lace. The third curl is carried round to the back part of the neck, as is also the lace which surmounts it. The back hair, after being tied, is divided into two parts and plaited in Grecian plaits. One of these plaits is fixed at the back part of the head, and the other is carried across the upper part of the forehead, like a coronet.' In the side view 'it will be observed that the disposal of the plaits presents precisely the effect of the antique diadem. The lace employed may be either black or white, but blonde is preferable to lace, being lighter. It may be observed that the edge should be either in scallops or vandykes, not straight. This coiffure . . . may be brought down low on each side of the face if desired.'

T   1850.

U, V   1849. Two views of the same coiffure. 'The front hair is arranged in smooth bandeaux on the forehead, descending at each side so as to completely cover the ears. The back hair is divided into several small twists, one of which is carried round the head in the manner of a turban. Below the twist are three rows of fancy French beads of a lozenge form, in imitation pearl. A single row of the same beads passes along the back part of the head, intermingling with the twists.'

W   1850.

X   1850.

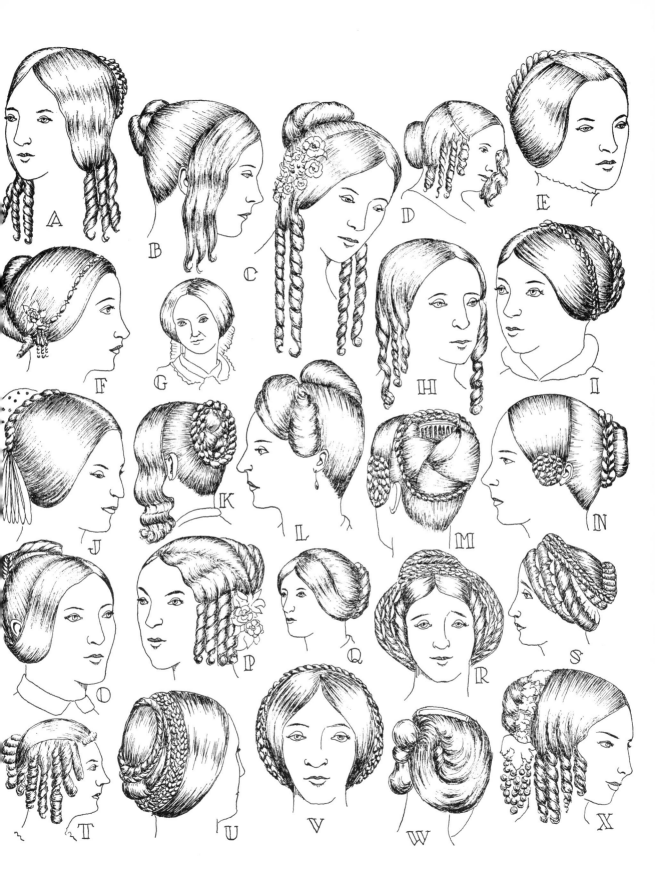

A

B

C

D

E

F

G

H

I

J

K

L

M

N

O

P

Q

R

S

T

U

V

W

X

PLATE 121 : NINETEENTH-CENTURY WOMEN 1851–1854

A   1851.

B-J, L   1852.

M, N   1853.

K, O-R   1854.

S, T   1854. Back and front. For parties. 'The front hair is parted horizontally on each side of the forehead into three distinct divisions, each of which is turned back and forms a roll. These *rouleaux* may be made either of the hair alone or by rolling it on small silk cushions, covered with hair-colored silk. In front they are divided by bandeaux of Roman pearls.' The back hair is 'entwined with the pearls very low on the neck and fastened by two pearl-headed pins of an antique bodkin pattern'.

In 1853 *Godey's Lady's Book* gave the following instructions for various ways of plaiting hair:

'*Grecian Plait* is woven as follows: Take a tolerably thin lock of hair; divide it into two equal parts. Take from the outside of the left-hand portion a very small piece of hair—about a sixth part—pass it over into the centre, and unite it with the right hand portion. Do the same from the right hand portion and pass it over into the centre and unite it with the left hand portion. Proceed thus, taking the small and even-sized lock alternately from the left and right hand portions until all is plaited. Be careful to keep this plait very smooth.

'*The Cable Plait*. Take three pretty thick strands of hair of equal size, place one in the centre. Take the left hand strand and lift it under the centre one and over it and back to its own place. Take the right hand strand and lift that under the outer one, and over it and back to its place. Work on thus alternately to the end. The best way of wearing this is to divide the back hair into two equal portions and then make two "cables" and having twisted them round each other, to wind this double cable round the head.

'The *Basket* or *Chain Plait*. Take four rather small strands of hair, plait with only three of these, weaving them over and under the fourth, which serves to draw the chain up, as in the way in which a plait of three is usually worked, taking first the left hand outside strand and working it under one and over the next until it takes the place of the right outside strand, which in its turn, is then worked to the left side, and so on alternately, always retaining one unmoved in the middle.'

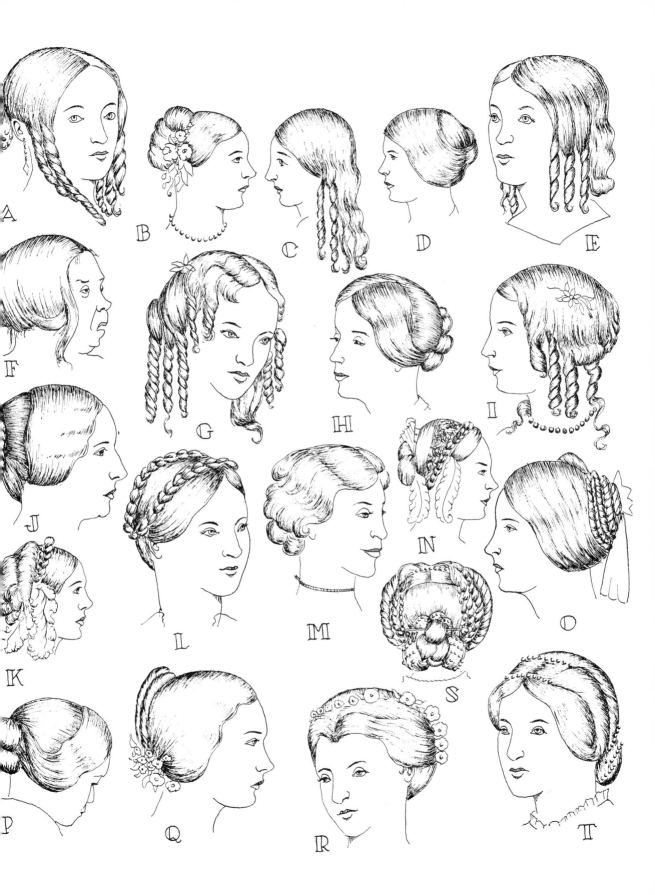

A
B
C
D
E
F
G
H
I
J
K
L
M
N
O
S
P
Q
R
T

PLATE 122 : NINETEENTH-CENTURY WOMEN 1854–1857

A   1854.

B   1854.

C   1855.

D   1855.

E   1855.

F   1855. Child.

G   1855.

H   1855.

I   1855. For evening wear.

J   1855.

K   1856. For evening wear.

L   1856. 'A simple head-dress for a school girl, intended for examinations, concerts, juvenile parties, etc. The hair is divided through the middle, quite to the neck and rolled *under* on each side, *cache-peigne* of natural flowers and foliage.'

M   1856. For evening wear.

N   *c.* 1856.

O   1856.

P, R   1856. 'The hair is parted so that nearly all is used in front, and this is subdivided into two parts. The bands are first puffed smoothly over the ears. The second division is then rolled *forward* over the ribbon. The ends turn under the comb. The remaining portion at the back is turned *across* the small ornamented comb and four ribbon loops placed so as to conceal all but the broad plait from view. The large roll forward is the newest point in the arrangement of the hair. It is sometimes drawn back instead of being parted on the forehead, and a heavy braid passed under it in place of the ribbon. This is also very new and effective.'

Q   Florence Nightingale.

S   1857.

T   1857.

Godey's had these suggestions about the fashions for 1856: 'In addition to many new coiffures composed of flowers, foliage, or feathers, we have seen several consisting entirely of pearls, coral, or jet. Those formed of a combination of flowers and ribbons may, however, be mentioned as among the most tasteful which have yet appeared. Others consist of several rows of excessively small foliage in crepe or velvet—the rows being disposed crosswise in the trellis or net manner. These nets of foliage are intermingled with lillies of the valley in gold or by bows of green gauze ribbon figured with gold, combined with the sprays of the flowers above mentioned. Head-dresses in the net form, like that we have just described, are also made in coral and pearls.'

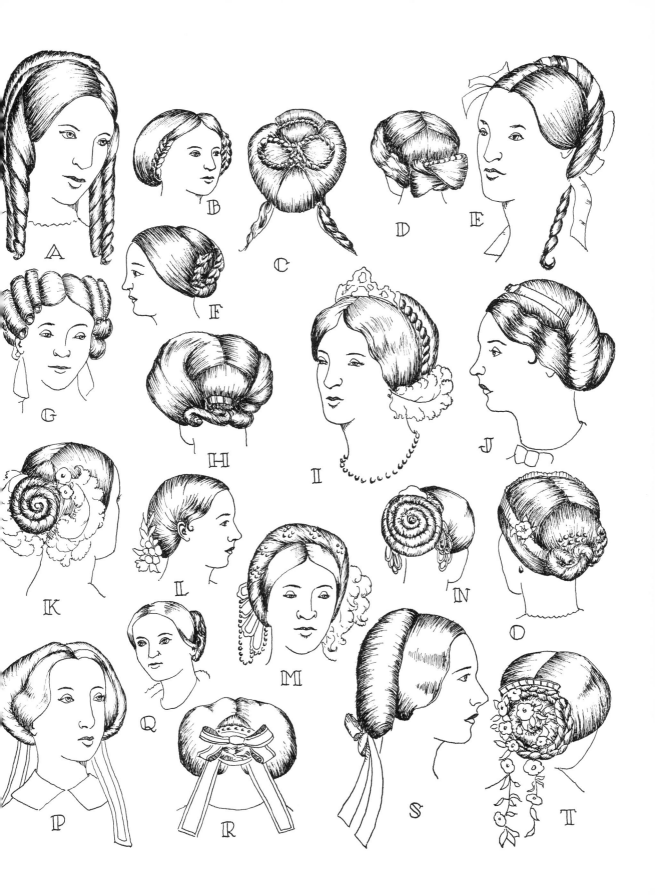

A B C D E F G H I J K L M N O P Q R S T

PLATE 123 : NINETEENTH-CENTURY WOMEN 1858, 1859

A 1858.

B 1858. Style worn in the French court.

C 1858. 'This ornament is at once new and tasteful. It is composed of large beads, etc. . . . It is to be found already at Bailey's and will be much in favor for the watering-place season, from its novelty and simplicity. It is kept in place by an arrow of gold or silver.'

D 1859.

E 1859.

F 1859.

G 1859.

H 1859, French.

I, J 1859, French. Back and front views. For evening wear.

K, L 1859, French. Front and back views.

M 1859, French.

N, O 1859, French. Front and back views. Inspired by portraits of Anne of Austria.

P 1859, French.

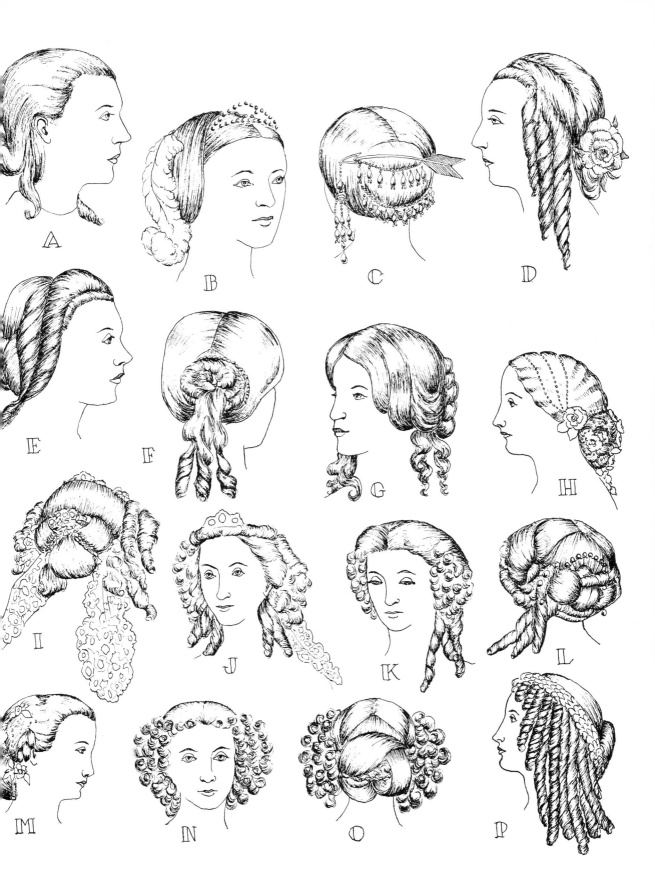

A

B

C

D

E

F

G

H

I

J

K

L

M

N

O

P

PLATE 124 : NINETEENTH-CENTURY WOMEN 1860

A   French. For evening wear.

B, C   Front and back views.

D   Fashionable coiffure for a soirée.

E   For daytime wear.

F, G   Back and front. 'La coiffure française'.

H   For daytime wear.

I, J   Hair style for a young lady. 'The whole head of hair is parted from the centre of the forehead to the nape of the neck. Then a transverse parting is made from ear to ear so that the hair is divided into four equal masses. The two portions of the front hair are arranged in plaitings of three, care being taken to comb the hair back from the forehead and to include all the front hair in the plaits. The plaiting of each portion of the back hair should commence just above the ear, and the ends must be carefully fastened by silk or very fine twist. The plait of back hair on the right hand side is passed across the nape of the neck, and the end is fastened by a hairpin under the root of the plait on the left side. The plait of the left side of the back hair is brought round to the right side and fastened in the same manner; and thus the two plaits cross each other at the back of the neck. The plaits of the front hair are then brought round to the back of the neck, where the ends are fastened under the crossing of the plaits of back hair.'

K   Fashionable coiffure for evening.

L, M   For wear at home.

N   Unfashionable style.

O, P   Style for ball or evening wear. 'In front this coiffure shows the hair disposed in three rouleaux, terminating in long ringlets, and also behind the ears are several ringlets of shorter length. The back hair is arranged in a cluster of five loops, to form which the hair is tied firmly at the back of the head and divided into five portions. The center loop at the back of the neck is very long and the two at each side of shorter length. The ends of the hair are twisted round the tie at the back of the head and concealed beneath an ornament of beads suspended from the top of the comb. Amongst the ringlets and rouleaux of the front hair are interspersed small stars and other brilliant ornaments, which, being fixed on elastic pins, are set in motion by every turn of the wearer's head, thereby producing a most elegant and showy effect. The same kind of pins are employed for fixing the tufts of white feathers, which add much to the grace and dignity of the coiffure. The jewelled agraffe worn in the centre of the forehead should correspond with the other ornaments of the headdress.'

Note: The descriptions are taken from *Godey's Lady's Book*.

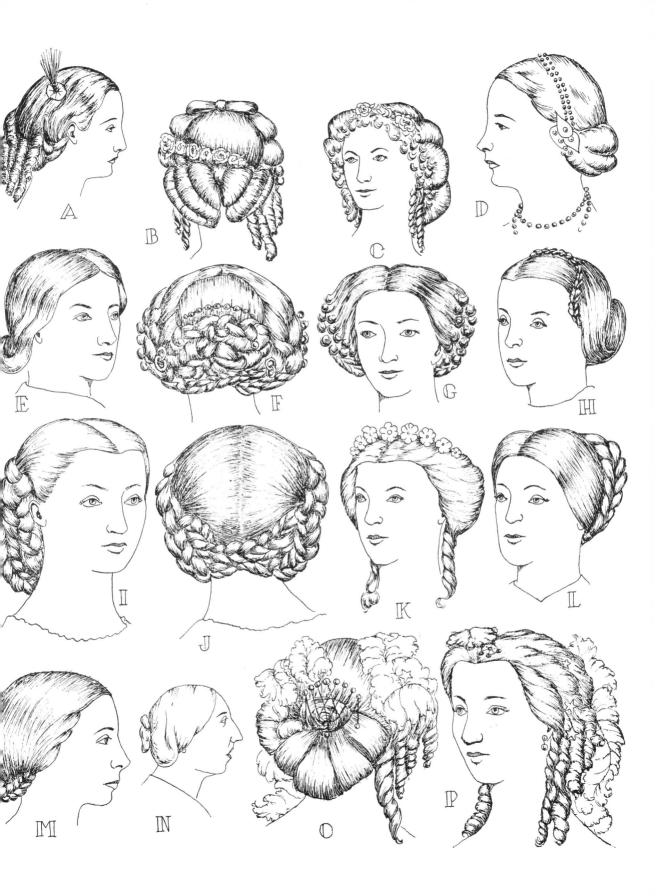

A

B

C

D

E

F

G

H

I

J

K

L

M

N

O

P

Plate 125 : Nineteenth-Century Women 1861–1863

A   1861.

B, C   1861, French. Front and back.

D, E   1861.

F, G   1861, French. Front and back.

H   1862. 'The front hair instead of being separated, as is usually the case, is taken as one strand. The braid is taken in the centre and plaited in a 3-plait. When it is plaited, turn the plait toward the back and comb the upper part of the hair over it. This will give the appearance of a roll and braid. If the roll is not becoming, turn the plait to the front and have it alone. The small lock at the end of the braid is intended to twist round the coil at the back and keep the braids firm.'

I-O   1862.

P, Q   1863, French. Front and back. 'The front coiffure consists of a full roll and a plait of three strands. The fall at the back can be of fake hair, pinned on, and the front plaits twisted round it.'

R   1863. 'The hair is arranged in two puffs on one side and the other in short frizzed curls.'

S, T   Back and front. 'The hair is parted very far back, almost to the neck, reserving but a small portion in which to catch the comb. The front hair is brushed off from the face and rolled forward over a fancy colored ribbon. A succession of rolls falls below this upper one and is carried to the back, where the fastenings are concealed by loops of ribbon which fall from the comb.'

Note: The descriptions are all taken from *Godey's Lady's Book*.

In 1862, according to *Godey's Lady's Book*, the new style for dressing the hair was 'a short rolled bandeau, which is generally waved. Upon this there is arranged a second bandeau turned back *à la Impératrice*, and the two are separated by small side combs, which are made in endless variety and give an air of piquant coquetterie to the head. When worn in the daytime, these small combs are made of light tortoiseshell, either with a row of small pearls, also in shell, very closely ranged together, or cut in clubs, points, or hearts for the evening. They are made of dead gold, either quite plain or studded with pearl, coral, steel, gilt, or even precious stones, according to the toilet with which they are worn. Sometimes the Greek design is worked in black enamel upon the dead gold. The comb at the back should correspond exactly with the side combs. Ivory combs are still worn, also shell with ivory ball tops. Among the prettiest shell are some with ball tops studded with tiny gilt stars.'

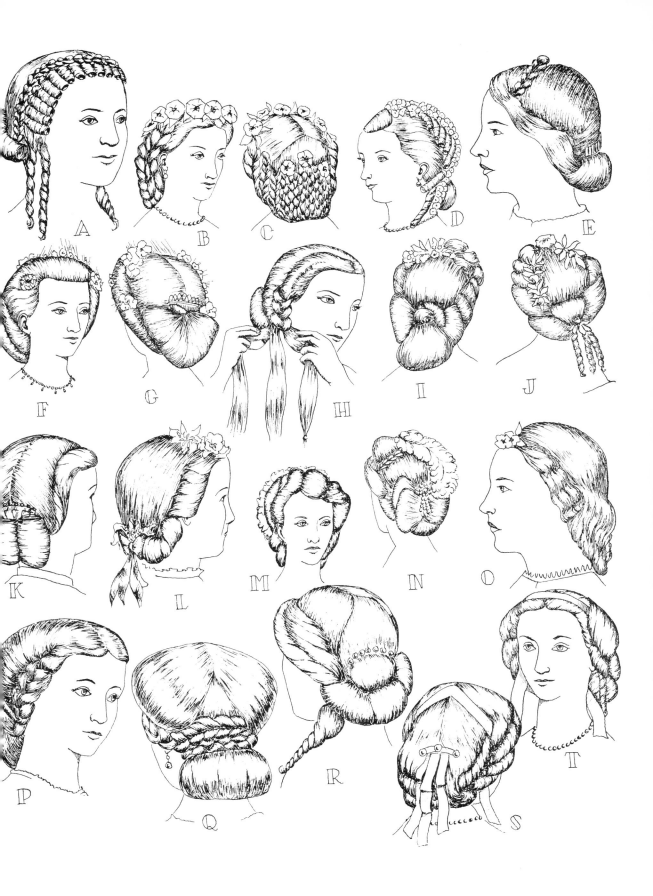

PLATE 126 : NINETEENTH-CENTURY WOMEN 1864, 1865

A   1864, French.

B, C   1864, French. Front and back.

D, E   1864, French. Back and front.

F   1864, French.

G   1864, French.

H, I   1864, French. Back and front.

J-M   1864, French. Chignons of false hair used to extend the natural hair and simplify dressing it. They were attached with a comb at the top and secured with hairpins.

N   1864, French. False curls attached to a hairpin. They could easily be stuck in wherever needed.

O, P   1864, French. Front and back.

Q-EE   1864–65, French. Chignons and braids of false hair.

FF, GG   1865, French. Front and back.

HH, II   1865, French. Back and front.

JJ, KK   1865, French. Back and side.

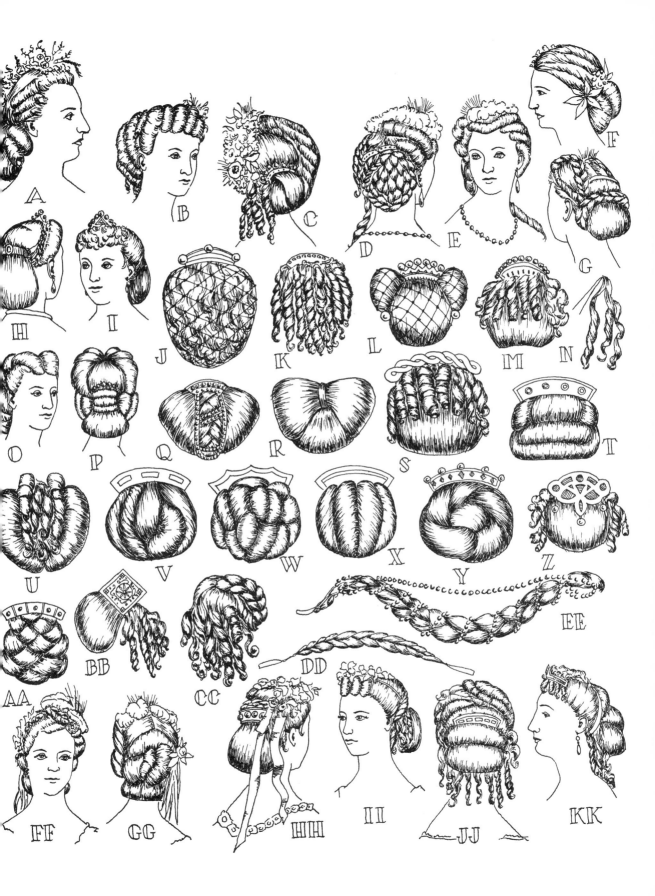

A

B

C

D

E

F

G

H

I

J

K

L

M

N

O

P

Q

R

S

T

U

V

W

X

Y

Z

AA

BB

CC

DD

EE

FF

GG

HH

II

JJ

KK

A   1866, French.

B, C   1866, French. Back and front. 'Make the middle parting and another across, not far above the forehead. The rest of the hair, having been tied behind, must be crisped and formed into a hollow roll. Next add a large tress, also crisped in hollow rolls, which must be placed one over the other. Divide the front hair into two parts on each side. Slightly crisp the upper one and apply a narrow velvet ribbon atop. Turn the ribbon round the hair as if to make an undulation with a double cordon. Push it back the same, without drawing too tight, then make a small puff on the temples with the ends. A small loop at top, behind the undulations. Add a ringlet and a few small curls at the sides. A trail of roses at the sides.'

D, E   1866, French. 'Make the middle parting, and then another across, about 4 inches from the forehead. Next form a small Mary Stuart on the temples and 2 curls on the forehead. The hair behind should be tied very low. Divide it into 5 parts and make them into loops rolled upwards like curls. Place a cluster of curls on the top of the head. Let a few of the small ones fall in front and the rest behind. Put a row of small curls to fall on the neck.'

F   1866, French. 'Separate a lock of hair on each side of the temples. Comb the rest *à la Chinoise* to the top of the head. Tie the back hair very tight. Put some very light small false curls over the forehead. Arrange a torsade in a round form behind with a small *cache-peigne* lightly curled in the middle. Place on the top of the head a small cluster of curls negligently scattered. Apply the ribbon as shown, and on each side of the chignon add a few curls on pins to complete the coiffure.'

G-J   1866, French.

K   1866, French. 'Separate a portion of the hair on the temples to make a small Mary Stuart. The remainder, combed back in the Chinese style and divided into five parts, is to be arranged in rolled loops, with a small addition of false hair. Lightly curl the hair in small rings just over the forehead. Now put a few large false curls on the top of the head.'

L   1866, French. 'Plain coiffure for home or city.'

M-W   1866–68, French. Chignons of false hair.

X, Y   1867, French. 'Make a parting to about four inches from the forehead and one across. Tie the back hair. In front, wave two locks so that the curls may keep their form naturally. Divide the hair on the temples horizontally, turn the waved lock back *à la chinoise*, raise the hair of the upper part of the temples above so that the waved lock may come between the two smoothed parts. Slightly crisp the top of the small bandeau to fill up the void between the front and the chignon. Behind, divide the hair into four parts, crisp it slightly and turn it to the left, placing the crisps in opposite directions to give the contour which completes the chignon. One of the rolls terminates in a ringlet a yard long.'

Z-II   1868, French. Coiffures, chignons, and combs.

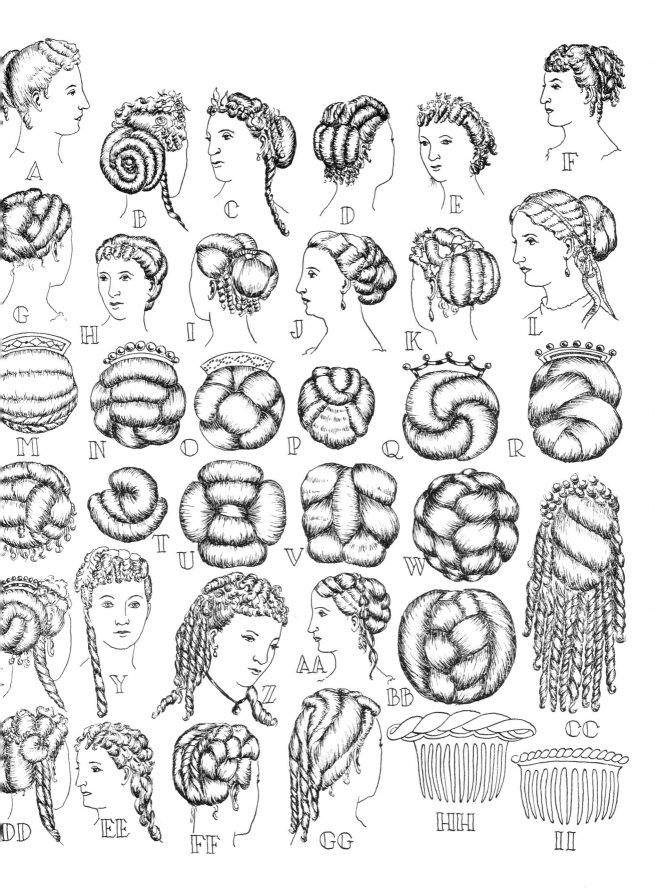

A

B

C

D

E

F

G

H

I

J

K

L

M

N

O

P

Q

R

S

T

U

V

W

X

Y

Z

AA

BB

CC

DD

EE

FF

GG

HH

II

PLATE 128 : NINETEENTH-CENTURY WOMEN 1869, 1870

A   1869, French. 'In front make two small marteaux with the comb, two relevés straight up from the roots on each side. A large *cache-peigne* completes the coiffure.'

B, C   1869, French. Front and back.

D   1869, French. Adapted from a style of the Middle Ages. 'This coiffure is composed in front of small superimposed bandeaux, while the hair behind is divided into four parts on each side and raised in loose torsades. Should the lady's hair be deficient in length or quantity, a few small tresses must be added. A comb inserted so deeply as to leave only its top visible completes this very original coiffure.'

E   1869, French. 'Part the hair three inches from the forehead. Take a lock on the top of the head to serve as a fastening. On each side make two relevés, and with the ends form a loop returning over them. Behind, two more relevés straight up from the roots. With the ends make diversified loops, and with three or four curls placed irregularly, the coiffure is completed.'

F-I   1869, French.

J, K   1869, French. 'Make a parting to three inches from the forehead, and another across some distance behind the ears. Make a foundation just on top of the head. With the front hair form a bandeau *à la vierge*, sloping off backward. Behind make limp loops interlaced, which must accompany the ears and rather low. Then, make in the middle a marquise chignon falling on the nape, and add a cluster of drooping curls.'

L   1869, French.

M   1869, French. 'Part the hair to about 4 inches in from the forehead, and also from ear to ear. After placing a small plat as a foundation, wave a lock on each side. Make a bandeau somewhat in the Russian style. The upper lock should be well crisped and turned inwards, the second less crisped and turned outwards, the waving very flat and sloping. The hair on the temples must also be turned outwards. Behind, divide the hair into 3 parts. Make 2 torsades rather low on the neck, and interlace them. Divide the third part, which is in the middle, into 2 portions; splice a plat to each and make a loose figure 8. A few curls of unequal length, a few flowers, and a diadem comb give a most pleasing finish to the coiffure.'

N-P   1869-70, French. Chignons of false hair.

Q   1869, French. 'The chignon is mounted on a wire ribbon. The mounting is round and about 4 inches in diameter. The centre is quadrilled. To make it you will require $3\frac{1}{2}$ ounces of frizzed hair from 24 to 30 inches in length. To execute it, roll the hair on itself, which is much more easily done when the hair is frizzed, and let 7 or 8 curls fall from the middle of the chignon.'

R-U   False hair.

Note: The quotations are all taken from *Moniteur de la Coiffure*.

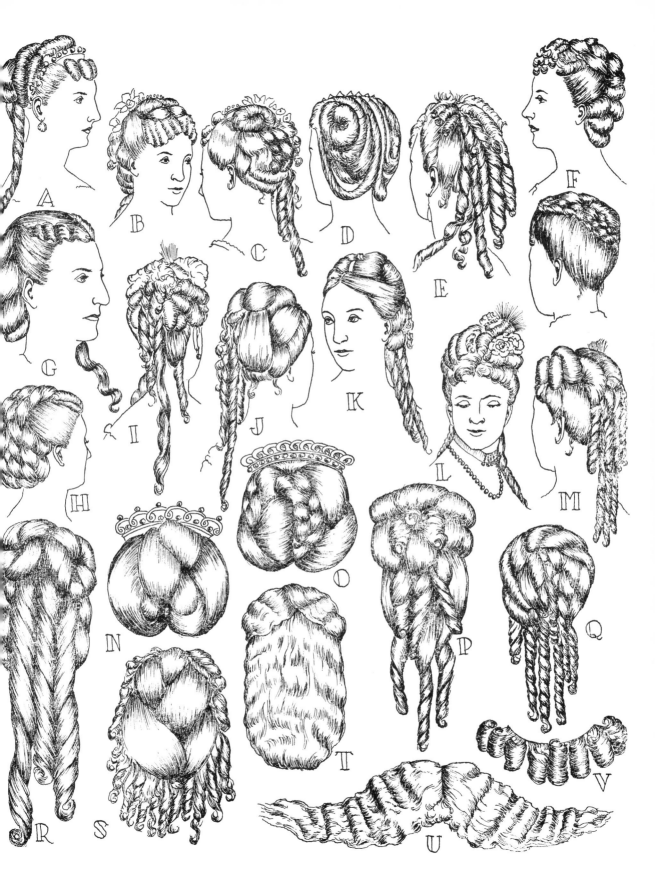

A

B

C

D

E

F

G

H

I

J

K

L

M

N

O

P

Q

R

S

T

U

V

PLATE 129 : NINETEENTH-CENTURY WOMEN 1870–1872

A, B, C   1870, French.

D   1870, French. 'Part the hair to 4 inches from the forehead. Make a side parting. Form a separation with the portion on the left. Wave the hair near the forehead. Then divide the rest into two parts and form a large torsade. Make a loop on top of the head and place the torsade upon it in order to imitate detached rouleaux. The side is raised by gently combing up from the roots. Below, a torsade prolonged on the neck. Right side, two relevés not too much turned and fastened behind. A few light curls complete the coiffure.'

E   1870, French. 'Divide the hair into two equal parts from the forehead to the nape. Take a small lock on top of the head, plait it, and roll it on itself. This is the support of the whole coiffure. Heat wave a lock large enough to make the bandeaux which are to be fastened on the plat, and preserve the ends. With the remainder of the hair make a large loop set up straight from the roots, and attach it to the plat with a pin. Add a cluster of long curls. With the ends of the four bandeaux, well crisped, or else with the rolls of crispings, make four loops, two of which come forward so as to join the bandeaux and form a whole. Two other loops are placed in the top of the head so as to conceal the origin of the curls.'

F, G   1870, French. False hair. Either one can be worn as a wig by combing the natural hair up into it from the temples.

H   1870, French. 'Make the partings to 3 inches from the forehead and from ear to ear. Plat the hair of the chignon and turn it on top of the head. Divide the front hair into two portions, wet it a little, then with the comb form a point on each side. Comb up the hair on the temples after crisping it slightly so as to form points. Take a plat of three branches 24 inches long and arrange it in interlaced loops. The right side is also made with a plat of the same length. Next add seven graduated curls.'

I, J   1871, French. Torsades of false hair.

K   1872, French. 'Make a parting at the side. Slightly wave the bandeaux, which must form two points on the right side and a wide undulation on the left. Add a Circassian plat in three strands and puffed out by means of a small lock of hair into the form of a diadem. On the opposite side a large waved lock comes and almost cuts the diadem in two. Behind, waved hair and curls turned on the fingers. Add an undulation, which comes to terminate the plat over the forehead.'

L-O   1872, French. Coiffures and false hair.

P   1872, French. 'This chignon is mounted on a rounded shape. With 60 grams of creoled hair 50 cm. long, make four torsades which go all around the chignon. With 15 grams of hair 45 cm. long mounted flat, make an undulation with the pin to form the middle of the chignon. Fasten to the mounting 2 descending plats and a long Alexandra curl in the middle between the 2 plats. May be worn out of doors or in the evening.'

Q, R   1872, French.

Note: All the quotations are from *Moniteur de la Coiffure*.

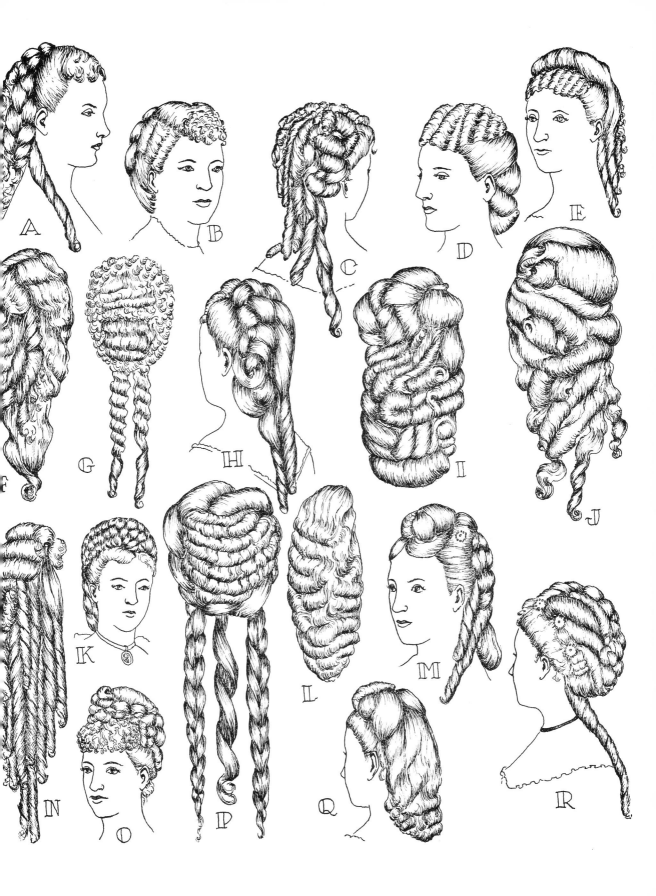

PLATE 130 : NINETEENTH-CENTURY WOMEN 1872, 1873

A, B   1872, French.

C   1872, French. 'This coiffure is wholly of false hair. Turn up all the hair *à la chinoise* and tie it at the top of the head. In front you must have 35 grams of frizzed hair 35 cm. long, and with it make 1½ metres of tresses to be sewn to a wire so as to form a lattice work 26 cm. long by 6 cm. wide. Make undulations on each side to form 3 points which fall over the forehead. Add a crisping across the middle of the mounting, and on it arrange the frizzed hair in small locks to form the waves. Make 3 torsades, each 30 grams, with creoled hair 60 cm. long, to be placed as shown. Then with about 15 grams of hair 45 cm. long, mounted flat in the English fashion, make undulations to the end of the hair, and cross it in the middle with the second torsade, then allow it to fall naturally. Make a small frisure on each side of the undulation. Insert a high comb above the second torsade and add a few curls. The back of the hair consists of a fancy chignon. The coiffure can be simplified by eliminating some of the pieces.'

D   1872, French.

E   1872, French. 'This coiffure is composed of a very light peruke without any cross parting. Make 2 undulations to fall over the forehead. Tie the hair of the peruke on top of the head. With this same hair, make several sausage curls over the forehead as seen in the plate. Make a *cache-peigne* on a quadrilled mounting with hair 50 cm. long and falling on the neck. An ordinary plat passes under the frisieres and runs up the side.'

F   1873, French. Torsade of false hair.

G, H   1873, French. Side and back.

I   1873, French.

J, K   1873, French. Side and back.

L   1873, French. Heartbreakers mounted on hairpins.

M, N   1873, French. Side and back.

O   1873, French. False hair which 'forms a coronet. It consists of very wide undulations mounted on a shape of net and wire with a large cravat bow behind and three long curls. The lady's own hair is passed through the middle of the coronet, and the hair dresser arranges it so as to harmonize best with the fake hair.'

P   1873, French. False hair 'mounted on a small round shape, is composed of four large and very smooth loops and a cravat bow with one loop turned upward, the other downwards. A *cache-peigne* made of eight long curls terminates the chignon. This *cache-peigne* may be worn alone by separating it from the chignon by merely cutting a few threads.'

Q, R, S   1873, French. False hair.

T   1873, French. 'Waved hair mounted on a comb having teeth at the sides only. Small curls are put in the middle to conceal the comb and fall over the parting.'

Note: The quotations are taken from *Moniteur de la Coiffure*.

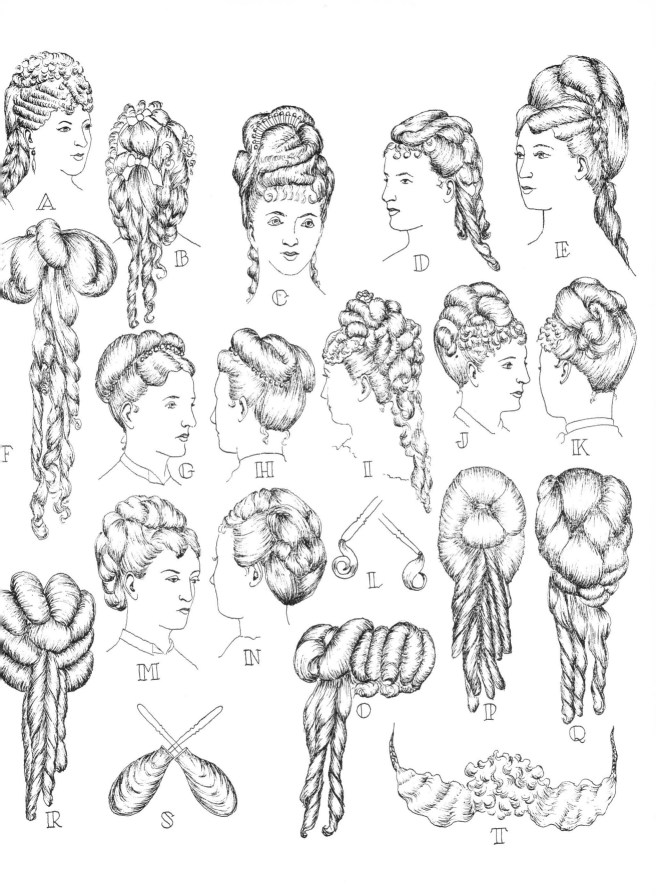

A

B

C

D

E

F

G

H

I

J

K

L

M

N

O

P

Q

R

S

T

Plate 131 : Nineteenth-Century Women 1874–1876

A   1874, French.

B, C   1874, French. 'Part the hair in front and from ear to ear. Tie a lock of hair on top of the head. Separate a small lock in front and frizz it with a small iron. Place it so that the bottom of the parting be covered by the hair of the side, hollow without, in a way to form deep undulations, which cannot be obtained either by the pin or by *bigoudis*. Comb the hair on the temples very high. Place a tress of 90 cm., make it into a bow turned on the head and rather high. Carry up the whole mass of hair on one part behind and make some marteaux loops.'

D   1874, French.

E   1874, French. 'This coiffure is wholly composed of false hair. All the lady's own hair must be combed up in front and behind and collected on the top of the head. Only the hair at the temples is to be left visible. To make the bandeaux you have only to lay flat on the forehead an applied bandeau. The rest of the coiffure consists of a chignon made to and mounted on a head shape or in several pieces if preferred arranged as follows: Front, 2 tails of 50 cm. or 55 cm. mounted as one branch and arranged as a twisted 8, in which passes another tress plat of 3 branches, plaited shorter. This part of the coiffure must be rather high. The back part is made of frizzed hair 40-45 cm. long, raised one above the other so as to form cascades with regular undulations and terminated by a long waved lock, arranged in three curls not frizzed.'

F, G   1874, French. Front and back.

H, I   1874, French.

J   1874, French. '. . . mounted on a wide-meshed and closely fitting gauze quilted with imperceptible slips of whalebone to give more firmness to the structure. It entirely covers the head and not a hair of the lady's own head is seen. It may be dressed either on the lady herself or on a wooden block. The first is preferable.'

K   1874, French. 'Hair plume. This original novelty, already so fashionably patronized, is composed of hair frizzed naturally. It is worn alone, as an aigrette, or in groups of two or three feathers. It may be added to all coiffures indiscriminately, for balls and evening parties, taking into account the color of the hair, of course.'

L   1874, French. Bandeau of false hair.

M-O   1875, French.

P-T   1876, French.

Note: All the quotations are from *Moniteur de la Coiffure*.

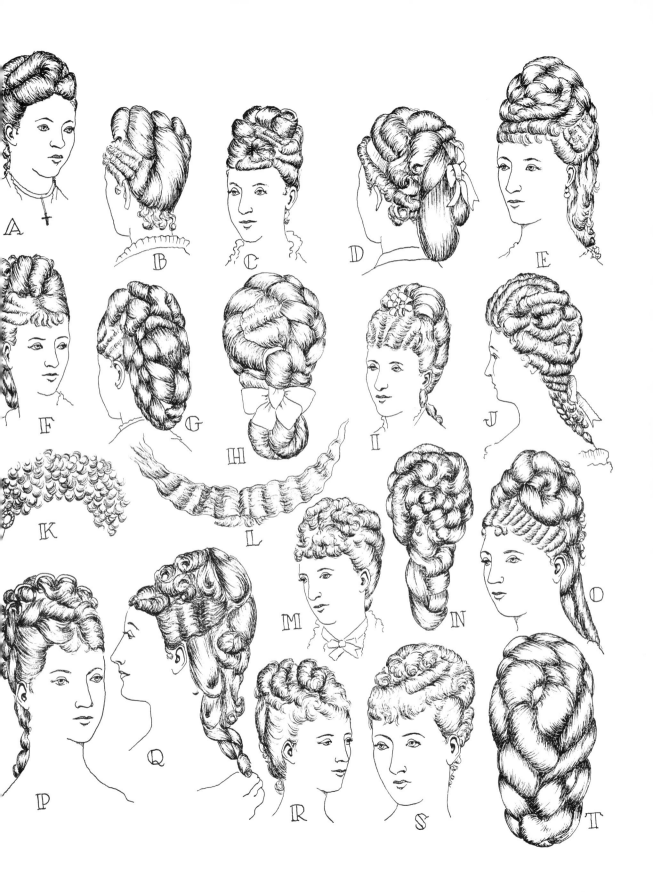

PLATE 132 : NINETEENTH-CENTURY WOMEN 1877–1879

A   1877, French. Back hair is a torsade of false hair.

B   1877, French. Hair at the temples is natural, but the rest may be a combination of various pieces of false hair.

C   1877, French. False hair on a foundation. The natural hair would be blended into it at the temples, while the front might be either real or false.

D   1877, French. This shows the use of the front piece shown in F below.

E   1877, French. Front hair is probably natural and the top and the back hair false.

F   1877, French. False front piece (see D above).

G   1878, French. False wave on hairpin.

H   1877, French. Natural front hair.

I   1878, French.

J, K   1878, French. Chignons for outdoor wear.

L   1878, French. Front may be false (see V below).

M   1878, French. Front probably false (see U below).

N   1878, French.

O   1878, French.

P   1878, French. Front hair natural.

Q   1878, French. Elaborate chignon for dinner parties or theatre.

R   1879, French.

S   1879, French.

T   1879, French. May be composed entirely of false pieces.

U   1879, French. False front piece which could be worn with M, N, or T above.

V   1878, French. False front piece which could be worn with L above.

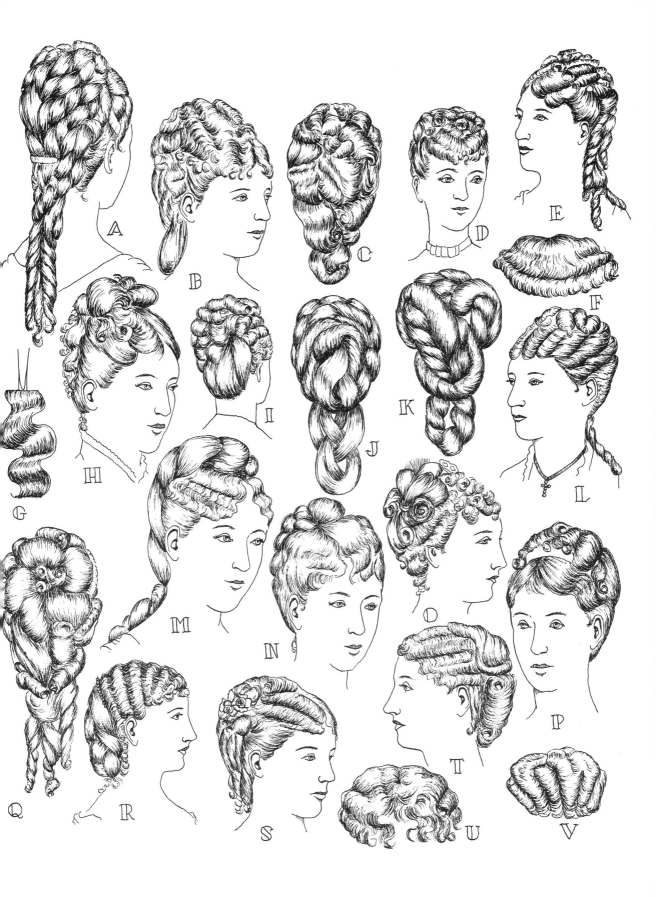

Plate 133 : Nineteenth-Century Women 1880–1883

A   1880. The comb used is shown below.

B   1880.

C   1881, French.

D   1881, French. The entire coiffure is probably composed of false hair pieces (see O below and the chignons on preceding plates).

E   1881, French.

F   1881, French. Torsade of false hair.

G   1881, French. Torsade and front piece of false hair.

H   1882, French. Torsade of false hair.

I, J   1882, French. Back and front.

K   1882, French. Front hair false, back hair partially natural.

L   1883, French. False curls.

M   1883, French. Front hair probably false (for back view see P below).

N   1883, French. False curls.

O   1883, French. False front piece (see D and G above).

P   1883, French. Chignon of false hair secured with large decorative pins (for front view see M above).

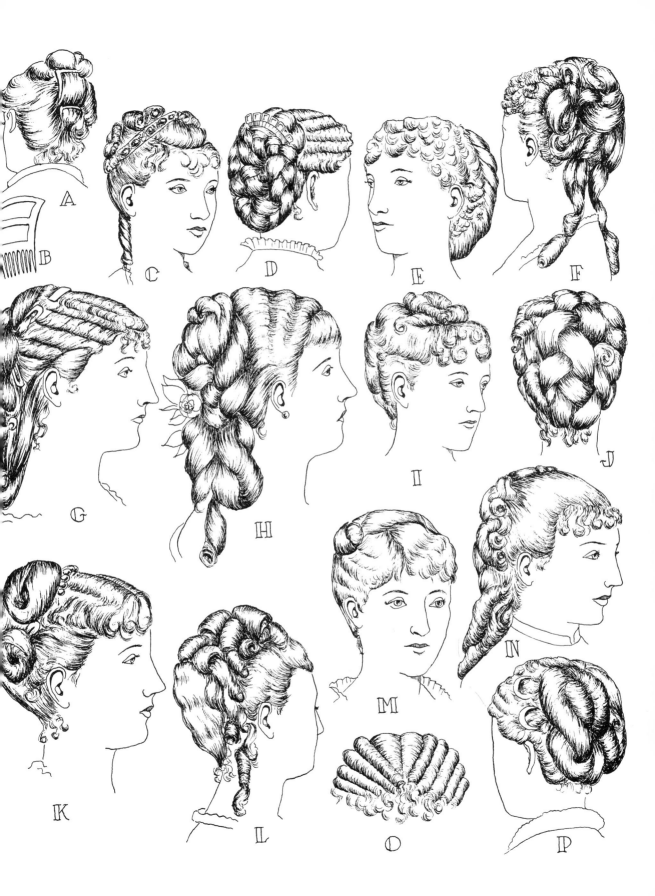

PLATE 134 : NINETEENTH-CENTURY WOMEN 1883–1886

A   Adelina Patti, 1843–1919.

B   1884, French. Top hair false, front and sides may also be a false piece or be composed of a number of frisette pins stuck into the natural hair (for back view see E below).

C   1884, French.

D   Dame Ellen Terry, 1848–1928.

E   1884, French. (For front view see B above.)

F   1884, French. Chignon of artificial hair.

G   1884, French. Chignon of artificial hair.

H   1884, French. This is essentially a partial wig since it covers the greater part of the head. The natural hair at the temples can be combed into it, and the front hair can be natural or false

I, J   1885, French. Front and back—the back hair is false.

K   1886, French.

L   1885, American.

M   1885, American.

N   1885, American.

O   1886, French.

P, Q, R   1886, French. P and Q show steps in making the torsade for the coiffure shown in R.

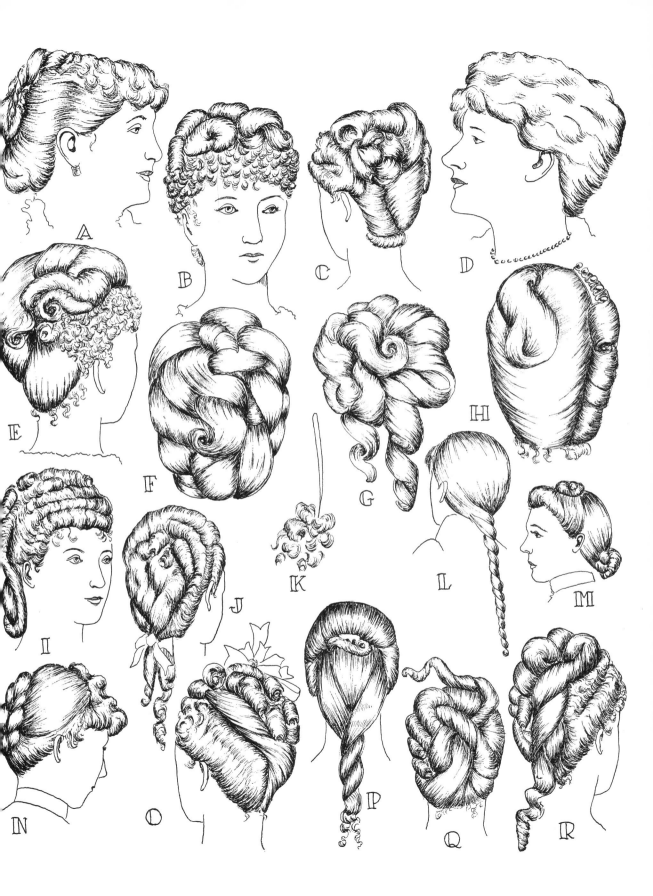

A

B

C

D

E

F

G

H

I

J

K

L

M

N

O

P

Q

R

PLATE 135 : NINETEENTH-CENTURY WOMEN 1886–1889

A   1886, French.

B   Wife of Ulysses S. Grant.

C   Daughter of Ulysses S. Grant.

D   1887.

E   1886, French.

F   1887, French.

G, H   1887, French. Back and front views of hair pieces mounted on long combs. These can be stuck into the coiffure wherever necessary.

I, J   1887, French. I represents a partially completed chignon, showing the construction. Note the comb at the top for attaching the chignon. The completed chignon, dressed and ready to wear, is shown in J.

K   1887, French. Chignon with decorative comb.

L, M, N   1888, French. L and M show steps in forming the torsade for the coiffure shown in N.

O   1888, French. Birds swooping in for a landing were very popular as hair decorations in this period. They were found even more frequently on hats.

P   1889, French.

Q   1888.

R   1889, French.

S   1888. 'A stylish high coiffure for dressy wear, in which the hair is all combed well forward on the top of the head and arranged in irregular soft coils, back of which is placed a bow made of faille ribbon 3 or 4 inches wide. The front hair is arranged in soft, fluffy curls.'

T   1888.

U   1889, French.

Note: All the quotations are from *Demorest's Monthly Magazine*.

In 1888 *Demorest's Monthly Magazine* reported on 'stylish hairdressing':
    'The most popular and general mode … of arranging the hair, is to pile it on top of the head in rolls, torsades, and puffs, to as great an altitude as a becoming effect will permit. A few short curls are added wherever they seem to find a suitable place, and the short front locks are curled in some one of the many styles which are devised to suit various types of face and contour of feature. Fringy and fluffy effects are passés, and the fashionable bang is for the most part an arrangement of decided curls and waves, loose and light in effect, but yet retaining their symmetrical form, whether lying flat on the forehead or curling softly over the temples.'

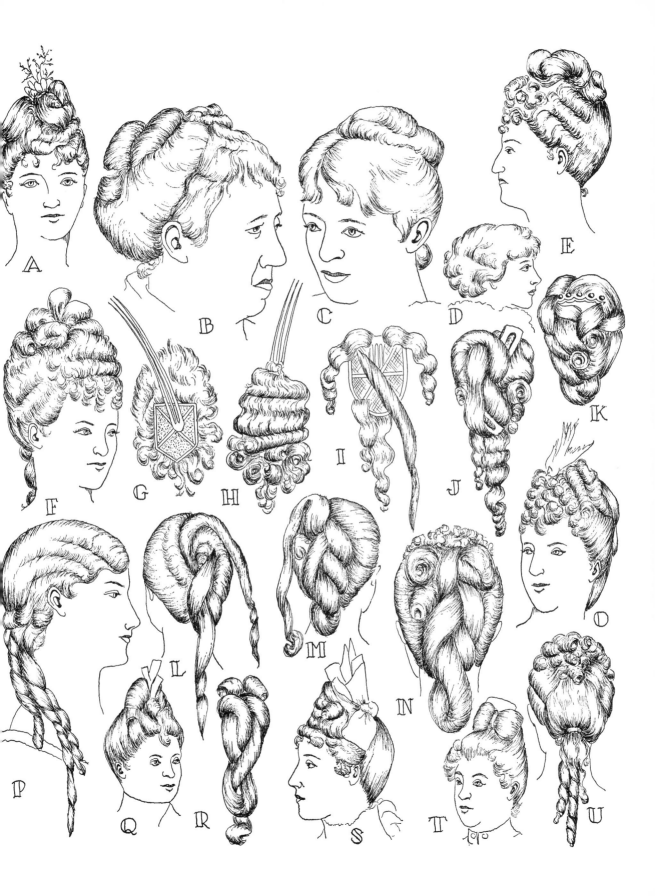

A

B

C

D

E

F

G

H

I

J

K

L

M

N

O

P

Q

R

S

T

U

PLATE 136 : NINETEENTH-CENTURY WOMEN 1890, 1891

A   1890, French. For evening wear.

B, C   1890, French. Front and back.

D   1890, French.

E   1890, French.

F, G   1890, French. Front and back.

H   1890, French. Front and back.

I   1890, French. Basic wig to which additional pieces can be added as desired.

J   1890, French.

K   1891, French.

L   1891, French.

M   1891, French.

N   1891, French. Frisette of false hair.

O   1891, French.

P   1891, French.

Q   1891, French. Decorative hairpins.

R   1891, French.

S   1891, French. Coiffure for a young girl.

T   1891, American. Isabel Mallon, writing in the *Ladies' Home Journal*, comments: 'Very few women can afford to wear their hair with such perfect simplicity. . . . The woman who can should never attempt any other style, for it is one that has been approved of by famous painters, and the arrangement is so absolutely simple that if it had nothing else, that would commend it.'

U   1891, American.

V   1891, American. According to Mrs Mallon, 'The locks have not been cut—they are only carefully arranged to simulate those that have. . . . It is only the woman who has fine light hair, rather than hair that is not very long, who can achieve it. The hair is curled all over the head and is then pinned down with hundreds of little lace pins close to it so that just the ends show. . . . Of course, it is impossible to arrange it oneself, but a helpful sister ought to be able to do it for you. No ornament is worn with such a coiffure, though if you have a great desire to carry out the Grecian idea, it would be in harmony to bind around it three fillets of white ribbon. Don't wear either gold or silver—leave them for older women, and let the young girls use the narrower ribbons.'

W   1891, American.

X   1891, American.

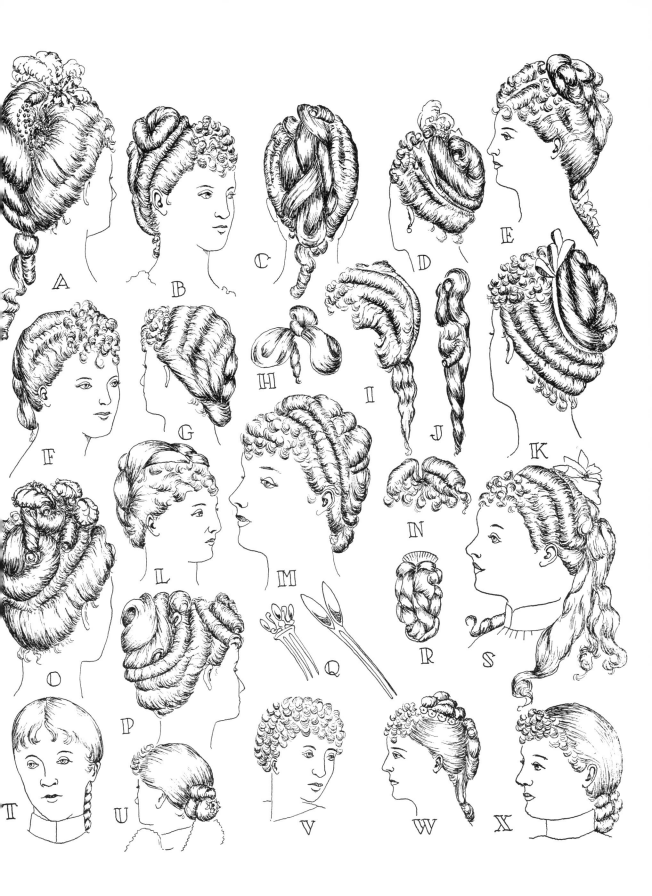

A

B

C

D

E

F

G

H

I

J

K

L

M

N

O

P

Q

R

S

T

U

V

W

X

PLATE 137 : NINETEENTH-CENTURY WOMEN 1891–1894

A 1891, American. Comment by Isabel Mallon in the *Ladies' Home Journal*: 'It is only becoming to women with oval faces and should not be attempted by the witching maid whose face is round and dimpled. The bang is short and fluffy, soft rather than frizzy. The hair at the sides and back . . . is drawn up to the top and fastened with lace pins. The band about the hair is of gold set with turquoises. It is necessary not only that the face should be oval, but the head must be well-shaped, so she must know her points who would dare it.'

B 1891, American. Mrs Mallon recommends this style for a 'piquant oval face with blonde hair', and she says: 'The hair is not very long and is, in front, cut in a short bang and fluffily curled. That drawn to the back has its ends curled and then combed out, while the usual black ribbon draws it together and forms an effective contrast of color. This mode of dressing the hair is one of the outcomes of a fancy of Sarah Bernhardt. . . . A clasp may be used instead of the ribbon, but the women who set the fashion think that the ribbon itself is in better taste. . . . How to curl it? Roll it over a lead pencil, then put the papers over that and pinch it carefully with an iron that is not too hot. In this way the hair is not injured.'

C 1891, American.

D 1892, American.

E American. Child.

F 1892, French. For evening wear.

G 1892, Finnish peasant.

H 1892, French. For evening wear.

I 1892, French.

J 1892, American. 'The front is cut so that when it is curled the bang looks slightly pointed, the centre curl coming right down, as it should, in the middle of the forehead. The remainder of the front hair is, after being crimped on a large iron, drawn back very loosely, the ends being turned up in long soft knots.'

K 1893, American.

L 1893, French.

M 1893, French. A 'new style hairpin'.

N 1893, French.

O 1893, French. Young girl.

P 1893, French.

Q-V 1894, American.

W 1894, French.

X 1894, American.

Y, Z, AA 1894, French.

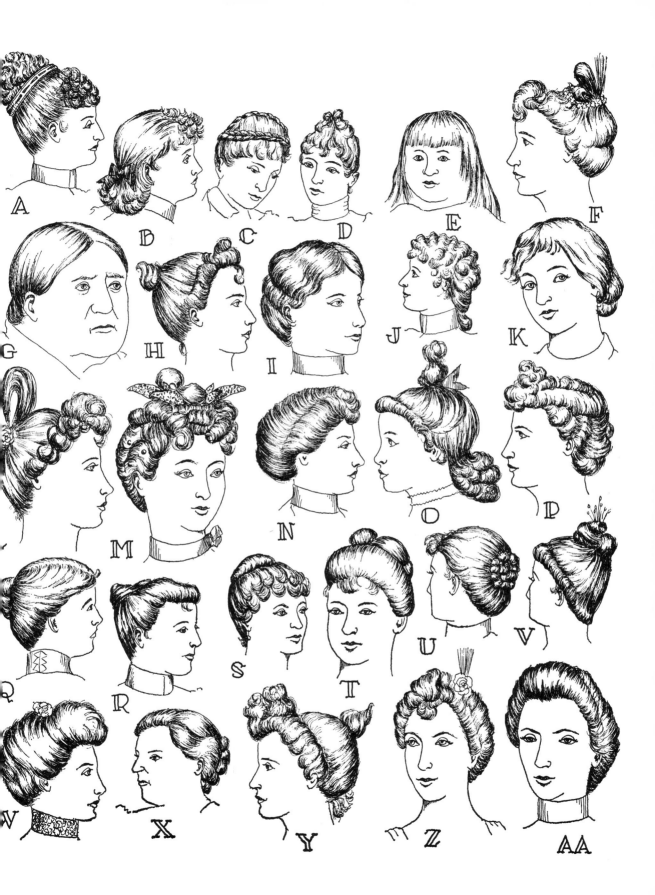

A B C D E F

G H I J K

L M N O P

Q R S T U V

W X Y Z AA

PLATE 138 : NINETEENTH-CENTURY WOMEN 1894–1897

A   1894, French. For afternoon wear.

B   American. Rose Hawthorne Lathrop, 1850–1926. Daughter of Nathaniel Hawthorne. After her husband's death in 1898, she became a Roman Catholic nun and later founded a community of Dominican nuns. The portrait was published in the *Ladies' Home Journal* in 1894 but may have been of a slightly earlier date.

C   1894, American.

D   1894, French.

E   1894, French. For evening wear.

F   1894, Italian.

G   1894, French.

H   1894, French.

I   1894.

J   1894, French. Hair style of Sarah Bernhardt.

K   1894.

L   1894, French.

M   1895, Dutch peasant.

N   1895, French.

O   1896.

P   1895, French. Worn with riding habit.

Q   1897.

R   1897, French. For evening wear.

S   1897, French.

T   1897, French. For evening wear.

U   1897, French. For evening wear.

V   1897, French. For evening wear.

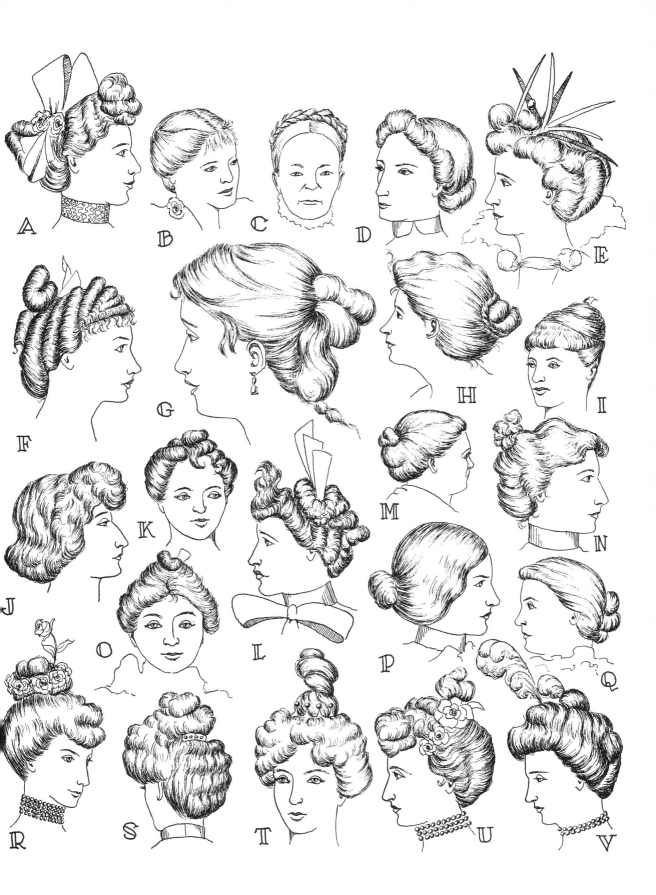

A   B   C   D   E

F   G   H   I

J   K   L   M   N

O   P   Q

R   S   T   U   V

PLATE 139 : NINETEENTH-CENTURY WOMEN 1897–1900

A   1897, French. For evening wear.

B   1897, French.

C   1897, French.

D   1897.

E   1897, French.

F   1897.

G   1897, English. Queen Victoria (for earlier portrait see Plate 119-D).

H   1898.

I   1898. Paris-inspired.

J   1898, American. Mrs Mallon considers this 'suitable for an elderly lady in the evening'. The front is 'in a regularly waved blouse roll'. There are two curls at the neck, and three jet combs are used.

K   1898, American. 'The short front hair is in three soft curls that fall well on the forehead, while the thick front lock, just back of them, is arranged in a high puff. The back hair is drawn up into a soft knot and tied into puffs with fillets of white satin ribbon. The hair at the sides and at the back below the knot is in large, very light waves.'

L   1898, French. For daytime wear.

M   1899, French.

N   1899, French. For evening wear.

O   1899, French.

P   1899, French. For the opera.

Q   1899, French.

R   1899, French.

S   1899, French. *Coiffure de bal.*

T   1899, French. For evening wear.

U   1899, French.

V   1899, French.

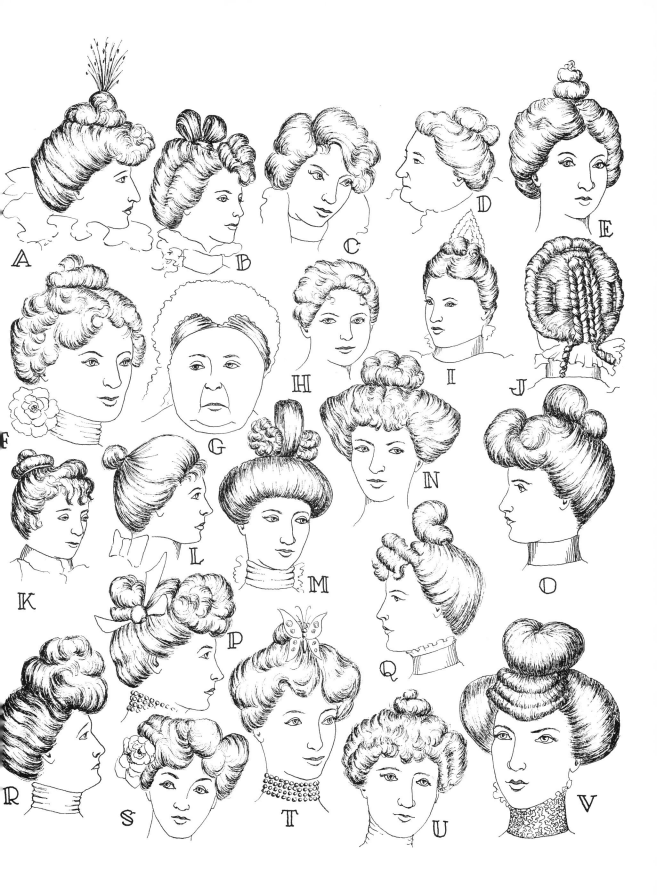

A B C D E

F G H I J

K L M N O

P Q R S T U V

13 · The Twentieth Century—Men

If the twentieth century should
remove whiskers from the face of
mankind, it will be glory enough
for one hundred years.

EDITH SESSIONS TUPPER

The first half of the twentieth century was, perhaps, the least colourful period in history for men's hair styles. Beards were unfashionable; moustaches, after the first decade, were not encouraged; and the hair was worn short. It was not until the second half of the century that there were some indications that another beard movement might be in the making.

THE EARLY YEARS (Plates 140-142)

Walter Shaw Sparrow, writing in 1901, when beards were on their way out, expressed the belief that 'a renewal of the old reverence for beards has ever been a sign of vigour in a nation, whereas general shaving in polished epochs has usually gone hand in hand with much social hysteria. That is why shaven people, after successful wars, after periods of militant awakening, have commonly put away razors with their swords, as we did after the Indian Mutiny. And in England, too, with the great dawn of the Reformation, the beard came to its own again, as during the energetic times of Edward III. We could no more spare the venerable beard of Knox, for instance, than we could think of Michelangelo in the act of modeling a shaven Moses.'

By the beginning of the twentieth century men had taken out their razors and were using them to shave more and more hair off the face. Older men often clung to their beards, and moustaches were still common. In fact, one of the strongest influences on fashions for men was the bristling moustache of the German Kaiser— not only in Germany, but throughout the Western world.

In the *Barbers' Journal* for 1902 there appeared an advertisement for the Kaiser Mustache Trainer: 'With patented flexible comb attachment, will train the mustache to any desired shape without inconvenience. Wear it 5 or 10 minutes after washing the face or at any convenient time and it will shape the mustache for all day, or if worn all night a few times the effect will be permanent. The stained and spotted vest and coat front caused by the drooping or straggling mustache is obviated. Results are astonishing and most satisfactory. They should be kept on sale in every shop for the convenience of customers and profit to the proprietor.' The price was fifty cents with a liberal discount to the trade.

Actually, the gadget was of German origin and was called originally a *Schnur-bartbinde* or moustache-binder. It was designed to keep the kaiser-style of moustaches pointing upward, and apparently it worked quite well. Constructed of silk gauze, two little leather straps, and two pieces of elastic web, it was pressed close to the face, covering the moustache, and was fastened behind the head (see Figure 116).

In the same year a Paris correspondent reported to the *Barbers' Journal* on conditions over there. 'In England one man in every three shaves himself. In France there is not one in forty who knows how to be his own barber. . . . Consequently, there are 6500 barbershops in the French capital; and it is estimated that there are about 25,000 persons more or less directly connected with the trade here.

'Perhaps in no city in the world is there such a vast and variegated category of tonsorial establishments. In some places you can have your hirsute incumberments removed for one cent, which is just the one-thirtieth of what you may be charged elsewhere for the same operation. The scale slides up and down according to locality —and to locality alone. . . .

'An infinite majority of the better class of shops in Paris charge 5 cents for a shave, 15 cents for a haircut, the same for trimming the beard, 15 cents for singeing, 10 cents for shampooing, and 20 cents for dyeing the hair, whiskers, or beard.'

In the usual Paris shop the customers sat in cane-seated armchairs (less convenient and comfortable, the Parisian barbers admitted, but much cheaper than more modern barbers' chairs) in front of mirrors and wash basins. There was invariably seated at a tall desk at the end of the room a woman who collected the fees and the tips as the customers left. The tips were pooled; and as the coins were heard dropping into the box, there was a chorus of *Merci, monsieur* from all the barbers. In some shops the same lather was used for several customers, and towels might be used on both face and hair of a dozen men before being discarded. When the shave was finished, the gentleman customarily washed his own face.

But perhaps the most interesting barbering establishment in Paris was to be found at the foot of a stone stairway leading from the Quai de Conti down to the river's edge, nearly under the arches of the Pont Neuf. A character named Old Jules was the barber; and, as the Paris correspondent reported it, 'his asking price for a shave was a cent, but I have been told he made a reduction in favour of his regular clients. . . . He would arrange his customers so that every man had a step to himself in the stone stairway leading up to the quai. When every man was in his place, Jules would go over to the river edge, fill a little tin soap-cup with water, and then start up the stairs. The man on the lowest step would be lathered first, then the man on the second, and so on all the way to the top. As he left each man, Jules would say, "Keep rubbing it." They all did. When he had lathered the man on the top step, the old barber would throw the tin soap-cup down to the "shop" and from his pocket would take a razor. Then he would go down the steps, shaving each man as he passed and rubbing his razor on a big apron he wore. It took him usually 40 minutes to get down the 22 steps, less than 2 minutes to a step.'

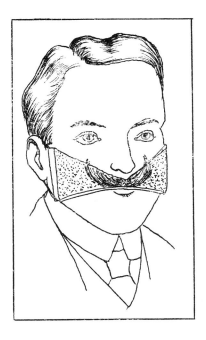

Fig. 116 : The *Schnurbartbinde* or moustache trainer

In 1903 in the *Chicago Chronicle* Edith Sessions Tupper set forth at least one woman's viewpoint on the wearing of beards:

'Welcome with joy the tidings that a distinguished physician has declared war on the beards of men, denouncing them as harbors of dirt and disease. If the twentieth century should remove whiskers from the face of mankind, it will be glory enough for one hundred years. . . .

'There are many kinds of whiskers and each set tells its tale. There are the opinionated whiskers. You know them, do you not? You see them on clergymen. They are long and narrow. Baer, the coal king, had opinionated whiskers. Dr. Parkhurst also. They announce as plainly as possible: "I am it. All else is dirt."

'I never saw a man wearing a Van Dyke beard who was not selfish, sinister, and pompous as a peacock. Many men consider this beard artistic. I believe artists do affect it. The man with the pointed beard takes himself very seriously.

'There are unctuous whiskers—long, broad, sweeping, plethoric—the whiskers of the Mormon elder. They usually fringe full, sensual, smug, hypocritical lips. Never trust such whiskers.

'There are the scholarly whiskers—close-clipped sideburns, affected by high churchmen and college professors. They are not so repulsive as chin whiskers and betoken much more refined tastes and lives.

'There are the close-clipped, respectable bank president whiskers, also worn by statesmen and some clergymen. They are the hallmark of probity, decency, and dullness.

'There are the whiskers of the anarchist—unkempt, matted, a ferocious setting for a savage face. Then there are the whiskers of the jay. But here language is feeble. There is such a wild, sloppy abandon to the whiskers of the rural districts, such a similarity to the wearers' own cornstalks and haystacks, that from afar they announce their use in life—that of choice tidbit to the hard-working gold brick man. . . .

'The imperial and mustaches are not so bad as whiskers. They give a man a soldierly air which is not unpleasant. If a man must wear hair on the face, let it be in this shape. A mustache often covers ugly teeth and lips, thereby proving a boon to mankind. . . . Heroes of novels by women as a rule sport long, blonde silky mustaches, which they are constantly curling and stroking. Ouida's beautiful guardsmen always have these lip adornments.

'Latterly, however, the Richard Harding Davis and Charles Dana Gibson men have set a new vogue, that of the smooth-shaven, stern-faced, dogged-chin chap. It has proved immensely popular and all classes of men have followed this fashion. So that nowadays it is difficult to tell coachmen from their masters or actors from clergymen.

'It is a cleanly fashion and one to be commended to all men with reasonably good features. There is a certain distinction about the clean-shaven man which the wearer of whiskers can never possess. Moreover, a smooth face is a stimulant to high thoughts. For behind walls and hedges and brambles of hair mean, low, cunning thoughts can conceal their traces, but they are blazoned forth on the open of a smooth cheek.'

In the following year an article in *Harper's Weekly* approached the whole matter from various angles and is worth quoting at some length:

'Nothing is presently plainer in a world that loves its little mysteries and likes to keep the observer in a state of tremulous suspense about a good many things, than the fact that it is beginning to shave again. It has always shaved, more or less, ever since beards came in some fifty years ago, after a banishment of nearly two centuries, from at least the Anglo-Saxon face. During all the time since the early eighteen-fifties, the full beard has been the exception rather than the rule. The razor has not been suffered to rust in disuse but has been employed in disfiguring most physiognomies in obedience to the prevalent fashion or the personal caprice of the wearers of hair upon the face, where nature has put it, for reasons still of her own. For one man who let nature have her way unquestioned by the steel, there have been ninety-nine men who have modified her design. Some have shaved all but a little spot on the upper lip; others have continued the imperial grown there into the pointed goatee; others have worn the chin beard, square cut from the corners of the lips, which has become in the alien imagination distinctively the American beard; others have shaved the chin and let the mustache branch across the cheeks to meet the

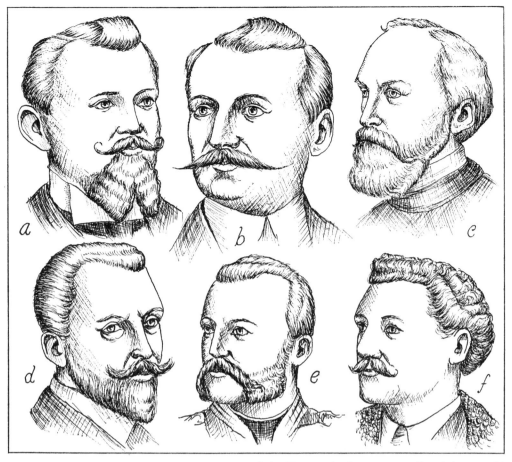

Fig. 117 : European styles of the first decade of the Twentieth Century: (a) Dr Acheray; (b) Louis Blériot (1872–1936); (c) Admiral Marquis; (d) Theobald von Bethmann-Hollweg, Chancellor of Germany 1909–17; (e) Grand-Duke Vladimir of Russia; (f) Signor Alvarez Quintero, Spanish dramatist

flowing fringe of the side-whiskers; others have shaved all but the whiskers shaped to the likeness of a mutton-chop; the most of all have shaved the whole face except the upper lip and worn the mustache alone. All these fragmentary forms of beard caricatured the human countenance and reduced it more or less to a ridiculous burlesque of the honest visages of various sorts of animals. They robbed it of the sincerity which is the redeeming virtue of the clean-shaven face, and of the dignity which the full beard imparted no less to middle-life than to age. . . .

'It is, to be sure, very dirty, and that is the best reason for reforming the beard altogether. To be perfectly frank, at the risk of being somewhat disgusting, we must own that the full beard collects dandruff, which plentifully bestrews the neckcloth and the waistcoat; but it is not filthier in other respects than the mustache, which sops itself full of soup and gravy and coffee . . . and is absurd besides. In the young, it is grown purely for vanity, with the hope of adding a certain fierceness to the innate sheepishness of the wearer's expression; in age, it forms the penalty of this vanity, for though the wearer would then gladly cut it off, he cannot do so without seeming to remove, in the consciousness of his friends, one of his features. . . . The mustache will probably survive every other form of beard because it is the most flattering to the vanity of the young.'

As to the current fashion, we are told that 'the flowing mustache, the up-and-out-branching, the deeply drooping, neither of these is now any more the mode than the mustaches which used to meet the fringing whiskers; and the barbers have even got a name for the close-cropped mustache which remains. They ask you if you want it stubbed. . . .

'The gain of manly beauty through the fashion of clean-shaving has not as yet, it must be confessed, been very great. Those who had not grown beards, of course, remained as they were, in their native plainness; but it is in the care of those who had worn beards that the revelations are sometimes frightful: retreating chins, blubber lips, silly mouths, brutal jaws, fat and flabby necks, which had lurked unsuspected in their hairy coverts now appear and shake the beholder with surprise and consternation. "Good heaven!" he asks himself, "is that the way Jones *always* looked?" Jones, in the meanwhile, is not seriously troubled. He is pleased with the novelty of his aspect; he thinks upon the whole that it was a pity to have kept so much loveliness out of sight so long. As he passes his hand over the shapeless expanses, with the satisfaction which nothing but the smoothness of a freshly shaven face can give, he cannot resist the belief that people are admiring him. At any rate, he has that air.'

The article goes on to point out that half a century earlier defenders of the beard had used as one of their chief arguments its contribution to health through keeping the wearer's throat warm and filtering the air entering the lungs and thus preserving him from consumption. 'But now that consumption is no longer consumption, but tuberculosis,' the article states, 'and is not hereditary but infectious, we believe that the theory of science is that the beard is infected with the germs of tuberculosis and is one of the deadliest agents for transmitting the disease to the lungs. . . . But nothing will persuade us, who grew up in the opposite theory, that thousands of human beings were not saved from consumption, before it was tuberculosis, by the air-sifting properties of the beard which now transmits the animate poison to the system it was given to protect.'

On this matter of microbes, Frank Richardson had this to say:

'A German scientist . . . estimates that 2,000,000 misanthropic microbes can find accommodation in "an average beard". This is bad hearing. But Monsieur Dachicourt, with cheery and perhaps—if one may say so with regard to a man with his vast reputation—speculative optimism, reduces the number (except on the West Coast of Africa—in particular, the district of the Congo) to a couple of thousand or so. Still, his figures are sufficiently alarming. It is no pleasing thing to feel that when one is talking to a bearded man one is in the presence of a huge invisible army which

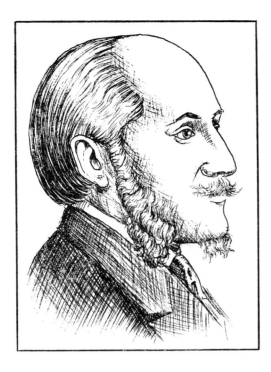

Fig. 118 : Edmond Rostand in 1913

may at any moment send forth a brigade, a battalion, a sergeant or two, intent upon the invasion of one's self. . . .

'It may be urged that persons who possess faulty dental apparatus can conceal the same with a moustache, and that beards are worn in order to protect weak throats. In this case they come under the category of "cholera belts" and "porous plasters". They are simply medical appliances, and people who require to wear them are clearly in so weak a state of health that they should not venture abroad.'

Mrs C. E. Humphry, in *Etiquette for Every Day*, published in London in 1904, writes that 'the great number of clean-shaven men in society has been a matter of remark of late. It is an instance of a radical change in a fashion whose processes are usually very gradual. There is not so much individuality about the shape and cut of the beard as there ought to be. . . . Regarded from merely the ornamental point of view, a beard of any kind is a mistake when a man possesses a well-cut chin. . . .

'Men with long faces should have round beards, if any. But if a man's face is abnormally round and fat, he should wear an "imperial", as the narrow, long variety of the Van Dyck beard is called. Oddly enough, it is the Americans who chiefly favour this form, though their faces, being long and narrow, need it less than any other. . . .

'The moustache, quite as much as the beard, has a wonderfully powerful effect upon a man's whole expression. The idea of virility, spirit, and manliness that it conveys is so great that it was a long time the special privilege of officers of the army to wear it, as characteristic of the profession of arms. It has now become general in almost all classes. . . .

'A man with a trivial nose should not wear a large moustache. Doing so will increase the insignificance of his insignificant nose. With a large nose, the moustache may be large too, but its ends should never extend further than in a straight line with the outer corners of the eyes. Sometimes the ends of a man's moustache are visible to persons walking behind him. This imparts to him a belligerent, aggressive air that makes small children refrain from asking him the time. . . . This ornament is full of expression. An artistic temperament is denoted by its soft silkiness of texture and curved droop at the corners. A lively vivacity, however it may be held in check by the "cultivated stoicism", as Carlyle phrased it, of the educated Englishman, may be plainly read in the moustache that actively bristles at the ends and turns neither up nor down. . . . The upcurled moustache bespeaks the dandy.'

In 1904 the kaiser moustache was still in favour since the *Barbers' Journal* carried an advertisement for Cosmetique Transparent—'To obtain the Latest Fad in Facial Adornment, the Kaiser Mustache. Contains no grease. Simply dip into water and apply to mustache and beard. Will keep same in shape for rest of day. Now used and for sale by all leading barbers.' The price was fifty cents (three shillings and sevenpence).

The hair was worn short, neatly trimmed, and parted—usually on the side. The centre parting was looked upon with some suspicion in certain areas of the United States. In the April 1904 issue of the *Barbers' Journal* a pronouncement from Texas was quoted to the effect that 'No man who parts his hair in the middle can ever carry Texas for the presidency'. The *Journal* pointed out that 'the dislike formerly entertained in New York and even in London to the practice of parting the hair of males in the middle has long since departed, as every man in the trade knows. How interesting that it survives in Texas. . . . Outside of Texas, the reproach of mannishness against a woman who parted her hair on one side and of effeminacy against the man who parted his in the middle has long since fled before the advance of civilization. Everyone wears his or her hair as he or she pleases subject only to the provisions of nature and to the Constitution of the United States.'

In England, according to Mrs Humphry, 'One man sweeps it back from his forehead; another brushes it down over his brow; a third allows the top part to fall about in every direction; while a fourth has all the lines of his hair running the same way, like those of a little brook.' This discussion is followed by the information that in the street a gentleman removes his cigar when passing a lady. Later Mrs Humphry points out that 'etiquette forbids a man to wear a wig, though it equally forbids a woman to appear without some sort of *chevelure*. If she is bald, she must hide her baldness. A man may grow long strands of hair where he can and train them from the sides across his baldness, but when even this fails he must e'en let things bide.'

But, in general, relatively little thought seems to have been given to hair on the head except to keep it neatly trimmed. Certainly no great conflicts or arguments raged over it. But hair on the face was another matter.

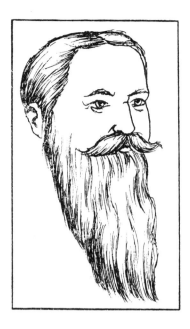

Fig. 119 : Olympian beard. French, 1912

In the autumn of 1906 the *North American Review* reported that word had just come from Rome to the effect that the waiters' union of that city had decreed that all waiters should wear beards. No reason was given, but presumably the clean-shaven face was looked upon, as it has often been throughout history, as a badge of servitude.

The *Review* pointed out, by way of contrast, that 'nowadays young men are almost invariably clean-shaven, and their elders are gradually yielding to the new fashion'. The editor shuddered at the 'contemplation of flowing beards in proximity to plates of soup. . . . Hairdressers', he admitted, 'have certain, though unsatisfying, excuse for utilizing their beards as convenient receptacles for their various combs, but a waiter has no such practical extenuation. In fact, the modern germ theory alone probably would suffice to deprive him of the privilege.'

In closing, the editor questioned whether or not the beard or moustache would ever again become popular. 'After all,' he concluded, 'women make fashion for men as well as for themselves, and the ticklishness inseparable from a growth of wiry hair in the vicinity of the lips, we are informed, has become in their view obnoxious.'

Along with those who become indignant or even belligerent about such matters and those who, taking themselves very seriously, cite religion or science in support of their claims, no matter which side they happen to be on, there are, happily, the satirists, who add a modicum of perspective to the conflict. One such was William Inglis, who in 1907 wrote a piece for *Harper's Weekly* entitled 'The Revolt Against Whiskers':

'Perhaps no greater evidence can be found of the sure and rapid growth of the aesthetic sense of the American people than the present revolt against whiskers.

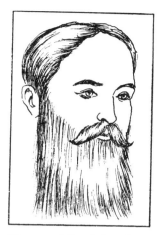 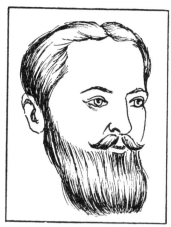 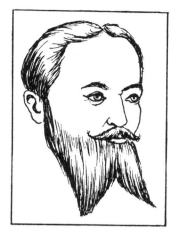

Fig. 120 : Miner's beard.   Fig. 121 : Square beard.   Fig. 122 : Forked beard.
French, 1912   French, 1912   French, 1912

Originating in Upper Montclair, New Jersey, a suburb of New York . . . the revolt has run like wild-fire over the land, leaped lightly across the Atlantic, and spread with marvellous rapidity throughout hirsutest England.'

Mr Inglis then explains that 'Mr. Cornish, a Democratic Assemblyman from Essex County . . . introduced in the New Jersey Legislature on April 1, a bill to tax whiskers. There was some sharp debate during which cowardly attacks were made upon the measure by low-minded persons . . . but at last right prevailed, and Speaker Elvins referred the bill to the Committee on Fish and Game.'

Returning to Mr Cornish, Mr Inglis continued: '"I made", he said, "many inquiries and collected much valuable data. Many whom I questioned were coarse and vulgar men, whose language to me when I politely asked the reason they wore whiskers is not fit to repeat. The majority said that they wore beards as a matter of economy, to save both barbers' fees and the cost of neckties."

'Mr. Cornish thought that an equitable schedule would be about as follows: Common or garden whiskers, $5 a year. Mutton chops, or Senatorial side fuzz, $10. Square chin and side pattern, $50. Red (of any design whatsoever), 20% extra. . . . Dundreary or lambrequin style, $8. Ministerial sideboards, $10. Imperials, paint-brushes, or ordinary camel's hair pencils, $30. Geometrical *retroussé* dusters, $50.

'A secret canvass of the Legislature reveals the fact that the members of both Houses are eager to tax the capillary microbe-carriers, but they fear reprisals. It is reported that even now groups of sturdy, burly men are gathering in the mountain fastness of Musconetcong, Peapack, Watsessing, and Pompton, resolved to take hideous revenge. The pen trembles to write of the ingenious and horrible tortures they purpose to inflict. Pale scouts bring in word that these vandals have bound

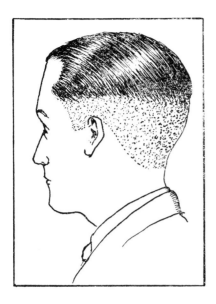

Fig. 123 : American military haircut, 1918

themselves by oath to weave their whiskers into lariats and therewith to rope and hang all legislators who vote for the tax. The barbarians were ever a cruel folk. . . .

'Enthusiasts for hygiene no less than lovers of the beautiful will be gladdened to hear that the good work is nobly advancing in England. That eminent capillary connoisseur, Frank Richardson, called Frank Whiskerson by *Punch* because he is the greatest living English authority on whiskers, is doing all he can to help the taxation plan.

'"It is the best thing in the world," he said in a recent interview. "The idea is splendid. It ought to be introduced in England at the earliest opportunity, but the taxes are not heavy enough. They should amount to £20 per whisker. I've never seen a man wearing a single whisker, but I don't see why it should not be done, just as a single eyeglass is worn. If men insist upon going about as if they were blots on the landscape I don't see why they should not pay a high price for the privilege."

'Mr. Richardson supplied the first official listing of known face furnishings. It is as follows: "Whiskers, ear guards, face fins, weathercocks, face fungus, holdalls, hearthrugs, cutlets, paint-brushes, and the whiskeret, mustaches, the inverted eyebrow, and the walrus." He said:

'"There is no reason why mustaches should not be taxed also. A modified mustache like an inverted eyebrow, such as I wear myself, might retail at a pound, whereas a walrus should not be allowed in the street until the man behind it had paid £20 to the government". . . .

'The owners and trainers of whiskers might fight the tax as sumptuary and unconstitutional, but they cannot prevail. For, as Paracelsus, or some other fellow, very truly said, "Whiskers have no friends."'

In 1907, in the midst of the controversy about the unsanitary aspects of wearing whiskers, a French scientist, taking the pragmatic approach, walked with two men, one bearded and one not, through the streets of Paris, the Louvre, and several large stores, completing the expedition on a crowded tram car. Then he had each of the young men in turn kiss a young lady with antiseptic lips. After each kiss, a sterilized brush was passed over the lips, then dipped into a sterile solution of agar-agar, which was quickly sealed and left standing for four days. At the end of that time, the solution from the shaven man was shown to contain relatively harmless yeast germs, whereas the one from the moustached man 'literally swarmed with malignant microbes'—tubercle bacillus, diphtheria and putrefactive germs, minute bits of food, a hair from a spider's leg, and other odds and ends. The obvious conclusions were drawn.

As we have seen, it was customary in many periods for men to perfume the hair and beard, and frequently this was more in the nature of a necessity than a luxury. But as Victorianism unfurled over the Western world like a smothering blanket, it was not considered proper for men to smell pleasant. It was quite permissible for them to smell of tobacco; but other than that, it was preferred that they should not smell at all.

This attitude was not easy to root out, but the early years of the twentieth century saw a beginning. In 1908 the *Barbers' Journal* reported that 'the custom by men of using extracts upon the handkerchief and of faintly scenting the hair and mustaches began anew in England about five years ago, after nearly a generation of abstemiousness in the matter of fragrance. This fashion has attained suddenly large proportions in this country. Whereas three years ago the big perfumers were engaged in merely supplying a staple amount of certain extracts and cologne water for men who have a way of clinging to their own fancies no matter what fashions rule, now they are vying with one another in the endeavor to produce some distinct novelty in fragrance which will captivate the masculine fancy. Enormous quantities of cologne water are being sold to men as well as an ever increasing quantity of extracts. So far sachets have been tabooed by them, save in rare cases; but there are men unable to resist the alluring, evanescent aroma of a dainty sachet.'

But it was not really until after mid-century that a wide variety of men's colognes with masculine names and masculine bottles began to flood the open market. And so long as they appeared to be designed exclusively for men, they met with very little resistance.

A newspaper article printed in the summer of 1912 and reprinted in the *Barbers' Journal* gives some interesting sidelights on the gentleman of the period:

'To begin with men like to smell sweet. Being ashamed to purchase perfume, they buy hair tonic. The shelf in front of every barber's chair looks like the buffet of a fancy drink fiend. . . . Having had his hair cut as he wants it, the man then has a shampoo. . . . There is the egg shampoo, the prepared egg shampoo, the tar shampoo, the patent preparation shampoo, and a combination of any of these shampoos, such as the tar and egg shampoo, and others. . . . After a man has been shaved and massaged, has had his hair cut and has been shampooed, he is ready for the finishing touches. All that has gone before is just a groundwork on which what is to follow is built.

'Suppose a man lacks color, his cheeks are white and have not the healthy peachy bloom of the simple life. The barber rubs his cheeks with rouge or a liquid preparation and colors them in this fashion.

'Suppose that the lips are not red enough or the skin on the lips is not soft, the barber rubs them with a lipstick or treats them with various softening and healing preparations.

'Suppose there are not eyebrows enough or those that are there are not dark enough. The barber either paints in new eyebrows or colors up the old colorless ones.

'Suppose the mustache is not quite brilliant enough or stiff enough. It is long enough, perhaps, but it drops and has not that jaunty, bristling, cock's-comb appearance that is admired in men's mustaches. The barber rubs it with a liquid preparation which makes it brilliant, stiff, bristly, and beautiful.

'Suppose any part of the facial geography is too red. The nose may be flowering like the scarlet geranium or the ears may be too encarmined. The barber treats the offending parts with a preparation which takes the color out of the skin.

'There are many other little processes, such as removing pimples and so on, that the man orders before the barber is through with his face. When all the small details have been attended to he usually has a rub with some sort of scented toilet water, and then the barber returns to the hair which was left tied in the towel after the shampoo.

'The towel is taken from the head, and the hair is found nearly dry. It may be necessary to curl the hair in front. This is done with a curling iron, just as the ladies' hair is curled. Any little fancy waves the customer wants are put in and then the hair is parted. The man is now released from the chair.

'There are hundreds of ways of making the part in the hair. Every man almost has ideas about how his hair should be divided. It must be parted at just such and such a place so as to cover a small bald spot; it must be parted over in this direction so as to show a high temple; it must be done this way or that way and the barber has to find the proper way after much experiment sometimes. . . .

'Having had his head and face beautified one would think that the man would be satisfied—satisfied, at least, that he had been made as pretty as the barber shop could make him. But not so. The modern barber shop has a manicure girl—many of them —and the modern man must have his fingers prettified before he trusts himself on the street alone. . . .

'The wig shop is a minor place in which the vanity of men is to be seen. Many men wear wigs, though women do not suspect it. Many men dye their hair too. More dye their mustaches.'

In the eighteenth and nineteenth centuries there were occasional forays into barbed verse on the subject of hair, usually women's. As a rule, it appeared when the styles got out of hand. But in 1912 a mild bit of doggerel turned up on the subject of men's hair:

> Some folks are proud because they're stout;
>   Some few rejoice at being spare;
> But few men care to talk about
>   Their hair.
>
> There are, I've noticed, men who wear
>   An unkempt mass upon the pate,
> Thick as a cottage thatch—the hair
>   I hate.
>
> There are, upon the other hand,
>   Some plastered polls with wash besprent;
> But I myself can never stand
>   The scent.
>
> The stuff that sticks on end, I find,
>   I view with equal lack of gush;
> It looks to me a meagre kind
>   Of brush.
>
> I never yet admired the nut
>   Cropped *à la mode* of ancient Gaul;
> It seems the most unkindest cut
>   Of all.
>
> I do not like the bardic style
>   (These are the men that should be shot);
> While curly fellows make me smile
>   A lot.
>
> And speaking broadly, I, for one,
>   Had I myself to suit my taste,
> I'd never let my coiffure run
>   To waste.
>
> But there! I have no choice, alack!
>   I'm, in the homely Scotch term, auld:
> I lost my hair some seasons back—
>   I'm bald!

Although the beard was no longer sanctioned by fashion in the United States, it was still worn in France. In 1912 a French barber discussed a few of the principal beard styles which were currently being worn and made a few suggestions for trimming:

'*The Olympian Beard.* . . . Leaving aside such excessive and remarkable growths as those of M. Louis Coulton, of Montlucon, (11 feet) or M. Jules Dumont, of Antryne (11 feet, 11⅘ inches), there are plenty of very long beards to be found; but barbers do not often get a chance to trim them. This form of beard is also known as the "patriarchal" or "flowing". The French painter Meissonnier, the Russian author Tolstoi, and many other famous men wore beards of this type. . . .

'*The Miner's Beard.* This form is met with most frequently and has been made familiar by the portraits of the Czar of Russia, Alexander III, King Leopold II of Belgium, and others. It sometimes descends entirely straight and sometimes in the shape of a fan, that is, a little wider at the bottom than at the top, but always is cut off squarely at the bottom. To trim it properly, draw it forward and brush it out flat, first on top and then underneath, supporting it during the brushing with the open hand held on the opposite side. It will be more elegant if it terminates rather thin than thick, but this thinness should be only at the extreme ends in order that it may not be too floating.

'*The Square Beard.* This is a classical form which requires to be rather thick in order to keep its shape. Its direction is straight forward. It requires frequent trimming, but exceedingly little is taken off each time. The operation, although long, consists mostly of brushing, combing, and pushing back in shape, that is, *dressing*. Sometimes, in order to give it more rigidity, it is crisped underneath, the top is stiffened with brilliantine, and the edges are strengthened with a hot iron. The beauty of this style depends upon the rigidity with which it holds its shape.

'*The Forked Beard.* This is not very stylish at the present time, but its vogue returns about every twenty years, and in the meantime, a certain number will continue to wear it. One must be exceedingly cautious in order not to ruin this form of beard, which is not obtained, as might be thought, by cutting out the center with the scissors, but by a continued shaping with the hand. The beard is just divided and then one trims with great judgment the hairs which project outside of the correct alignment all around the two points, and only these. Some dandies, after having had their beards trimmed in this manner, have them moistened with an atomizer and allow them to dry in this form or have them dried with hot air from a hair drier and do not comb them thereafter; but if properly executed, this beard will retain the shape which it is given. If, however, in spite of the instructions just given, the beard is combed strongly forward and shaped with the scissors, the cut parts will not furnish the necessary support to the points.' (See Figures 119-122.)

The insanitary procedures in use earlier in both French and American barbers' shops have already been mentioned. But apparently the outrage of contemporary writers had not fully taken effect, for in 1912 the following paragraph appeared in a Nebraska newspaper:

'There ought to be a law in Nebraska and every state compelling barbers to use only clean hot towels on men's faces. At present the same towel is used over and over again upon face after face. The public is entitled to this protection against the possible spread of disease and against this uncleanliness. Today barbers in Nebraska use the same hot towels for a number of customers. Unless you demand it, you are very apt to get a towel on your face that has been used on a good many other men's faces ahead of you. You have no way of knowing whose face the towel was used on before you. Aside from the insanitary feature, the practice is unclean. It is filthy.'

In the war years there were very few beards, and the remaining moustaches were usually rather small. Brophy attributes the toothbrush moustache of the First World War to unhygienic conditions in the trenches. Just as they kept the hair cropped short 'in order to reduce the nesting area for egg-laying lice', they kept their moustaches cropped also.

Perhaps the most distressing development in the United States during this period was the type of military haircut in which the head was clipped close all around, leaving the hairline at approximately eyebrow level. This was something like the bowl cut of the early fifteenth century except that the hair which remained on top was cut fairly close. This style was worn by men who had never been in the army, and it was regularly inflicted on children. It is possible that in both cases the practical triumphed over the aesthetic, the hope being that the shorter the hair was clipped, the longer before the next trip to the barber. The style was never fashionable; but it persisted for many years among those who cared nothing for fashion, especially in small towns and in more rural areas. (See Figure 123.)

THE TWENTIES (Plate 142)

In 1920 the *Barbers' Journal* carried a news item from Cleveland: 'It's here at last—the eyebrow plucking parlor for men. James Macaluse, proprietor of a barber shop at East 115th Street and Superior Avenue, announced his intention of conducting a plucking establishment in connection with his regular tonsorial work. "I've had a number of men come in recently and ask where they could get their lashes drooped or their brows weeded out and run into nice curves," he said. "I'll practice on the first one, and then after a time I'll get the knack of pulling 'em out gently," he said.'

But apart from this rather newsy bit, there was really not much of interest to report in the way of tonsorial developments. Probably the most intriguing item in the December issue of the *Journal* was contained in a very short paragraph:

'We were very sorry to hear of the experience of Mr. Aubrey Stearns of San Francisco. We hope, however, that he was not greatly inconvenienced by his unpleasant experience.' The item was headed 'Too Bad'.

In 1921 the editors did find a mild development to write about. According to them, 'The once furiously popular military haircut, in which the clipper moved the neckline up as near the crown as possible, is as good as dead . . . partly because it

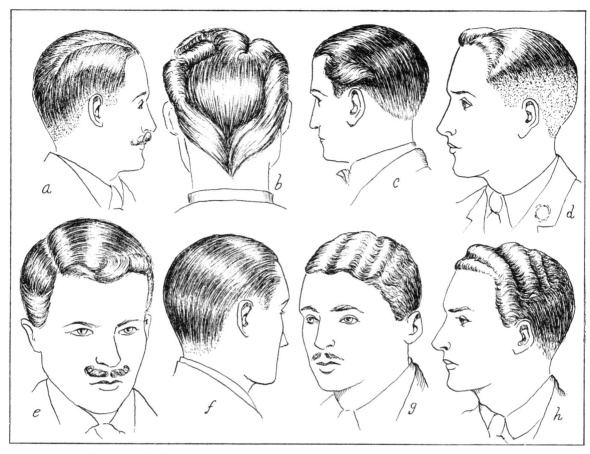

Fig. 124 : English hair styles of the 1930s: (a) Major; (b) Regent; (c) Argent; (d) Military;
(e) Coif; (f) Manchester; (g) Chester; (h) Gloster. (The terminology is Foan's)

became moribund in the east and the boys who went east and noted its condition
came back and turned thumbs down in the west. Its waning is also part of the general
tendency among so many men who went to war to get away from military things
as much as possible.' But the *Journal* was over-optimistic. The popularity of the
military haircut may have subsided, but it did not die out. Even as late as the 1960s
it was not unknown in rural areas of the United States.

The *Journal* admitted that 'Styles in haircuts vary little, and with the return to the
regular everyday haircut, about the only choice a customer has is between having it
cut long or having it cut short. As between these two styles, the "long" group is
leading. . . . The style in which the hair is left long on top and brushed straight back
or parted is gaining in popularity all over the country, especially in big cities.

'Another tendency reported by barbers is that the little Charlie Chaplin nose
affair is vanishing. Its once proud wearers have allowed it to spread to the full
width of the mouth or have banished it altogether. More have done the latter because
the mustache is less popular in 1921 than even in 1920.'

The thin, pencil-line moustache of the late 1920s apparently got its impetus in Hollywood, though the style was hardly a new one, having been worn by Charles II several centuries earlier.

It was more or less customary in 1922 to part the hair on the left side. However, as Alfred Stephen Bryan pointed out in a column on 'Correct Dress for Men', many men, 'because their hair is thinning along the temples, prefer to part it in the centre. This is a matter of no consequence, but it is an affair of some consequence that the hair be kept short and that it shows a lustre which denotes habitual care.'

Lustre, in fact, became exceedingly important in the twenties with the patent-leather look popularized by such film stars as Rudolph Valentino and George Raft. Valentino also created a sort of vogue for sideburns, but they were never fashionable and never really quite respectable.

However, with the very flat, plastered-down hair, there arose in some quarters a vogue for a rather stiff wave, which looked artificial and usually was.

It was reported in June 1922, that the latest fad in Boston was the marcel wave for men. 'They are', said the article, 'lining up now with the blondes with bobbed hair for the hot iron applications to the flowing locks in the beauty parlors. The secret leaked out recently when Mrs. C. M. Lamping-Nolan, who has done enough hair to reach from Boston to China, admitted that some of the smarter young men of the town are acquiring curly locks with which nature never endowed them.'

One of the operators added further details: 'Men who have what we call a natural line marcel the best. By the natural line I mean the manner in which the hair falls from the forehead. Most all blondes have their hair waved, or more properly speaking, marcelled.' She then explained that men had their hair done to make them 'look prettier' and that they were much braver about it than women, who tended to cringe at the approach of the hot iron.

It can be seen on Plate 142 that there was a certain variety in styles during the twenties. But in the United States, as a rule, beards were worn only by elderly men, whereas young men wore no facial hair at all. Neat, conservative moustaches were acceptable when worn by middle-aged or elderly men and were considered rather distinguished. Moustaches which were not neatly trimmed were considered old-fashioned; and though tolerated when worn by one's gardener, they were thought somewhat eccentric when worn by one's friends. Moustaches which were too full and too carefully waxed or too thin were looked upon in middle-class circles as affectations and therefore open to suspicion.

Although most men wore the hair short and usually straight and flat, men in the arts often wore it longer and fuller. The centre parting was still worn occasionally, but the side parting was preferred. The flat, gleaming pompadour was worn throughout the twenties. The hair was sometimes marcelled, it is true; but this was never considered quite proper by the middle classes. In general, the hair was supposed to be short and neat and that was all.

THE THIRTIES (Plate 143)

The patent-leather look was considered *passé* in the thirties; the pompadour was not fashionable; and the hair was seldom parted in the centre. Although it was still worn short, any natural wave was allowed to have its way instead of being plastered down. Sometimes it was even encouraged—surreptitiously, of course.

In the *Art and Craft of Hairdressing*, published in London in 1936, Foan showed two styles of wavy hair which could be achieved with proper cutting and judicious use of comb and water (Figure 124 *g* and *h*). Although the names of the various hair styles shown were originated by Foan, he claimed that they had been adopted by other hairdressers and were in general use when the book was written.

Conservative moustaches were still worn occasionally by older men but seldom, at least in the United States, by 'respectable' young men. Figure 125 shows some of the styles being worn in England. It is perhaps significant that beards, though rarely worn, were sometimes being written about.

In an article published in *New Outlook* in 1934, it was noted that men of the preceding generation had looked upon whiskers with scorn and amusement. 'They were either the mark of dotage or the badge of effeminacy, depending on the age of the stubborn ones who might cling to them in spite of advancing thought. A veteran of the Mexican War, for example, might hold fast to a chin concealer if he so desired, for after all the old must be occasionally indulged. Frenchmen could wear whatever shape or kind of beard the Latin taste favored. . . . But no-one else. A young American man with a beard laid himself open to any charge his saner neighbors might lay against him, and naturally enough, no American wore one.' Moustaches were acceptable 'provided they were kept out of harm's way by a strict discipline of wax, hot irons, and daily trimming. But the face proper, up to and above the ears, had to be kept clear.'

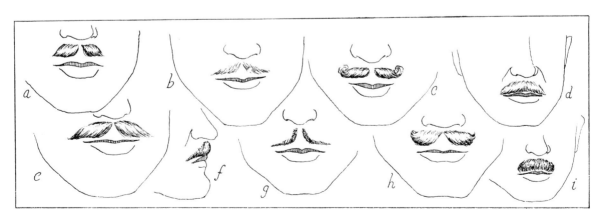

Fig. 125 : English moustaches of the 1930s: (a) Consort; (b) Shadow; (c) Guardsman; (d) Major; (e) General; (f) Military; (g) Coleman; (h) Captain; (i) Regent. (The terminology is Foan's)

New Outlook laid the credit or the blame squarely on the shoulders of King C. Gillette and his safety razor. No doubt Mr Gillette made the whole thing less painful; but men had been shaving off and on since the Egyptians, as custom dictated, without Mr Gillette's assistance or encouragement.

In view of the widespread beardlessness, the magazine was distressed to learn that Rumania had not kept up with the latest fashions, but the editors were relieved to note that she was now coming round and had actually put beards under government control. 'Every beard in Rumania,' they informed their readers, 'now requires an official permit, which must be paid for. The announcement was made not long ago, and to see that everyone heard it, mounted couriers were sent to every village and town, where the proclamation was read to the people. . . . The government was not primarily interested in revenue, but in bringing Rumania at last into line with a clean and modern world.'

Ernest Boyd, a bearded defender of the beard, writing in the *New Statesman and Nation* in August 1935, expressed the opinion that 'a bearded man in America enjoys all the privileges of a bearded woman in a circus'. He looked forward, however, to the time, which even then seemed to be in the making, when beards would again abound. Others were dismayed at the prospect.

The Forties (Plate 144)

The only notable change in this decade was that wavy hair was not only acceptable but fashionable, and the slightest wave was encouraged. The straight-haired often managed a slight wave with comb and water or occasionally, though never openly, with the help of a professional hairdresser. Even when the hair was worn straight, it was often cut and combed to give it a certain fullness. Men's hair fashions were being set by young film stars and entertainers, the fashions were copied by teenagers and college students, and thus the styles were established.

Beards were rarely seen in the United States and moustaches only occasionally, but perhaps the very lack of them piqued the interest of writers. Edith Effron, writing in 1944 in the *New York Times Magazine*, stated that the beard 'is the American male's greatest inhibition. The 1944 woman generally shares the opinion of Shakespeare's Beatrice, who, in *Much Ado About Nothing*, declares: "Lord, I could not endure a husband with a beard on his face; I had rather lie in the woolen."' As for the moustache, Miss Effron suggested that 'it plays many roles today: South American suavity, French affectation, Sicilian villainy. It is Chaplin-pathetic, Hitler-psychopathic, Gable-debonair, Lou Lehr-wacky. It perplexes. It fascinates. It amuses. And it repels.' She felt that men wearing moustaches in 1944 did so for purely practical reasons, and she quoted the results of a poll taken by the *New York Post* in 1944 showing that 'mustache-wearers feel their adornment to be economically advantageous, inspiring of confidence, dignified, distinctive, mature, and refined'.

In the same year Dr Marion Smith, an anthropologist of Columbia University, expressed her opinion that men who were wearing moustaches were non-conformists. Dr A. A. Brill, a psycho-analyst quoted by Miss Effron, was not quite so concise in his opinion: 'America is a young country. We are young in many ways and we don't like to assume the burdens of age. The mustache is a symbol of maturity, and the American who doesn't care to grow older shaves it off. That's why the ideal of this nation is a clear-cut, clean-shaven youth. Frequently young men grow mustaches in order to look older, but as they gain in years, they shave them off or cut them down in size. Unconsciously, these men wish to wipe out the signs of age. In general,' he concluded, 'it is a sign of bad adjustment if you do not follow the style of your country. The waxed mustache—or the mustache shaved in an artificial pattern—is an affectation in America.' Finally, he decided that 'apart from all that . . . it's just a matter of taste'. Miss Effron pointed out that Dr Brill was wearing a small white moustache and a tiny goatee.

In her investigation of moustaches by way of the barbers, Miss Effron discovered that most of them considered men wearing moustaches difficult to deal with, and she quoted one as saying, 'They're fussy as old maids. You can't hardly ever please them.' Another barber listed the four most prevalent types of moustache in America as the 'waxed-pointy kind', the 'Clark Gable type', the 'Dewey one', and the 'drooping mustaches'. Women, she found, did not care for any of them.

THE FIFTIES (Plate 145)

In this decade we find not only a wide variety of hair styles, ranging from the popular crew cut to the long Elvis Presley style and finally to the Caesar cut, but also a sprinkling of beards and moustaches among the less conservative element.

In the January 1950 issue of *Barbers' Journal* there was an article on 'fan waving' —using a comb and a hair dryer to develop and shape a wave in men's hair. Barbers were beginning to call themselves hair stylists, and the more expensive shops were adding hair colouring and permanent waving to their other services.

The *New York Times Magazine* pointed out in December 1954 that a few male models were appearing in advertisements wearing moustaches. 'Is this evidence', inquired the magazine, 'that the mustache is also returning to the common lip?' The great majority of barbers questioned on the subject were convinced that it was not.

But in the autumn of 1955 *Look* noted that beards were to be seen increasingly on young men on the street, in offices, in restaurants, and in night clubs. 'Young wearers', concluded *Look*, 'have apparently rebelled, decided to save the estimated two-thirds of a year spent during the adult male's life grimly wielding the razor.' The article stated flatly that the most popular style was the Vandyke.

Late in 1956 *Life* reported that the 'flattop' hair style had become so popular with men that a Wisconsin barber had attached his electric clippers to a telescoping arm which could shear off the hair with geometrical precision. He estimated that thirty to forty per cent of his patrons requested the 'flattops'.

With the increase in attention to men's hair, and the improved techniques in wig-making, it is not surprising that more and more men began to wear hairpieces. This development also undoubtedly was spurred on by the number of film and television actors who were known to wear them.

Late in 1958 a New York wig-maker reported that since 1954 there had been a 750 per cent increase in the sale of men's hairpieces and that about 75 per cent of these were in the ivy league style and were sold to men under thirty-five. A few months later *Time* reported that Sears, Roebuck were sending out thirty thousand catalogues 'in discreetly unmarked white envelopes', advertising their 'career-winning toupees', ranging in price from $109.95 (£40) to $224.95. Both long-haired and close-cropped models were available. Late in 1959 a New York firm, called Hairlines Inc., reported that young businessmen accounted for about 40 per cent of their sales.

THE SIXTIES (Plates 146, 147)

The trends established in the fifties continued to develop in the early sixties along with an increased consciousness of style. A greater variety of styles was worn than in the previous decades, and considerably more time and attention were given to the hair. This was reflected in the barbers' shops, some of which took on a very chic look and offered such inducements as razor cutting, tinting, and permanent waving. A few of the more exclusive establishments even supplied their customers with hair-pieces. One Madison Avenue barber charged $25 for styling the hair and provided for the convenience of its customers (mostly executives and actors) a mask called Sudden Youth.

In November 1963 *Time* reported on two new male beauty parlours in New York: 'The big news in the skin game is that it's getting masculine to be feminine. The leathery look in men is Out. Creams and cleansers, powders and pomades, hair-tinting combs, face-tightening masks, nail lacquers, hair sprays and sweet-smelling stuff in all sizes, shapes and prices are booming in the male market, and the cosmetics industry is rushing to repackage its female products into something for the boys. ... Beautician Aida Gray has branched out from her female trade in Beverly Hills to open two masculine beauty parlors ... where she has facilities for facials, massages, instant skin-tanning and eyebrow tinting. "In the past year or year and a half," chirps chic, French-born Aida, "there's been a tremendous rise in men's cosmetics. I got into the male line when I discovered that about 50% of my customers had husbands who were using their beauty creams. We sell green powder for ruddy skin and blue powder for sallow skin. We don't sell them powder puffs, of course." Manufacturers and retailers were reluctant to try to explain the shift in male habits,

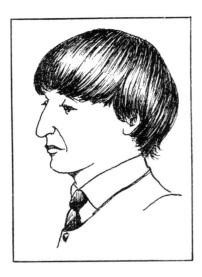

Fig. 126 : Beatle haircut, 1964

though they were quick to take advantage of it. As one busy and happy buyer put it, "Men have just decided not to smell like men any more. They want to smell good."'

The hair was still being worn relatively short and neatly trimmed and was still rarely parted in the middle. Partings were sometimes quite low on the side. The Caesar cut gained enormously in popularity and was worn by many college men and fashion-conscious young men everywhere. It was, however, strictly a young man's cut and was not considered suitable for older men, though undoubtedly it was influential in bringing their hair forward a bit. In England the so-called *English cut* (Plate 145-U-AA) was still very much in evidence. It could probably not accurately be described as either fashionable or unfashionable. Like chips with everything, it was simply there. The wildly eccentric hairstyle of Liverpool's Beatles (see Chapter 14) appeared to be a runaway development of the Caesar cut. Sideburns were not worn, except by an occasional eccentric.

But the most notable development was the increase in the number of beards. In the 1961 edition of *The Manual of the Associated Master Barbers and Beauticians of America* there was to be found, for the first time in many decades, a chapter on beards, including a special chart of twenty-one styles. In 1963 Kent Brushes made available, also for the first time in many decades, a Moustache-and-Beard-Good-Grooming-Brush, five and a half inches long. Moustaches, even rather full ones, were sometimes worn without beards, though in general young men preferred small beards with or without hair on the upper lip.

The increased interest in beards was no deterrent to the shaving industry. According to Edward T. Ewen, writing in the *New York Times Magazine*, American men bought about 3,700,000,000 razor blades a year along with 18,000,000 razors and 6,000,000 electric shavers at a total cost of nearly $300,000,000—the equivalent of more than a hundred million English pounds. Manufacturers of electric shavers regularly brought out new models, each one a little larger than the one before. In the early sixties shaving soap, brush-on creams, and brushless creams had all given way in popularity to aerosol lathers. The introduction by an English firm of a coated stainless-steel blade, giving about four times as many shaves as the conventional kind, represented perhaps the most significant advance in blade shaving since Gillette's invention of the safety razor in 1895. Although the Gillette company seemed unenthusiastic about offering the public a blade which would give four times as many shaves for only three times the price, the shavers themselves were delighted; and American men bought seven million of them in 1962. Gillette eventually joined its competitors by offering a stainless-steel blade. But a slight reduction in profits was a minor worry of manufacturers compared to the threat, however remote, of a revival of beards. Mr Ewen concluded his *Times* article with a word of comfort for the shaving industry:

'Fortunately for Schick, Remington, Gillette and company, beards today are very much out of fashion, worn for the most part only by beatniks, aging philosophers, free-lance magazine writers and Mitch Miller. Once thought of as a sign of the virile male, beards in general are now considered a sign of the chinless nonconformist—which is exactly the way that everyone inside the shaving industry would like everyone outside the shaving industry to keep on thinking.'

Although there were many who, like Mr Ewen, scoffingly discounted the signs of a developing interest in beards as a manifestation of the lunatic fringe, claiming that beards were not compatible with computers and space travel, there were others, fewer in number, who gleefully—or gloomily—predicted another bearded age.

PLATE 140 : TWENTIETH-CENTURY MEN 1900–1910

A   American. Stephen Crane, 1871–1900. Novelist, journalist, poet.

B   American. Grover Cleveland, 1837–1908. 22nd U.S. president.

C   1901, English.

D   English. Sir Henry Irving, 1838–1905 (for earlier portrait see Plate 102-O).

E   1900, English.

F   1904. Mark Hambourg. Russian pianist.

G   1903, American. William Gillette, 1853–1937. Actor and playwright.

H   1905, American. Arnold Daly.

I   1905. Joseph Conrad, 1857–1924. Novelist.

J   1903, Russian. Czar Nicholas II, 1868–1918.

K   1905, American. Victor H. Metcalf. Secretary of Commerce.

L   1905, American. E. A. Hitchcock. Secretary of the Interior.

M   1905, American. Maurice Hewlett. Writer.

N   1905, American. Booth Tarkington, 1869–1946.

O   1905, American. James Wilson. Secretary of Agriculture.

P   1904, English.

Q   1905, American. Henry Miller, 1860–1926. Actor-manager (for earlier portrait see Plate 105-U).

R   1905, American. H. A. Van Alstyne. Engineer.

S   1905. Heinrich Conreid. Director, Metropolitan Opera.

T   1908, German. Ludwig Ganghofers. Writer.

U   1907, English.

V   English. George Meredith, 1828–1909. Novelist and poet.

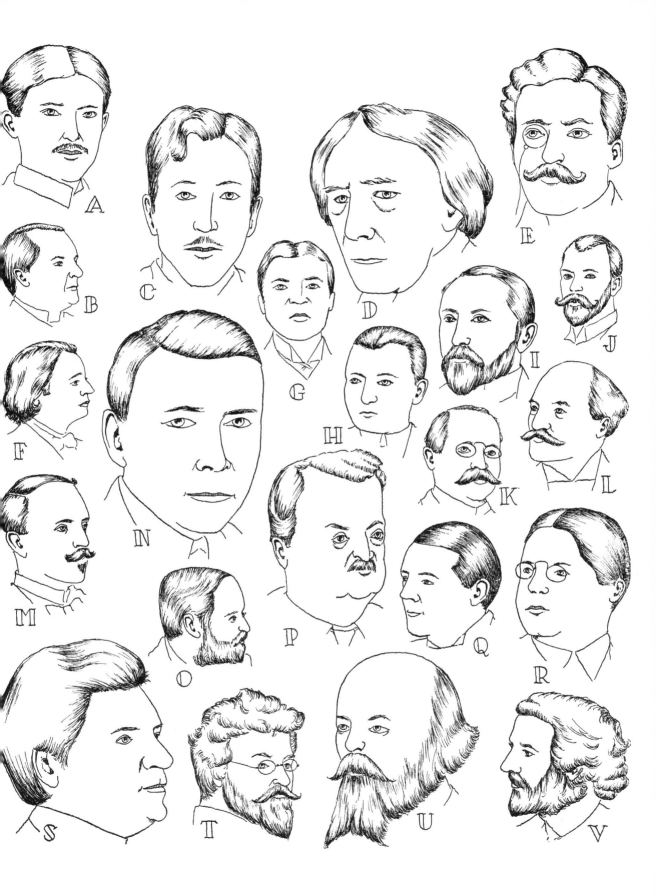

PLATE 141 : TWENTIETH-CENTURY MEN 1900–1915

A Émile Verhaeren, 1855–1916. Belgian poet and dramatist.

B John Philip Sousa, 1854–1932. American bandmaster and composer.

C Henrik Ibsen, 1828–1906.

D O. Henry (William Sydney Porter), 1862–1910.

E Piotr Kropotkin, 1842–1921. Russian anarchist.

F Miguel de Unamuno y Jugo, 1864–1936. Spanish philosopher.

G Georg Morris Cohen Brandes, 1842–1927. Danish writer.

H Rupert Brooke, 1887–1915. English poet.

I James Bryce, 1838–1922. English historian and politician

J 1911. American actor.

K 1911. American actor.

L 1912, American. Guthrie McClintic. Stage director and producer.

M 1910, British.

N 1912, American.

O 1914. American actor.

P 1914. American actor.

Q King Albert I of Belgium, 1875–1934.

R 1915. Robert Harron. American film actor.

S 1914, Charles Chaplin.

T 1915, British. *Walrus* moustache.

U 1914, John Drew.

———————

See also the European hair and beard styles in Figures 117-122.

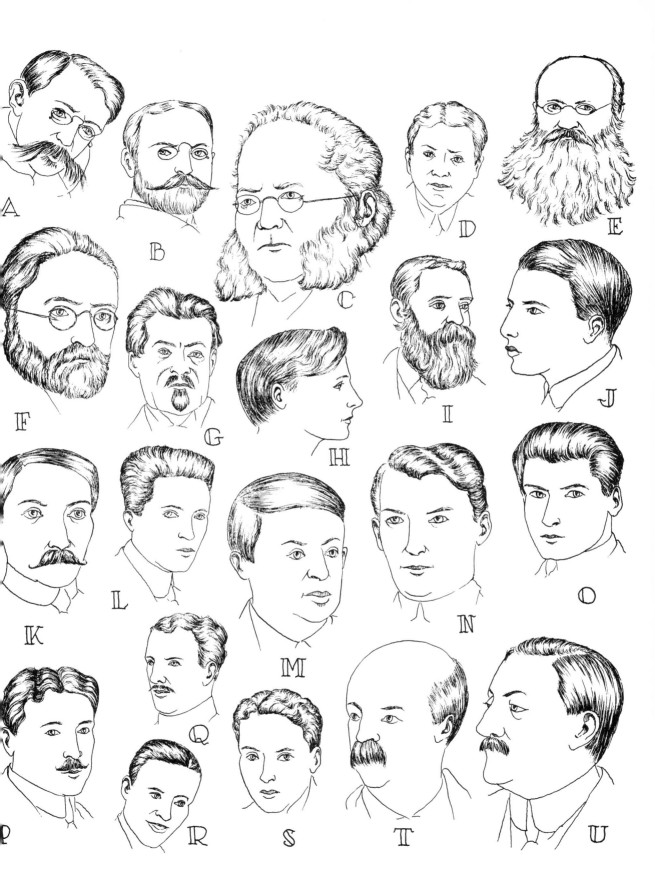

A　B　C　D　E

F　G　H　I　J

K　L　M　N　O

P　Q　R　S　T　U

PLATE 142 : TWENTIETH-CENTURY MEN 1915–1930

A   Woodrow Wilson, 1846–1924. 28th U.S. president.

B   1917. American boy.

C   1918, British.

D   1919. American singer.

E   1916, British.

F   1919, American.

G   Vladimir Ilyich Lenin, 1870–1924.

H   1920, American.

I   Joyce Kilmer, 1886–1918.

J   Rudolph Valentino, 1895–1926.

K   c. 1922. American senator.

L   1929. John Barrymore.

M   1924. American actor. The *Barber's Journal* called this the *Student style*.

N   1925. American boy.

O   c. 1925. American reformer. *Walrus* moustache.

P   1927, American.

Q   English. John Drinkwater, 1882–1937.

R   1930, American.

S   1926. American actor.

T   Calvin Coolidge, 1872–1933. 30th U.S. president.

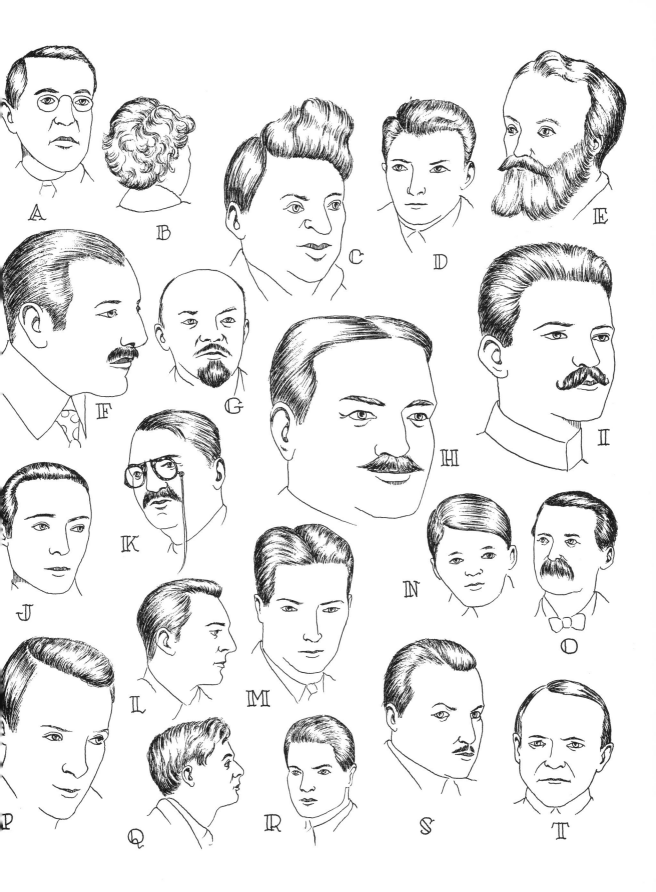

A

B

C

D

E

F

G

H

I

J

K

L

M

N

O

P

Q

R

S

T

PLATE 143 : TWENTIETH-CENTURY MEN 1930–1940

A   William E. Haskell, 1862–1933. American journalist.

B   1931, British.

C   1932, British.

D   1931, British.

E   1932, British.

F   1931, English. John Gielgud.

G   1933. American actor.

H   1935, British.

I   Norman Douglas, 1868–1952. English writer.

J   1935. Will Rogers. American humourist.

K   Adolf Hitler, 1889–1945. *Toothbrush* moustache.

L   1937. American actor.

M   1938, American. W. C. Fields.

N   Sir Anthony Eden. Born 1897.

O   Walter Damrosch, 1862–1950. German-American conductor, composer.

P   1940. American college boy.

See also the English hair styles and moustaches in Figures 124 and 125.

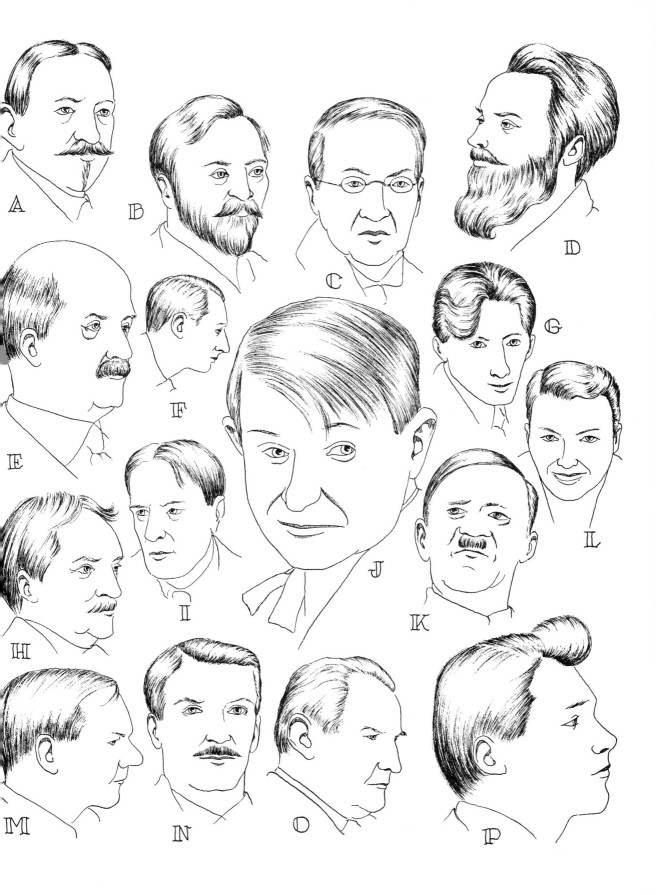

A B C D E F G H I J K L M N O P

PLATE 144 : TWENTIETH-CENTURY MEN 1940–1950

A   British. George Bernard Shaw, 1856–1950.

B   1940, American.

C   1940, American.

D   1940, American.

E   1940, American.

F   1940, American.

G   1941. American film actor.

H   1940, American.

I   English. James Hilton. Novelist.

J   1941, Russian. Josef Stalin, 1879–1953.

K   1941, American.

L   1947, American. Paul Kelly. Actor.

M   1941, American.

N   1945. American actor.

O   1948, American. Jackie Cooper. Actor.

P   1947. American actor.

Q   1946, American. Chris Alexander. Actor-dancer.

R   1948. American actor.

S   1948, American. Gene Nelson. Dancer.

T   1949, American. John Lund. Actor.

U   1950. British writer.

V   1950. American writer.

W   1950. British writer.

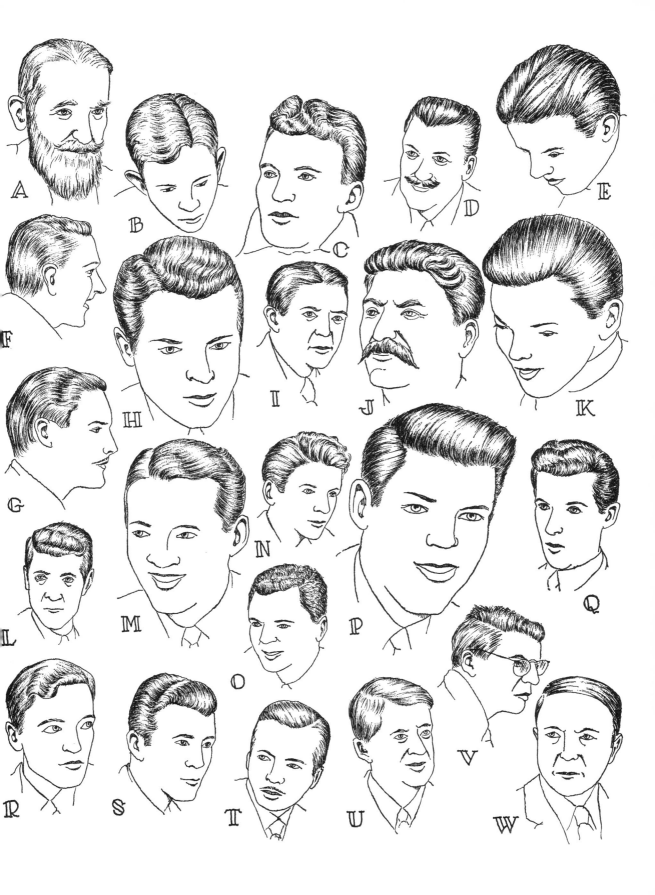

PLATE 145 : TWENTIETH-CENTURY MEN 1950–1960

A   1950. American actor.

B   1950. American actor.

C   *c.* 1950. American college professor. Writer.

D   1951, American. Frank Albertson. Actor.

E   1951. American actor.

F   *c.* 1952. American writer.

G   1953, American. Mitchell Erickson. Actor.

H   1952, American. Ray Stricklyn. Actor.

I   1953, American. Carleton Carpenter. Actor.

J   1953, American. Orson Bean. Actor, comedian. *Crew cut* (see also P below).

K   1954, American. *Madison Avenue cut.* Hair about an inch long, flat on top and sides. Usually combed to the side or slightly forward, then brushed back in front.

L   *c.* 1955. American writer.

M   1954, American. James Dean. Actor.

N   1956, American.

O   *c.* 1956, American.

P   1956, American. *Crew cut.* A popular style with college men and sometimes with older men who hoped it would make them look younger. A still shorter cut, not so stylish, was known as the *butch cut.*

Q   1956, American. *Elvis* style. Long hair, rising in a high wave in front, usually worn with sideburns. Worn by Elvis Presley, American entertainer (see also 146-B).

R   *c.* 1957. American writer.

S   *c.* 1957. Australian writer.

T   *c.* 1958. Austrian writer.

U   *c.* 1958, British. *English cut.* Hair long on top and sides, full over the ears and in back, and combed back from the forehead.

V   *c.* 1958. American writer.

W   *c.* 1959, American. John Steinbeck.

X   *c.* 1959. American writer.

Y   *c.* 1959. American writer.

Z   1959. American actor.

AA   *c.* 1959. British writer. *English cut.*

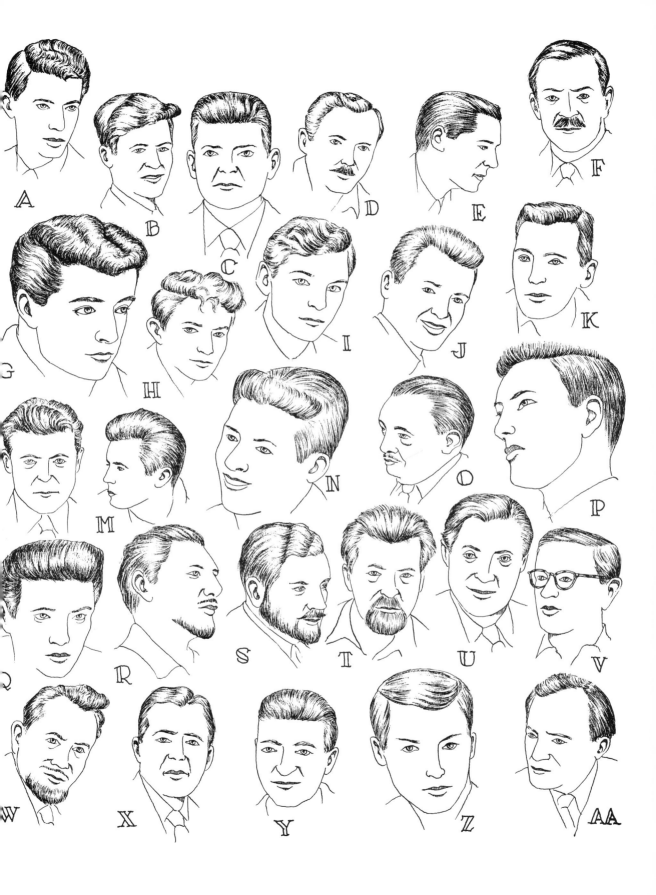

A

B

C

D

E

F

G

H

I

J

K

M

N

O

P

Q

R

S

T

U

V

W

X

Y

Z

AA

PLATE 146 : TWENTIETH-CENTURY MEN 1960, 1961

A   1961, English. (Sketched in London.)

B   1961. American college student. *Elvis* style (see also 145-Q).

C   1960, American. Jim Kirkwood. Writer.

D   1961. American college student.

E   1961, American. Bobby Rydell. Popular singer.

F   1961, American. Raymond Burr. Actor.

G   1961. American college student.

H   1961, French. *Caesar cut*. Hair combed down over forehead. Very popular with young men. (Sketched in Paris.)

I   1961. American college student.

J   1961, English. *Caesar cut*. (Sketched in London.)

K   1961, American. Eccentric style. (Sketched in Greenwich Village.)

L   1961, American. *Caesar cut*. (Sketched in Chicago.)

M   1961. American foreign correspondent.

N   1961, American.

O   1961, French. *Caesar cut*. (Sketched in Paris.)

P   1961, English. Teddy boy. (Sketched at Marble Arch in London.)

Q   1961, French. *Caesar cut*. (Sketched in Paris.)

R   1961, French.

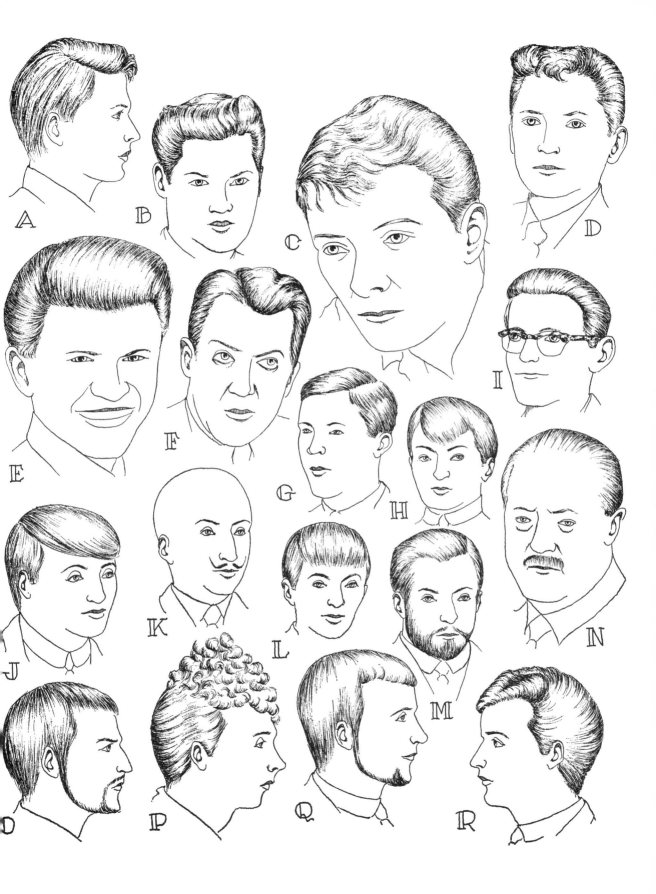

Plate 147 : Twentieth-Century Men 1962, 1963

A   Tennessee Williams, born 1914. American playwright.

B   American. (Sketched in New York.)

C   German student. *Caesar cut.*

D   American hairdresser.

E   English. (Sketched in London.)

F   American. Mitch Miller. Conductor.

G   John F. Kennedy. 35th U.S. president.

H   English. (Sketched in New York.)

I   American businessman.

J   American. *Caesar cut.* (Sketched in New York.)

K   American. (Sketched in Greenwich Village.)

L   American student. *Flat-top crew cut.* When the hair was of normal length on sides and back, as it is here, the style was sometimes called the *Detroit*, the *Dutch*, or the *California* cut.

M   American. (Sketched in New York.)

N   French. Small *Vandyke* beard. (Sketched in Paris.)

O   English. (Sketched in London.)

P   American writer.

Q   American pianist.

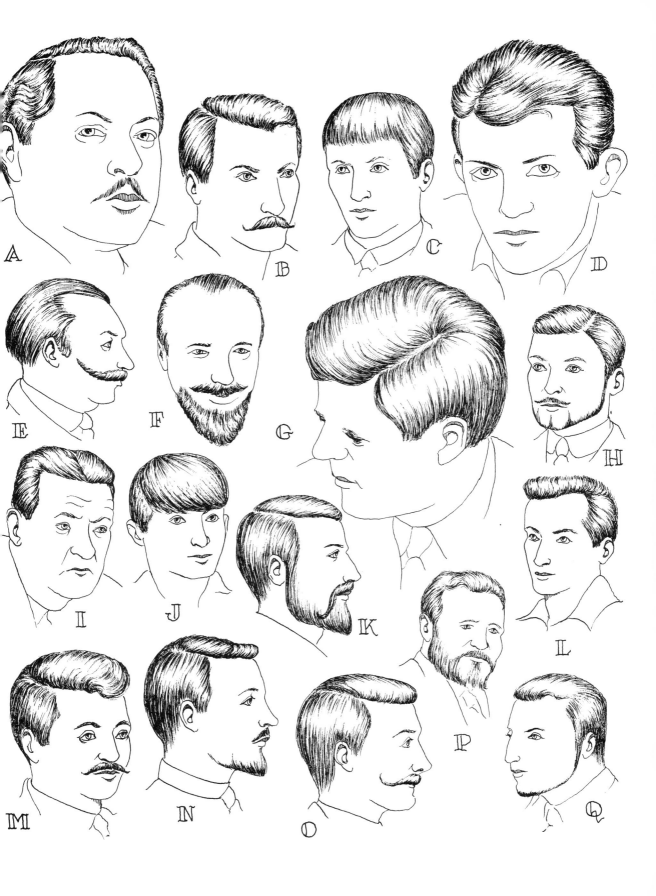

14 · The Twentieth Century—Women

It is quite likely that some day
in frenzied haste, casting all caution
to the winds . . . I shall flee to a
coiffeur and come out a shorn
lamb to join the great army of
the bobbed.
                    MARY PICKFORD 1927

The twentieth century provides a kaleidoscope of hair styles for women beginning with the towering Gibson-girl pompadour, passing through the incredibly ugly, emancipated bob, and reverting early in the second half of the century to the excessive coiffures reminiscent of the late eighteenth century. The hairdressers achieved a prominence they had not enjoyed since the days of Marie Antoinette, and they vied furiously with each other to create new styles. But in the end it was who wore the styles that really mattered. With the coming of moving pictures, Hollywood stars automatically set the styles. Garbo, Mary Pickford, Colleen Moore, Jean Harlowe, Clara Bow—any one of them had more influence than Queen Mary, Mrs Vanderbilt, or Grace Coolidge. Later, European stars became equally influential. And, except for Jacqueline Kennedy, it was the film stars who continued to influence the trend. There were occasional attempts by hairdressers and publicists to launch new styles, such as the Cleopatra look, coming on the crest of an enormous amount of publicity about the film; but these did not always prove popular. Women were frequently told in the newspapers and magazines how they were going to be wearing their hair next season, whether they liked it or not. Sometimes they wore it that way, and sometimes they did not. The only sure thing was that they would be wearing it differently.

1900–1910 (Plates 148, 149)

In March 1900 the beauty editor of London's newspaper for ladies, *The Queen*, wrote: 'The tendency of the present day as regards hairdressing is towards a somewhat *négligé* style, conspicuous for a studied carelessness which, while the very opposite of anything approaching disorder, is equally far removed from the set regularity of outline distinctive not so long ago of the fashionable coiffure. The waves of hair at the sides and back are full and arranged in broken rather than in fine and stiff lines, while the curled fringe is replaced in many instances by a full pouf or a series of rather large, lightly rolled curls.'

It was the custom of *The Queen* to heap upon its advertisers regular and enthusiastic praise. In April readers were told, probably not for the first time, that Eugène

Morphy of Oxford Street could be absolutely depended upon for skilfully made hair pieces: 'His Marcella fringe points to the latest direction of fashion; three curls, frizzed rather than curled, fall on to the forehead in front, while the rest of the hair is skilfully waved. His Parisian knot for the back of the head is equally judicious and can be arranged with the least expensive of his switches. He can be absolutely relied on for those aids to a good appearance which are so valuable; for example, the pretty pins made of tortoiseshell, with diamond tops; the excellent waving irons, such as the Rapid, which can be heated either by gas or spirit; the rose bloom for the cheeks, either pink or flesh colour, and stimulating hair lotions so good for the head. His pomades are nutritive, and the walnut pomade is darkening as well as strengthening to the hair.' The editor then describes a Morphy court coiffure with the hair 'divided down the centre, the sides, being loosely arranged, coming slightly over the ears. Some frizzed curls lighten the parting. At the summit of the coiffure a large loop is supported at the sides by a few soft marteaux, the plumes and veil in the rear.'

In both England and the United States Paris was still considered the hub of the fashion universe. One did not barge blindly ahead with new fashions but waited patiently—or impatiently—for news from Paris. In May *The Queen* reported that 'Hairdressing over in Paris seems to alter little, the front being usually parted slightly to one side, held with a diamond comb, while the waves are large. The ornaments seem to be of three kinds, either the outstretched wings of a bat-like shape in tulle spangled with silver or diamonds, aigrettes of divers shapes entirely made of diamonds, or a double bunch of flowers. . . . Forget-me-nots, small pink roses, or pale violets are alike successful when used to decorate the hair. The large bunches of two sizes, mounted flat, are used on either side of the erect knob. . . .

'Fringes, or, more correctly speaking, their various substitutes, are the only point in hairdressing about which there is just now much novelty to chronicle. The back hair manifests little variation beyond the fluctuating tendency of the coil or knot to assume a higher or lower position, and this, after all, is more a matter of taste than a rule of fashion.'

According to the August 25 issue of *The Queen*, a great many women were wearing transformations, as wigs were euphemistically called; and both *The Queen* and its advertisers seemed to be waging a joint campaign to persuade even more of them to do so. A December issue carried twenty-four advertisements for hair and hair products—transformations, toupées (for women), fringes, clusters of curls, switches, dye, shampoo, curlers, tonic, depilatories, and so on. The fashion editor described a new device being promoted by one of the advertisers.

It was 'half-frame, half-toupée—for dressing the hair in the raised Pompadour style which it is at present the aim of fashionable hairdressing to achieve. The new addition certainly partakes of some of the best points of both frame and toupée, for while it gives the form produced by the one, it has all the lightness of the other, and at the same time renders it possible for the coiffure to be composed for the main part of the wearer's own hair. First there is a light foundation of invisible hair net, made so as to fit easily to the head. On this is mounted an uncrushable Pompadour dressing of natural, wavy hair, with a fringe as full or as slight as may be wished. The natural hair is brought out through the opening between the fringe and the Pompadour, and combed back over the latter, with which it mingles in a perfectly imperceptible manner. . . . The fringe is by no means an indispensable part of the arrangement, as the convenient device can be adapted for a Pompadour coiffure pure and simple either without a fringe, with a few curls at the temples, a centre curl, a side parting, or, indeed, with any variation of the fashionable style that may be required.'

In this first year of the new century the problem of colouring the hair was still in women's minds, as it had been for several thousand years. A slightly puzzled editor wrote in *The Queen*:

'It is extraordinary of late years how grey and white hair has come into vogue. Quite young women are seen with white hair, and no doubt this is due in a measure to the fact that to be in the fashion of past years they dyed their tresses golden, auburn, or any other hue that prevailed, and this has whitened the tresses when the colouring passed away. But it is absurd to think that any hair on the head can be bleached. It is said to have been done by Americans in America and in Paris, but though we have devoted a good deal of time both in New York and in the French capital to ascertain how this can be done, we have never been able to discover anybody who will undertake to do it. The price of white and grey artificial hair is often very high, and it is quite easy to bleach it off the head. . . . Combs are still worn, but not so much for ornament as use, to give a rounded form to the hair and push it forward or down in the nape of the neck.'

In July 1901, on the other side of the Atlantic, the *Delineator* brought its readers up to date on the latest styles:

'Dark hair should be smoothly dressed while light or blond hair should be loosely arranged in soft waves and fluffy curls. . . . The soft, loose waves which are almost universally becoming and quite as popular as they have been for some time, provide the first step in dressing the hair. There are many different ways of procuring the desired effect, the curling or crimping irons being most generally used, though great care should be exercised that the irons are not rough or overheated, else they will destroy the beauty of the hair. An excellent plan is to wrap each lock to be waved in paper, to protect it. . . . A low forehead permits the wearing of the high, soft Pompadour, which remains in popular favor, while the face with a high forehead is improved by an outline of tiny curls. The part at the centre still has its adherents, though that made at the left side of the loose Pompadour is more popular.

'Misses of fifteen or sixteen years of age will arrange their hair in a braid with the end brought up underneath and tied with a ribbon bow—black velvet ribbon being preferably used—or, in a loose knot placed low at the back with curling ends falling at the nape of the neck, is another mode.

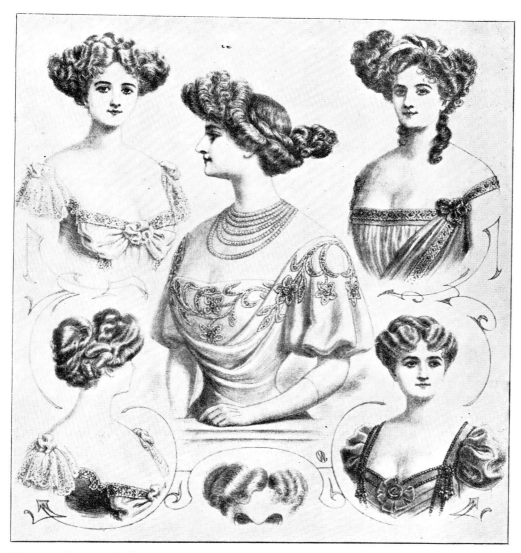

Fig. 127 : Fashionable French styles of 1908. Coiffures by M. Camille Croisat

'The woman who appreciates correctness in every detail of her toilette suits her coiffure to the occasion, and while with street costume she may wear her hair in a half-low knot or braids wound round the back of the head, she will arrange it high on the head and introduce some of the numerous dainty hair ornaments and pins when attired in evening dress.'

The reader with scanty hair is assured that 'there are all sorts of artificial means provided to overcome this deficiency, and so perfectly do they match both in color and the quality of the hair as to defy detection. One of the newest styles for dressing the hair for ceremonious occasions is the Transformation . . . made of naturally wavy hair. It is circular, very narrow, and follows the outline of the head, and forms long waves from each side of the front, which is a bang effect with a curl at the centre and a soft Pompadour back.' The editor adds that there are 'innumerable accessories for dressing the hair elaborately for ceremonious functions, and no fashionable woman considers her wardrobe complete without many of these. Care, however, should be taken to avoid excessive decoration.' A few fashionable ornaments are described—'a delicate pink Japan rose, bearing iridescent spangles over each petal and maiden-hair fern in graceful sprays at each side . . . two thick sprays of violets on each side of a large fluffy bow of gauze ribbon with satin ribbon edge . . . back and side combs made of carved tortoise-shell.'

In 1902, with Victoria gone and Edward soon to be crowned, emphasis in *The Queen* quite naturally shifted to hair styles suitable for the coronation. But in the excitement the old reliable advertisers were not forgotten: 'Already that successful exponent of the science of hairdressing, Mr Nicol, has brought out at his much frequented establishment, 50 Haymarket, a coiffure of natural wavy hair, which, under the name of the Coronation transformation, is designed with a view to the fashionable festivities or courtly function for which it is likely to be called into requisition. . . . The new transformation or toupée (for it can be mounted in either form) [is] quite the most recent development of the self-dividing transformation so greatly in request ever since its introduction a season or so back. The strong point of this artistic aid to the coiffure is its adaptability to any and every style of fashionable hairdressing, and this attractive quality is more than ever characteristic of its newest form, in which it is equally suitable for an arrangement as a Court coiffure or a simple morning dressing, to be worn with a knot of hair set high on the head or a coil resting low down on the neck.'

In a subsequent issue titled ladies were reminded that their hair styles should be designed with the knot on top of the head, not at the back, in order to keep the coronet from slipping off.

In general, English and American styles were very much the same since both came from Paris. The differences, such as those provided by occasional coronations, were minor.

Annie Kellet, writing in the *Ladies Home Journal* in 1903, informed her readers that the tendency to wear the hair low was quite marked. 'There is a good reason for this, as the low coiffure is in harmony with the hats and gowns which are worn this season. . . . The coils of the hair are arranged to appear large and loose; the effect, therefore, is much softer than it was last year.' In discussing pompadours, she suggested that it was sometimes necessary to roughen the inside slightly to give it sufficient fullness. This is what, in the 1960s, was called 'teasing' the hair.

From the *Barbers' Journal* of 1904 we glimpse the male viewpoint of women's fashions: 'At present . . . women do not, as a rule, part their hair in the middle or at all. They roll it and tousle it into the nearest attainable imitation of a jute mop projecting from the forehead.'

In general, during the first decade, the hair was very full and loose with emphasis on width rather than height, though there were some topknots. Pads, false hair, and combs were used in profusion.

In the early years of the century in London Karl Nessler, a German hairdresser, was perfecting his invention of the permanent wave. When, in 1904, he was able to electrify the device, it became sufficiently practical that he was able to advertise 'Nestlé Permanent Waving'. It was under the name of Charles Nestlé that he later established himself with great success in New York. The first permanent waves required an exhausting twelve hours to complete and were enormously expensive. It was not really until after the First World War that they became generally popular.

In the autumn of 1908 Mrs Ralston wrote in the *Ladies Home Journal* that 'the arrangement of the hair has been gradually changing for a year and now has quite another look than formerly: it is lower, softer, and conforms more to the shape of the head. Hair ornaments likewise have changed, some being low and others high. . . . Tulle bows may be used for the theatre or in the evening when a hat is not required, and are so simple to make and so pretty and airy that every girl should have one. . . . Some of the prettiest of these bows are of two colors, one over the other: silver-gray and pink are charming, or a soft blue and white; or again gold or silver gauze ribbon could be used. Place them rather high on one side of the head—the exact position depending on the arrangement of the hair and what is becoming.'

1910–1920 (Plates 149-151)

The second decade brought a reaction against the exaggerated, heavy coiffures requiring the use of pads and false hair to give them the proper shape. In 1911 the *Ladies Home Journal* interviewed six prominent, unnamed women to try to get an answer to the burning question, 'Can a woman's hair be done simply?' The answer was apparently an unqualified *Yes!* The *Journal* reported:

'In all of these six cases these women have found it possible to wear their hair simply without resorting to the use of the unsanitary and ridiculous "rat" or "puff". And in four of the instances cited the women have themselves confessed to the writer that they "have not much hair". But, as one of these women said: "I would

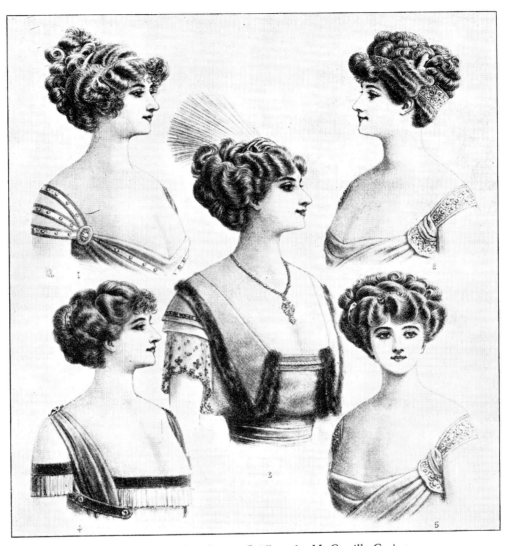

Fig. 128 : Fashionable French styles of 1911. Coiffures by M. Camille Croisat

infinitely rather go without hair if need be than live a lie to myself, my husband, and my children.''

'It is this fact that so many women fail to see, that in the wearing of shams they are living a lie not only to themselves but also to those nearest and dearest to them. And in far more instances than women imagine they have lost something of their subtle womanhood, something of the respect that they crave and would have in the eyes of husband and children, by their assumption of the sham, of whatever nature, in their toilet. A husband recently said to the writer: "My respect for my wife fell immeasurably when I saw she was of the kind to resort to shams in her dress." . . . The step from the wearing of a lie to the acting of a lie is not a long one. . . . The question for a woman to decide is not . . . "Would I look better if I wore this sham or that imitation?" The real question for her to ask herself is . . . "Am I going to live a lie?"'' It is probably safe to say that a good many readers decided they were.

However, the rats were on their way out, and the hair was beginning to conform to the shape of the head (see Plate 150). In 1913 Mary Atherton described the new trend in the *Ladies Home Journal*: 'We have with us a stylish coiffure made up of bang, ear-lappet, and a coil of some sort at the back of the head; a style capable of charming things when properly treated, rigidly hideous in unintelligent hands.' The ear-lappet refers to any hair brought over the ears. 'One virtue it invariably has, this coiffure of today', Miss Atherton continues, 'no matter who uses it or how, it is small. At last we have a fashion that restores the head to its proper size; but like everything else, the present-day coiffure has the defects of its virtues. If bang and lappet concentrate on nose, eyes, and mouth, they emphasize these features impartially, whether they are ugly or beautiful. So if we are going to use the present coiffure successfully, let us use it sensibly.'

Having got rid of the excess width, women started very shortly to increase the height of the coiffure. But the bulk of the hair extended back and upward from the crown, rather than being set statically on top of the head.

In March 1916 the *Journal* reported that the coiffure of the season was distinguished by 'just a little less tension, more indulgence toward the need of the features resulting in softer waves, a few natural puffs and coils and beautiful pins and combs correctly posed. . . . The high coiffure loses some of its stateliness and the more youthful low arrangements have added charm when adorned with the new pins in pretty and unique dagger designs, adaptations from fern leaves, and the new chignon combs, all exquisitely studded with brilliants and colored stones.'

There was an additional note in June: 'Not for everyone are the hairdressings which droop over the ears and with cunning curls, caress the cheeks. Smooth and close, without a single wavering hair over brow or ears, are other coiffures. . . . For formal occasions hair ornaments are not of the elaborate character which has been fashionable. One or two slender bar pins, varying but little in size from the lace pin of the daytime, are worn, and small, brilliant-headed pins with square or Doric shaped tops, often incrusted with sapphires, emeralds, rubies, or amethysts, frequently complete a coiffure.'

After the war a few brave souls bobbed their hair; and others, not so courageous, turned theirs under to make it look as much like a bob as possible. The bob was a daring new thing, undoubtedly a manifestation of the emancipation of women. But it had been a hundred years since women cut off their hair, and the decision to take such an irrevocable step was not an easy one to make. It rested with the film stars to lead the way.

1920–1930 (Plates 152-154)

In England long hair, neatly waved, was still fashionable; and transformations (never referred as wigs) were popular. In the March 6th, 1920, issue of *The Queen* there were eleven large advertisements for transformations (at an average price of seven guineas) and fifteen advertisements for conditioning, colouring, removing, and restoring hair. There was also a beauty page which each week ran a large engraving of a transformation available from one of the advertisers, accompanied by an enthusiastic description.

But real hair or false, a neat, well-defined parting was essential. According to *The Queen* in January 1920, 'Fashions come and fashions go, but the charm of the parting continues its triumphant way. . . . At one time the hair falls away severely from it, leaving a long clear line running right across the top of the head. So was the Madonna parting of the early days of the war, the severity of which was in keeping with the spirit of the time. Now the reverse is the case, and little tendrils of hair break merrily from the coiffure, putting all severity aside, while the parting appears as a cleft between rising bands of crisp, waved hair, or as a division forming naturally in a riot of curls.'

On March 27 *The Queen* took notice of a slight change in the styles:

'There are three outstanding features of the new coiffures. The first is the prevalence of partings, but partings placed for the most part in unexpected positions. There is decided piquancy in such placing, and big opportunities for artistic and original developments. Sometimes these partings start at the side from the crown by the head towards the forehead in orthodox fashion and continue their way until the front is nearly reached, when they turn abruptly towards the centre, with something of the effect of the question mark, so that the little fringe . . . falls from the parting on one side, losing itself in the ordinary long hair on the other. Sometimes the parting will run deliberately parallel to the forehead instead of at right angles to it. . . . Sometimes, again, the parting will cut like a clear, cleft line, for quite a short distance at the side, inclining sharply either to the centre or the region of the ear as the case may be. But almost certainly there will be a parting somewhere, equally with the hair rising, full and vital from it, for anything like flat hair is anathema.

'A second characteristic of the season's coiffure is the swathing of the neck with the hair, as it were. For no longer is it brushed upwards, disclosing the roots or curly tendrils clinging around them, nor carried back to be lost in chignon or twist. *Au contraire*, the long, full tress, charmingly waved for the most part, is folded from temple to temple, so that the neck appears swathed with hair. . . .

'This swathing . . . leads on to . . . the return of the classic knot. . . . For if the hair be drawn around in this really new fashion, it follows that the long hair must be arranged in some such fashion, unless, of course, the fact of having long hair at all is to be suppressed, as was the case some years back, when the hair were simply swathed round with the ends tucked in, a fashion completely *passée* now. There is considerable latitude in the placing of the knot, as well as its form. Sometimes, indeed, a few nice fat curls replace it, and indications of a return to curls are not wanting. . . . But wherever we place it, the knot, coil, chignon, curls, or whatever it may be must stand well away from the head, providing the novel silhouette on which after all the modishness of the coiffure so largely depends.'

Late in January, on a page of 'Answers to Correspondents', there was one answer addressed simply to 'Iris':

'I am afraid both tongs and pins are proving detrimental to your hair, which is becoming so thin in front. Could you not give it a rest for the time by wearing a toupet, and meanwhile give nourishment and massage to your own hair to improve its growth? . . . If, however, you will not take such wise steps as these, I should advise the use of tongs, kept as cool as possible, with constant applications of a nutritive agent, such as Rowland's Macassar oil, to the roots of the hair to counteract in some degree these mischievous effects.' It is interesting to note that the only alternatives are false hair or cool tongs. The possibility of wearing the hair uncurled is not even considered.

The revival of wigs, no matter what they were called, can undoubtedly be traced directly to the fashion for neat, well-defined, deep waves in the hair. Such a hair style was difficult to achieve and to maintain, and too strenuous efforts to do so probably resulted in a good many disasters which required covering up. The popularity of the wig at this time was made possible by the fact that it could be made to look completely natural. The current styles concealed all roots of the hair, both front and back—except for those along the parting. And they could be made seemingly to grow out of the scalp by means of a *drawn parting*, for which two layers of silk gauze were used, the hairs being knotted into the under layer and then drawn through the upper layer—a technique requiring considerable time and skill. Women did not flaunt their wigs, as they had in the eighteenth century and as they would in the 1960s. They wore them, but they preferred that nobody know it. Even the coming of the bob did not put an end to the wigs, which continued to be made in all the latest styles.

With the twenties the popularity of the bob spread quickly. There was still a feeling that it might be a passing fad; and if the fad passed, what then? This

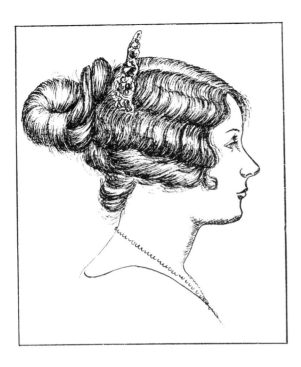

Fig. 129 : Unbobbed Englishwoman of 1923

undoubtedly kept many women away from the barbers' shops. But there were still large numbers of them who were willing to take the chance.

In January 1923 the *Barbers' Journal* issued the latest report on the bob. It was, they said, 'shearing short all the beautiful golden, brown, and black tresses. Women-folk young and up to fascinating, fatal forty are shedding their respected glory of great pitiful waving locks and spiralled curls in dainty beauty shop baskets and on the barber's shining linoleum.

'The close snip rage is raging worse than ever, and soon, if no indignant act of providence intervenes, masses of soft, lustrous feminine braids so much admired of man since the ape gave him his start, will be seen alone on elderly mothers and their surviving mamas.'

About this time there were rumours that the bob was on its way out; but in the autumn of 1923 the Paris correspondent of the *London Hairdressers' Weekly Journal* reported a sudden revival of interest, throwing the leading coiffeurs into a frenzy of uncertainty.

Irene Castle was generally credited with introducing the bob into the United States. But in 1924 a man named Henderson supplied his version of the origin of the bob:

'Bobbing in theory and practice has been worked into a science by a dean of the art and a high priest of bobdom, Signor Pierro Raspanti, who claims credit for having sheared the first locks that set women off on the bob-haired trail and opened up a special line of business for his trade. That was in the days when even Irene Castle's hair was long. A celebrated artist, a woman past the second blush of youth, came to the little room where Signor Raspanti presided over manicure tables and

hairdressing chairs in a New York department store. She demanded a bob. . . .
"Ten years from now, mark my word, half of the women will wear their hair short."

'Signor Raspanti was conquered. A vogue was started that has far exceeded the prophecy of its originator. This was an event on the calendar of the man who now cuts women's hair all day long. A dozen men under him work at it from the opening until the closing of the shop while women by scores wait in line. 3500 are clipped there every week; hundreds are turned away. Soon, Signor Raspanti predicts, there will be no long locks to sever, since already 90% of the young women and 50% of their elders, without age limit, have joined the ranks of the bobbed. . . .

'"Never, never will women wear their hair long again," he insists. "That is only a dream of the hair dressers. . . . There was a time when I had to have smelling salts on my table here, so many women felt faint when they saw their hair was gone. I remember one Frenchwoman who cried and cried. She declared she would not go home; her husband would kill her. I was almost as distressed as she was. I would have given anything to put that hair back where it was. But it was too late. That was the way with many of them then, but it is no longer so. Nowadays they only rejoice in the freedom of bobbed hair."'

The bob was, of course, a great boon for the barbers since most women preferred to have their hair cut by experienced barbers rather than hairdressers. And the barbers lost no time in exploiting the new source of revenue. In 1924 the following advertisement appeared for the Tri-City Barber Schools, one branch of which was located on the Bowery in New York:

'The Boy Bob has the beauty parlors going. The boy bob is a taper haircut. Barbers can cut them. This has increased the barber's receipts wonderfully. . . . By permitting our students to Shave from 15 to 25 customers per day, from 5 to 10 Hair Cuts right from the first day they enroll, saves from two to three years' time. With our enormous business we can teach the most backward student in a very short time. We pay a cash commission to anyone who will bring or send us a student.'

With encouragement coming from all sides, except from within their own families, usually, more and more women succumbed to the temptations of short hair; and in the spring of 1925 Julia Hoyt wrote: 'It certainly begins to look as if "woman's crowning glory" is soon going to be a relic of the past. I can picture that some fifty or a hundred years from now, paintings and photographs of women with long flowing hair or with complicated and magnificent coiffeurs [sic], will be exhibited as amusing and interesting curiosities.

'I read in the paper the other day that 2000 women are having their locks shorn every day. One still hears many arguments, for or against this custom. Those who are against it are almost invariably either the older women, who do not feel they can adopt it, or men. These people still feel that it is wrong because, first, it's new, and therefore must be wrong and second, because they've had "woman's crowning glory is her hair" drummed into them ever since they can remember and have grown to firmly believe it.

'Well, speaking for myself, I had an enormous amount of "woman's crowning glory", and as far as I can now tell, I'll spend the rest of my life with the small amount of my crown that is with me now. I well remember the day, four years ago, that I had my hair cut. It was a very hot day. My hat, as usual, was cutting my forehead in two, owing to the large knot of hair at the back of my head, and my head was dripping from the heat. I walked into a hair dresser's establishment and said: "Cut off my hair." I must say that the first snip of the scissors gave me a shock, like a cold bath or taking gas. However, the first moment was the worst. As my head began to feel cooler and lighter, I derived an enormous amount of pleasure from seeing the long pieces of hair fall to the floor.'

Miss Hoyt then reported that women in Paris were beginning once again to show their ears. 'Some years ago,' she said, 'there were all sorts of rumours about a famous beauty, Clio de Mérode—that she had been born without ears, that they were deformed, etc.—all because she was the first woman of that period to cover her ears. Now we speak of showing them as an extraordinary and revolutionary fashion. Ears that are little and well shaped and pink (of course a little rouge can accomplish the latter requirement) are charming, but in general I cannot see that they are much help to a woman's looks.'

Celia Caroline Cole, writing in the *Delineator* in 1925, warns that the bob is not for everyone, especially those with straight hair. 'If straight hair is left long,' she suggests, 'it can be gracefully draped. In fact, one of the most thrilling heads we know has long, straight black hair, parted in the center and drawn like black velvet curtains down on either side of the head with the face looking out, mysterious and serene, between these soft and unforgettably lovely curtains.'

For long hair she suggests 'a gay, rollicking coiffure . . . shoulder length, sweeping around the part on the side to a fetching little bun over one ear.' She adds that 'the part in the middle is as smart for bobs as for long hair and the "curtain" effect can be achieved just as effectively'.

In 1925, on her return from Paris, Mary Brush Williams rushed to the hairdresser's, which turned out to be rather crowded. 'The girls were sitting on the floor', she reported in the *Ladies' Home Journal*, 'on one another's laps, and in the operating chairs, where they were strung up on the permanent-waving apparatus. Nearly all of the hair was short, and the first thing the girls did when released was to comb it until that lying on the left of the part rose to meet that lying on the right of the part like an aureole.' Mrs Williams was terribly distressed and said so. 'Coming as I had so recently from the seat of all fashion,' she said, 'it struck me how *démodé* that style of hair arrangement was over much of the world.' She added that 'long hair and short alike are left in primeval straightness. Moreover, it is not only uncurled and unfluffed, but it is made to shine. What is of further importance, I suppose this to be more than a passing fancy of fashion, which is to take its place with short skirts, collarless necks, and other styles that have come to stay.'

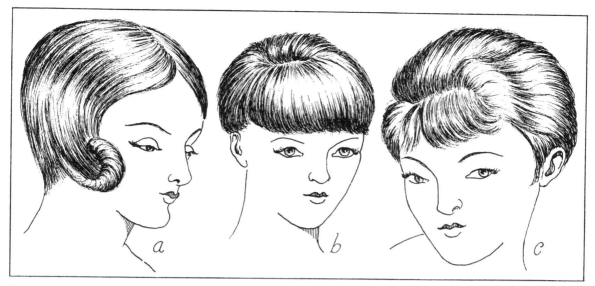

Fig. 130 : Fashionable American styles of 1926: (a) Orchid bob; (b) Coconut bob; (c) Moana bob

In a report to the readers of *Good Housekeeping* in the spring of 1926, Nora Mullane was clearly happy over the state of the hair:

'How pleasant they are to look at—the proud, smoothly-coiffed, youthful, brave bobbed topknots of today, hair brushed and clipped until it outlines charmingly the line at the back of the head! So different they are from the grotesque shapes and sizes we have seen since the twentieth century ushered in the towering pompadour. Here is freedom and simplicity and a lightness of head. . . . Hats are easy to buy, head-aches from hairpins and heavy coils disappear, and hairdressing takes less time—though more thought.' However, she warns the older women and those with large, less-than-perfect features or big heads that they might do well to keep their hair long.

The various styles of bob were usually named. The Chesterfield, the Horseshoe, the Orchid, the Moana, the Garçon, the Gigolo, the Carmencita, the Coconut—all these were popular in 1926. Three of them are illustrated in Figure 130. The *Garçon* was known in England as the *Eton crop* and in America as the *boyish bob* (Plate 153-F). According to London hairdresser Gilbert Foan, it was worn during its short vogue in England chiefly by fashionable mannequins and their imitators as well as a few mannish women.

The wig-makers were keeping up with the bobbed styles, though they had doubled their prices. *The Queen* for October 6, 1926, carried a full-page advertise-ment by Maison Nicol in New Bond Street showing a transformation available for fifteen guineas. A 'toupet for front or top of the head only' started at seven guineas. Shingled heads were twenty guineas and up. 'Whether the Postiche be a Trans-formation, a Shingled Head-dress or only a small Torsade to wear at neck over hair that is shingled or otherwise, it is certain to be the best that money can buy and to prove an immediate success. . . . Please write today for a Descriptive and Illustrated

Catalogue. This will give much interesting information both regarding the various postiches and also will tell you about the new exclusive system of permanently waving a lady's own hair without the use of any electric heaters (where this is preferred to wearing a natural wavy postiche). A visit to our showrooms would be esteemed and would help you to make a wise decision.'

The October 13 issue included an engraving of a wig from Maison Georges in Buckingham Palace Road, combining 'tidiness and softness. . . . It well justifies its name—La Naturelle—composed as it is of natural wavy hair with a side parting absolutely indistinguishable as artificial. It will be noted that the ears are partially shown, a characteristic of the latest modes.'

The electric permanent waving machines were at this time being superseded by a steam process, and a home permanent waving outfit was available from Marcel in Oxford Street.

In December 1926 *The Queen* considered the question of suitable coiffures for the elderly woman, which seemed to be 'something of a problem these days. Not a few have found a solution to it in the universal shingle, and often with an unexpected and somewhat surprising measure of success.' But the writer also warns that 'for a middle-aged or elderly woman to fall a victim to the shingle merely and solely because it is the fashion and suits her daughters and their friends is a mistake and often a fatal one. The younger women today are so well groomed, heads are so sleek, hair waves so becomingly set, that the older women should certainly be on their mettle not to look less well turned out, nor to have that unkempt appearance about the coiffure which, in hair that has lost or is losing its colour, is so woefully unbecoming and also so ageing in appearance.'

Although the bob unquestionably precipitated some tense moments in the home as well as in the beauty shop, there were occasionally more serious consequences. It was reported in the spring of 1926 that a Missouri woman filed a petition for the return of her six children, who were currently living with a guardian. When the oldest girl, aged twelve, was asked by the judge if they wished to return to their mother, she answered, 'No. We don't believe Mother is a Christian woman. She bobs her hair, and the Bible says in the eleventh chapter of First Corinthians that a woman should not cut her hair. She wears jewellery and bright clothes. A Christian woman shouldn't do these things.' The three older children were placed in private homes 'with Christian influences'.

Objections to the bob on religious grounds were by no means confined to Missouri. In the same year there was in circulation in England a tract entitled '*Bobbed' Hair: Is it well-pleasing to the Lord?* Although the author was less vituperative than the seventeenth century's Reverend Thomas Hall, whose target was long hair worn by men, he was equally serious about the whole matter and equally certain of the infallibility of his own opinions. He began mildly enough:

'Will our sisters in Christ—the younger ones especially—suffer a few words of exhortation and entreaty? A new fashion has come into the world that knows not

God, and many who do know Him are following it. The new fashion is called "bobbing" the hair! . . . No Christian would willingly grieve the Lord, and assuredly none would knowingly disobey His word. But "evil is wrought by want of thought as well as want of heart!" . . . The human family, having thrown off God, is a seething mass of restlessness and discontent (Isa. lvii. 20-21). No satisfaction can be found. Nothing pleases the mind long, so that those who cater for the world's amusements and fashions have to keep their brains continually on the rack in order to provide something fresh. But why should Christian women fall victims to all this? . . . Has God's word nothing to say concerning these things? Let us turn to 1 Cor. xi. 3-16. In verse 15 we read, "If a woman has long hair, it is a glory to her: for her hair is given to her for a covering". This one passage should suffice for all who wish to please God. . . . In verse 6 we are told that it is "a shame for a woman to be shorn or shaven". The new word "bobbed" is only another way of saying shorn.'

The word *bobbed* was, of course, not new at all, having for some time been applied to horses' tails. But the distressed author was in no mood to be deterred by facts. 'A "bobbed" woman', he thundered, 'is a disgraced woman! Surely a very serious consideration for all who fear God! What will the Lord say to our sisters about this when we all stand at His judgment seat?' Reminding his readers of the woman who wiped the feet of Jesus with her hair, he asked: 'Where would our present-day defaced sisters have been in such a scene? What services could they have rendered the Lord in their unnatural condition? . . . How strangely ill at ease our poor shorn sisters would have been had they been present in the Bethany home that day! . . . The refusal to utter the word "obey" in the Marriage Service, the wearing of men's apparel when cycling, the smoking of cigarettes, and the "bobbing" of the hair are all indicative of one thing! God's order is everywhere flouted. Divine forbearance tolerates the growing evil for the present, but the hour of Divine intervention in judgment approaches fast.'

But twentieth-century women were not to be deterred by the fear of divine intervention any more than seventeenth-century men had been. There were more immediate doubts and fears to be reckoned with.

Like most women, Mary Pickford wrestled with the question of whether or not to bob her hair. Unlike most women, she wrestled in print. In April 1927 she had this to say: 'I could give a lengthy and, I think, convincing discourse about long hair making a woman more feminine, but there is some doubt in my mind as to whether it does or not. Of one thing I am sure: she looks smarter with a bob, and smartness rather than beauty seems to be the goal of every woman these days. Whenever I go to the theatre and see the rows of heads in front of me, I send up a little prayer of thanksgiving that we no longer have to view great masses of false hair, curls, and puffs of various shades, and that dreadful abomination once known as the "rat". But I can not confess to any liking for shaved necks. They are dreadful and take away all charm and femininity from the most attractive woman.'

Miss Pickford then gives the various reasons why she has not bobbed her hair—

her family, her maid, her fans—all would be distressed and shocked. But at the end of her article she says, 'Now, after giving all these arguments against the bob, I feel the old irresistible urge, and it is quite likely that some day in frenzied haste, casting all caution to the winds, forgetting fans and family, I shall flee to a coiffeur and come out a shorn lamb to join the great army of the bobbed.' And that, of course, is what she eventually did.

Not to be outdone, the *Ladies' Home Journal* a few months later asked Lynn Fontanne to speak to the women of America about making themselves beautiful. Cosmetics had gained acceptance of a sort along with bobbed hair, but there still remained some doubt in the minds of many that it was quite respectable. Miss Fontanne minced no words on the subject:

'In sending out this bulletin to American women, I want first of all to ask you to make up your faces. Study makeup. Put it on your faces frankly, boldly—but with artistry. Don't mind what your husbands say. Let them object as loudly as they please. . . . They'll get used to makeup after a while, just as they are getting used to short hair. Not only getting used to it but admiring it and being proud of their wives for being in the know. Short hair not only calls attention to the beautiful shape of one's head, it is chic, which is another way of saying it is a symbol of youth, of the desire to be charming and attractive and of this day and age. . . . Long hair is dangerously on the edge of frumpishness.'

With the bob and the wider use of cosmetics came an increased interest in dyeing the hair. Henna had been used widely since before the war and was considered acceptable by some, not quite respectable by others. But hair-dyeing was no longer the hush-hush matter that it once had been.

In February 1928 one of the leading articles in *Good Housekeeping* was entitled 'Shall I Dye My Hair?' It was written by a physician who concluded that the only safe and effective dye on the market was henna. 'It may seem a sweeping statement', he wrote, 'to say that there is not one single dye known today which combines effectiveness with harmlessness, yet it is literally so. However reluctant one may be to admit that so far science has not found the way to aid men and women in their combat with gray hairs, it is imperative that the truth be made known to the thousands upon thousands of people who are dealing with or contemplating the use of these dangerous materials. In New York City the danger inherent in the general field of dyes was all too definitely demonstrated by the great number of toxic poisonings which were brought to the attention of the health authorities. The result was that an amendment to the Sanitary Code of the city was passed in 1926 prohibiting the use of noxious hair dyes and cosmetics.' He added that the law had very little effect. In concluding the long and detailed article, the physician said that 'it would be unduly pessimistic to think that it will be impossible for scientists, who have already wrested so many secrets from the earth, to wrest this one—how to dye human hair safely, effectively, and permanently. It is a piece of research that will be done, because the need for such a product is a widespread and human need.'

In March 1928 Ruth Murrin announced happily in *Good Housekeeping* that 'girls are going to look like girls this year'. She gave credit for this to the more feminine styles in clothes. 'It was obvious at once', she said, 'that sleek, close-cropped boyish heads arose oddly from these feminine gowns. They looked like flowers grown on the wrong stems! Immediately came the cry for a new coiffure—one that would retain the convenience and freedom of short hair and that would gain the grace and distinction of long hair. A bob that looked like long hair—that was what everybody wanted.' So that is what everyone got (see Plate 154-N).

Miss Murrin pointed out that femininity was not to be confused with frizziness, that the hair must still be shining and well-cared-for. She made one exception, however—'the curled-all-over, Greek-god effect; but this style will not be worn by many, for it is becoming only to certain small, piquant young persons and to girls whose hair has naturally an incorrigible curl.'

The coiffure was expected to follow the shape of the head with no bulges. Marcels or permanents were to be flat and loose.

Miss Murrin reported on the new 'half-bob', explaining that 'there are two kinds, one which some of the young girls in their teens have adopted, and one which older women like. Girls who are letting their hair grow reach that halfway stage when their hair is neither long nor short, and they have the ends—just the ends—curled in big, round curls around the head from ear to ear. This style is very attractive for youngsters, but rather trying, I should think, for older people. Some older women, who hesitate to go the whole way and cut off their hair entirely, are having the front hair bobbed and leaving the back long so that it can be done in a neat chignon at the nape of the neck.' Women who preferred short hair during the day sometimes added a fake chignon for evening.

The barbers, not surprisingly, continued to extol the virtues of the bob and did not take kindly to any suggestion that it might ever go out of style. In February 1929, Ralph M. Murphy, a hairdresser and cosmetician, wrote rapturously on the subject:

'Nothing is fashionable and beautiful unless it is becomingly striking and smart to the individual. And where could we find this better illustrated than in the "sculptured bob"? . . . Wherever we find a woman of style, we find the smart fashionable bob in a Marie Antoinette, a La Paloma, or a French Swirl—bob creations that are outstanding features among the leading hairdressers and artists. Make a mental picture of a woman whom we could term a "fashion plate" with a tall, willowy figure, sheer hose, dainty French-heeled slippers, short skirts, a soft, delicate chiffon frock with a Marie Antoinette French bob—a bob that makes Madame exquisitely beautiful and feminine. This creature is very good to look upon. But, on the other hand, picture the same woman with long, heavy hair piled up on her head in a knot. Immediately this coiffeur [*sic*] subtracts 98% from her appearance, and there is very little left to attract. . . . The trouble with most women who claim to be tired of bobbed hair is that they go to the nearest barber or hairdresser and take a chance instead of patronizing an "artist". The person who knows how to make them fashionable—different—individually different so that they may have a job of distinction—a healthful creation of which they can be proud. . . .

'If you ask a woman who is letting her hair grow why she is letting it grow, she will answer, "Oh, I want to be different". If she is past sixteen, she cannot afford to be different, for her age is against her. . . . My professional yell is, "The bob forever" and I know there are thousands and thousands more with me!'

In April of the same year Joseph de Silvis wrote, 'The bob will either bring out the natural charms of a woman or it will make her look frightful. It is all in the way in which it is cut. It would be superfluous for me to mention why the bob can never go out of style. The reasons are the same that men will never go back to long beards. . . . If we take a good look at those who are starting to let their hair grow, we feel sorry for them. They give us the impression of being in mental agony. They are fidgety and develop a terrible nervous condition. They do not know what to do with their hair. They build a veritable wire fence around it, that is all useless. No matter what they try they look awful.'

Two months later Mr de Silvis, who, according to his own admission, was the 'only creator of hair bobbing styles in America', told how the windblown bob came about. 'One hot day in July 1928', he said, 'I was resting and refreshing my tired old bones on the sands of Atlantic City Beach . . . when my artistic subconscious guided my eyes toward a very beautiful female whose hair was artistically disarranged by the soft breeze. . . . I turned to my wife and asked her if that head of hair suggested anything to her. "Yes, it looks foolish to me with that wind blowing all around," she replied. "That's it!" I exclaimed. . . . It is the Windblown Bob."' And was it a success? 'I'll say it was,' answered Mr de Silvis, 'and it is still going strong. Its popularity is phenomenal.' (See Plate 154-R-S.)

Mr de Silvis then suggests that the style is best adapted 'to young, slim girls, preferably those with a slight wave in their hair or those who have a flat permanent wave'. He adds that it never looks good on very straight or very curly hair and that it also never looks good on very tall or very fat women.

But once the right head of hair for it has been found, either a natural neck-line or a point is cut and tapered up gradually. The hair is 'shredded' in layers from the top down and the ends tapered irregularly, the hair being moulded to follow the contour of the head. Then the hair is set and dried and the ends 'disturbed' with a fine comb to achieve the windblown effect. This style, according to Mr de Silvis, could be worn with or without a parting.

Then George E. Darling took his turn in trying to refute persistent rumours that the bob was on its way out. 'Go to any theatre, stand at any busy street corner, visit the most fashionable shops, sports events, offices, schools, or anywhere women congregate and you will find an overwhelming majority sporting bobbed hair. Visit the most far flung hamlets, the greatest cities, the urban or suburban districts, and you will find that the bob is still supreme. It is not a hair style that is preferred by only one class of women—it is the choice of all. . . .

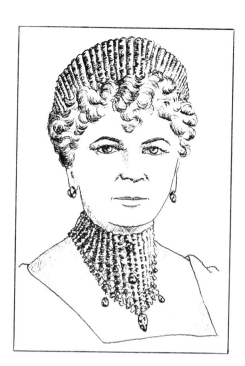

Fig. 131 : Queen Mary in 1934, wearing a
conservative hair style,
unaffected by the latest fashions

'Why do . . . people . . . say the bob is going out? They have been shouting that from the housetops for years. In fact, ever since the bob came in. . . . If they were hurting only themselves no-one would mind them. But no, through their ravings they are trying to tear down and destroy one of the greatest professions in this country. Before the bob became the accepted style, there were less than 11,000 beauty shops in America and a woman rarely entered a barber shop except to have her youngster's hair cut. Today there are more than 40,000 beauty shops in operation in the United States alone. And almost every barber shop in the country caters to women as well as men. . . . What was it that made the beauty and barber profession as great and as prosperous as it is today? The Bob.' But the short bob had passed its peak, and women were thinking about longer hair.

1930–1940 (Plates 155, 156)

In the summer of 1930 a New York hairdresser estimated that thirty per cent of his clients were experimenting with longer hair and that the rest had decided against it for the moment. 'But', he said, 'those thirty per cent are tremendously powerful in their influence—society women between the ages of eighteen and thirty-five. Business and professional women, in the main, are not going in for longer hair no matter how young they are.'

Betty Thornley, writing in *Colliers*, hastened to assure her readers that longer hair did not mean 'the Greta Garbo semi-bob. This was', she said, 'an amusing fashion for those who could wear it, but so many women who couldn't made disastrous

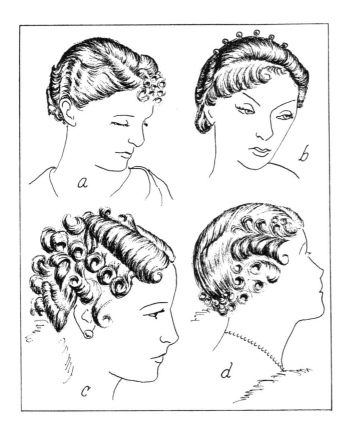

Fig. 132 : Fashionable English styles of 1935:
(b) and (c) are 'transformations'

attempts that it has been considerably discredited. There is nothing windblown or arty about the reigning daytime variants of the long-short coiffure.'

In speaking of bobbed hair, Miss Thornley made it clear that the boyish bob was a thing of the past. 'Severity of any kind just doesn't exist. . . . Straight hair—like really long hair—is something so infrequently seen that it must be classed as a personal idiosyncrasy. The bob of today, like the modified length, is based on the wave.'

In the same year fake pin curls on wires were sometimes worn during the day with hats; and in the evening, in order to give the effect of longer hair, fake chignons were worn or sometimes even wigs, which were always referred to as 'transformations'.

In January 1931 the editor of *The Queen*'s beauty page paid a visit to the beauty and hairdressing shop of M. André Hugo in Sloane Street. 'What struck me most', she reported, 'was his ingenious new device for dressing growing hair. This is a small oblong-shaped appliance with a hole at each end. The hair is divided down the centre and one portion is pulled through each hole, then these ends are crossed over to form a figure of eight, and the ends are tucked in, so that the result is a very fashionable and distinctly neat looking little bun on the nape of the neck. The price for this is the very moderate sum of half-a-guinea.'

The following month she wrote that the question of whether to wear the hair long or short 'has in most cases been settled in favour of longer tresses, but in the meantime there are those troublesome growing ends to be dealt with, which the well-groomed woman dreads. The Maison Stewart . . . has very successfully found a solution to this problem, and their little postiche of curls, made specially for this purpose, are really delightful. If you have not the features for curls and you prefer something a trifle more severe, little twists of hair, Grecian knots and thick, soft plaits that clip on to the back of the head in such a way as to be perfectly secure and absolutely undetectable can be obtained very cheaply.'

In the *Woman's Home Companion* for November 1932 Hazel Rawson Cades noted that the fashion of the moment 'favors shorter hair, flatter waves, a breaking up of surfaces by the use of flat curls and little ringlets—and as much forehead as possible. The long curls on the neck are *démodé*. The favored line is a natural one— quite feminine but neat. It may be cut rather short . . . with a second layer of longer hair just above it. . . . The hair is shadow waved . . . and the ends of the hair are really bent back to give a crisp flat effect which intensifies the smart simplicity of the hairdressing.'

In the mid-thirties Gilbert Foan designated the *Ten-inch bob* as one of the most popular of the new longer bobs in England. Waves and clustered curls, he noted, were coming back, along with centre partings. Fringes were no longer popular. The vogue for the centre parting was, he felt, influenced by an exhibition of Italian paintings in London in 1930.

In May 1934 *The Queen* reported that the coronet plait was 'one of the most favoured modes of the season. It may be had with a roll of curls attached to go across the nape of the neck, fitting closely over the ends of the shingle. . . . The flat unwaved effect across the front is one of the new modes most in favour at the moment. . . . Exquisite neatness . . . is the hall-mark of true elegance. . . . The sculptured effect . . . is representative of the most approved modes worn at present by the well-dressed Parisienne.' Transformations were still being advertised by a few determined wig-makers and still cost fifteen guineas. Permanent waving was available in one of the better known salons from £2 12s. 6d.

In February 1936 Ruth Murrin assured her *Good Housekeeping* readers that 'today there is a style for every type. Your hair may be any length from four to five inches down to your waist—whatever pleases you. You may part it on the side, or at the back of your head, in the middle, or not part it at all. You may wear it in curls or loose waves or straight as an Indian's. You may bare your forehead or camouflage it with a fringe. You may brush your hair behind your ears or hide them under a froth of ringlets.' With all this latitude Miss Murrin had one or two cautions: 'Don't slant your hair down across your forehead; it dates you badly. Don't choose a bushy coiffure or one that makes your head look big; such a coiffure is not smart, and it ruins the line of a hat.' She then suggested studying the coiffures of the film stars for new ideas. 'For example,' she suggested, 'Ginger Rogers sometimes arranges her red-gold locks in a fluffy long bob that almost touches her shoulders, a style which is not practical for you or me. It is too long and would prove a nuisance with fur-collared coats. But you might start with the basic idea of this arrangement—side part, hair brushed back behind the ears and ending in fluffy curls. . . . If your face is thin, try the center part so attractive in the natural, unstudied coiffures of Eleanor Powell and Gladys Swarthout.'

According to *The Queen* in June 1937 the trend in hair was upward—'towards off-the-face styles that are so alert-looking and youthful, with flat curls high up in the waves, a cluster of curls on the forehead, softening that dead line at the neck. Emphasis, too, on sleekness. Bizarre effects are banned, for women have found them both impractical and uneconomical.'

In the same periodical it was reported in 1939 that Vasco of Dover Street had used Raeburn's portrait of Lady Scott Moncrieff as the inspiration for a new hair style 'in which the curls are grown long at the front, parted in the centre, and drawn forward over the forehead. The hair at the back is arranged in thick Victorian ringlets, falling softly on the nape of the neck, and the whole effect of this unusual coiffure is one of gracious dignity and charm. The Edwardian influence is still apparent in the upward sweep of the hair at the sides. This is a style which is, above all things, individual—it can look striking and lovely on the right person, but the curls lying flat on the forehead are not always easy to wear, and so with this in mind Vasco has not forgotten the less original but always popular coiffure in which the curls are clustered becomingly on the top of the head. The Victorian motif is retained at the back, but the swept-up sides are fall, rolled over in a big soft curl.'

In general, during the latter part of the decade, the hair tended to be swept back from the forehead and temples in a slight wave and worn fairly long on the neck with rolls or curls, exposing all or part of the ears.

It should perhaps be noted that the thirties saw the passing, after nearly half a century, of the marcel, a landmark in hairdressing. Marcel himself died in 1936 at the age of eighty-four.

1940–1950 (Plates 156-159)

The early part of the decade was marked by an influence straight out of Hollywood. *Life*, in November 1941, was specific in pinning down the moment of birth of the new style:

'The 49th minute of the movie *I Wanted Wings* is already marked as one of the historic moments of the cinema. It was the moment when an unknown young actress named Veronica Lake walked into camera range and waggled a head of long blonde hair at a suddenly enchanted public. . . . Veronica Lake's hair has been acclaimed by men, copied by girls, cursed by their mothers, and viewed with alarm by moralists. It is called the "strip-tease style", the "sheep-dog style" and the "bad-girl style" (though few except nice girls wear it), but to most movie-goers it is simply the Veronica Lake style' (Plate 156-E). *Life* then informed its panting readers that 'Miss Lake has some 150,000 hairs on her head, each measuring about .0024 inches in cross-section. The hair varies in length from 17 inches in front to 24 inches in back and falls about 8 inches below the shoulders. For several inches it falls straight from the scalp and then begins to wave slowly.' *Life* closed its brief summation of essential Lake-data with the intriguing information that 'her hair catches fire fairly often when she is smoking'.

The fad for wigs, which blossomed in the late 1950s, was foreshadowed considerably earlier. An article in *Colliers* in July 1941 stated that 'bangs on a comb, stately coronets of braided hair, luscious chignons mounted on hairpins, and gleaming cascade bobs on an elastic have gone to the heads of the nation to the tune of ten million dollars' worth of hair goods a year. It's an industry that may hang by a hair but definitely is on the crest of what looks like a permanent wave.' It was also pointed out that 'across the counters of department stores and chain stores, in beauty parlors and even in millinery shops, women are buying hair goods for fun rather than necessity, casually trying them on right out in the open as though they were hats, shamelessly proud of the invisible combs to which the clusters of curls are attached'. One wig, of course, always leads to more; and the article pointed out that to have two or three was common, whereas some women 'have as many as ten wigs for use on any occasion'. At the same time the average cost was estimated at about fifty dollars, with some wigs running as high as $350. Roughly five million dollars' (about two million pounds') worth of hair was being imported annually, and not more than five per cent of the hair used in wigs was supplied by American women.

In the spring of 1943 *The Queen* reported with evident pleasure that 'The United States have followed our lead in popularising short hair styles, which have proved themselves to be attractive, practical, and easy to manage. . . . For the past year or so, even before the United States entered the war, American women have been turning more and more to short hair, abandoning the shoulder-length bob popularised by motion picture stars. Long hair, and even the long bob, is troublesome to keep neat, impractical for the working woman, whether she devotes her time to home defence work or is employed in a munitions or aircraft factory. . . . The short hair cut can be beautiful and becoming. . . . The hair is cut to a uniform three inches all over the head, then softly waved, and the curls brushed loose. The woman who wears this type of hair can take care of it easily at home and keep it neat through a long working day.' In 1943 there were no advertisements for transformations.

Reporting in the summer of 1945 on the trend toward topknots, *Life* pointed out that 'it took nine years for women's hair to move up off the neck and shoulders to the very top of the head in the current fashion variously called the doughnut, sausage, or topknot hairdo'. Their estimate of nine years was based on the first show held by the American Hair Design Institute in 1936, at which a few upswept hairdos were shown. Shortly after that, according to the *Life* article, 'some models, actresses, and women who make fashion their business, timorously began pushing up the hair. They started at the back, brushing the hair slightly forward and sideways.

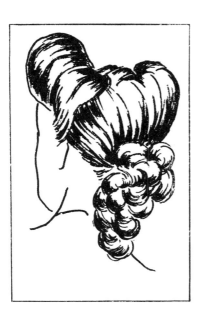

Fig. 133 : Fashionable English style of 1945,
with false curls added at the back

Gradually the brush strokes took in more and more of the hair and by last winter all the hair—front, sides, and back—was brushed up from the roots into a roll or mass of curls at the top. As a result, many women this summer look a little like Madame Recamier or yesteryear's washerwoman.'

Early in 1946 *Life* predicted that a change in women's hair styles was coming, but they indicated that the experts were still unsure how radical it would be, though all seemed to agree that shorter hair was inevitable. 'Hairdressers Paul of Charles of the Ritz and Michel of Helena Rubinstein', reported *Life*, 'are sick of the long-haired, cocker-spaniel look, are plumping for short bobs and are cutting customers' hair to the minimum whenever they get a chance.' Most women, according to *Life*, were adopting a wait-and-see attitude about the whole thing.

In the summer of 1947 T. Vasco Ltd of London stated in a full-page advertisement that 'In answer to numerous esteemed enquiries received on Cold Perms: Monsieur Vasco presents his compliments and wishes to inform you that Cold Perms of his own invention are now done at his establishment on any length and quality of hair with great success'.

In December 1949 the beauty editor of *The Queen* decreed that in view of the high rising necklines and small tight-fitting hats, the hair had to be worn short. 'A sleek well-groomed head is an integral part of the contemporary silhouette and as yet there are no indications of any change in the spring and summer collections. . . . Short hair is here to stay—for the next six months at any rate. This should be welcome news, for nothing is more practical during the summer months, and almost without exception short hair, provided it is skilfully styled, gives a youthful appearance. . . . Light streaks are again fashionable. These can be tinted to match an evening dress—the colour can be washed out next day. . . . Find the style that suits you, look after it, and enjoy the freedom of short hair for as long as fashion will let you!'

In March 1948 (see Plate 158) Dawn Crowell of *The Ladies' Home Journal* informed her readers that hair was moving forward over their ears in 'wide waves, pretty rolls, or soft curls. Refreshingly different from the skin tight arrangements of yesterday, these new hair-dos will flatter most faces—play up femininity. A few inches cut from a long bob allows shorter ends to curl up or under, gently breaks a too-severe hairline, maintains a well-groomed look. Front hair can comb into bangs or curls or brush aside into high waves.' In September *Good Housekeeping* reported that the new styles were smooth and simple and that unless one had naturally curly hair, 'the crown should be kept straight and the ends permanented just enough to turn up or under nicely. The ends should not be thinned out but left thick and lush.' Perhaps one of the most popular and enduring styles of the period was the feather cut (Plate 158-I), which satisfied the desire of many women for shorter hair, was relatively easy to take care of, and was flattering to most faces.

It is interesting to note that although the marcel had, at least among the fashion-conscious, disappeared with the thirties, a book published in 1948 in London by the Hairdressers' Registration Council, devoted an entire chapter to the technique of marcel waving. Evidently a good many English women were sticking to their marcels.

Although styles in the forties came and went, as usual, and the hair was up and down, fashion standards seemed less rigid; and there appeared to be a greater emphasis on individual freedom in choosing the most flattering style. Those illustrated on Plates 156-159 show an extraordinarily wide range for a single decade. And most of them were conservative enough so that they did not go out of style quickly. Emphasis seemed to be largely on bringing out the beauty of the hair and using it to its fullest advantage to point up the beauty of the face, as opposed to that of the twenties and the early sixties, when fashion was everything, and beauty was largely forgotten.

1950–1960 (Plates 160-162)

The fifties brought long hair, short hair, coloured hair, false hair, and eventually wigs. Hair was becoming increasingly important, and everything possible was done to change it, if not to beautify it.

In February 1950 a great jump forward in hair colouring was made with a preparation which bleached, shampooed, and dyed permanently in one operation. This was quickly followed by another short, one-step process. As a result, women developed an experimental urge and began streaking their hair with blonde, silver, red, and bluish tints. They even used artists' water colours for temporary streaks to match shoes, dresses, and accessories. By mid-summer, it was reported, the fad was picking up speed. Then the advent of liquid colour which could be sprayed on made possible a practical, temporary colour change. This invention, called Color Sprā, was a special boon to actors. Later it was packaged in push-button spray tins, which proved even more convenient.

In November *Life* reported a dramatic jump from the short shingle to the chignon. But as *Life* pointed out, hair does not always grow quickly enough to follow the fashion; and when that happens, the answer lies in false hair, most of which is usually obtained from Balkan peasants. A New York firm in late November reported a five hundred per cent increase in the custom hair piece business since summer.

'Thanks to improved processes,' said *Life*, 'dyed hair no longer looks as artificial as it did years ago, and thanks to changed social ideas, it no longer automatically labels a woman as "fast". But until recently the time and money involved have kept most women from getting their hair dyed. Their latest encouragement to try it is a new product. . . . Selling for two dollars, it enables a woman to change the color of her hair at home simply by painting the dye on. The danger of streaking, which has always made home bleaching a risky venture, is averted by a catalyst in the dye which stops color oxidation when it has reached a maximum intensity—about fifteen minutes. . . . On the basis of beauty parlor statistics . . . there are ten million women in the U.S. who would like their hair dyed.'

A year and a half later *Life* reported that since the development of home hair dyes, about one woman in five had taken to some kind of touching up. 'Now the ancient practice of hair powdering', said *Life*, 'has been brought back to produce a hair tint that can be safely worn to the beach. Instead of the flour used in the eighteenth century, the new product is a tinted metallic powder derived from an odd source: the aluminium dust inhaled by miners to coat their lungs as a protection from coal gas.' But, added *Life*, 'it is subject to smudging and, if used in large doses, will shower the wearer's shoulders. But it is useful for dressing up the hair for a special occasion with this season's popular streaks.'

In 1950, according to *Time Magazine*, there were manufactured about 10,000 permanent-wave machines and about 45,000 driers. In the United States in 1951 there were about 127,000 beauty parlours, employing 350,000 people and patronized by 3,750,000 women. It was estimated that four out of every ten American women coloured their hair. This year marked the death of Karl Nessler, inventor of the permanent wave, at the age of seventy-eight.

In December 1952 streaks were still being worn in the hair. According to *McCalls*, 'A gold streak is a dramatic accent in brown, dark blonde or red hair . . . used to highlight a wave, accent curls over the temples. This type of glitter comes in liquid form, goes on with a brush, washes out in the next shampoo. . . . A silver streak gives an air of elegance and distinction to a simple arrangement of dark or graying hair. Try the powder shine that sprays right on the hair from a squeeze bottle, stays there until you brush it out or shampoo it out. . . . Gold or silver sparkles look like stardust. . . . The glitter comes in a shaker-top bottle. Sprinkle generously—it clings firmly through the evening if hair is first sprayed with a light fixative.'

In 1954 *Life* reported that during the previous year about fifteen tons of hair had

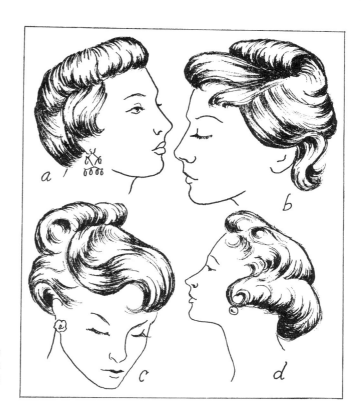

Fig. 134 : Fashionable English styles of 1955:
(a) (the *cube cut*) and (b) are from
advertisements in *Queen*; (c) and (d)
are from fashion pages

been imported at about a dollar an ounce, the price depending on colour and quality. Most of it would be used for women's hair-goods. But then in the midst of all the rage for chignons and false hair came the reaction—first the poodle clip, then the Italian cut. In mid-summer 1953 *Life* reported that 'when the stars of Italian movies shown in the U.S. began to sport short, shaggy haircuts that looked a little messy but were undeniably interesting, they touched off a ground swell of imitative barbering that this summer is equalling last year's poodle clip. . . . The Italian cut is shaggy but sculptured, with deep waves on the crown, spit curls framing the fore-head and cheeks and a carefully ragged nape. . . . Like the poodle, this haircut requires constant clipping.' (See Plate 161-I.)

But then came the aftermath. 'With the coming of spring fashions,' *Life* announced early in 1954, 'thousands of tousle-topped women are confronted with the question: "What to do with an old Italian hairdo?"' One answer, *Life* suggested, was a plastic or metal band, plain or decorated, which pulled the front hair back smooth and let the back hair fluff up and out.

However, the short styles were by no means out of fashion. In fact, they became even shorter with the butch cut (Plate 161-J), a passing fad in the summer of 1954, and the gamin style (Plate 160-L), which was more popular and lasted considerably longer. It was clearly not for everyone; and though it was considered very chic for a while, hardly anyone really liked it—with, perhaps, the exception of the very few, such as Jeanmaire (Plate 160-L), to whom it seemed to be suited.

In 1955 *Look* reported that as a result of the new Empire look in fashions, hair was being worn long again—Empress Josephine style with spit curls.

In reporting in the summer of 1956 on the new bouffant hair style (as much as 14 inches wide), *Life* described it this way: 'More exaggerated than anything seen since women hid rats in their hair at the turn of the century, this new style is a completely smooth hairdo evolved by cross breeding last year's page boy hair style with this spring's outsize hat. The bouffant look is basically a thick page-boy hairdo, 8 to 10 inches long, which has been puffed out at the sides and lacquered in place. . . . The new hair style rules out any possibility of hats; but wearers can decorate their widespread tresses with giant hair bows, jewels, or feathers.'

In the early spring of 1957 *Life* reported a rush of teen-age girls in Grand Rapids, Michigan, to have their hair cut in the style worn by Elvis Presley—a tuft in front of the ear and several locks hanging over the forehead. In the six weeks preceding the article more than 1,000 girls had been clipped *à la* Presley. The beautician responsible for the fad estimated, perhaps somewhat optimistically, that 75,000 girls would have similar cuts during the next year. The fad went unacknowledged by the fashion world.

For the wider coiffures, large wire mesh rollers were developed for use in setting the hair (Plate 161-O). These attained enormous popularity and by the sixties seemed to be used by practically all women. Unfortunately, in the United States they were occasionally worn on the street as well as in the privacy of the home—with a rather astonishing electronic effect, to say the least.

Undoubtedly the most memorable hair fashion event of 1958 was the use of wigs by Givenchy for the spring showings in Paris. When the short-haired models needed more hair to go with the new fashions, Carita obligingly solved the problem by making wigs for them. The idea seemed to appeal to women of fashion not only as a means of quick and frequent changes in hairdo, but as a practical time-saver; and the style, with the help of the usual promoters, began to catch on.

At the end of the decade the bouffant look, which was paving the way for the distortions of the sixties, was still fashionable. And even then ominous lumps were beginning to appear on female heads.

THE SIXTIES (Plates 163-167)

Once again, as they had been two hundred years earlier, women were at the mercy of their hairdressers, who vied with each other in developing new styles. It was a deadly serious game; and they played it as if their professional lives were at stake, as no doubt they were. The hairdresser whose creations appeared on the most famous women was considered top man, and he commanded top prices.

The professional hairdresser in this period, which is thought to have begun about 1952, achieved a status hardly matched by the indispensable coiffeurs of the late eighteenth century. Late in 1961 *Life* pointed out that the hairdresser had become 'a personage sought after, showered with gifts, lavishly entertained'. This had become, said *Life*, the age of the hairdresser—witness, the New Yorker who always took her hairdresser to Europe and another who had her own private phone in a salon. George Masters, a young Hollywood hairdresser, charged $75 (about £27) for a home call, *Life* reported, earned $65,000 a year, and had been given an expensive automobile by grateful clients. In 1963 he was lured to New York, where he planned to work nine months of each year.

Colour, thanks to new scientific developments, ran riot. It was estimated in an article in *Cosmopolitan* in June 1960 that one out of three American women coloured their hair at a cost of 45 million dollars spent in drugstores and 250 million in beauty parlours. 'The day of the mousy blonde has passed,' said *Cosmopolitan*, 'as has the era of the platinum blonde, the carrot-topped redhead, the shoe-polish brunette.' They pointed out that the modern woman's hair turned Just Peachy, Copper Blaze, White-Minx, Chocolate Kiss, Fuchsia, Honey Doux, Bordeaux, Fury, Frivolous Fawn, or even Tickled Pink; and, they added, 'if you're ever wondering what happened to your dear old gray-haired granny, she turned Night Silver, True Steel, Silver Blue, Mink, or Smoky Pearl'.

In addition to the all-over solid colouring, various techniques were used either to make the hair more natural or to add interest. *Drabbing*, as one might suspect, referred to a process of toning down bright colours, especially the reds and yellows, by the use of a white or champagne-coloured rinse. *Frosting* involved bleaching small strands of top hair all over the head. This was normally used when the body of the hair was dark. *Tipping* was the same process on the front of the head, while *streaking* meant bleaching in several broad streaks starting at the hairline around the face.

A down-on-the-ranch opinion of the two-tone hair colour was overheard on a train out of St Louis: 'I saw this gal yesterday in the bus station in Tulsa—looked like a skunk—black on both sides and white stripe up the middle. Couldn't make up her mind what she wanted to be.'

In 1959, with the bouffant hair style still at its peak, the hairdressers, the press, and probably the film publicists for *Cleopatra* seemed to be conspiring to force the Egyptian look on the public (Plates 164-J, 165-I). Women were told flatly that they would be wearing it, models were photographed with it, and it was even promoted on television. Beauty salons stocked wigs in order to be ready for the demand. On February 27 *Look* presented two modern Egyptian hairdos created for them by Michel Kazan—the 'Cleopatra Coif' and the 'Nefertiti'—and gave instructions for dressing them. 'Superimpose two such famous glamour girls as Elizabeth Taylor and Cleopatra', said *Look*, 'and you are in for a beauty boon.' They were certain that the combination was 'bound to inspire a new Egyptian look every bit as sweeping as the recent tousled B.B. and pale-lipped Italian looks'. But somehow the Egyptian look never really got off the ground in quite the way it was intended to, though its influence was felt in modified form.

As in the eighteenth century, the desperate hairdressers latched on to any event or idea or personage to inspire a new hair style. Whereas in the earlier period it was battles, queens, goddesses, parks, gardens, and eventually even executions, in the twentieth century it was films (*Cleopatra, Marienbad*), plays (*Oliver*), insect dwellings (beehive), food (brioche, mushroom, artichoke), and famous and beautiful women (Jacqueline Kennedy, Brigitte Bardot).

In March of 1962 *Newsweek* had some blunt words about the current fads, especially among teen-agers: 'Hold the hair straight out, tease it with a comb until it gets frizzled, then comb some of the outside hair over this big mess of frizzled-up hair and set it in place with a cloud of hair spray. This creates the bouffant, a hairdo filched from eighteenth-century France, whose tortured variations—mushroom, flip, French twist, chemise, French roll, artichoke, and bubble—began sprouting a few years back. In the adult world, which has moved on to the Cleopatra look, it's now a bit passé. But among U.S. teenagers, bouffants are proliferating as fast as the toadstools they resemble.'

Chicago teachers estimated that seventy per cent of the girls wore bouffant styles. A Detroit counsellor complained about schoolgirls who could barely get through doorways. And occasionally girls had to be spoken to because the students sitting behind them were unable to see the teacher. One Los Angeles teacher felt there was a correlation between extreme hair styles and low grades and suggested that the poorer students simply wanted to excel at something.

In discussing the towering hair styles of the eighteenth century, we mentioned the astonishing practice of leaving the hair untouched—often for months at a time—and the revolting results when the construction was finally dismantled. The twentieth-century mind finds this difficult to believe, let alone understand. Yet in 1962 in Canton, Ohio, a high school girl kept a bouffant, teased hairdo intact without combing for several weeks until a classmate sitting behind her in school noticed blood on her neck. An investigation by the doctor revealed the source of the trouble to be a nest of rather lively cockroaches that were thriving in the darkness, warmth, and apparent security of their new home.

In September 1962 *Time* noted that 'depending on which foreign film actress was in vogue, U.S. women over the past few years have tangled their hair until it swelled out to blimp proportions or plastered it down on their skulls as if it were Saran Wrap. Now hair is headed in the only remaining direction: up, up, up.' The new coiffures, intended strictly for evening but occasionally seen during the day, seemed to be inspired by the 1830s look and were achieved not with wigs but with false pieces pinned to one's own hair, which might be relatively short. Hairdresser Adrian called the new style 'practical and elegant. That's what the new look's all about. You're having lunch in town and you've got this gala to go to at night, so you put the hair piece in a bag and take it with you, and with four hairpins you've got your elegance.' Sometimes the soaring hairpieces matched the natural hair; sometimes they were of contrasting colour or colours—peach and deep gold, lavender to ash blonde, etc. Frequently, straight, smooth pieces were combined with wavy, curly, or even frizzy ones. Prices of Adrian's pieces ranged from $75 for the solid colours to $500 (£178) for the more splendid, multi-colour creations.

Even feather wigs were being worn for the first time since the eighteenth century and were considered to be 'especially elegant at the cocktail hour'. The *Post* reported that for dressy evening wear Alexandre of Paris had invented 'a clean, upswept coiffure with a mass of curls or a Danish-pastry bun whirled at the top. The secret ingredient is a *postiche*, or hairpiece, pulled like taffy into an elongated shape.' They further reported other creations which 'look as if Boy Scouts had got their hands on ropes of lacquered hair and were inventing fantastic knots of them'.

Vogue also predicted elaborate high styles for evening with lots of false hair but simple styles for day wear with enough hair to work with in the evening. Colouring was expected to continue in importance.

In November 1961, in an article on the comeback of the wig, the *New York Times Magazine* reported that 'A copywriter in a New York advertising agency chooses her wigs to match her clients. For those in the fashion business she pops on a super-bouffant job in blond, while for conferences with a publisher of religious books she wears a nondescript model in brown. Her own hair is strictly for sleeping on.'

By 1963 wigs were well established and were clearly more than just a passing fad. A New York wig-maker estimated that 1½ million wigs, worth 25 million dollars, were being worn. Sears, Roebuck believed that 6½ million women were wearing wigs or hairpieces. A year earlier *Newsweek* had quoted an estimate of 225,000 to 500,000, exclusive of those wearing them out of necessity. Prices ranged from about $5 for the cheapest synthetic hair wigs to more than $500 for high-quality human hair. Better synthetics sold for about $50, while human hair was usually at least $300 (£125). Prices had been rising sharply because of the increased demand for hair, which cost as much as $350 a pound. As usual, blond and grey were more expensive than darker hair. According to the U.S. Department of Commerce, approximately $100,000 more was spent on importing hair in 1962 than in 1961. Although wig prices were prohibitive for many customers, pay-as-you-wear wigs were attracting some of them. Wig-making establishments had mushroomed from perhaps a hundred in the late 1950s to thousands by 1963. And wig accessories, such as cases (costing as much as $150), wig blocks, wig cleaner, etc., helped to establish wig making as a major industry.

Wigs were worn both for convenience and for covering up what was usually called 'problem' hair. Although there seemed to be a growing tendency to match the wig to one's own hair colour, many women still preferred to have several wigs in a variety of styles and colours for various occasions. And instead of spending hours at the beauty shop under the dryer, they simply dropped off their hair there and picked it up later at their convenience. No stigma was attached to wig-wearing; and the human hair wigs, when properly dressed, were so convincing that it was not usually possible to tell whether they were real or not. This led to much speculation by other women as to whether or not certain friends or celebrities were or were not wearing wigs—not that they objected. They merely wanted to know. It was even possible to purchase wigs of bleached white human hair, which could be tinted as often as one wished with a temporary rinse.

In addition to full wigs, false hairpieces were also worn, as well as streaks, spit-curls, and widow's peaks. Figure 135 illustrates what Saks Fifth Avenue called *wigbands*—hair 'mounted on a band of rayon velvet . . . in 24 shades to blend or contrast with your own hair. . . . They're sewn—not glued—on to strong, cool, porous mesh and then mounted on a snug-fitting stretchy band in assorted colors'. They were promoted in a full-page advertisement in *The New York Times* in August 1963, and they sold for $65 and $75.

At the same time a human-hair wig of weft sewn to a coarse net foundation with a black velvet band covering the front edge was selling for 150 francs ($30 or 10 guineas) in Paris. The French version was a complete wig, and the hair was not sewn to the band, which could be removed if desired. Wigs without the band and with more hair were usually at least 300 francs. The band wig in various versions was worn in London, Rome, and other world capitals, as were other styles, no matter what their origin. The partial or complete wig with a front band, probably because of its practicality and relatively low cost, achieved considerable popularity and was still being sold and worn in 1964. But this was only one of many styles following the general trend.

A popular recording (fleetingly popular, at any rate) was called *I Dig Her Wig*, and in the United States the NBC-TV staged a Why-I-Want-a-Wig contest. Eventually the wigs would go; but for the moment business was booming.

In October 1963, James Ridgeway, writing in the *New Republic*, estimated that before the year was out 45,000 wigs would be purchased in Washington, D.C., which he considered the 'wig capital of the world', and that between two and five million women in the United States were wearing wigs. Handmade wigs were selling from $250 to $750 (or as high as 250 guineas); and in 1962, reported Mr Ridgeway, 175,000 pounds of hair were imported from Italy alone. The total amount was probably comparable to that imported a hundred years earlier when chignons were in fashion. Even poodles were reported to have been seen wearing wigs.

In the seventeenth and eighteenth centuries valuable wigs were snatched off the heads of their owners in the streets of London. In 1963 in Washington the technique was somewhat more sophisticated. A woman would buy a 'human hair' wig for $100 or more, making a small down payment and signing a contract for the remaining payments. On opening the wig box at home, she would find a cheap yak or synthetic-hair wig, perhaps not even of the colour she had chosen. By the time she returned it to the wig shop, the negotiable contract would have been sold to a finance company, which, under law, had no responsibility for the wig but was able to collect payment for it, even to attaching funds from the woman's bank account if necessary. The only recourse was to sue the company, and that would cost far more than the wig.

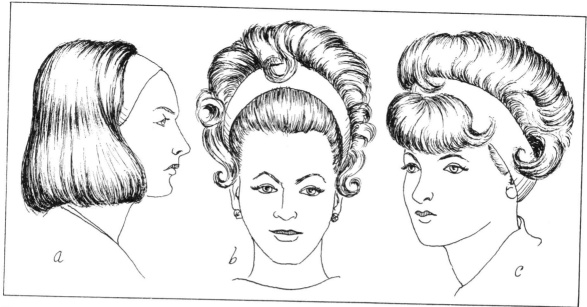

Fig. 135 : Partial wigs or *wigbands*: (a) page-boy style attached to band; (b) natural front hair combined with partial wig on band; (c) false bangs and back hair attached to band, natural side hair showing in front of band

Eventually the mania for false hair extended to the eye-lashes. Although false eye-lashes had been worn for many years, their use outside the theatre was not exactly flaunted. But suddenly in 1964 they became almost a necessity for the fashionable woman, who was ready for a change from the painted Egyptian eyes but was not ready to give up what *Time* called the Big-Eyed Look. Beauty salons began hiring 'falseticians' to help their customers with their eye-lash problems. A variety of new eye-lashes appeared, some of them—costing up to $20 or £7 and lasting two or three weeks—designed to be attached, one by one, to the customer's own lashes. Some were made of human hair, some of mink, and some (at $80 a pair) of sable. Real enthusiasts were known to wear as many as three pairs at once.

In February 1964 there occurred a curious phenomenon which had some passing impact on the world of hair. The United States, after ample warning, was invaded by four young Englishmen who, in their way, caused nearly as much stir as the invading British nearly two hundred years earlier. They were, however, received with considerably more enthusiasm; and the near riots they caused were expressions of an adulation nobody could quite explain. The four, emanating from Liverpool, were known as the Beatles; and although they billed themselves as singers, whatever it was they did was more or less drowned out by the hysterical screams of their fans.

Their one claim to fame, however transient, lay, like Samson's, not so much in their talent as in their hair. All four wore their hair in a modified fifteenth-century cut, completely obscuring their foreheads. Coming, as they did, at the height of a wig cycle, the result was, not surprisingly, a flurry of Beatle wigs. According to *Time*, they were being sold 'by the hundreds of dozens'. A manufacturer of novelties, appearing on television, claimed to have made and sold thousands of them. Established wig-makers in New York were getting frequent calls for them. Department stores featured them in window displays. And everybody talked about them.

That the wigs were sold seems certain. Who wore them is less clear. Certainly they were not in evidence on the streets of New York. Presumably they were bought by teen-agers and their indulgent parents, worn wherever teen-agers wear such things, and then, eventually, discarded along with other passing fancies. Perhaps, like the outmoded eighteenth-century wigs, some of them were used for dustmops.

The adult world of fashion was, as we have seen, far from immune to similar fads. In February 1963 *Vogue* enthusiastically endorsed the Oliver haircut, which they described as 'roundly-shaped hair, nibbled at the edges, tumbled on to a face of melting piquancy'. The inspiration was the musical version of *Oliver Twist*, an extraordinary success first in London, then in New York.

In August, in a roundup of opinions from hairdressers in the world's fashion capitals, *Vogue* concluded that the coming style for day wear would be 'hair short enough to clear the new collars . . . close enough to the head to be described as "small" . . . moving into curviness; turning into the nape of the neck; fringing from the crown of the head into bangs'. For evening wear eleven of the twelve hairdressers interviewed wanted 'something dazzling'. Rene of London wanted more movement, a sculptured effect, and less sleek hair, slightly longer, with chignons for evening; Alexandre of Paris voted for short hair for day with fanciful hair ornaments for evening; and Filippo of Rome preferred the side hair 'going up like plumes' in the daytime and an immense postiche on top of the head for evening.

What actually was worn by the fashion leaders in 1964 was a narrow hairdo, high at the crown, the height achieved by teasing the natural hair or wearing a postiche. The hair could be worn either up or down. It was more likely to be down during the day, up in the evening. Bangs (not too heavy) sweeping across the forehead and even cutting through an eyebrow were fashionable (see 'Fashionable' style, Figure 1).

Early in 1964 Lois Long, writing for *The New Yorker*, reported on the current trends:

'Hair much sleeker and closer to the head for daytime (you can pin on hairpieces to create fantastic effects at night). . . . Most of our best hairdressers will make up switches (that's what women *used* to call them) and other appendages to match your hair and to add temporary glory to the coiffure. But Lilly Daché, always thorough as well as adventurous, would prefer to have you start a complete wardrobe (or headrobe?)—bicycle clips with bangs attached or with poufs atop them, *postiches*, foller-me-lads curls, ponytails, and the like. In her Wig Whimsey studios . . . there are practitioners who can coordinate partly artificial hairdos (made of real hand-knotted hair, though) with one's facial contours so as to improve or enhance them, just as hats are supposed to do. Mme Daché swears that small hairdos can be made up in a day, full wigs in two or three days.'

A do-it-yourself article in *Family Circle*, a magazine designed primarily for the

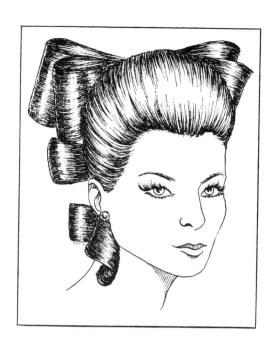

Fig. 136 : High-fashion style of 1964, with stiffly
lacquered bows of false hair

middle-class housewife or career girl, included a number of practical suggestions for simple, fashionable-conservative hair styles, which once again, except for an occasional slight bump at the crown, followed the natural shape of the head. Emphasis was on colour, natural sheen, and just enough wave to emphasize the beauty of the hair. Here are a few of the suggestions:

'Hair is *cut soaking wet*, taking into consideration the natural tendencies of the hair, with no thinning or tapering (except for bangs). . . . When hair is evenly dried so that any remaining moisture can be hardly felt, *comb the hair till it meshes into the lines of the hair style.* As you comb, bring out the natural tendency of the hair to turn up or under, to curl or to lie flat. If a few clips are needed to control the hair, put them in place and leave them for about 10 minutes. Hair that is cut, dried, and combed in this fashion will be wearable without further setting.

'If a woman does nothing more with her hair, says stylist Victor Vito, she should look for a good haircut and seek the lift of hair coloring. Hair coloring adds body to the hair and does more than an elaborate hair creation to brighten a woman's looks. . . .

'Setting on large rollers gives an elegant side-part flip-end hairdo—ideal for the working wife or for any dress-up occasion. . . . In line with today's hair fashion, the hair is kept slightly shorter at back than at the sides. . . . Bangs are kept long . . . and are cut unevenly. Most bangs are shortest at the middle of the forehead and are tapered to be longest at the temple to blend into the curve of the side hair. . . . Straight hair should not be tapered at the ends; you need all the thickness and weight you can get at the ends if the hairdo is to keep its shape and move beautifully with you. . . .

In England the Beatles, the Rolling Stones, the Pretty Things, and similar groups seemed to be having at least a passing effect on the hairdos of impressional teen-age girls, whose consuming ambition in life, at least for the moment, was often merely to touch the hair of one of the singing idols. Sometimes they even tried to look as much like the boys as possible, and for a while it was not always easy to tell which was which. In September 1964 the *New York Times Magazine* ran six pictures of young, long-haired Britons with an indispensable caption indicating which were boys and which were girls.

That it was the girls who were emulating the boys and not the other way around is indicated by a Lancashire lad's reply to a question about his long hair: 'My bird [girl friend] wears her hair short. I don't want to look like a girl, so I have my hair long.' Like Samson, the young Englishmen, in spite of the elegant dress of a group known as the Mods, considered their long hair a mark of virility. It could also be of considerable assistance professionally. According to Anthony Carthew in the *New York Times Magazine*, Brian Jones of the Rolling Stones put it this way: 'My own mother thought I was ridiculous at first. But I told her about all this money we're earning, and she saw the point.'

In February 1964 *Home and Country* showed two fashionable styles by London hairdressers. Both were chin-length bobs, fairly flat on the sides, with a high crown, the smooth front hair cutting across the forehead (see Plate 167-K).

In April, Eleanor Nangle, writing in the *Chicago Tribune*, emphasized the general acceptance of false hair in the world of fashion: 'No one bats an eye now when a woman, complimented on how pretty her coiffure is, says, "It's not mine, dear; it's my wig". Or, when complimented on its color, says "It's a new tint, sunset gold with a splash of apricot frappe".' She illustrated her point with photographs of three new high-fashion hairdos from Elizabeth Arden featuring lacquered bows of false hair—a curious blend of the styles of the 1770s and the 1830s (see Figure 136). Although hair styles are seldom repeated in precisely their original form, they are frequently reflected decades or even centuries later in a slightly altered version. The beehive (fifteenth-century Italian), the bouffant style (late eighteenth century), the Egyptian look, and stiffened hair bows all were fashionable within the space of a very few years in the mid-twentieth century, when styles worn by the fashion leaders changed with astonishing rapidity.

In the sixties most of these forays into the past seemed to be for the purpose of searching out the eccentric rather than the beautiful. The late summer of 1964 brought, along with continuing race riots and shooting wars, a few Parisian models with shaved hairlines (fifteenth century) and bald heads (ancient Egyptian). The idea, which originated with couturier Jacques Esterel, was received on the other side of the Atlantic with reactions ranging from disbelief to revulsion. Actress Bette Davis, whose own hairline had been shaved when she played Elizabeth I, condemned the fad on purely practical grounds—the scalp itches when the hair starts to grow back in.

Perhaps the whole idea got its impetus from the new and deliciously scandalous topless bathing suits for women. At any rate, it was duly noted by the press, as it was intended to be; but hardly anybody (except, perhaps, an apparently desperate fashion designer and some naturally-bald women) expected or wanted anything to come of it beyond a little flurry of publicity.

About the same time history was repeating itself in quite a different way. Not only were robbers relieving well-stocked wig shops of their merchandise, but petty thieves, who couldn't be bothered with the complexities of planning a robbery or of substituting cheap wigs for expensive ones in what were supposed to be legitimate transactions, adopted the more direct sixteenth and seventeenth century method of simply snatching a wig from a convenient head and disappearing into a crowd. In New York a woman subway rider reported to the police that as the train stopped and the doors opened, a singularly ungallant gentleman, who was standing nearby, snatched her $125 wig and vanished through the doors as they slid shut.

But wig snatchers and bald fashion models, though providing a touch of piquancy, were hardly typical of mid-twentieth century life. Throughout history, as we have seen, women have never ceased to devote considerable time and attention to their hair, sometimes with disastrous consequences. But never before had it been possible to do so much so easily and with such gratifying results.

The vast majority of women, even those relatively low in the social scale, visited beauty shops occasionally, most of them regularly. Shelves in the stores were stocked with safe preparations and gadgets for washing, conditioning, bleaching, tinting, dyeing, and curling the hair, many of them specially blended for a particular type of hair—fine, medium, course, dry, oily. They were available at prices practically all women could afford, and they could be used at home in a relatively small amount of time. Newspapers, magazines, television, and radio all conspired to keep the hair problem before the public, and there were several magazines on the stands devoted exclusively to hair.

Gone were the days when only royalty and the social élite could afford the time and the money to maintain their hair in the latest fashion. There were simply no long hours available for weaving the hair into hundreds of tiny braids, no slaves to whip when a curl went wrong, no social and economic barriers to dressing the hair in the latest fashion. In the mid-twentieth century even high school girls could and sometimes did wear styles popularized by Jacqueline Kennedy or Brigitte Bardot. Hair was no longer just woman's crowning glory—it was big business. And the taste-makers intended it to stay that way.

PLATES 148-167: THE TWENTIETH CENTURY – WOMEN

PLATE 148 : TWENTIETH-CENTURY WOMEN 1900–1905

(Although all of the styles on this plate appeared in American publications, those marked 'Fashionable' were in most cases probably of French origin. Those not so marked have been taken from advertisements, story illustrations, and portraits.)

A-F   1900, American. Fashionable.

G   1900, American. Young girl.

H   1900.

I, J   1900, American. Young girl.

K, L   1903, American.

M   Ethel Barrymore, 1879–1959.

N   1903, American. Fashionable. 'Suitable for a debutante.'

O   1903, American. Fashionable. 'Coil with new-style hairpins.'

P   1903, American. Fashionable. 'Pompadour with undulations.'

Q   1904, American. Fashionable.

R   1904, American. Fashionable.

S   1904, American.

T   1904, American.

U   1904, American. Fashionable.

V   1905, American. Fashionable. For evening wear.

W   1905, American.

According to Annie Kellet, writing in the *Ladies' Home Journal* for 1903, the correct way to make a pompadour is to 'divide the hair in the centre of the head back of each ear; divide the front hair into 3 parts, front and sides; then put it up in 3 separate parts, the front first and then the sides. To make the pompadour firm, either use a roll or a crepee, or rough the hair underneath. The very large pompadour is going out of style, or rather it is still worn large at the sides, but not so large over the face.'

Miss Kellet then suggests that 'The correct way for a young girl to dress her hair, when she is wearing a short walking skirt, is to have it arranged in a braid with ribbon bows. The hair when arranged in this way should lie close to the head and not show a division between the pompadour and the back hair. In order to get this style, the pompadour should be parted from the crown of the head an inch back of the ears, giving a slanting appearance to the side of the head. The pompadour is then carried to the top of the head and fastened with 3 combs; then it is braided until it reaches the under hair, where the 2 parts are braided together. The plait when finished, instead of being turned over as is generally done, is slipped through from underneath and carried to the top, where a ribbon bow is tied. A second bow is tied at the nape of the neck.'

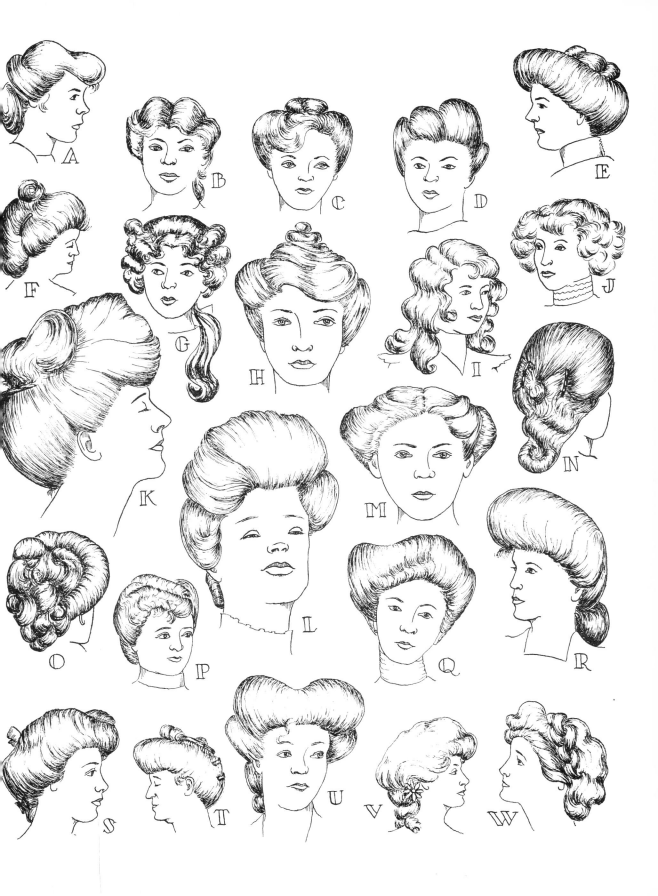

PLATE 149 : TWENTIETH-CENTURY WOMEN 1905–1912

(The styles marked 'Fashionable' appeared on the fashion pages of American publications and were often of French origin.)

A, B   1905, American.

C-H   1906, American. Fashionable.

I   1907, American. Fashionable. According to Mrs Ralston in the *Ladies' Home Journal*, the hair styles in 1907 were showing 'greater softness and irregularity of outline'.

J   1907, American. Fashionable. Suitable for evening wear. 'Hair is parted at one side and drawn loosely across the brow, twisted, fastened with a small comb at one side to puff it out loosely, and then gathered in with the coil and arranged at the top of the head. This coil should be toward the back and kept quite flat and low to conform to the contour of the head. A bandeau of jet or some bright stones is worn across the front of the coil to give the coronet shape.'

K   1907, American. Fashionable.

L   1907, American.

M, N   1908, American. Fashionable. In this year Mrs Ralston reported that 'the side part with the low, flat line has now quite replaced the pompadour. The back hair is also soft and loose and brought well forward back of the ears so that it shows from the front. It is arranged in puffs which are made by dividing the hair into strands—as many strands as you want puffs—then starting at the ends, roll it toward you over your first two fingers and lay it flat against the head, catching it with a pin, top and bottom. Three puffs are a pretty number, the centre one being a little higher and fuller than the two side ones. . . . Combs are now placed at each side of the head to hold the hair securely, and a large one is placed in the back, either above or below the soft knot.'

O   1910, American.

P   1908.

Q-U   1910, American.

V, W   1910, American.

Y, Z   1912, American. Fashionable.

See also the French styles in Figures 127 and 128.

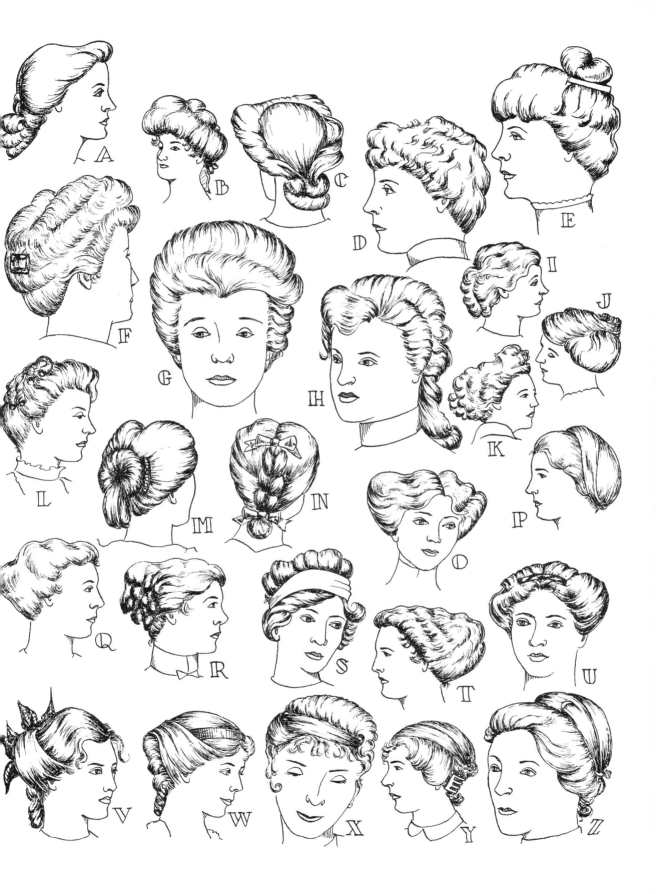

PLATE 150 : TWENTIETH-CENTURY WOMEN 1912–1915

(Those American styles marked 'Fashionable' appeared in the fashion pages of American publications and in many cases were of French origin.)

A, B   1912, American. Fashionable.

C-F   1913, American. Fashionable. According to Ida Cleve Van Auken, writing in 1913 in the *Ladies' Home Journal*, 'The elaborate hair ornaments now being worn in the evening are typical of the orientation of the moment and serve as an offset to the simple style of hair dressing prevailing. The general tendency in all arrangements of the hair is to follow the natural shape and contour of the head.'

G   1913, American. Fashionable. Coiffure partially completed. 'The lower back hair portion is tied to make a firm foundation.'

H-K   1913, American. Fashionable.

L   1913, American. First step in arranging the hair. 'When a side parting is used, the hair is divided into 4 parts.'

M   1915, American.

N   1915, American. Style suitable for a young girl.

O   1914, American.

P   1914, American. Fashionable.

Q   1914, American.

R   1915, American. Young girl.

S   1914, American. Fashionable. This is designated as a coiffure for a young girl.

T, U   1914, American. Fashionable.

V   1914, French. Fashionable.

W   1915, American. Fashionable little girl. *Dutch cut.*

X, Y   1914, French. Fashionable.

According to the *Ladies' Home Journal* for September 1914, 'No longer do we see the contour of the head in the new high coiffures, although it must be said that there is no exaggeration of height but an effect of harmonious proportions in the formal arrangements. Once again we are in the midst of the pompadour but a very different pompadour from what we have previously worn—with flat, low lines in front, gradually rising toward the crown of the head in graceful, wavy lines. To heighten the effect an exquisitely shaped tortoise shell comb in fan shape, studded with sapphire-blue stones, may be used.'

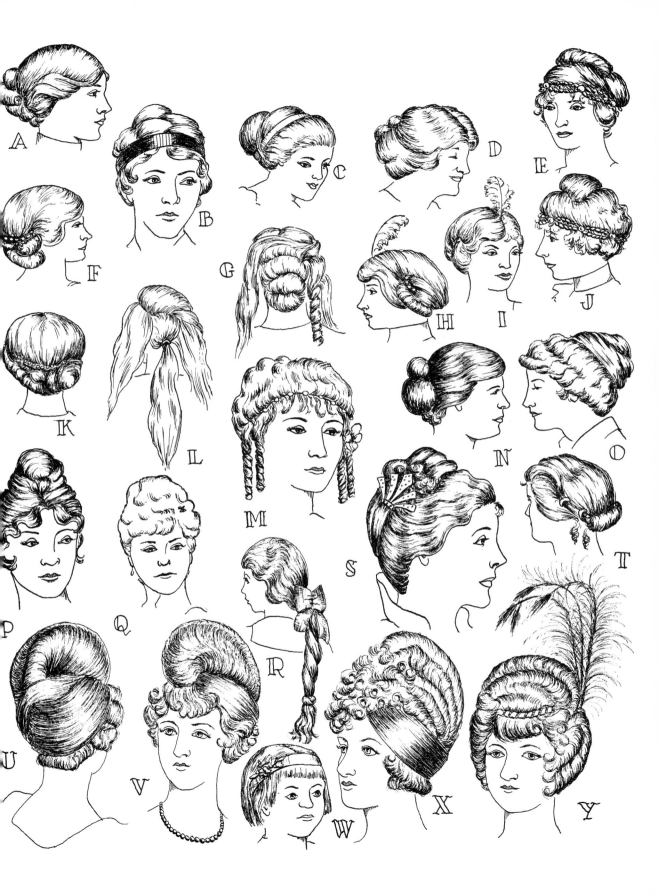

A

B

C

D

E

F

G

H

I

J

K

L

M

N

O

P

Q

R

S

T

U

V

W

X

Y

PLATE 151 : TWENTIETH-CENTURY WOMEN 1915–1920

(Although all of the styles in this plate appeared in American publications, many of the ones marked 'Fashionable' were undoubtedly of French origin. The ones not so marked appeared in advertisements, story illustrations, or portraits.)

A   1915, American. Fashionable.

B   1917, American. Little girl.

C, D   1917, American. Front and side.

E   1917, American.

F   1917, American. Fashionable. 'It would seem that a compromise had been made between the high coiffure of old and the more recently favored low coiffure, for the fashionable hairdressing of the evening stops just below the top of the head, though it is far above the position where the low coiffure coiled itself. Conspicuously high are the exquisitely carved and often brilliantly sparkling combs of Spanish genre. . . . One is impressed with the beautiful deep waves in the well coiffed hair, not only seen in the evening but under the smaller crowned hats of the daytime.'

G   1917. American child.

H   1917, American.

I   1917, American. Fashionable.

J   1917, American.

K   1917, American.

L   1917. Fashionable combs.

M   1918, American.

N   1918, American.

O   1918, American. Fashionable. 'One does not need to be demure to wear this madonna-like hair arrangement, but we can safely say that it will not fail to make you appear that way.'

P   1918, American. Fashionable. 'If you want to exploit the most modish coiffure, draw your hair up high à la pompadour and close at the sides, then twist it into a soft high roll at the back of the head.'

Q   1918, American. Fashionable. 'There are those women who require just such a high, formal coiffure as this one, twisted into a loop, caught with a tortoise pin. It is as necessary to the evening costume as an ostrich-feather fan.'

R, S, T   1919, American. Fashionable.

U   1919, American. Hair turned under to look like a bob.

V   1919. 'From Paris comes news that a new coiffure has been created at last. It is very, very low. . . . If you are young enough to wear an ingénue frock of sheer organdie, try to persuade your hair into this fluffy coiffure. It is coiled low in back with a fringe in front. Place over it a flower bandeau.'

W   1919, American.

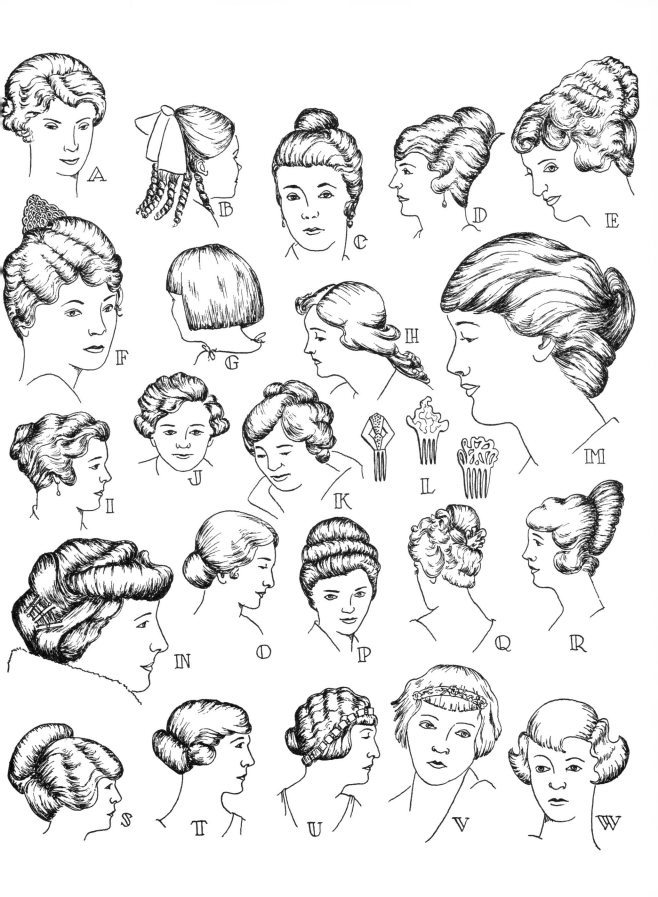

(The styles marked 'Fashionable' are taken from the fashion pages of American publications and are in many cases of French origin. Styles not so marked are taken from advertisements and illustrations.)

A   1920, American.

B   1920, American.

C   1920, American. Little girl.

D   1920, American.

E   1920. American screen actress.

F   1920, American. Fashionable young lady.

G   1920, American. Fashionable young lady.

H   1920, American. Fashionable.

I, J   1920, American. Fashionable. Front and back.

K   1922, American.

L   1923, American. Fashionable.

M   1923, American. Fashionable.

N   1923, American.

O   1923, American.

P   1923, American. This appeared in an advertisement for a permanent wave at $15.

Q   1923, American. Fashionable, for evening wear.

R   1923, American. Fashionable.

S   1923, American.

T   1923, American.

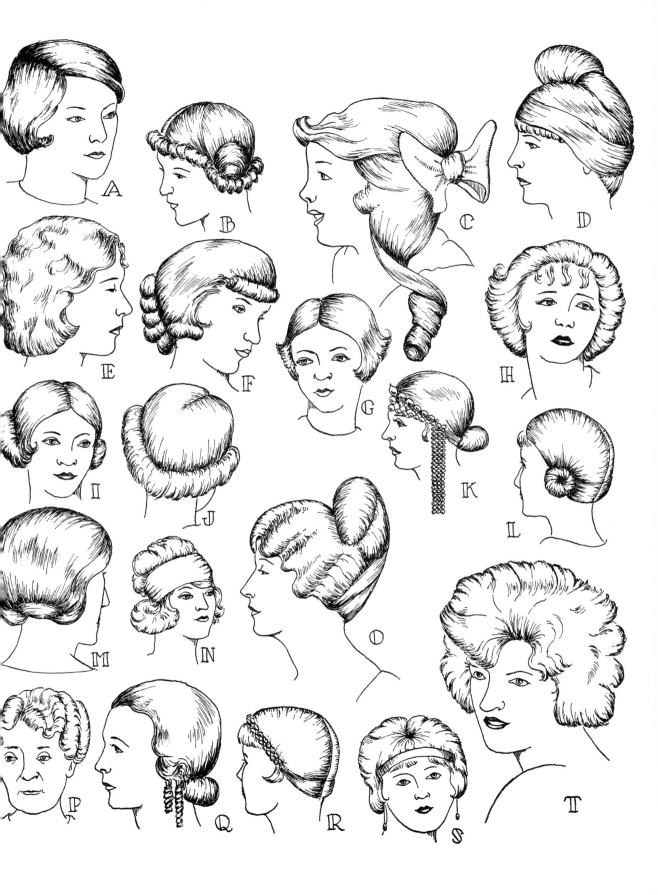

A B C D

E F G H

I J K L

M N O

P Q R S T

Plate 153 : Twentieth-Century Women 1924–1929

A   1924. American screen actress.

B   1925. American screen actress.

C   1925, American. Fashionable. *Shingle*. According to Celia Caroline Cole in the *Delineator*, 'the line of the hair at the side should follow the line of the chin to the ear. If the hair grows so that a point can be made in the center of the back, have your barber cut it to a point. Paris isn't doing the point much, but it is becoming to most American women, especially if they are past their youth: a lovely sloping curve from behind the ear down to the sharp little point. . . . If you can't have a point, have a curve. Don't have a straight line.' Provided a woman has a well-shaped head, the hair, says Miss Cole, 'is cut close to the head in the back about a third of the way up from the nape of the neck and from there on it is longer. The whole aim is to have a beautiful line for the back of the head—that loveliness one finds in the head of a young boy. If the hair is thin or the neck scrawny . . . the smart hair-dresser does not cut the hair close to the nape of the neck, but cuts it in one length from the crown to the nape, thinning the ends with a razor so that it will not stand out. The hair is then waved and brushed flat to the head.' (See also F below and 154-E.)

D, E   1925, American. These are from an advertisement for a hair preparation and are labelled 'Authentic Parisian Styles' (see also J below).

F   1925, American. Fashionable. *Boyish bob*.

G   1925. American screen actress. *Wave bob*. Cut straight around the head, then waved up at the ends for fullness. Also worn with bangs.

H   1925, American. Fashionable.

I   1925, American. Fashionable. *Egyptian bob*.

J   1925, American (see D and E above).

K   1925, American. Fashionable.

L   1927, American.

M   1927. Lynn Fontanne (for later portrait see 157-L).

N   1927. Greta Garbo.

O   1927, American.

P   1927, American. *Charleston cut*. Very fashionable in 1925.

Q   1928, American. Fashionable.

R   1928, American.

S   1928, French.

T   1928, American.

U-Z   1929, American.

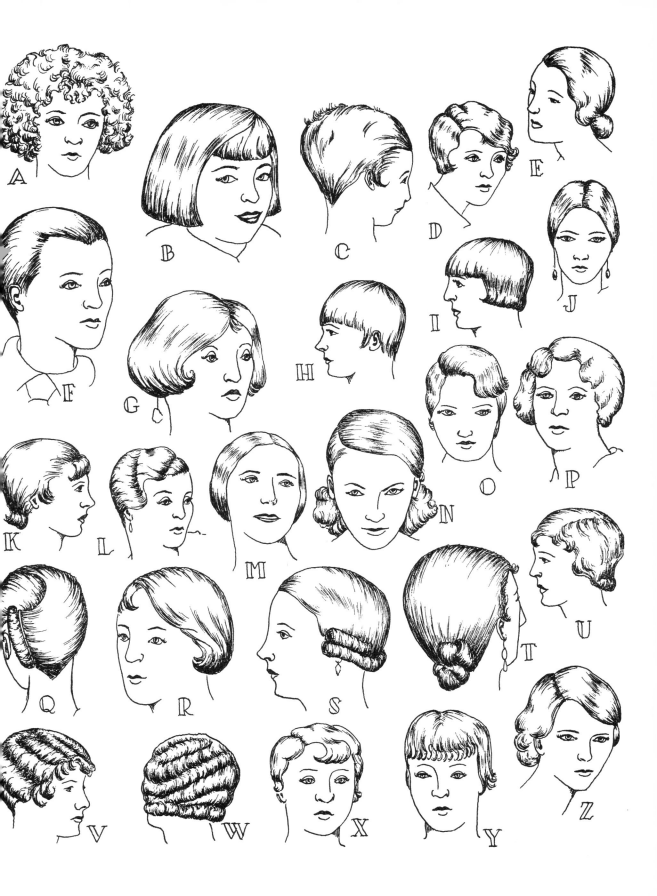

PLATE 154 : TWENTIETH-CENTURY WOMEN 1924–1929

A 1924. *Old English bob* with bangs.

B, C 1924. *Egyptian bob.*

D 1925.

E 1925. *Mannish bob.*

F 1925. According to Celia Caroline Cole, writing in the *Delineator* in 1925, 'To be *modée* and exciting and to look like an illustration in a novel, the hair should be either shingled or dressed so close to the head that it looks like paint. No more large, gnome-like heads. They're small and chic and Greek now. A darling little head on the top of a slender, supple body not at all concealed by its extremely simple frock—that is she! Far more like a boy than a woman. And, by the way, the difference between the boyish haircut and the shingle is only in the gradation in the back: the boyish is a bit shorter at the crown. And a whisper: the old straight bob is very *démodée.*'

G 1925.

H 1925. *Marcelled bob.*

I 1925.

J 1925. *Charleston cut.*

K 1925. Writing in the *Ladies' Home Journal,* Mary Brush Williams reported on the current fashions: 'Like so many items of international consequence, the news broke over us in Paris gradually: Dry, crisp, fluffy hair is "out of luck and out of fashion"; locks sleek and shiny are the thing. . . . The coiffure is now more likely to be carefully laid out and planned like a formal garden, with straight, close-cut lines in the back and perhaps a staircase of waves gently, oh, very gently marcelling up either side of the forehead, and all held sparklingly in place with a splash of brilliantine.'

L 1925. *George White Scandals bob.* Variation of the wave bob, with the wave on one side. Cut straight around and waved slightly at ends for fluffiness.

M 1927.

N *Antoine bob.* According to Ruth Murrin, 'They have practically tabooed the "hanging bob" which persisted so long, and now short hair must be worn long at the sides and trained back as though it were long hair. Ears are not so bold as they have been; they are partly or entirely covered. A curled and tendrilly softness characterizes the hair that frames the face, which emphasizes sweetly fine features and delicate skin. . . . In the back the hair is often straight, but some wave from the ears forward is needed by most faces. The part on the side is more popular than one in the middle because it is more generally becoming and lends itself so well to the swirl in back. The swirl is favored by the smartest coiffeurs because from the front and side it gives bobbed hair the effect of being long. . . . This means that the hair is longer on one side of the head than on the other, is brushed over the ears to the back, and is trained to stay in place.'

O 1927. *Gilda bob.*

P 1927. *Soubrette bob.*

Q 1927. *Faun bob.*

R, S 1929. *Windblown bob.*

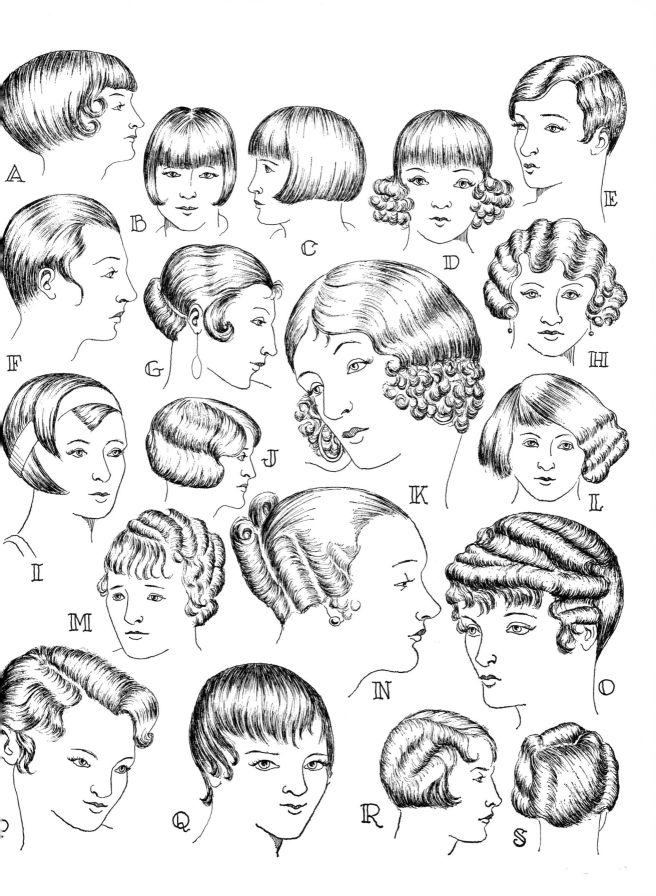

A

B

C

D

E

F

G

H

I

J

K

L

M

N

O

P

Q

R

S

PLATE 155 : TWENTIETH-CENTURY WOMEN 1930–1938

A-F   1930, American. According to Betty Thornley, writing in *Collier's*, 'The hair is invariably longer at the sides than it used to be, and most coiffures have small, flat, turned-up ringlets here, sometimes carried back to a point behind the ears and pinned; in others the ringlets are brought across the back of the neck. Those who don't go in for curls may choose an arrangement in which big flat waves cover the ears, come forward along the jawline, and swirl together in back—not so different from last year's bob except that it's longer all over and gives much the effect of the chignon versions when considered from any but the rear elevation. Some older women like an up-and-backward arrangement in which the ears are uncovered, and the swirl gives the feeling of the old French twist.'

G   1932, American. Mrs Herbert Hoover.

H   1932, American.

I   1932, American. Mrs Eleanor Roosevelt.

J-L   1934, American.

M   1935, American.

N, P   1937, American.

O, Q, R   1938, American.

In 1931 Charles Boch, in a radio address, informed his listeners of the current trends in hair styles: 'For the newest ways of hairdressing you should let your hair grow until it is an inch and a half or two and a half inches long at the neck line. This hair is then rolled in a long single roll across the nape of the neck or it is worn in a group of ringlets. The front hair is kept comparatively short and arranged softly around the face. The real secret of the new coiffures is to keep the hair properly thinned out. . . . This year the hair styles permit women real scope for individual arrangements. If the hair grows in a beautiful line across the forehead or if you have one of those highly prized widow's peaks, by all means wear the hair off the forehead in a soft arrangement of waves. As for the ears, if they are well shaped, show them by all means. Otherwise, hide them.'

Writing in *Collier's* the following January, Elizabeth Boutelle also favoured the soft roll in back and said that one way to 'give it a 1932 twist is to arrange it in two graduated rolls instead of one. . . . Double or single, this year's version is not worn low on the neck like the old one, but always follows the natural hair line'. She also indicated that 'instead of being waved down on to the cheek in a line perfectly parallel to the part, the hair should be worn long enough to give the effect of having been brushed back and then pushed forward into a soft wave, with the emphasis on the sweep away from the temples'.

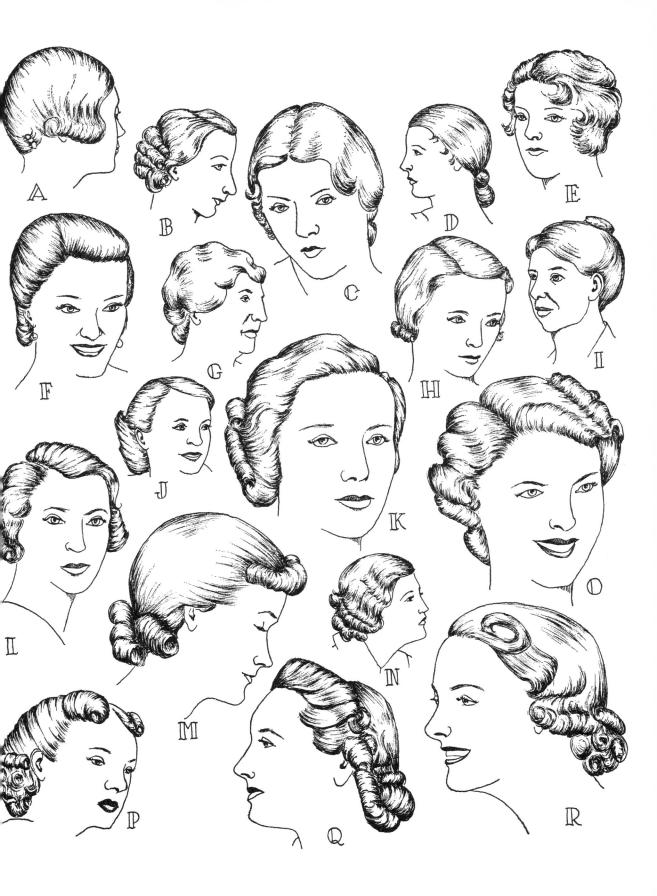

A

B

C

D

E

F

G

H

I

J

K

L

M

N

O

P

Q

R

PLATE 156 : TWENTIETH-CENTURY WOMEN 1939–1942

A   1939, American.

B   1939, American.

C   1939, American.

D   1940, American.

E   1941, American. Fashionable. Side parting, hair long and slightly waved, partially concealing one eye. Style popularized by Veronica Lake.

F   1940, American.

G   1940, American. Fashionable.

H   1941, American.

I   1941, American.

J   1941, American.

K   1941, American.

L   1942, American. Fashionable.

M   1942, American.

N   1942, American.

O   1942, American. Fashionable.

P   1942, American. Fashionable.

Q   1942, American. Fashionable.

R   1942, American. Fashionable.

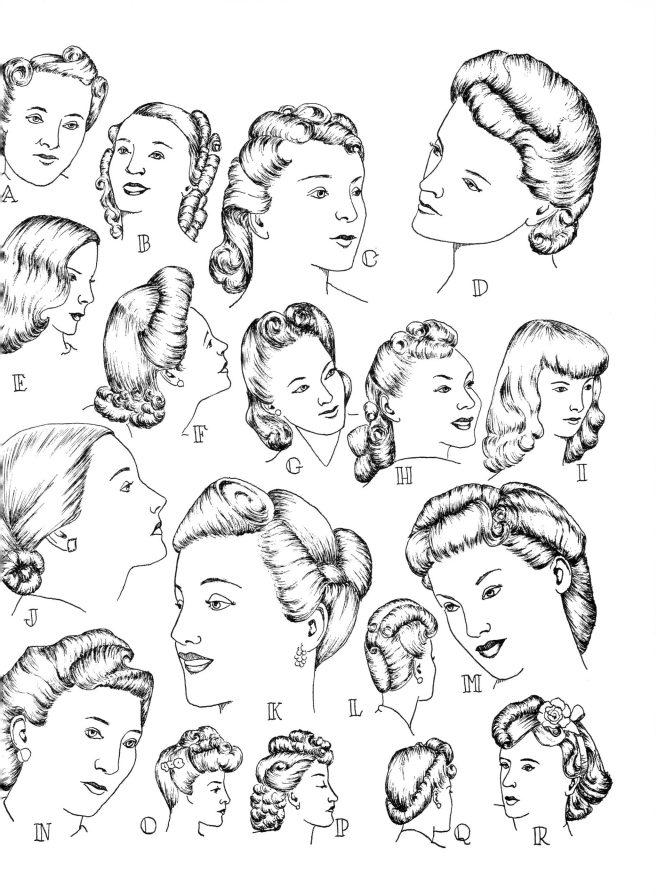

A

B

C

D

E

F

G

H

I

J

K

L

M

N

O

P

Q

R

PLATE 157 : TWENTIETH-CENTURY WOMEN 1943–1945

A   1943, American.

B   1943. American screen actress.

C   1943, American.

D   1943, American.

E   1944. Ruth Gordon.

F   1944, American.

G   1944. American screen actress.

H   1944, American.

I   1944, American.

J   1944. Gertrude Lawrence, 1898–1952.

K   1945. American actress.

L   1945. Lynn Fontanne (for earlier portrait see Plate 153-M).

M   1945, American.

N   1945, American.

O   1945, American. Fashionable.

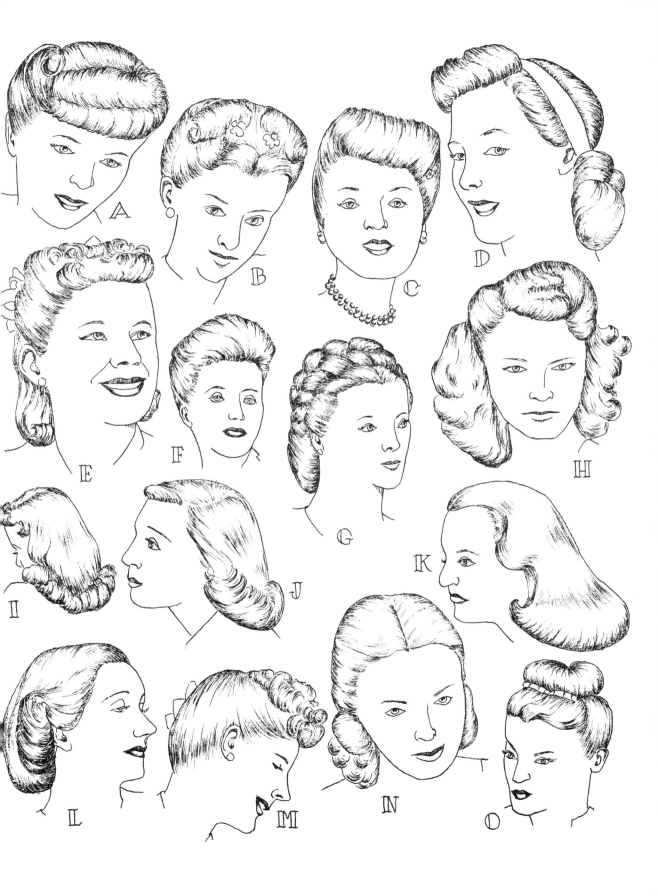

Plate 158 : Twentieth-Century Women 1945–1949

A   1945.

B   1945. For evening wear.

C-H   1947. Dawn Crowell's late summer report for 1947 in the *Ladies' Home Journal* was, as usual, enthusiastic: 'The circular wave from a centre part is news. . . . It can continue in soft short curls or romantic shoulder length locks. A wide taffeta ribbon that ties in a bustle bow adds femininity to a "tailored" head. Braids belong to any age but must be manipulated to make the most of *your* face! Flowers, real or make-believe, turn into evening chignons. Scarf rings, pearls, and pins lead new lives on top of beautifully groomed heads.'

I-N   1948.

O, P   1949.

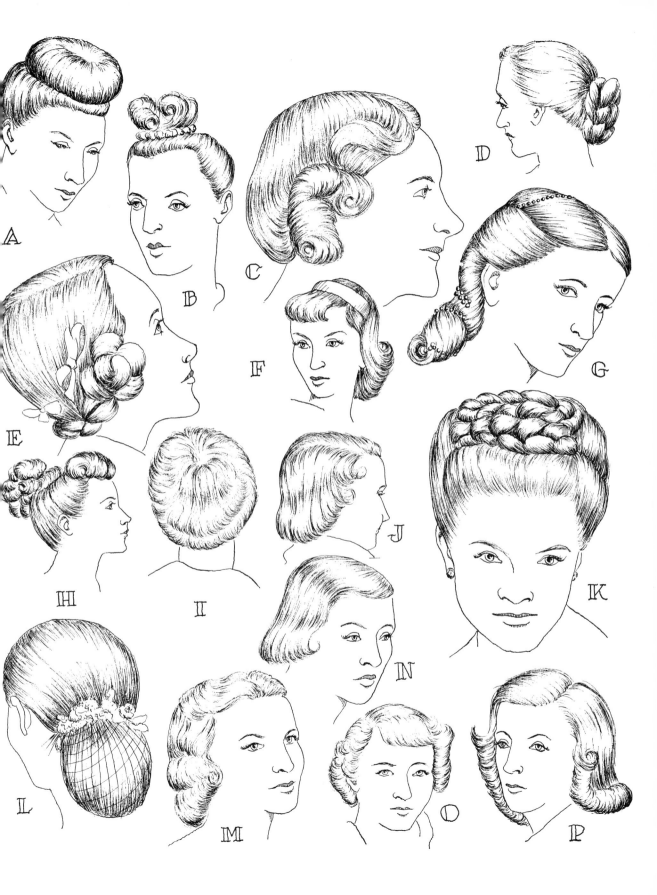

A

B

C

D

E

F

G

H

I

J

K

L

M

N

O

P

PLATE 159 : TWENTIETH-CENTURY WOMEN 1946–1949

A 1946, American.

B 1946, American.

C 1946, American.

D 1946, American.

E 1946, American.

F 1947, American. For evening wear.

G 1947, American.

H 1947, American. Fashionable.

I 1947, American.

J 1947, American. Fashionable.

K 1947, American.

L 1947, American.

M 1948, American. Fashionable.

N 1948, American. Fashionable.

O 1949, American.

P 1948, American. Fashionable.

In the autumn of 1946 *Good Housekeeping* was very permissive in its attitude toward hair styles, suggesting several possibilities:

'If you want a radical change from the updo you have been wearing . . . if you like to wear a new style before everybody else does . . . if you dislike hairpins but don't mind frequent trips to the hairdresser to keep in trim . . . one of the new shorter cuts, with or without the silky bang, should suit you to a T.' But for the woman who had let her hair grow and liked it that way, *Good Housekeeping* suggested she leave it long. For the woman addicted to frequent changes in style, they suggested an in-between length. If, on the other hand, 'a clear uncluttered air is what you aim at . . . if you like the kind of coiffure you can wash and set yourself without too much difficulty . . . if you prefer to get variety with the help of a net and a ribbon rather than by frequent changes of hair style . . . if updos and curls make you appear a little strange to yourself .. then you probably should cherish a smooth and shining page boy'.

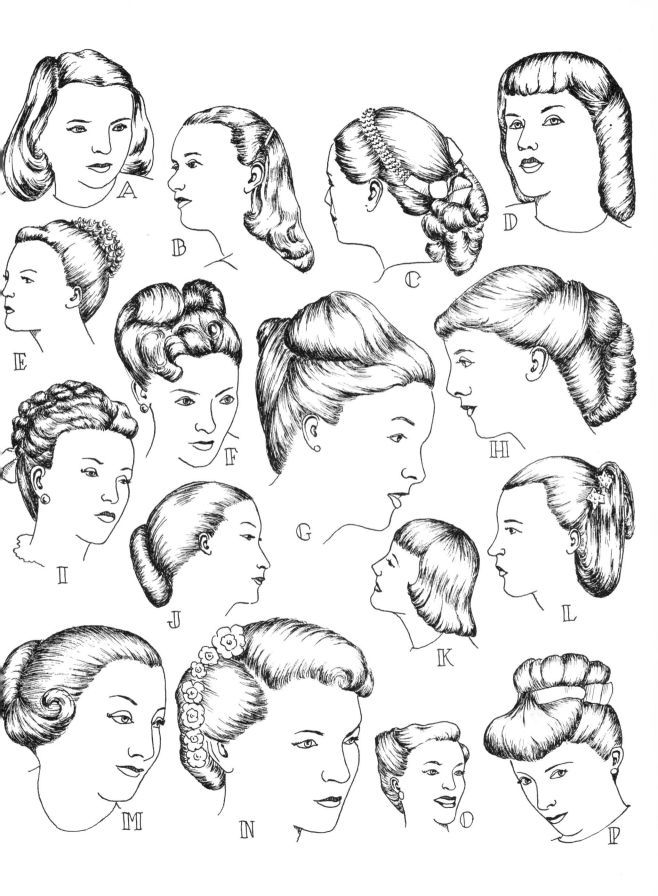

A

B

C

D

E

F

G

H

I

J

K

L

M

N

O

P

PLATE 160 : TWENTIETH-CENTURY WOMEN 1950–1956

A, B   1950, American. Fashionable. Front and back. 'Make forward pin curls at temples; alternate, turning curls reverse and forward around head.'

C   1950, American. Fashionable. '3 large forward pin curls on each side, 6 in back.'

D, E   1950, American. Fashionable. Back and side. 'Sweep hair back from face, fasten with combs just behind ears. Comb remaining hair off neck; arrange in curls.'

F   1951, American. Fashionable.

G   1951, American.

H   1952, American.

I   1953, American. Fashionable.

J   1954, American. Fashionable young lady.

K   1954, American.

L   1954, French. Zizi Jeanmaire. Singer and dancer.

M   1955, American. Fashionable.

N   1955, American.

O   1956, American.

P   1956, American.

Q   1956, American.

R   1956, American.

In 1956, according to *Good Housekeeping*, the hair was generally being worn longer. 'The boyish cut is gone. With that exception you may have your own length, from an inch or two below the nape to just about the shoulder. The newest coiffures are wider; but if you prefer a top-lofty effect, by all means wear it.

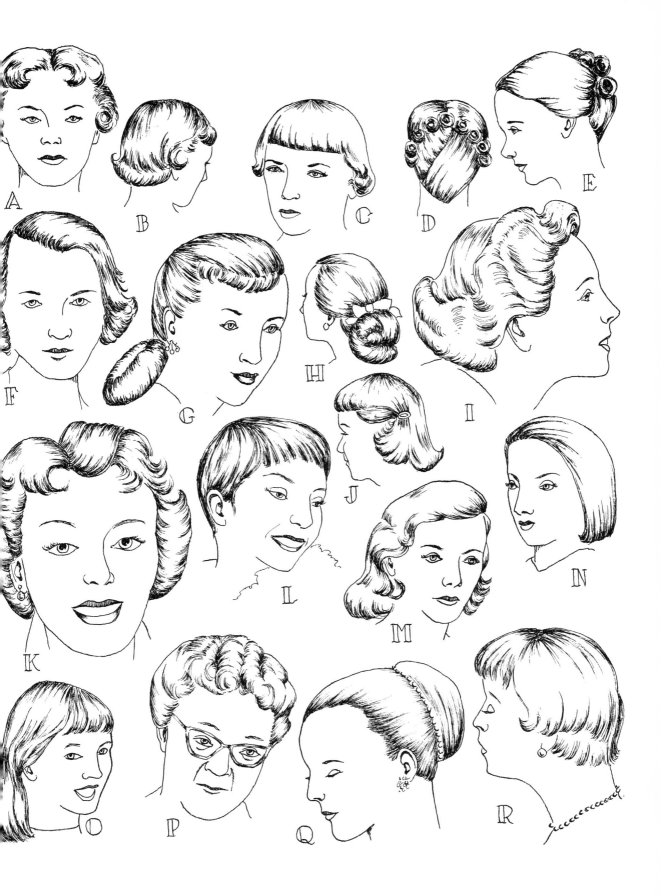

A

B

C

D

E

F

G

H

I

J

K

L

M

N

O

P

Q

R

PLATE 161 : TWENTIETH-CENTURY WOMEN 1950–1957

A   1950.

B   1950.

C   1950. False hairpieces.

D   1950. Hair in pin curls.

E   1950.

F   1951, American.

G   1951, American child.

H   1952, American child. 'Wavy hair makes a fine pony tail, a hairdo both neat and charming. It can be side or middle-parted or have no part at all.'

I   1953. *Italian cut.*

J   1954, American. *Butch cut.* Worn in the summer of 1954.

K, L   1954. Decorative head bands.

M   1954.

N   1954.

O   1956. Hair in $1\frac{3}{4}$-inch curlers.

P   1956.

Q   1955.

R   1957. *Feather cut.*

S   1957. In mid-year *Good Housekeeping* indicated that hair was going up and that the trend was toward piling it on top of the head. However, they also referred to the feather cut (R) as 'the hairdo that continues year after year to be the top choice of millions of women'.

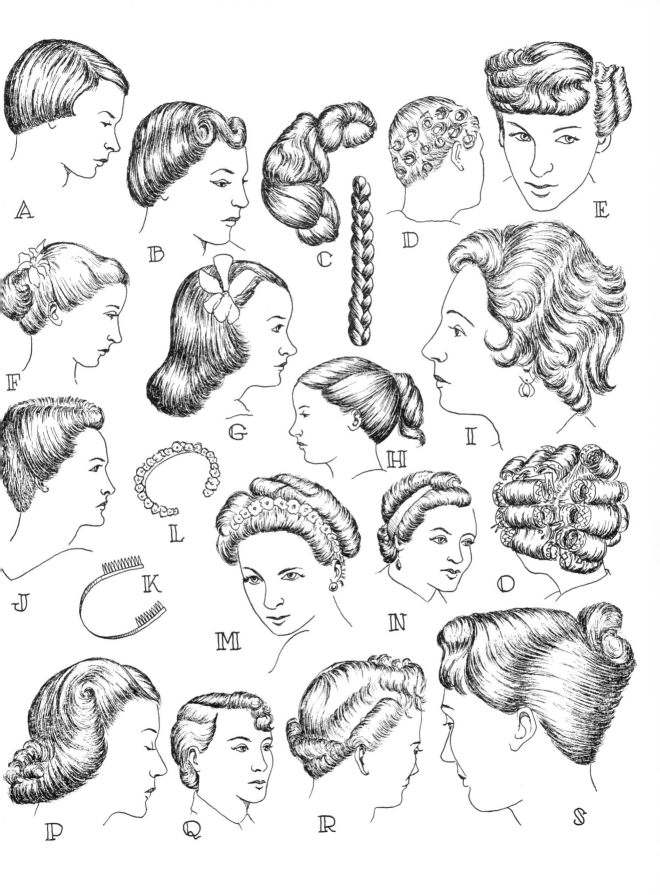

A

B

C

D

E

F

G

H

I

J

K

L

M

N

O

P

Q

R

S

A   1957. American child.

B   1957. American child.

C   1957, American. Fashionable.

D   1957, American. Fashionable.

E   1957, American. Fashionable.

F   1958, American. Fashionable.

G   1958, American. Fashionable.

H   1958, American. Fashionable.

I   1958, American. Fashionable.

J   1958, American. Fashionable.

K   1958, American. Fashionable.

L   1959, American. Fashionable.

M   1959, American. Fashionable. *Beehive* style.

N   1959, American. Fashionable.

O   1959, American. Fashionable.

P   1959, American. Fashionable.

Q   1959, American. Fashionable.

R   1959, American. Fashionable. *Beehive* style.

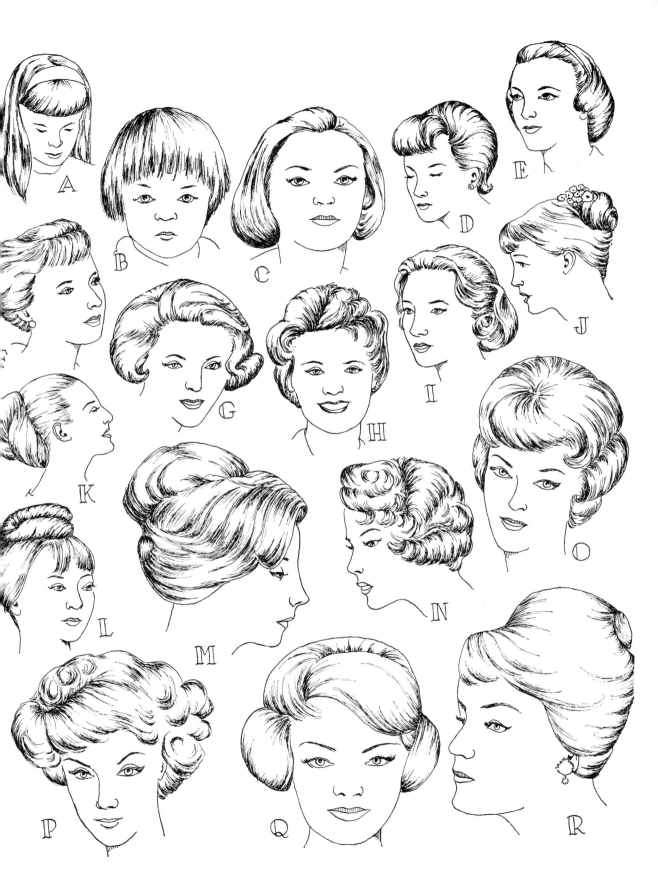

A

B

C

D

E

J

G

I

H

K

L

M

N

O

P

Q

R

PLATE 163 : TWENTIETH-CENTURY WOMEN 1960, 1961

(All of the styles on this plate were fashionable in the years indicated. Most of them were taken from fashion pages or fashion advertisements. A few were sketched from life.)

A 1960, American. Note that the hair is slightly puffed up over the crown, distorting the natural shape of the head.

B 1960, American. *Beehive* style.

C 1960, American.

D 1960, American.

E 1960, American.

F 1960, American.

G 1960, American. Wig.

H 1960, American.

I 1960, American. Wig.

J 1960, American.

K 1960, American.

L 1960, American.

M 1960, American.

N 1961, American. Conservative-Fashionable.

O 1961, American.

P 1961, English. (Sketched in London.)

Q 1961, French. (Sketched in the Paris Metro.)

R 1961, English. (Sketched in London.)

S 1961, American.

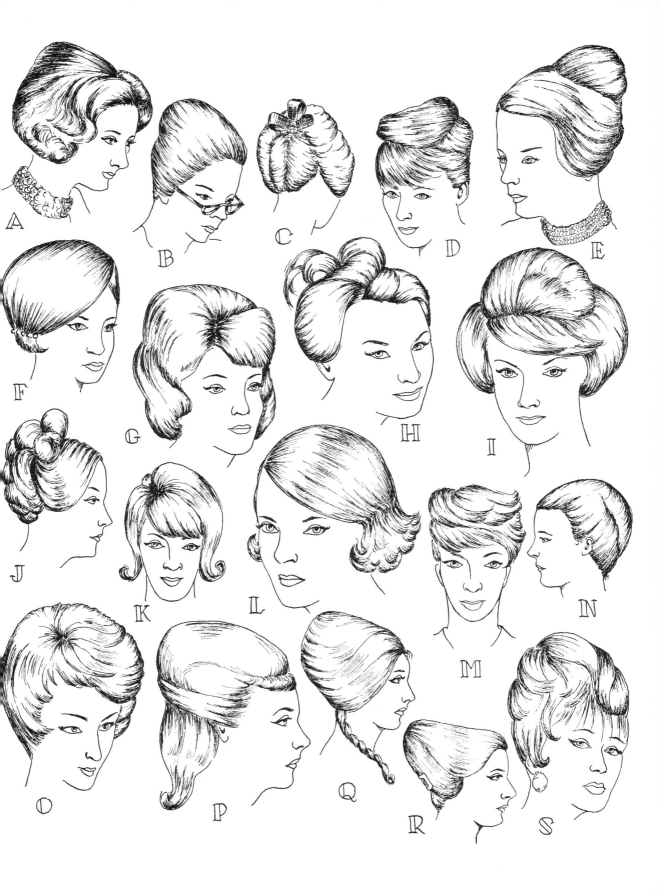

A

B

C

D

E

F

G

H

I

J

K

L

M

N

O

P

Q

R

S

PLATE 164 : TWENTIETH-CENTURY WOMEN

(All of the styles on this plate were fashionable in 1961 and into 1962. Some were taken from fashion pages and fashion advertisements, some from photographs of prominent people, and some were sketched from life.)

A   1961, French. *Guiche* style. Usually worn with smooth, short hair. Latest fashion in Paris for winter, 1960–61.

B   1961, American.

C   1961, American. *Beehive* style.

D   1961, American. Jacqueline Kennedy style.

E   1961, American shopper. *Beehive* style. (Sketched in Chicago department store.)

F   1961, American. (Sketched in New York.)

G   1961, American.

H   1961, American. Natural hair.

I   1961, American. Natural hair.

J   1961, American. Early example of the *Egyptian* style.

K   1961, American. Natural hair.

L   1961, American.

M   1961, American. Natural hair, with fake *postiche*.

N   1961, American.

O   1961, American.

P   1961, American. Natural hair done up on twenty rollers.

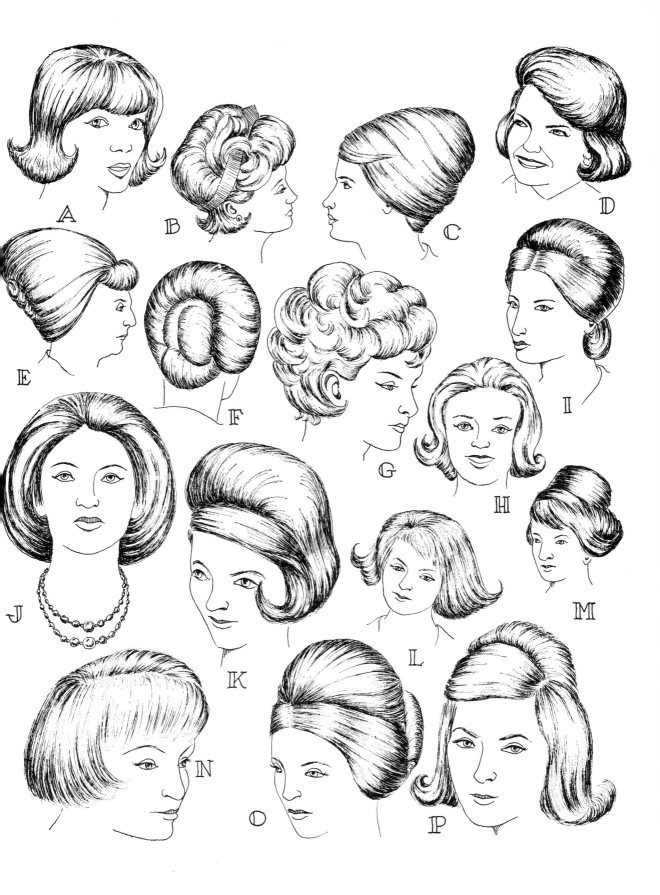

A

B

C

D

E

F

G

H

I

J

K

L

M

N

O

P

PLATE 165 : TWENTIETH-CENTURY WOMEN 1962

A   Natural hair teased.

B   Natural hair, *bubble* style.

C   Natural hair.

D   Hair set on large rollers, then combed out, teased, and brushed.

E   Natural hair teased.

F   Mrs Leonard Bernstein. Evening coiffure.

G   Natural hair teased for bouffant effect.

H   Elizabeth Ashley. *Marienbad* style.

I   Wig. *Egyptian* style.

J   Natural hair.

K   For evening wear.

L   Jacqueline Kennedy. *Brioche* style.

M   Natural hair or wig.

N   Wig.

O   Wig.

P   Natural hair with pieces added.

Q   Natural hair.

R   Natural hair or wig.

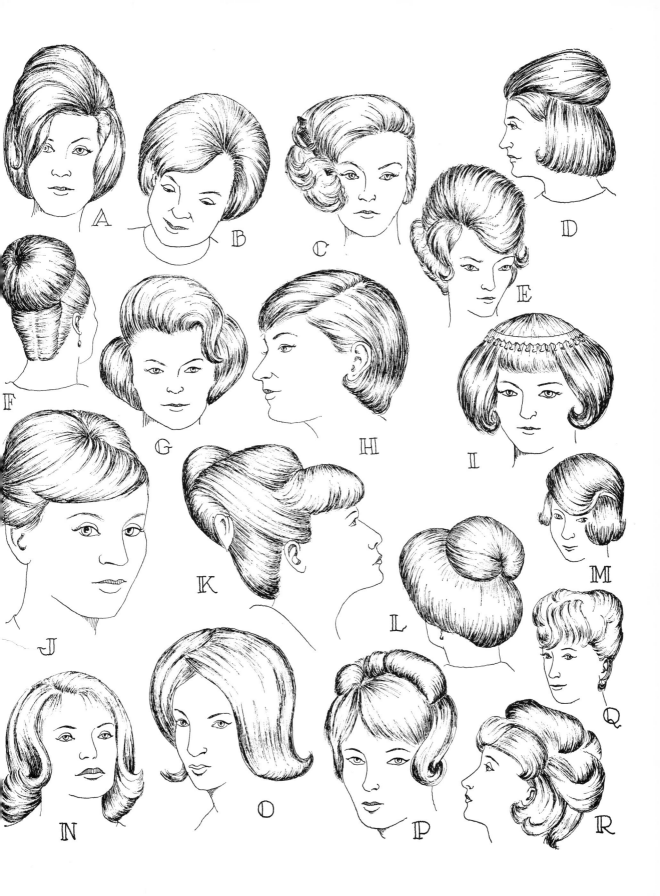

A

B

C

D

E

F

G

H

I

J

K

L

M

N

O

P

Q

R

PLATE 166 : TWENTIETH-CENTURY WOMEN 1962, 1963

A   1962.

B   1962, American. *Egyptian* style. Natural hair set on rollers and teased.

C   1962. Italian film actress.

D   1962, American. False topknot.

E   1962, French. High fashion model. False topknot. Such extreme fashions were rarely worn except by high fashion models in order to set trends.

F   1962. High fashion model.

G   1962.

H   1963.

I   1963.

J   1963, American.

K   1963, American. *Guinevere* style. Inspired by the Broadway musical *Camelot*.

According to an article in the *Saturday Evening Post* in October 1962, the 'bouffant look is "out", in clothes and coiffures. The elongated, Modigliani look is "in", from thigh-length jackets to spiralling hairdos. As one fashion commentator describes it, a woman must look like "a single, long-stemmed flower suspended and effortless, swaying in the wind".' More specifically, the *Post* announced that 'the familiar souffle hairdo has been superseded by a new, cropped, caplike look for the hair'. This hairdo, said the *Post*, 'makes it easy for the fashion sophisticate to change styles at will either through wigs (still all right despite an ominous popularity) to wig-type hats that suit a temporarily manic mood'.

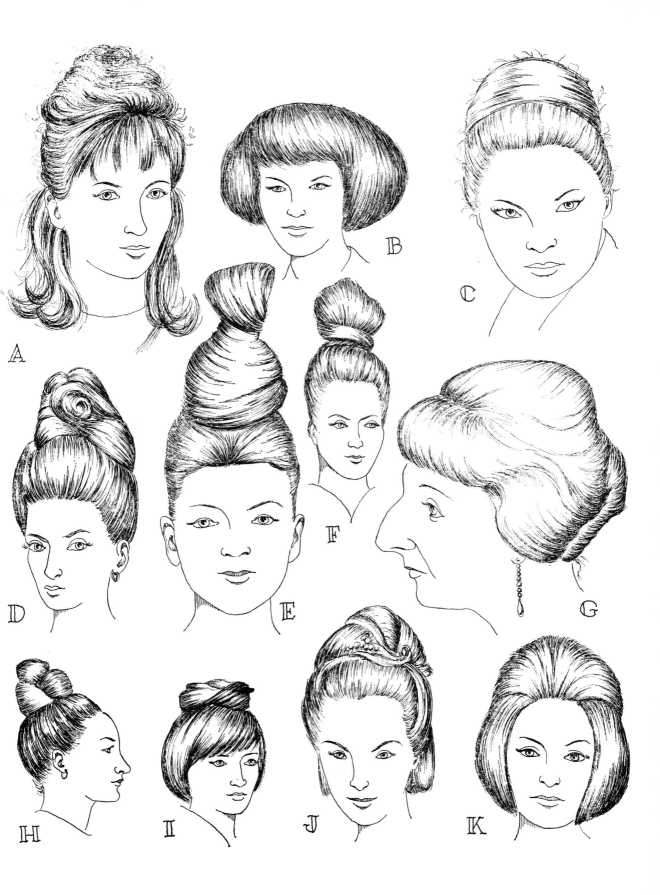

A

B

C

D

E

F

G

H

I

J

K

Plate 167 : Twentieth-Century Women 1963, 1964

A 1963, New York. For evening wear. The topknot is false.

B 1964, London. Debutante.

C 1963, American. A fairly extreme version of a style suitable for natural hair or wigs.

D 1963, Chicago. 'Visible waves are absent (though a foundation permanent, just to give body, is often an essential under-cover ingredient) and there isn't the trace of a curl. All is silky smoothness and subtle shaping.'—*Chicago Tribune*.

E 1964, London. Suitable for day or evening wear.

F 1964, American. A very popular style.

G 1964, American. The large bow is attached to a ribbon encircling the head. Small, flat bows were more commonly used to decorate the hair, especially on wigs.

H 1964, London. Note similarity to men's styles of the late fifteenth century.

I 1964, New York. Back hair is false.

J 1964, London. (Similar to F above.) A fashionable and popular style.

K 1964, London. Fashionable and popular.

L 1964, London. Fashionable arrangement for evening.

M 1964, London. High fashion model. The front half seems to be derived from the 1840s and the back from Pisanello.

N 1964, London. High fashion model. Coiffure for evening wear. This is an extreme style, created perhaps by an over-enthusiastic hairdresser. It may or may not have been worn in public, but it did appear in *Queen*.

O 1964, London. An extreme style for evening wear. Note similarity to some of the styles of the 1820s.

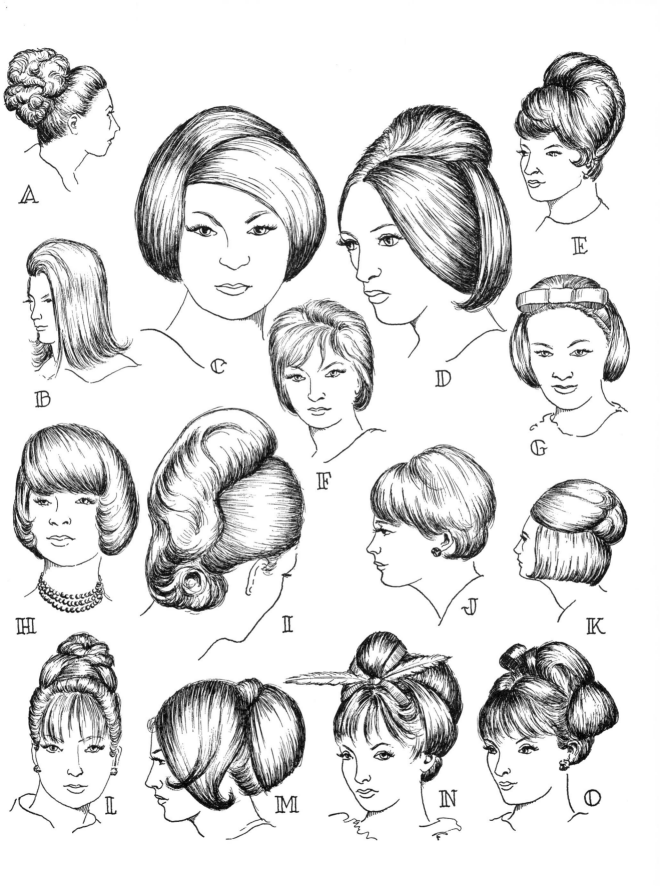

A

B

C

D

E

F

G

H

I

J

K

L

M

N

O

Supplement 1965-1978

MEN (Plate 168)

In the years between 1965 and 1970, while the Beatles were bringing about a revolution of sorts in popular music, they were also sparking a revolution in men's hair styles, which grew gradually longer—not just a few men's, but most men's. As early as 1966 a Yale oarsman noted that even crew men didn't wear crew cuts any more. The revolution, as a glance at history should enable one to predict, was not entirely peaceful. Militant short-haired conservatives watched with alarm and occasionally reacted with violence as sideburns crept down the cheek, skin on the neck disappeared, along with foreheads and even eyebrows, boys carried hair brushes to school, men began visiting male beauty parlours, and a musical called *Hair* made theatrical history.

In 1966, reports Bruce Jay Friedman, a New Jersey school committee decreed that boys with duck-tail or Beatle hairdos would not be admitted to classes. The opposition picketed, then capitulated and had their hair cut. In 1968 a private school in the Eastern United States kept its collective mind and its doors closed to the change in boys' hair styles, insisting upon, 'no shaggy-dog hairdos, hair trimmed reasonably close and on a slant, back and sides; hair never to reach collar level; sideburns no lower than about the middle of the ear; no bangs; hair brushed back from the forehead; no beards or feeble attempts'. The headmaster of another private school blocked the school doorway, refusing admittance to all long-haired boys until he had cut off their Prince Charles bangs. His reasoning, crisp and to the point, must have seemed to him irrefutable—'Sloppy hair, sloppy thinking'.

A school principal in Pennsylvania was moved by a court decision to be more charitable. Faced with the court's support of the right of an eighteen-year-old student to wear his hair touching the back of his shirt collar (see Plate 168-F), a violation of school regulations, the principal, backed by the Board of Education, arranged for a two-way telephone hookup between the school and the boy's home. Thus the winner of the school's only National Merit Scholarship was able to continue his class work without contaminating the other students.

Unrest flared up in other parts of the country as well. In Los Angeles a boy was convicted of disturbing the peace for refusing to cut his hair. In Texas a university professor, whose son was barred from school on account of his long hair, demanded to know if a boy had to forfeit his civil liberties in order to get an education. An increasing number of court decisions indicated that he did not. Yet on May 7, 1970, a fifteen-year-old student was admitted to a California hospital in serious condition as a result of being scalped by two self-styled 'patriots', who objected to his long hair as being un-American.

Elsewhere, in the larger cities of most Western countries and on college campuses, men's hairdos ranged from medium short to very long, and upon occasion grew into giant feather-light puffs. None the less, long hair was still controversial among conservatives who resisted the lessons of history. On August 3, 1969, as reported by *Commonweal*, the mayor of San Miguel de Allende, Mexico, 'instructed his police to seize all long-haired males found on the plaza, take them to police headquarters and there forcibly to shave them'. This was done to a number of boys. Three of the boys' fathers, who protested the action, were also seized and forcibly shaved. Reaction was mixed, but the mayor received an astonishing number of congratulations for his presumably illegal action.

Beards, moustaches, and long hair were banned by law or regulation in Cuba, Argentina, Greece, and Disneyland. And the beauties of the American countryside were set off by large red, yellow, and blue billboards with the exhortation to 'Beautify America, Get a Haircut'.

Wigs and toupees were worn increasingly. According to *Newsweek* in 1967 $1\frac{1}{2}$ million American men wore some kind of hairpiece—an increase of more than four hundred per cent in ten years. Hair plugs (small pieces of skin with healthy hair transplanted from the back of the head to the front) provided a natural growth of hair for the partially bald and financially solvent. An average transplant was reported to cost as much as $2,500 (£1,041). In a new process called hair weaving, the false hair was tied directly to the wearer's own and tightened three or four times a year.

Wigs were worn both to conceal baldness and to cover one's natural hair. Business men who were required to keep their hair short sometimes wore long-haired wigs for social occasions. Long-haired men with part-time jobs requiring short hair found that short-haired wigs solved their problem, as did a New York hair stylist who tucked up his shoulder-length hair under a short-haired wig to go apartment hunting. 'They say you can live anywhere you want', he explained. 'Well, you can't if you have long hair.'

The development of synthetic stretch wigs contributed enormously to wig wearing among men, and by 1970 they were buying them at men's beauty salons and trying them on openly at department store wig bars.

During this time, beards, both real and false, were worn by a small minority and seemed to be generally accepted with good-natured tolerance, sometimes even with admiration. The style was individual—there were no rules of fashion. But the beards were generally short and fairly conventional (Plate 168-G-J). False ones were readily available in both department stores and men's hairdressing salons. The popularity of moustaches can probably be traced to the Beatles' growing them. Like long hair, they met with considerable resistance, particularly among more conservative businesses, which frankly warned applicants that moustaches would not be welcome. A counsellor for a Midwestern American employment agency, according to *Newsweek*, expressed the firm opinion that 'Bankers don't have mustaches'. And by and large, American bankers didn't. In any case, some men, perhaps even bankers, did wear false moustaches on their days off or for going out in the evening.

WOMEN (Plates 169, 170)

For a while, as men's hair got longer, there seemed to be some attempt on the part of women to distinguish between the sexes by keeping their hair either shorter or longer than men's, but by 1970 it was clear that the sexes were, in many ways, merging. There were uni-sex clothes, uni-sex hair styles, and uni-sex wigs. There were evidences of it even in 1965 with Vidal Sassoon's chunky, masculine-looking hair styles (Plate 169-E), not unlike the current Beatle-inspired hairdos for men. In 1966 Sassoon, operating primarily from his New York salon, was still making news and multiplying clients with his increasingly geometric hair styles, which could easily pass for wigs (Plate 169-J). In 1970 he introduced The Veil—a thin screen of long hair hanging over the face.

But other stylists and other women preferred more feminine hairdos with an abundance of curls or flowing locks, most of them false. The feminine look was particularly in evidence in 1968, with great masses of Shirley Temple curls (Plate 170-C) or demure wisps of hair framing the face (Plate 170-D).

In the autumn of 1966 falls came into fashion and remained as standard equipment for women who wanted longer hair but preferred not to wear a complete wig. Pinned or clipped to the hair at the crown and covered by one's natural hair, the fall could fill out a page boy, hang over the shoulders in natural waves, be sprayed into stiff exotic conformations, or be piled on to the head in curls, puffs, or braids. Long falls of European hair sometimes cost as much as $600 (£250), whereas synthetic ones could be bought for as little as $10 (£4). Less rigid fashions and the development of inexpensive, natural-looking synthetic hair made it possible for women to vary their hair styles with the time of day if they liked and to build a wardrobe of wigs without bankrupting their husbands.

In July 1969 *Vogue* reported on Mrs Graham Mattison's current hair collection—a mini-wig, a short half-wig, a long fall, a small Cadogan, a thick braid, a huge bow of hair, a long wavy switch, skinny braids, and small clusters of curls. Another use of false hair was in the fashionable streaking—glueing on the streaks instead of bleaching strands of the natural hair. The streaks were available from New York wigmaker Bob Kelly in packets of twenty.

It was estimated in 1968 that wig sales in the United States amounted to more than $500 million a year (over £200,000,000), a rise of more than 1,000 per cent in nine years. Wigs ranged in price from about $8 (£3) to $1,000 (£400). Stealing wigs had become increasingly profitable since ounce for ounce the more expensive ones could be worth five times their weight in gold.

Wigs got involved with the law for other reasons as well. A New York Civil Court judge handed down a decision in favour of a plaintiff whose blonde wig had been ruined by a careless hairdresser. In announcing his decision, the judge quoted Pope:

> The meeting points the sacred hair dissever
> From the fair head, forever and forever!
> Then flashed the living lightning from her eyes. . . .

And, the judge added, rhyming his own couplet with a judgment fairer, one hopes, than his meter:

> A judgment in Small Claims Court should soothe her sighs.

According to *Forbes Magazine*, most of the wigs were sold by beauty salons and by department stores, where wig counters proved to be thirty or forty times as profitable as cosmetics counters. In the larger American cities and their suburbs it was estimated that up to 80 per cent of the women owned some kind of wig or hairpiece.

The enormous demand for human hair, which European markets could no longer supply, provided India with a new export business. For centuries the enormous piles of black hair sacrificed to the Lord Venkateswara ('We humble ourselves before you, Lord Venkateswara. We will shave our heads and offer our hair in masses of black clouds') were burned by the priests. But in 1966, the Indian government, belatedly aware of a good thing when it finally realized its potential, set up a hair-processing factory in Madras. Six months later, according to *Newsweek*, the factory's eight hundred workers were turning out twelve thousand wigs a month.

In the fall of 1969, despite a lack of conformity in hair styles, *Vogue* managed to pin the latest hair fashions down to three but refused to take sides. There was long hair, sleek and smooth and pulled back (Plate 170-I); very short hair, clipped short with sideburns (Plate 170-N); and, oddly enough, a revival of the Gibson girl poufed style (Plate 170-J). Perhaps the most unusual hair style of the period was the Afro (Plate 170-F) which blacks, both men and women, evidently wore as a symbol of racial pride and which sometimes grew to what must surely have been the most enormous hairdos since the eighteenth century. The style caught on, and Afro wigs in various colours were worn by both blacks and whites. In 1970 the newest hairdo was the Ape—short on top, long in back, looking, as *Time* put it, like nothing so much as 'a wet mop . . . after a hard day on the kitchen floor'.

Throughout the last half of the decade hair styles were remarkable for their variety, as shown in the following plates. Most of these are derivative of earlier styles from the ancient Greek to the late Victorian. It is perhaps indicative of the times that hair styles, both men's and women's, were eclectic, demonstrating, by and large, a curious blend of past fashions and present freedom of expression.

MEN (Plate 171)

Within a few years, however, false moustaches were no longer needed, even by bankers. More real moustaches were now being worn, and by the end of the decade they had become fairly commonplace. Beards, though less popular than moustaches, were considered a matter of individual taste.

And so, actually, were hair styles. Men were becoming increasingly conscious of hair fashions in the 1970s and began having their hair 'styled' instead of 'cut'. And to help them maintain their fashionable hairdos, blow-driers, which many fashion-conscious men came to consider indispensable, were manufactured in a variety of shapes and sizes. And as if this weren't enough—and for some men it obviously wasn't—Vidal Sassoon marketed a six-piece 'Air Styling Comb and Brush Kit', including a natural boar-bristle attachment for brushing, a wide plastic spike brush for styling and scalp massage, and an aluminium hot-comb for straightening the hair.

At the beginning of the decade styles were medium or long, straight or naturally wavy, and covering at least part of the ears. Centre partings were becoming more popular. The 'Mark Spitz look' (centre-parted hair, full and brushed back, with a neat moustache) was perhaps the most popular of the straight-hair styles.

The revolution in men's hair styles, which was now going on, had begun in the 1960s with a rebellion against short hair. Then, in the early seventies, some of the avant-garde rebelled against long hair and cut their hair short. Other men preferred a short, curly style known as the 'Greek-boy look'. (For men whose hair did not fall naturally into ringlets, permanents were available.) The practical advantage of the style was that it required very little care. For busy men who had resigned themselves to spending as much time on their hair as their wives did, this was reason enough for switching to a curly permanent. And a number of them stayed with it even when the popularity of the style declined. Still others, satisfied with their long hair, simply kept it, along with the blow-driers.

Thus, at the end of the decade men were wearing their hair long or short, straight or curly, parted or not parted—as it pleased them. And they were not only wearing their own hair the way they wanted to but they seemed to be content to let others do the same.

WOMEN (Plates 172, 173)

The 1970s began with the ragged-looking, very un-feminine 'Ape' (a style copied by some men) continuing to be worn. But by 1972, though still seen, it was out of fashion. It had become, according to Vidal Sassoon's artistic director, 'a phenomenal bore, making everyone look like a stamped-out replica of everyone else'.

The more drastic of the new styles ranged from short and sleek, with every hair in place, to a casual, schoolboy crop. Short-short crops were occasionally seen, and short, brushed-back styles were popular. The new styles were evidently related to the new trend towards more sportswear in women's clothes. Shaggy, unkempt hairdos simply did not look right.

Fads came and went. The newest one in 1972 and 1973 was painting the hair. The paint could be brushed on in stripes or sprayed on in patterns. The stripes (painted on with a lightening fluid) were allowed to dry, then shampooed out for a natural two-tone look. For patterns, stencils were cut and held in place over a flat, smooth hairdo. The decorative pattern or design was created by spraying a temporary hair colour onto the stencil, using a different stencil for each colour. The painted pattern was, of course, even more temporary than the colour spray it was put on with, since it obviously would not survive combing.

Permanent waving increased in popularity in the second half of the decade, culminating in what was called the 'stack perm', which required attaching dozens of permanent wave rods to a scaffolding of chopsticks on top of the head, creating an effect, before the paraphernalia was removed, reminiscent of the towering French *fontange* hair styles of the late seventeenth century. The technique was designed for women with long, straight hair who wanted only the lower part of it curled.

In the mid-seventies popular styles tended to be rather feminine, ranging from medium short to medium long and from slightly waved to tightly curled. The hair might be brushed back off the forehead, draped across it, or nearly concealing it with fluffy bangs. Some styles were trimmed fairly close to the head at the back; others were cut full and hung nearly to the collar. Sometimes the hair was combed forward from the crown and curled back just above the eyebrows. It might be side-parted, centre-parted, or not parted at all. Full, waved sideburns were incorporated into some of the styles. Buns and knots were fashionable and might be placed high, low, centre, off-centre, just above the forehead, or on the side, with long wisps of hair hanging casually around the face and shorter ones at the neck.

By the end of the decade the fashionably careless look had given way to neater, sleeker, more sophisticated styles, with a simple roll or a gentle wave, perhaps set off by a single jewel, a feather, a flower, or a fancy comb.

The material in this chapter is not referred to in the Sources or the Index.

PLATE 168 : TWENTIETH-CENTURY MEN 1965–1970

A 1965. *Sosh* style. Always carefully combed and greased.

B 1965. *Caesar* style. Popular with children and teen-agers.

C 1965. *Surfer* style. Washed frequently, never greased, usually looked windblown.

D 1966, American. University student.

E 1966, English. Working class.

F 1966. Hair style of an Ohio student whose expulsion from school resulted in one of the first court cases testing the right of a U.S. citizen to wear long hair.

G 1968, American. False beard and moustache. Natural hair. Ready-made false beards, moustaches, and sideburns were available in a variety of styles, singly or in sets. The good ones were hand-made and were applied to the face with spirit gum.

H 1968. Full sideburns with moustache.

I 1968, American. False sideburns. Most men who wanted long sideburns grew their own unless prevented from doing so by a conservative employer.

J 1968. False beard.

K 1970, Italian.

L 1969, French. Dress designer.

M 1970. *Afro* style. (See also Q and U below.)

N 1970. Natural hair and moustache.

O 1970, French.

P 1969.

Q 1969, American. College student with *Afro* style in blond hair. Also available in various colours of wigs.

R 1969.

S 1970.

T 1970. *Natural* style.

U 1970. *Afro* style.

V 1970, American.

W 1970. Stretch wig of synthetic hair.

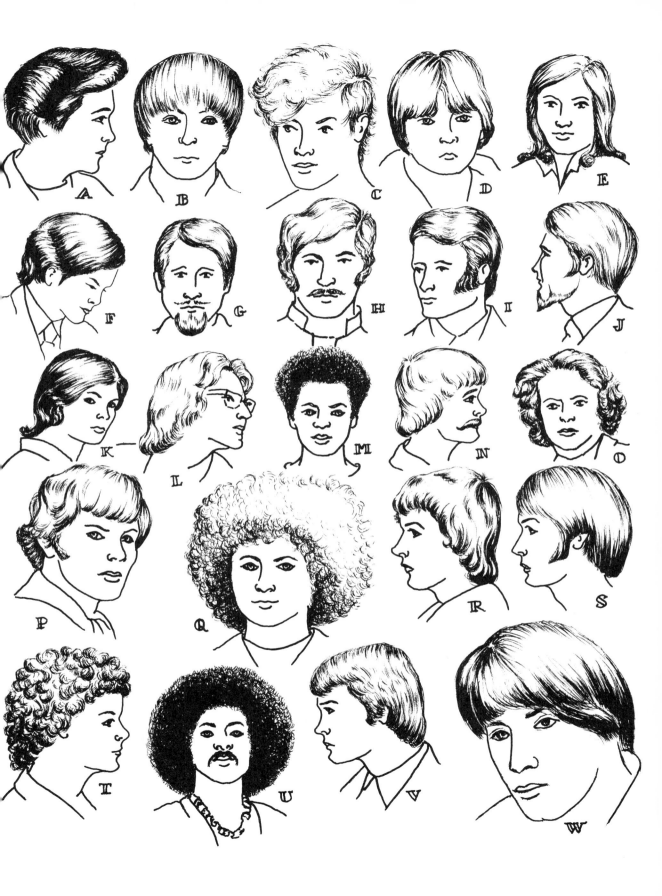

PLATE 169 : TWENTIETH-CENTURY WOMEN 1965–1967

A   1965, New York. Hair style by Mr Alfonso of Bergdorf-Goodman.

B   1965. Natural hair.

C   1965. Natural hair, teased in back.

D   1965. Crown-pouf hairdo. Top hair 5 inches long, ends tapered; hair set with large rollers and pincurls; back hair feathered at crown.

E   1965. Hair style by Vidal Sassoon.

F   1966. Real and false hair combined.

G   1966. Michel Kazan hairdo with false curls.

H   1966. Natural hair poufed at crown.

I   1966. Natural hair with fall.

J   1966. Vidal Sassoon geometric style.

K   1966. Wig.

L   1966. Natural hair with fall.

M   1967, New York. Dynel chignon worn with natural hair. Price of 32-inch chignon, $14.98 (£6).

N   1967, New York. Twenty-four inch fall worn over natural hair. Price of fall, $125 (£50).

O   1967, New York. Page boy style, with hair poufed from centre crown. Styled by Mr Kenneth.

P   1967. Natural hair with false curls.

Q   1967. Human-hair wig. Price, $29.95 (£12). Matching wig for men available.

R   1967, New York. Natural hair styled by Mr Alfonso of Bergdorf-Goodman.

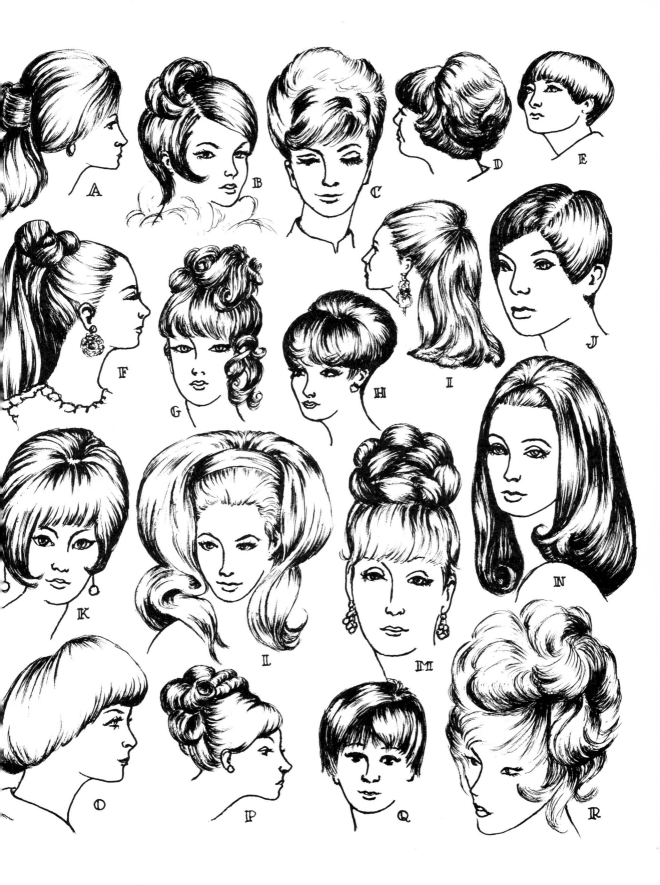

A 1968. Natural hair.

B 1968. Natural hair with fall.

C 1968. *Shirley Temple* style. Wig.

D 1968. Natural hair, poufed at crown.

E 1969. Short clipped natural hair.

F 1969. *Afro* hair style.

G 1969. Natural hair, possibly with false topknot.

H 1969. Natural hair with fall.

I 1969. Natural hair with false topknot.

J 1969. Natural hair poufed in Gibson girl style, topped with false curls.

K 1969. Natural hair.

L 1969. Wig.

M 1970. Style known as the *Ape*. Hair short on top, long in back, with a shaggy look. Could be either straight or curly.

N 1970. Close clipped style with sideburns.

O 1970.

P 1970. Natural hair with long fall.

Q 1970. Natural hair. Front and crown set with large rollers, back and side with medium ones. Hair is brushed back and held with elastic, then ends are back brushed to make pouf, which is shaped with the fingers.

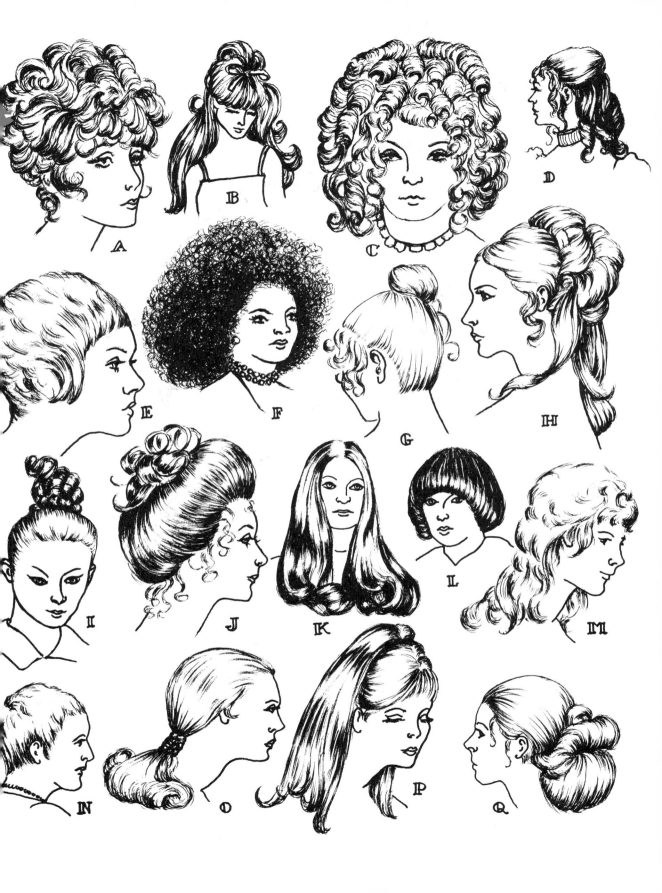

A

B

C

D

E

F

G

H

I

J

K

L

M

N

O

P

Q

A   1971. Popular style for young men.

B   1971.

C   1972. More conservative style than B.

D   1972. The *Mark Spitz* look. Named after the Olympic swimming champion. An extremely popular American style. The hair style was also worn without the moustache.

E, F   1973. Popular styles.

G   1973. Fashionable young men's style.

H   1974.

J   1975.

K   1975. Fashionable curly look.

L   1975.

M   1976. *Crew cut*. Adopted by some fashion-conscious men as a reaction against long hair.

N   1976. Braided style, called *cornrowing*, which replaced the *Afro* in popularity.

O   1976. Very fashionable style.

P   1976. Fashionable young men's style with centre parting.

Q   1976.

R   1977.

S   1977. Casual young men's style.

T   1978. Popular curly style. The moustache with turned-up ends was much less popular with young men than the ones shown in D, F, K, M, and O.

U   1978. Popular style.

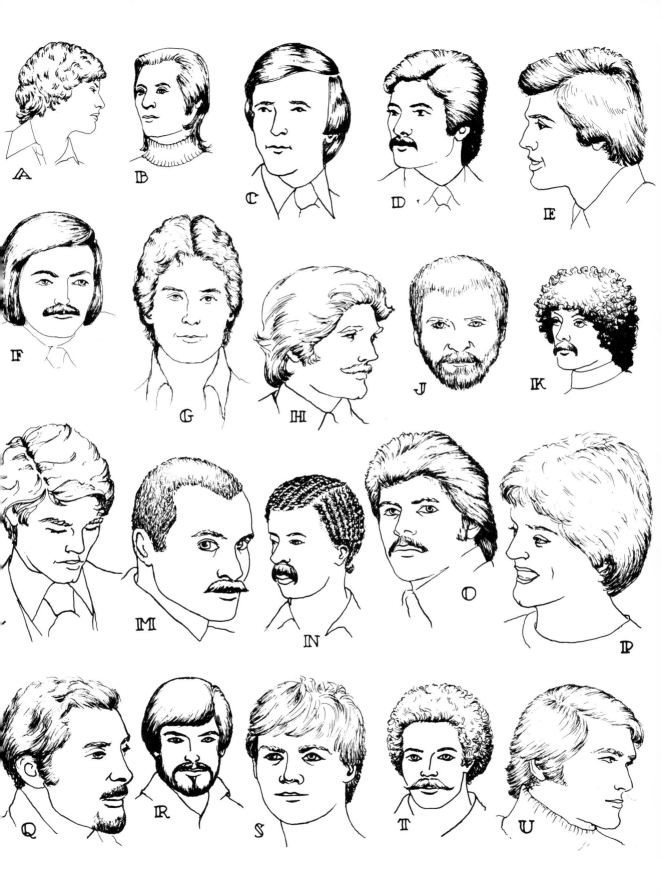

A

B

C

D

E

F

G

H

J

K

M

N

O

P

Q

R

S

T

U

A   1971. Fashionable style.

B   1971. Natural hair with curled ends. Fashionable style.

C   1972. Fashionable style.

D   1972. The *Zelda*. Adaptation of a twenties' style.

E   1973. *Cornrowing* style, which replaced the *Afro* in popularity.

F   1973. Natural hair or wig.

G   1973. Natural hair or wig.

H   1974. Natural hair.

J   1974.

K   1974.

L   1974. Natural hair.

M   1974.

N   1975. Natural hair with topknot braid of false hair.

O   1975. *Wedge cut*. Also known as the *Dorothy Hamill*, after the Olympic skating champion.

P   1975.

Q   1975. The *Chinese look*. Note similarity to the *Zelda* (D, above).

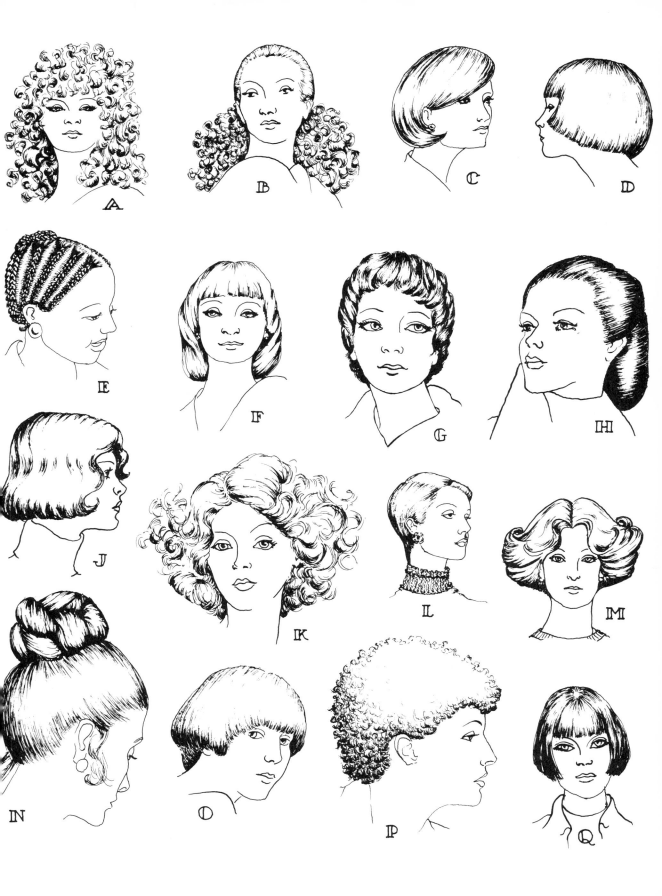

A

B

C

D

E

F

G

H

J

K

L

M

N

O

P

Q

A 1975. Fashionable style.

B 1976. Fashionable style.

C 1976. Fashionable style.

D 1976.

E 1977. Asymmetrical look.

F 1977. Fashionably dishevelled look.

G 1977. Natural hair with false braids, which were used in a variety of fashionable styles. They were often decorated with ribbons, flowers, or simulated pearls.

H 1977. Fashionable asymmetrical look.

J 1977. High fashion asymmetrical style.

K 1977. A curly style popular with the fashionable and the unfashionable.

L 1978. Fashionable look.

M 1978. Natural hair with false pouf.

N 1978.

O 1978. Individual style, incorporating braids and naturally wavy hair. (Sketched on a New York subway.)

P 1978. Fashionable look.

Q 1978. Fashionable look.

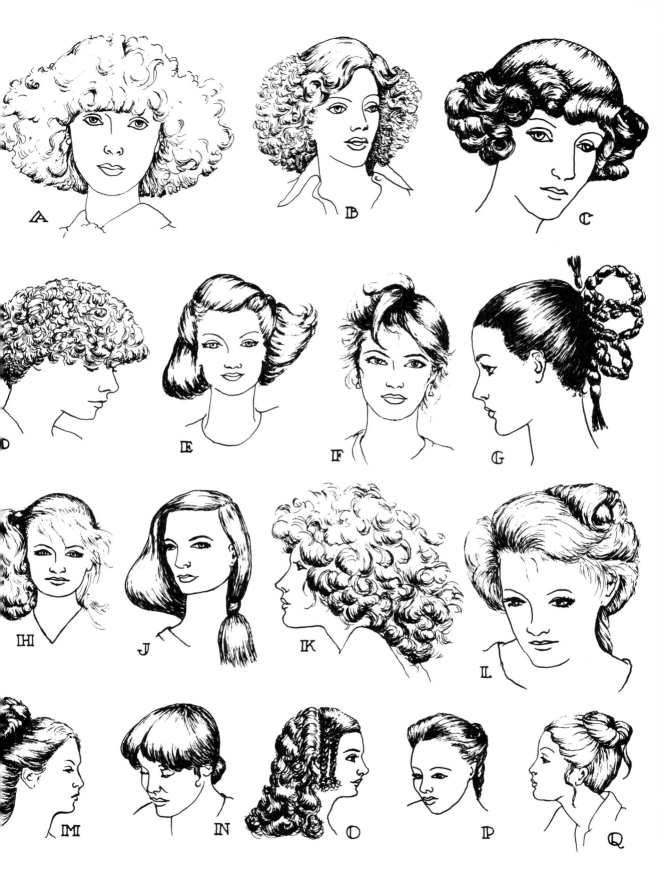

A

B

C

D

E

F

G

H

J

K

L

M

N

O

P

Q

Sources

Museums and Libraries

Amsterdam—Rijks Museum
Chicago—Art Institute, Public Library
Copenhagen—Museum of Applied Arts and Crafts, Museum of Danish Theatrical History, National Museum, Ny Carlsberg Glyptotek, State Art Gallery
Florence—Uffizi Gallery
London—British Museum, National Gallery, National Portrait Gallery, Tate Gallery, Victoria and Albert Museum, Wallace Collection
New York—Frick Collection, Metropolitan Museum of Art, Public Library
Paris—Musée Carnavalet, Musée de Cluny, Musée de l'Homme, Musée du Louvre, Musée des Monuments Français
Ravenna—Sant'Apollinare Nuovo
Rome—Vatican museums
Stockholm—National Gallery of Art
Venice—Palazzo Ducale, San Marco
Washington—Library of Congress, National Gallery of Art
Public libraries in Boston; Cleveland; Richmond, Virginia; Louisville, Kentucky; Elgin, Illinois

Books and Periodicals

Académie de Coiffure
All the Year Round
American Mercury
Andrews, William—*At the Sign of the Barber's Pole*; J. R. Tutin, Cottingham, Yorkshire, 1904
Antiques Review
Art and Archaeology
L'Art et la Mode
Art of Beauty; London, 1825
Art of Beauty, edited by 'Isobel'; C. A. Pearson, London, 1899
Ashdown, Mrs Charles Henry—*British Costume During Nineteen Centuries*; Nelson, London, New York, 1953
Atlantic Monthly
Barbers' Journal
Barker, William—*A Treatise on the Principles of Hair-Dressing*; J. Rozea, London, c. 1786
Barton, Lucy—*Historic Costume for the Stage*; W. H. Baker, Boston, 1938

Bastard, Auguste—*Costumes de la Cour de Bourgogne sous le Règne de Philippe III dit le Bon*

Beaumont and Fletcher—*Elder Brother*; 1637

Bechtel, Edwin de Turck—*Jacques Callot*; G. Braziller, New York, 1955

La Belle Assemblée

Bénard, Robert—*Perruquier Barbier*; Paris?, 1761?

Bentley's Miscellany; London

Bertelli, Donato—*Le Vere Imagini et Descritioni delle piu Nobilli Citta del Mondo*; Apud Donatum Bertellū, Venetijs, 1578

Binder, Pearl—*Muffs and Morals*; George G. Harrap, London, 1953

Blum, André—*Histoire du Costume en France*; Hachette, Paris, *c.* 1924

Boehn, Max von—*Modes and Manners*; G. H. Harrap & Co. Ltd, London, 1932–5

Boissard, Robert—*Mascarades*; 1597

Brenzoni, Raffaello—*Pisanello, Pittore*; L. Olscki, Firenze, 1952

British Museum Quarterly

Brophy, John—*The Human Face*; Prentice-Hall, New York, 1946

Brough, Robert Barnabas—*The Moustache Movement*; London, T. H. Lacy, 18—

Bulwer, John—*Anthropometamorphosis: Man Transform'd; or, The Artificial Changeling*; Printed for J. Hardesty, London, 1650, 1653

Burchard, L'Abbé de Bellevaux—*Apologia de Barbis*; Typis Academiae, Cantabrigiae, 1935

Burlington Magazine

Burton, Robert—*Anatomie of Melancholy*; Printed by John Lichfield and James Shert, for Henry Cripps, Oxford, 1621

Calabi, Augusto—*Pisanello*; G. Modiano, Milano, 1928

Cambridge Antiquarian Society Proceedings

Campbell, Mark—*Self-Instructor in the Art of Hair Work*; M. Campbell, New York, Chicago, 1867

Canel, A.—*Histoire de la Barbe et les Cheveux en Normandie*; A. Lebrument, Rouen, 1859

Challamel, Jean—*The History of Fashion in France*; S. Low, Marston, Searle & Rivington, London, 1882

Chambers's Journal

Child, Theodore—*Wimples and Crisping Pins*; Harper & Brothers, New York, 1895

Coletti, Luigi—*Pisanello*; A. Pizzi, Milano, 1953

Colliers

Colliers Encyclopedia

Connoisseur, The

Cornhill Magazine

Coronet

Cosmopolitan

Costumes Parisiens

Croisat—*Les Cent-un Coiffeurs de Tous les Pays*; L'Éditeur, Paris, 1836–8

Cunnington, C. W., and Phyllis—*Handbooks of English Costume*; Faber & Faber, London, 1952–9

Dalton, Ormonde M.—*Byzantine Art and Archaeology*; Dover Publications, New York, 1961

Dandré-Bardon, Michel—*Costume des Anciens Peuples*; A. Jombert, Paris, 17—

Darly, Mary—*Comic Prints of Characters, Caricatures, Macaronis, &c.*; Mary Darly, London, 1776

Davenport, Millia—*The Book of Costume*; Crown, New York, 1948

Day, T. A., and Dines—*Illustrations of Medieval Costume in England*

Delineator

Demorest's Monthly Magazine

Diderot, Denis—*Encyclopédie ou Dictionnaire Raisonné des Sciences, des Arts, et des Métiers*

Dobson, Austin—*The Works of William Hogarth*; G. Barrie & Son, Philadelphia, 1900

Donelan, Daniel D.—*Figaro in All Ages*; The Varriale Publication, New York, 1927

Doran, John—*Habits and Men*; R. Bentley, London, 1855

Du Chastel de la Howarderie, Albéric—*Syracuse, ses Monnaies d'Argent*

Dulaure, Jacques Antoine—*Pogonologia or a Philosophical and Historical Essay on Beards*; R. Thorn, Exeter, 1786

Duplessis, Georges—*Costumes Historiques des 16e, 17e, 18e Siècles*

Duruy, Victor—*History of Greece*; Estes & Lauriat, Boston, 1890-1

Duruy, Victor—*History of Rome*; C. F. Jewett, Boston, c. 1883

Eclectic Magazine

Elliot, Frances—*Old Court Life in France*; Putnam, New York, London, 1893

Éloffe, Madame—*Modes et Usages au Temps de Marie Antoinette*; F. Didot et Cie, Paris, 1885

English Illustrated Magazine

Enlart, Camille—*Manuel d'Archéologie Française*; A. Picard, Paris, 1904-29

Erdmannsdörffer, B.—*Mirabeau*; Velhagen & Klasing, Leipzig, 1900

Etherege, George—*Man of Mode*; H. Herringman, London, 1676

Evelyn, John—*Fop-Dictionary*; London, 1690

Evelyn, John—*Mundis Muliebris; or the Ladies Dressing Room Unlock'd and Her Toilette Spread*; 1690

Evelyn, John—*Numismata*; B. Tooke, London, 1697

Evelyn, John—*Tyrannus; or, the Mode* (Ed. from the edition of 1661) B. Blackwell, Oxford, 1951

Every Saturday

Fairholt, F. W.—*Costume in England*; Chapman & Hall, London, 1846

Famous Composers and Their Works; J. B. Millet Co., Boston, 1900

Ferrario, Giulio—*Il Costume Antico e Moderno*; V. Batelli, Firenze, 1823-30

Fletcher, J. S., and Massinger, Philip—*Queen of Corinth*, 1618

Foan, G. A.—*Art and Craft of Hairdressing*; Pitman, London, 1936

Fosbroke, Thomas—*Encyclopedia of Antiquities*; J. Nichols & Son, London, 1825

Fraser's Magazine

Frazer, James G.—*The Golden Bough*; Macmillan, London, 1890

French Engravings of the Eighteenth Century (Widener Collection)

Galérie des Modes et Costumes Françaises

Gallery of Fashion

Garsault, François Alexandre Pierre de—*Art du Perruquier*; Paris, 1767

Gentleman's and London Magazine

Gentleman's Magazine

Gentleman's Magazine of Fashions

Gentlemen's Fashions

Geszler, J.—*Die Moden des XIX Jahrhunderts*; E. Berté, Wien, 1897

Gibbs-Smith—*The Fashionable Lady of the Nineteenth Century*

Gilchrist, Peter—*A Treatise on the Hair or Everybody her own Hair-Dresser*; the author, London, *c.* 1768

Godey's Lady's Book

Goldscheider, Ludwig—*599 Self Portraits*; Phaidon Press, Vienna, 1937

Goldscheider, Ludwig—*Roman Portraits*; Allen & Unwin Ltd, London, 1940

Gombrich, Ernst H.—*The Story of Art*; Phaidon Publishers, New York, 1951

Goncourt, E. L. A.—*La Femme au XVIIIe Siècle*; Paris, 1882

Good Housekeeping

Good Society; George Routledge & Sons, London, 1869

Gough, Richard—*Sepulchral Monuments of Great Britain*; London, 1786

Grand-Carteret, John—*Les Élégances de la Toilette*; A. Michel, Paris, 1913

Grande Encyclopédie

Granger, James—*A Biographical History of England* (5th edition); W. Baynes & Son, London, 1824

Green Bag, The

Greene, Robert—*Quip for an Upstart Courtier*; John Wolfe, London, 1592

Habits of Good Society: A Handbook of Etiquette for Ladies and Gentlemen; J. Hogg & Sons, London, 1859

Hairdressing and Beauty Culture; Pitman, London, 1948

Hall, Thomas—*Comarum, the Loathsomnesse of Long Haire*; N. Webb & W. Grantham, London, 1654

Hammerton, J. A. (Ed.)—*Wonders of the Past*, Putnam, New York and London, 1923–4

Harleian Miscellany; R. Dutton, London, 1809

Harpers Bazaar

Harpers Weekly

Harrison, William—*Description of England*; Trübner, 1877–81

Hartley, Cecil B.—*The Gentlemen's Book of Etiquette*; G. W. Cottrell, Boston, 1860

Haswell, Charles H.—*Reminiscenses of an Octogenarian of the City of New York*; Harper & Brothers, New York, 1896

Hefner, J. de—*Costume du Moyen-Age Chrétien*

Heyck, Ed.—*Florenz und die Medici*; Velhagen & Klasing, Leipzig, 1909

Heyck, Ed.—*Friedrich I*; Velhagen & Klasing, Leipzig, 1901

Heyck, Ed.—*Kaiser Maximilian I*; Velhagen & Klasing, Leipzig, 1898

Hind, Arthur M.—*Early Italian Engraving*; Knoedler, London, 1938–48

Hobbies

Hogarth, William—*Analysis of Beauty*; Printed by J. Reeves, London, 1753

Holland, Henry—*Heroologia*; Arnhem?, 1620

Holland, Vyvyan—*Hand-Coloured Fashion Plates 1770–1899*; Batsford, London, 1955

Holme, Randle—*Academy of Armoury*; Chester, 1688

Hope, Thomas—*Costume of the Ancients*; W. Miller, London, 1812

Horizon

How to Arrange the Hair (by one of the Ladies' Committee of Almanacks); Partridge, London, 1857

How to Behave, a Pocket Manual of Republican Etiquette; Fowler and Wells, New York, 1857

Humphry, Mrs C. E.—*Etiquette for Every Day*; Grant Richards, London, 1904

Hurll, Estelle M.—*Portraits and Portrait Painting*; L. C. Page, Boston, 1907

Hutton, Henry—*Follie's Anatomie* (from the original tract printed in 1619); Percy Society, London, 1842

Hygeia

Independent, The

Infantry Journal

Inglis, William—'The Revolt Against Whiskers' (in *Harpers Weekly*, 1907)

Ireland, Samuel—*Graphic Illustrations of Hogarth*; R. Faulder & J. Egerton, London, 1794–99

Irish Quarterly Review

Jode, Peeter de—*Theatrum Principum*; Antwerp, 1651

Journal des Dames

Kaemmerer, Ludwig—*Chodowiecki*; Velhagen & Klasing, Leipzig, 1897

Kelly, Francis—*Historic Costume*; Batsford, London, 1925

King, Moses—*Notable New Yorkers*; Bartlett & Co., New York, Boston, 1899

Kings and Queens of Ancient Egypt; Hodder & Stoughton Ltd, London, 1925

Knickerbocker

La Croix, Paul—*Directoire, Consulate, et Empire*; Firmin-Didot, Paris, 1885

La Croix, Paul—*Histoire de la Coiffure*; Seré, Paris, 1851

La Croix, Paul—*Les Arts au Moyen Age*; Firmin-Didot, Paris, 1880

La Croix, Paul—*Moeurs, Usages et Costumes au Moyen Age*; Firmin-Didot, Paris, 1871

La Croix, Paul—*The Eighteenth Century*; London, 1876

La Croix, Paul—*XVIIe Siècle, Institutions, Usages, et Costumes*; Firmin-Didot, Paris, 1875

Ladies Dictionary; J. Dunton, London, 1694

Ladies Home Journal

Ladies Magazine

Lady's Friend

Lady's Magazine

Lady's Pocket Magazine

Lafoy, John B.—*The Complete Coiffeur*; New York, 1817

Lambert, George—*The Barbers' Company*; T. Brettell & Co., London, 1882

Lang, August—*Zwingli und Calvin*; Velhagen & Klasing, Leipzig, 1913

Lanté, Louis Marie—*Costumes des Femmes Françaises du XIIe au XVIIIe Siècle*; C. Tallandier, Paris, 1900

Laran, Jean—'La Coiffure des Femmes à la Fin du Règne de Louis XIV' (in *Societé de l'Histoire du Costume*, vol. 2)

Laver, James—*Clothes*; Horizon Press, New York, 1953

Le Clerc, Jean—*Le Spectacle de la Vie Humaine*

Ledwich, Edward—*Antiquities of Ireland*; S. Hooper, London, 1791–5?

Legros—*L'Art de la Coëffure des Dames Françoises*; Boudet, Paris, 1768, 1769

Lehrs, Max—*Geschichte und Kritisher Katalog des Deutschen, Niederländischen, und Franzö-sischen Kupferstichs im XV Jahrhundert*; Wien, 1908–34

Leisure Hour

Leloir, Maurice—*Histoire du Costume de l'Antiquité à 1914*; E. Henri, Paris, 1933–49

Leon, Ernestine F.—'Bob vs. Knob in Imperial Rome' (in *Art and Archaeology*, 1927)

Lester, Katherine M., and Oerke, Bess V.—*Accessories of Dress*; Manual Arts Press, Peoria, Illinois, 1940

Lester, Katherine M.—*Historic Costume*; Manual Arts Press, Peoria, Illinois, 1942

Life

Lippincott's Monthly Magazine

Living Age

London Chronicle

London Magazine or *Gentleman's Monthly Intelligencer*

Lyly, John—'Midas' (1591), in *The Dramatic Works of John Lilly*; Smith, London, 1858

Mademoiselle

Magazine of Art

Manoni, Alessandro—*Il Costume e l'Arte detta Acconciature nell'Antichità*

Marbot, Jean Baptiste Marcellin, Baron de—*Memoirs of Baron Marbot*; Longmans, Green & Company, London, 1892

Marcks, Erich—*Elizabeth von England*; Velhagen & Klasing, Leipzig, 1897

Mariette, Pierre Jean—*Traité des Pierres Gravées*; Paris, 1750

Marneffe, Alphonse de—*Les Cheveux, la Barbe, et la Moustache*; La Table Ronde, Charleroi, 1939

Masciotta, M.—*Autoritratti dal XIVo al XXo Secolo*; Electra, Firenze, 1949

McCall's

Mentor

Merrifield, Mrs—'Dress as a Fine Art' (in the *Art Journal*, March, 1853)

Meyrick, Samuel R., and Smith, Charles H.—*Costumes of the Original Inhabitants of the British Islands, from the Earliest Periods to the Sixth Century*; T. McLean, London, 1821

Mitchell, Edwin Valentine—*Concerning Beards*; Dodd, Mead & Co., New York, 1930

La Mode Feminine 1490–1900; Éditions Nillson, Paris, 1926

Le Moniteur de la Coiffure

Le Moniteur de la Mode

Morazzoni, Giuseppe—*Il Libro Illustrato Veneziano del Settencento*; U. Hoepli, Milano, 1943

Morazzoni, Giuseppe—*La Moda a Venezia nel Secolo XVIII*; Milano, 1931

National Cycopedia of American Biography

Nessler, Charles—*The Story of Hair*; Bino & Liveright, New York, 1928

New Outlook

New Statesman and Nation

New York Times Magazine

Newsweek

Norris, Herbert—*Costume and Fashion*; J. M. Dent & Sons Ltd, London, 1924

Nugent, D. Rothe de—*Anti-Titus ou Remarques Critiques sur la Coiffure des Femmes au XIXe Siècle*, 1813

Oettingen, Wolfgang von—*Daniel Chodowieckes Handzeichnungen*; J. Bard, Berlin, 1907

Once a Week

Osburn, William—*Ancient Egypt*; S. Bagster & Sons, London, 1846

Otis, H. (pseud.)—*Pictorial History of the United States*; W. P. Hazard, Philadelphia, 1860

Outing

Palmerlee, Grace—'The Coiffure of Roman Women as Shown on Portrait Busts and Statues' (in *Records of the Past*, May, 1910)

Pepys, Samuel—*Diary and Correspondence*; Bell and Daldy, London, 1867

Perfect Etiquette; or How to Behave in Society; E. G. Rideout & Co., New York

Piattoli, Giuseppe—*Raccolta di Quaranta Proverbi Toscani*; N. Pagini e G. Bardi, Firenze, 1786–8

Pictorial Review

Piesse, G. W. S.—*The Art of Perfumery*; Piesse & Lubin, London, 1862

Piton, Camille—*Le Costume Civil en France du XIIIe au XIXe Siècle*; E. Flammarion, Paris, 1913–15

Planché, J. R.—*History of British Costume*; London, 1834, 1839

Pratt, Ellis (E. P. Philocosm)—*The Art of Dressing the Hair*, 1770

Procter, Richard Wright—*The Barber's Shop* (revised edition); A. Heywood, Manchester, 1883

Prynne, William—*The Unlovelinesse of Love-lockes*; London, 1628

Queen, The

Quicherat, J. E.—*Histoire du Costume en France*; Paris, 1877

Racinet, A. C.—*Le Costume Historique*; Firmin-Didot, Paris, 1888

Rambaud, René—*Les Fugitives*; Société d'Éditions Modernes Parisiennes, Paris, 1954

Reader, The

Records of Fashion

Records of the Past

Redfern, W. B.—'Hair and Wig Powdering from Early Days' (in *Cambridge Antiquarian Society Proceedings*, October 18, 1909)

Rees, Abraham—*Cyclopedia*

Renan, Ary—*Le Costume en France*; Paris, 1890

Repository of the Arts

Repton, John Adey—*Some Account of the Beard and the Mustachio Chiefly from the Six-teenth to the Eighteenth Century*; London, 1839

Reynolds, Reginald—*Beards*; Allen & Unwin Ltd, London, 1950

Rhead, G. W.—*Chats on Costume*; F. A. Stokes, New York, 1906

Robida, Albert—*Yesteryear*; Scribner's, New York, 1891

Rosenberg, Adlof—*Friedrich August von Kaulbach*; Velhagen & Klasing, Leipzig, 1910

Rowland, Alexander—*The Human Hair*; Piper Bros., London, 1853

Rowlandson, Thomas—*Characteristic Sketches of the Lower Orders*; S. Leigh, London, 1820

Ruppert, Jacques—*Le Costume*; R. Ducher, Paris, c. 1930–1

Saturday Evening Post

Saturday Review of Literature

Scheffler, Karl—*Bildnisse aus Drei Jahrhunderten*; Karl Robert Langewiesche, Leipzig

Schmidt, Minna M.—*400 Outstanding Women of the World and Costumology of their Time*; Minna M. Schmidt, Chicago, 1933

Science of Shaving, The (by 'Homo Sum'); Cambridge, 1931

Scientific American

Seeck, Otto—*Kaiser Augustus*; Velhagen & Klasing, Leipzig, 1902

Shaw, Henry—*Dresses and Decorations of the Middle Ages*; W. Pickering, London, 1843

Southey, Robert—*The Doctor*; Harper & Bros., New York, 1836

Spahn, M.—*Philipp Veit*; Velhagen & Klasing, Leipzig, 1901

Sparrow, Walter Shaw—'Hirsute Adornments and their Lore' (in *Magazine of Art*; 1902)

Speculum

Speight, Alexanna—*The Lock of Hair*; London, 1871, 1872

Steinmann, Ernst—*Botticelli*; Velhagen & Klasing

Stéphane—*L'Art de la Coiffure Feminine*; La Coiffure de Paris, Paris, 1932

Stewart, James—*Plocacosmos, or the Whole Art of Hairdressing*, London, 1782

Strutt, Joseph—*A complete View of the Dress and Habits of the People of England*; R. Faulder, London, 1786

Stubbes, Philip—*The Anatomie of Abuses*; Richard Jones, London, 1583, 1585

Tait's Edinburgh Magazine

Temple Bar

Thatford, Gilbert S.—*Thatford's Illustrated Styles of Cutting and Dressing the Hair*; Baker, Godwin & Co., New York.

Thiers, Jean B.—*Histoire des Perruques*; Avignon, 1777

Time

Todd, Capt. Frederick P.—'The Ins-and-Outs of Military Hair' (in the *Infantry Journal*; March–April, 1940)

Tomes, Robert—*The Bazar Book of Decorum*; Harper & Brothers, 1877

Town and Country

Turberville, A. S.—*English Men and Manners of the Eighteenth Century*; Clarendon Press, Oxford, 1926

United Service Magazine

Urzidil, Johannes—*Wenceslaus Hollar*; Dr R. Passer, Wien, 1936

Uzanne, L. O.—*Fashion in Paris*; W. Heinemann, London, 1901

Uzanne, L. O.—'Weapons and Ornaments of Women' (in *Cosmopolitan*; 1906)

Vanbrugh, John—*The Relapse; or, Virtue in Danger*; T. Johnson, London, 1877

Vanity Fair

Vecellio, Cesare—*Habiti Antichi e Moderni*; Firmin-Didot, Paris, 1859–60

Verheiden, Jacob—*Portraits of the Reformation*, 1602

Villermont, Marie, Comtesse de—*Histoire de la Coiffure Feminine*; Renouard, Paris, 1892

Viollet-le-Duc, Eugène—*Dictionnaire Raisonné du Mobilier Français*; Paris, 1872

Vogue

Walkup, Fairfax Proudfit—*Dressing the Part*; F. S. Crofts and Co., New York, 1938

Waters, John—'On Beards' (in *Knickerbocker*, 1850)

Weiss, Hermann—*Kostümkunde*; Ebner & Seubert, Stuttgart, 1862–4

Westminster Review

Whole Art of Dress, The (by a Cavalry Officer); E. Wilson, London, 1830

Wickenhagen, Ernst—*Geschichte der Kunst*

Wilcox, R. Turner—*The Mode in Hats and Headdress*; Scribner's, New York and London, 1959

Wilkinson, J. G.—*Manners and Customs of the Ancient Egyptians*; London, 1837

Wilson, Erasmus—'A Popular Treatise on the Skin and Hair' (in *Westminster Review*, 1854)

Wilton, Mary M.—*The Book of Costume*; H. Colburn, London, 1847

Woman's Home Companion

Works of William Hogarth, The; Baldwin & Cradock, London, 1835–7

Wright, Thomas—*A Caricature History of the Georges*; J. C. Hotten, London, 1867

Young, Sidney—*Annals of the Barber-Surgeons*; Blades, East & Blades, London, 1890

Zemler, Charles de—*Once Over Lightly*; New York, 1939

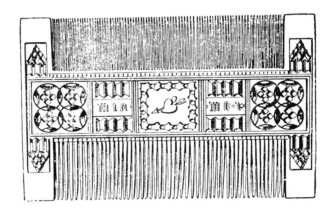

Index

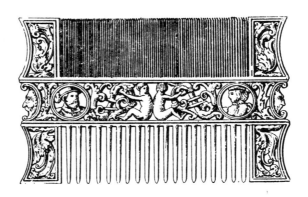